Ear, Nose and Throat Simplified

Third Edition

Bachi T Hathiram
Professor and Head
Department of ENT and Head and Neck Surgery
Topiwala National Medical College and
BYL Nair Charitable Hospital
Mumbai, Maharashtra, India

Visiting Consultant
Sir HN Reliance Foundation Hospital and
Medical Research Center, Mumbai, Maharashtra, India

Vicky S Khattar
Assistant Professor
Department of ENT and Head and Neck Surgery
Topiwala National Medical College and
BYL Nair Charitable Hospital
Mumbai, Maharashtra, India

Visiting Consultant
Sir HN Reliance Foundation Hospital and
Medical Research Center, Mumbai, Maharashtra, India

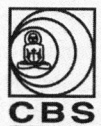

CBS

CBS Publishers and Distributors Pvt Ltd

New Delhi • Bengaluru • Chennai • Kochi • Kolkata • Mumbai
Bhopal • Bhubaneswar • Hyderabad • Jharkhand • Nagpur • Patna • Pune • Uttarakhand • Dhaka (Bangladesh)

Ear, Nose and Throat Simplified

Third Edition

ISBN: 978-93-88178-80-8

Third Edition: 2019

First Edition: 1999
Second Edition: 2002

Published by Satish Kumar Jain and produced by Varun Jain for

CBS Publishers and Distributors Pvt Ltd

4819/XI Prahlad Street, 24 Ansari Road, Daryaganj, New Delhi 110 002, India.
Ph: 23289259, 23266861, 23266867 Fax: 011-23243014
Website: www.cbspd.com e-mail: delhi@cbspd.com; cbspubs@airtelmail.in.

Corporate Office: 204 FIE, Industrial Area, Patparganj, Delhi 110 092, India
Ph: 4934 4934 Fax: 4934 4935 e-mail: publishing@cbspd.com; publicity@cbspd.com

Branches

- **Bengaluru:** Seema House 2975, 17th Cross, K.R. Road, Banasankari 2nd Stage, Bengaluru 560 070, Karnataka, India
  Ph: +91-80-26771678/79 Fax: +91-80-26771680 e-mail: bangalore@cbspd.com

- **Chennai:** 7, Subbaraya Street, Shenoy Nagar, Chennai 600 030, Tamil Nadu, India.
  Ph: +91-44-26680620, 26681266 Fax: +91-44-42032115 e-mail: chennai@cbspd.com

- **Kochi:** 42/1325, 1326, Power House Road, Opposite KSEB Power House, Ernakulam 682 018, Kochi, Kerala, India.
  Ph: +91-484-4059061-65 Fax: +91-484-4059065 e-mail: kochi@cbspd.com

- **Kolkata:** 6/B, Ground Floor, Rameswar Shaw Road, Kolkata-700 014, West Bengal, India
  Ph: +91-33-22891126, 22891127, 22891128 e-mail: kolkata@cbspd.com

- **Mumbai:** 83-C, Dr E Moses Road, Worli, Mumbai-400018, Maharashtra, India
  Ph: +91-22-24902340/41 Fax: +91-22-24902342 e-mail: mumbai@cbspd.com

Representatives

- **Bhopal** 0-8319310552
- **Jharkhand** 0-9811541605
- **Pune** 0-9623451994
- **Bhubaneswar** 0-9911037372
- **Nagpur** 0-9021734563
- **Uttarakhand** 0-9716462459
- **Hyderabad** 0-9885175004
- **Patna** 0-9334159340
- **Dhaka (Bangladesh)** 01912-003485

Printed at: Goyal Offset Printers, GT Karnal Road, Industrial Area, Delhi, India

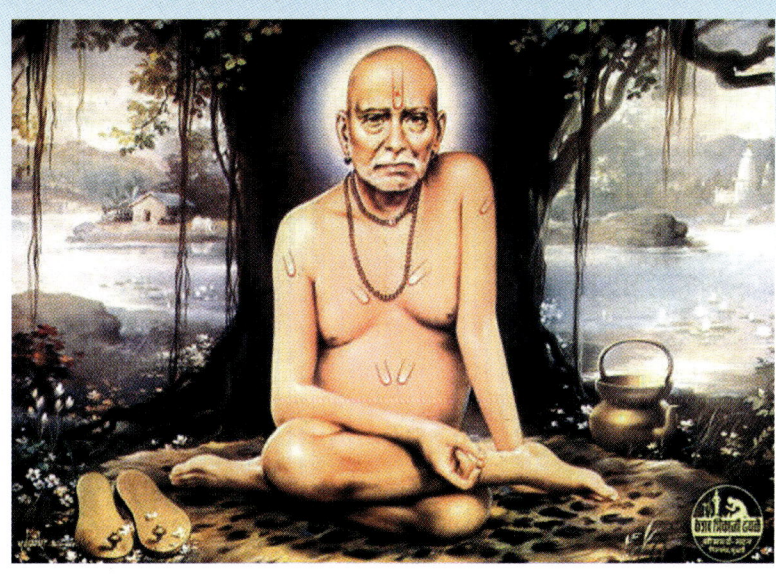

Shri Swami Samarth

to

My father, Adi Dinshaw Mistry—who taught me the value of hard work and loyalty
My mother, Viloo Adi Mistry—for her selfless love and caring
Both my parents and mamma—for their blessings and encouragement
My husband, Tempton—always loving, caring and encouraging
My miracle and happiness, Karishma and Khushi—for making life worthwhile
Rustom, Khushru, Firozee, Sharon, Jenaifer, Zenia,
Travis and Hazel—for believing in me and being with me

—Bachi T Hathiram

My father, Subhash Chandra Gyanchand Khattar—my support
My mother, Veena Subhash Khattar—my encouragement
My grandparents, Gyanchand Khattar, Mohandevi Khattar,
Vas Dev Pawa, Tulsidevi Pawa—who indulged me
Shalu, Sameer, Sehar and Sia—my indulgence
My family, friends, teachers and students

—Vicky S Khattar

Forewords to the Third Edition

It is my pleasure and honour to have been asked to write the Foreword for the third edition of the textbook written by Dr. Bachi T Hathiram and Dr. Vicky S Khattar. The first two editions have been very well received by students as well as practitioners which have prompted them to come out with the third edition. The authors have covered the entire spectrum of ear, nose, throat, diseases as well as their treatment and have included the recent advances in the various fields of ENT in this book.

There are chapters on Anatomy and Physiology of the ear, nose, larynx, etc., and this is very systematically followed on a clinical examination, the various symptoms, as well as the various diseases affecting each of these organs. This is followed by the treatment protocols involved in the management of these conditions, and there is an additional chapter on the recent advances in the various aspects of ENT.

The authors need to be complimented for the meticulous care that they have taken in putting the various chapters together, making them as simple to understand for the undergraduate students as well as for the practitioners. The text is further supported by excellent pictures and diagrams which make it easy to understand the various aspects of ENT disorders.

I am sure that this book will be of great value to students in enhancing their knowledge of ENT and for practitioners in understanding the various aspects of ENT diseases and treating their patients in a more meaningful manner.

Padma Shri Prof. (Dr). Milind V. Kirtane

It is a pleasure to write the Foreword for the third edition of the textbook written by Prof (Dr) Bachi T. Hathiram and Assistant Prof (Dr) Vicky S. Khattar. With number of undergraduates increasing and the student teacher ratio widening, a student finds it very difficult to acquire clinical knowledge. In such circumstances the topics covered by the two authors are of great help to the students. All the chapters are written with great care so that the students can get oriented with the topics. The book will not only help the students to face the examiner well but also add to their knowledge. The illustrations presented in the book are very vivid.

The chapters on anatomy and physiology are extremely important for the undergraduates which are described very well along with clinical symptoms and their management. The surgical procedures described in the book are of great importance and are described in simple language for the benefit of the reader.

The section on Recent Advances is an excellent addition to the book. Students need to have the knowledge of hearing aids, cochlear implants, etc. which they will gain from chapters under the section.

The book comprises 62 chapters which have covered all aspects of otorhinolaryngology for undergraduate students and the MCQs at the end of text will be of great help to them. I am sure all undergraduate students as well as teachers will benefit from this book.

Prof. (Dr.) Ashutosh Pusalkar

Foreword to the First Edition, 1999

This latest book, written by two otolaryngologists from the TN Medical College and BYL Nair Hospital in Mumbai, lives up well to its title and it will be welcomed by those for whom it has been written, namely undergraduate medical students, trainee specialists and primary care doctors.

The anatomy and physiology of each region are discussed in clear terms, with an emphasis on clinical applications; and for each region, the main symptoms are discussed before the conditions occurring in each region are described in a more formal way. The principles of some of the commoner surgical procedures are discused and there are useful chapters on recent advances.

Throughout the book, the text is written in a simple, synoptic style, and it can be highly recommended as an introduction to this expanding specialty.

John Ballantyne, CBE, FRCS
Emeritus ENT Surgeon
Royal Free Hospital
London

Message from the Dean, Second Edition, 2002

It gives me great pleasure to write a message as Dean TN Medical College and BYL Nair Ch. Hospital, for the second edition of this textbook 'ENT-SIMPLIFIED' by Dr. Bachi T Hathiram and Dr. DS Grewal.

The authors have written this edition in a simple and easy-to-remember style that one associates with this textbook. There are new chapters added keeping in mind the changing trends in examinations and the advances in the field of ENT. The book contains separate sections on instruments, operations and MCQs as well as recent advances, making it complete for theory and practical exams. It would be an added advantage to the department and college libraries of teaching institutes.

This textbook is written especially keeping the student in mind. I am sure it will prove invaluable to the undergraduate student as well as to the diploma and degree student. Consultants and teachers would find it as a useful addition to their resources.

I wish the authors success in their venture.

Dr. (Mrs.) Sharadini Dahanukar,
TN Medical College and BYL Nair Ch. Hospital

Message from Dr. N L Hiranandani, First Edition, 1999

It gives me immense pleasure to write a few words for this textbook named 'ENT SIMPLIFIED' which is the first of its kind from our department. I have known the authors since a long time and both are extremely academically oriented. The book is an outcome of months of hard and dedicated work on their part.

I am sure this book will be of great use not only to undergraduate students but also to postgraduates and teachers of ENT. It is concise and very much to-the-point at the same time giving an explanation for most clinical features thus increasing the understanding of the reader. The chapters on instruments and operations as well as the diagrams are especially note-worthy and well written.

The entire book is clinically oriented without being monotonous or boring thus, making interesting reading. I am sure it will be of great help to all students especially for reproduction during exams and I recommend it for MBBS, DLO, DORL, AST (BSc and MSc) students and teachers as well as for general practioners.

Dr. N L Hiranandani
Hon. Professor; Department of ENT
TN Medical College and BYL Nair Ch. Hospital

Preface to the Third Edition

It is indeed a great pleasure to present the third edition of this popular ENT textbook to the students. This textbook has been written after a long hiatus during which we have gone through every aspect of this rapidly advancing field and tried to incorporate the salient features keeping in mind the gruelling schedule of the undergraduate students of medicine today.

We are sure that this edition will also prove invaluable to the postgraduates, since we have maintained the simple format of text as well as diagrams, making it easy to remember and replicate in the exams. From the very outset, this book has aimed to 'simplify' the subject, making it interesting and palatable to the novice and undergraduate students, and even practitioners of medicine as a ready reckoner. Its flavour lies in its lucid presentation and stardardisation of the format in each chapter.

Despite the field undergoing a metamorphosis in the past decade, the book prides itself in its content, which although not exhaustive, simply attempts to 'introduce' the enchanting world of ENT to the reader, and spur them for further reading; simultaneously retaining its status as a comprehensive textbook for the undergraduate syllabus. We are extremely grateful to our Dean Dr. Ramesh Bharmal who has been a source of constant encouragement.

We express our heartfelt gratitude towards our residents, who since the previous edition have been involved in various stages of development of this edition. They have proved to not only be a constant source of inspiration, but also encouraged us from time to time to pursue our academic efforts. We would like to mention each and every one of them as below:

Shobhit Srivastava, Santosh Davis, Minal Shroff Modi, Rajeev T, Prashant Sharma, Ankit Jain, Deepanjali Kulkarni, Atul Tekade, Hemant Nemade, Harshad Nikte, Reema Rai Shetty, Parag Watve, Harshal Sonavane, Anjoo Choudhary, Alok Nema, Balagopal Kurup, Supriya Rode Kadam, Hemant Sharma, Sanket Dani, Ankit Jain, Sunil Khot, Snigdha Devane, Diptarka Bhattacharyya, Lubna Sayed, Sobhana Chandran, Sohil Gala, Ruchi Shah, Pravin Rajgadkar, Rachana Mehta, Pallavi Singh, Vinayak Chandran, Raksha Dabhekar, Ashwinikumar Gaikwad, Ashwini Mastud, Sreena Dev, Snekha Dominic, Priyanka Aage, Aarti Pawar, Sidrah Mirza and Vishnu K S.

Bachi T Hathiram
Vicky S Khattar

Preface to the Second Edition

We, the authors of this book are delighted to present the second edition of our textbook 'ENT Simplified'. The favourable response of the students and teachers of various institutions to its first edition was most encouraging and it gives us great pleasure to present this new edition.

Due to the tremendous strides made in the advancement of the subject by intense research and keeping in mind the changing curriculum of the students which requires more exposure to MCQs and recent advances in our field, a separate section on MCQs and chapters such as cryotherapy in ENT, radiotherapy, AIDS in ENT have been added, still maintaining the simple, explicit and easy-to-reproduce character, which has been the hallmark of this book. The second edition has also incorporated many useful suggestions of our students and each comment has been received with utmost attention.

We are very grateful to our Dean Dr. (Mrs.) Sharadini Dahanukar for the encouragement and support that she has given us throughout our endeavour.

We are especially thankful to Dr. Santhosh Davies and Dr. Minal Shroff, for their patient and meticulous help, Dr. Sanjay Chalbria was most helpful with improvement in various chapters and we are grateful for his constant support. Dr. Neelam Sathe, Dr. Lovneesh Kumar, Dr. Rahul Mehta, Dr. Kaushal Sheth, Dr. Alok Mohorikar, Dr. Pravin Sonwatikar and Dr. Shobit Shrivastav deserve a special thanks for their suggestions and cooperation which helped us for this editon. We are also thankful to Dr. Mohd. Hashmi for his help.

Though the book is aimed especially for the undergraduate student, it will act as a guiding light to the postgraduate students and also practising doctors. We are sure our colleagues will continue to use it for teaching and guiding students as in the past.

Bachi T Hathiram
DS Grewal

Preface to the First Edition

In this day and age, there are several textbooks on ENT, however, a book with simple language, explicit and easy-to-reproduce diagrams and most importantly, keeping in mind the busy schedule of undergraduate students (MBBS, nursing, audiology and speech therapy), general practitioners and ENT residents is the need of the hour.

We have attempted to keep in mind the need for a simple, self-explanatory book which makes the subject of ENT easy to grasp and easier to recollect. Even though topics such as salivary glands, tracheobronchial tree, oesophagus and neck are included in the ENT syllabus, we have not included these in our book since they are given full justice in any standard surgical textbook.

We are extremely grateful to our Dean, Dr. (Mrs.) KD Nihalani for her encouragement and support without which the publication of our book would not have been possible. We are also ever-grateful to Dr. LH Hiranandani for his guidance as well as for giving us one of the best and most sophisticated ENT department which gives us the best opportunity for academic work in addition to other routine ENT activities. We are greatly honoured and thankful to Prof. John Ballantyne for patiently going through our book, giving valuable suggestions and for writing the Foreword to our book. We are especially thankful to Dr. Paresh Tankwal, Dr. Dinaz Irani, Dr. Vijay Jagasia, Dr. Ninad Gaikwad, Dr. Manish Patankar, Dr. Anurag Singhal, Dr. Vinita Joshi, Dr. Nilam Sathe, Dr. Trupti Manjrekar, Dr. Neha Shah, Dr. Ritu Aggarwal, Dr. Ashwin Diwedi, Dr. Rohan Walvekar, Dr. Lovneesh Kumar, Dr. Kaushal Sheth and Dr. Rahul Mehta for helping us in the writing of this book. Mrs. Alka Kondar and Mrs. Pratibha Patil of our department have been very helpful from time to time.

We shall be ever grateful to M/s. Bhalani Book Depot who were the mastermind behind the conception and creation of this book. Mr. Rajesh Bhalani has been a constant source of encouragement to us.

The simple and easy to reproduce diagrams are due to the efforts of our artist, Mr. Pramod Mahajan who most patiently and meticulously reproduced ideas on paper. Mr. SN Chalke has been a great help in the preliminary typing. The credit for all the photographic work goes to Mr. SS Patil and Mr. MB Dabholkar of our photography department.

We are sure this textbook, as its name suggests will make understanding and recollecting ENT much simpler.

Bachi T Hathiram
DS Grewal

Contents

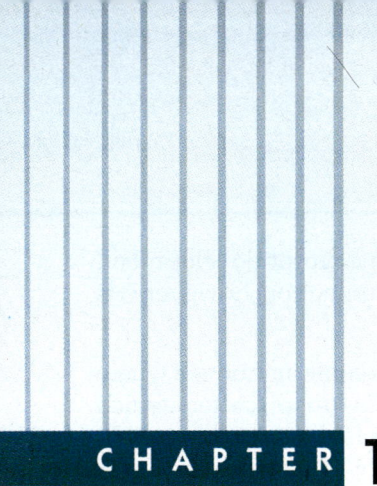

CHAPTER 1

Examination of the ENT Patient

INTRODUCTION

Proper history taking is the most important part of any medical examination. The same is true for ENT examination (an idea about the various diseases can be had from the history elicited from the patient). For example, a person whose house is located close to the railway tracks and who has developed impaired hearing over a period of time is probably suffering from noise-induced hearing loss. Similarly, a patient who complains of recurrent sneezing and watering of the eyes for a long period of time has probably got allergic rhinitis.

EQUIPMENT FOR ENT EXAMINATION

The basic equipment required for ENT examination may be categorised into two types. These are:

- Illuminators
- Instruments for examination

The various equipments used for examination are also used for performing minor procedures and surgery of the ear, nose and throat.

Illuminators

Proper illumination is one of the most important prerequisites for ENT examination. Proper visualisation of the ear, nose and throat requires a special type of illumination which focusses light at the point of examination or surgery. Various different kinds of illuminators have been developed and are used regularly by the ENT surgeons.

Bull's eye lamp and head mirror   The Bull's eye lamp consists of an electric bulb of 100 watts housed in a metal cage. The cage is placed on a stand whose height and position can be adjusted according to the needs of the consultant surgeon. The cage has a metallic cover with a convex lens on one side which makes the rays of light parallel. This parallel beam falls on the head-mirror worn on the head of the examiner. The mirror reflects the light at the appropriate place and brightly illuminates the area to be inspected.

The head mirror consists of a concave mirror which diameter is 9 cm and has a central aperture of 2 cm diameter. It converges the rays of light at a focal point which is 20 cm (focal length). The aperture of the mirror is kept in front of the right eye of the examiner and this allows the examiner to have a binocular view of the structures to be examined. The source of light is kept behind the left shoulder of the patient. Mirror is worn on the head with the help of an adjustable head band.

Bull's eye lamp and the head mirror are the most commonly used sources of illumination in ENT (Fig. 1.1A).

Electric headlight   In this illuminator, the source of light and the mirror to focus the light are so made that they are worn on the head of the examiner. The source works either on electricity or battery (Fig. 1.1B).

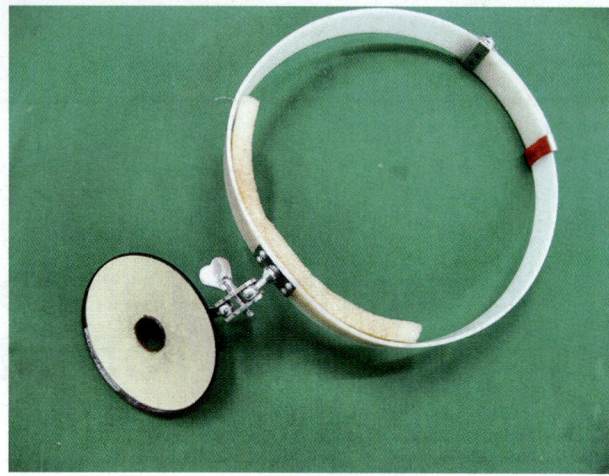

Fig. 1.1A: Bull's eye lamp and head mirror

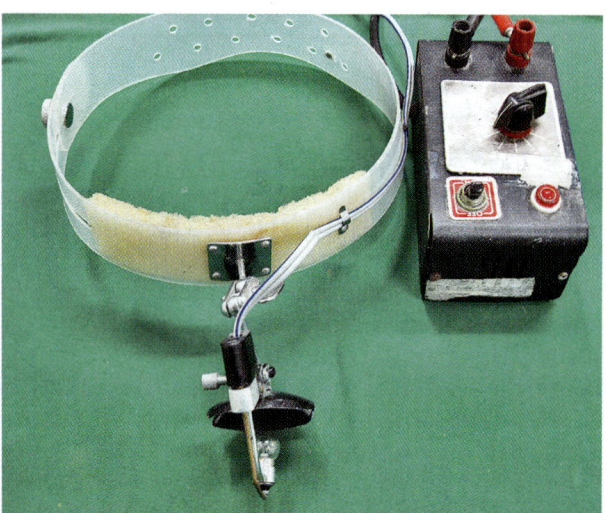

Fig. 1.1B: Electric headlight

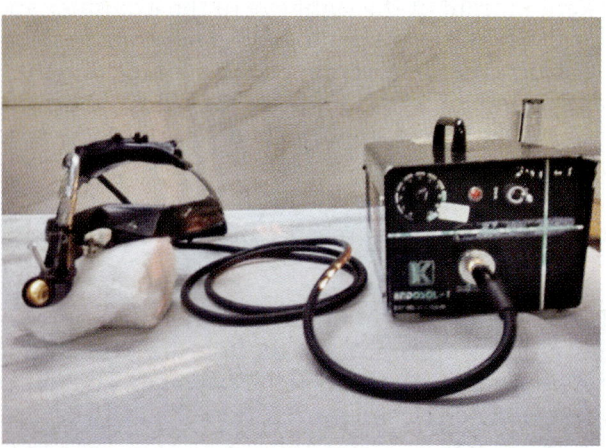

Fig. 1.1C: Fibre-optic headlight

Fibre-optic headlight This is a recent development. It provides extremely good illumination, however, it is expensive (Fig. 1.1C).

Otoscope This is a self-illuminating instrument where the source of light is a bulb which runs on battery which is loaded on the handle. There is a convex lens which helps in examination of the ear with a magnification of 2X (Fig. 1.1D).

Otoscopes may be fitted with a rubber tubing and bulb which can be used for Sieglisation, called 'pneumatic otoscopy' when performed using an otoscope. This allows the examiner to get an idea about the movement of the eardrum, presence of a labyrinthine fistula and this may also be used to introduce powdered medication into the middle ear through a perforation.

Surgical microscope This is best for examination and surgery as it enables the examiner to visualise minute details under high magnification. It is mainly used for ear surgery but also can be used in nose and laryngeal surgery, e.g. ethmoidectomy, removal of vocal cord nodules by microlaryngoscopy, etc. (Fig. 1.1E)

Others Rigid sinuscope (nasal endoscope) is being extensively used in diagnosis of diseases of the nose. It has a fiberoptic source of light and built-in optics for visualisation. Similarly a direct flexible or rigid laryngoscope illuminates and also helps in visualisation of the larynx. Oto endoscope is used for diagnosis of ear

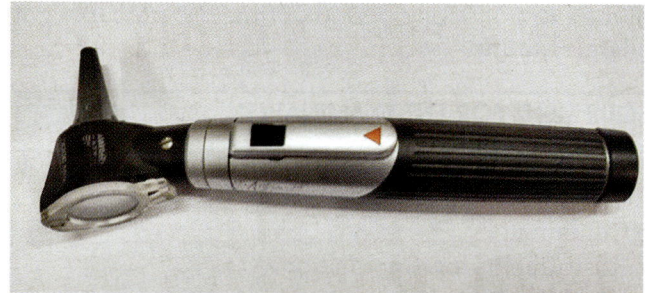

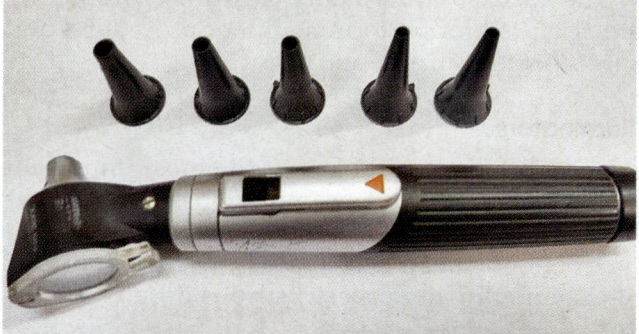

Fig. 1.1D: Otoscope

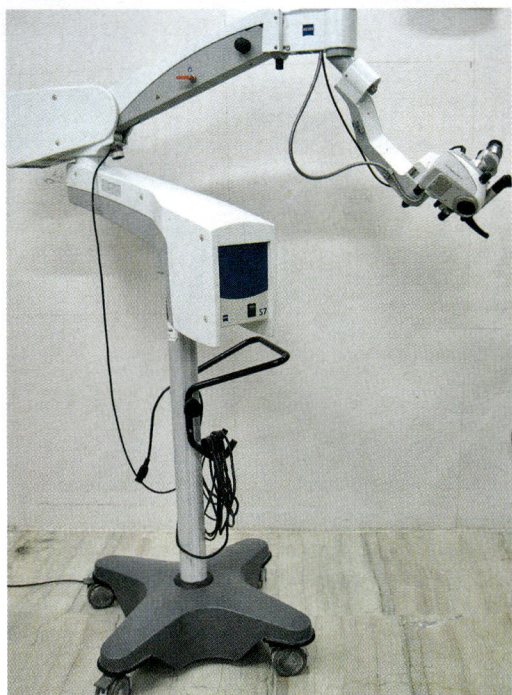

Fig. 1.1E: Surgical microscope

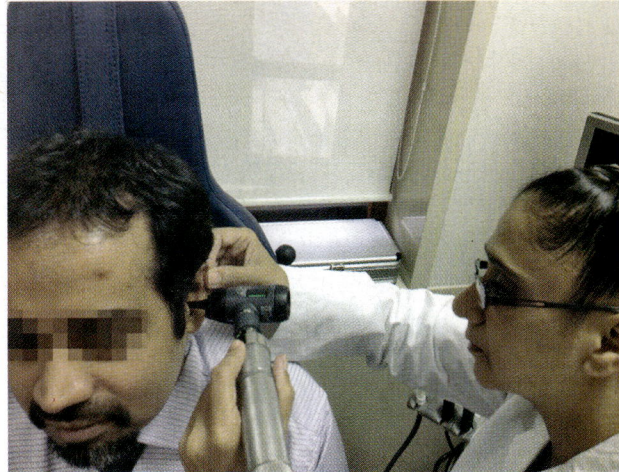

Fig. 1.2A: Examination of ear with otoscope

disease as well as for surgery. It helps to see the areas difficult to visualise by microscope. Also nasal and oto endoscopes are available in various angulations of lens, thus further improving vision during surgery. Diagnostic sinus endoscopy and fiberoptic laryngoscopy can be done as OPD procedures.

Instruments for Examination

These have been dealt within details in specific chapters.

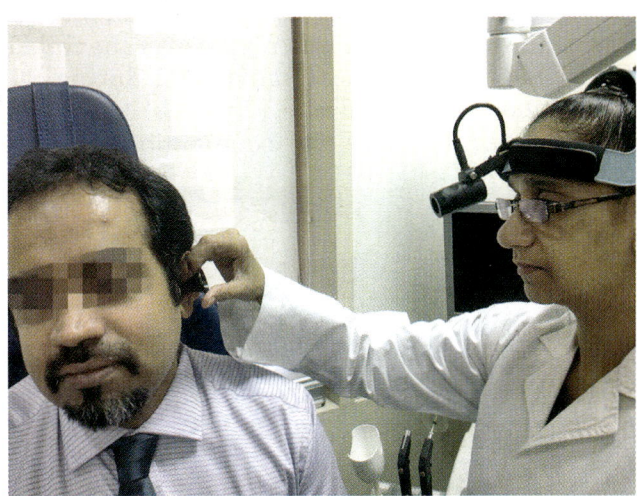

Fig. 1.2B: Examination of ear with speculum using on electric headlight

POSITION OF THE PATIENT AND EXAMINER

Patient is asked to sit on a chair which should preferably be an ENT examination chair. The examiner sits facing the patient. The Bull's eye lamp is placed behind the left shoulder of the patient. Examination of the neck is best carried out when the examiner stands behind the patient with the patient's neck flexed. (Fig. 1.2 A, B, C and D)

EXAMINATION OF CHILDREN

A cooperative child can be examined without any difficulty. Taking the child into confidence is a very important aspect of the examination. An uncooperative child is examined by asking the parent to take the child on their lap in such a way that the legs of child are held firmly between those of

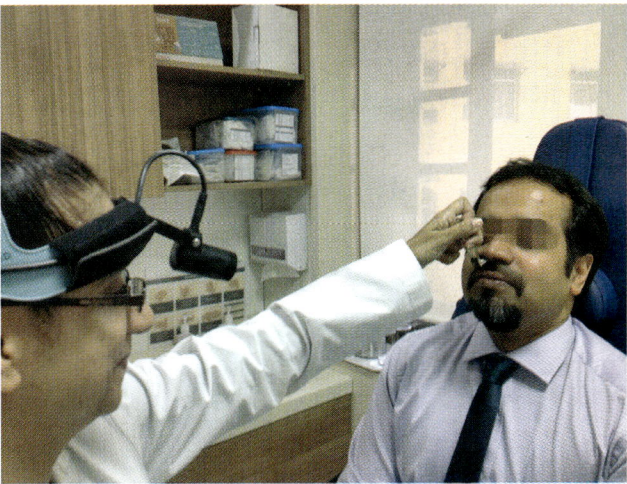

Fig. 1.2C: Examination of nose using a fibre-optic headlight

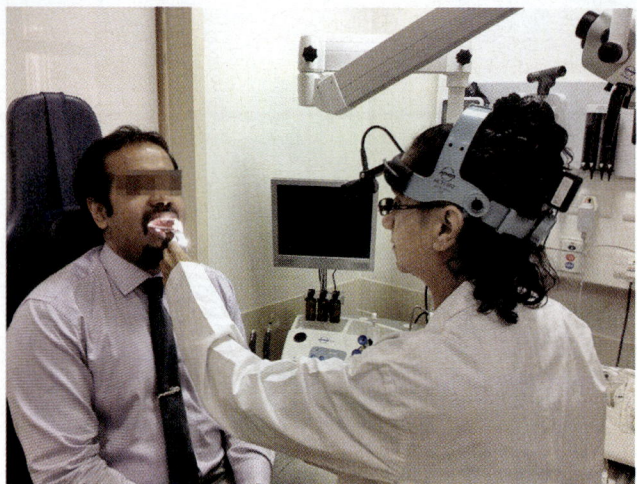

Fig. 1.2D: Examination of throat using a fibre-optic headlight

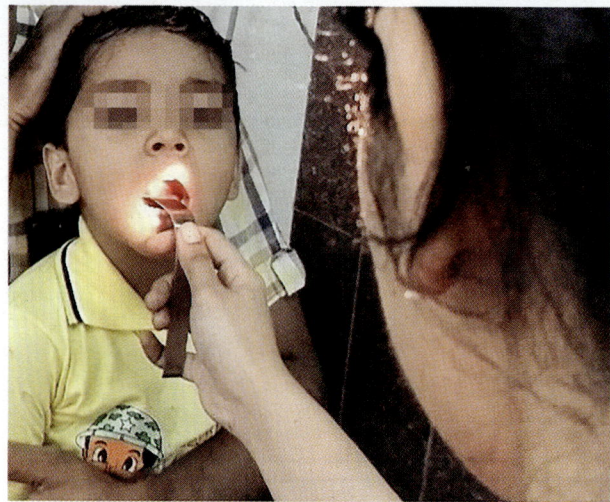

Fig. 1.3B: Examination of throat

the parent. The parent fixes the hands of child with her one hand and places the other hand over the child's forehead to prevent head movement during the examination (Fig. 1.3A, B and C).

In most of the cases, the examination can only

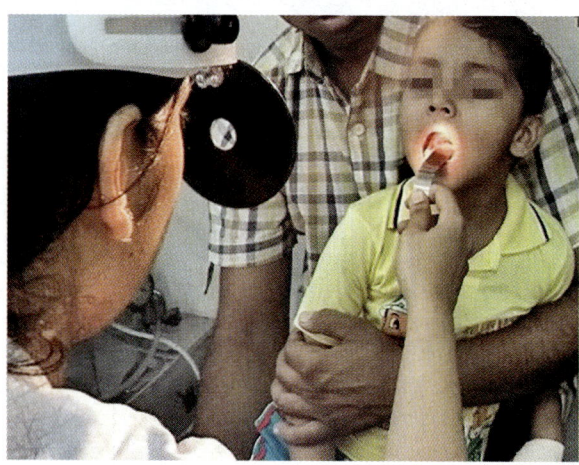

Fig. 1.3C: Examination of throat using Bull's eye headlight

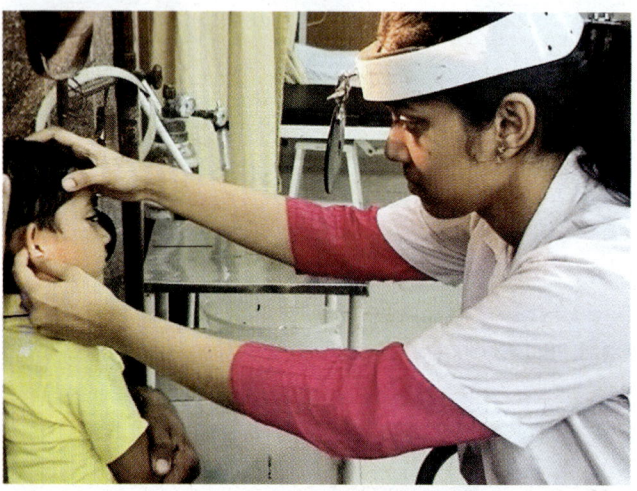

Fig. 1.3A: Examination of ear using a Bull's eye headlight

be carried out with illumination. Instruments are generally not required as the child does not have hair in the ears or nose and the anatomical positions of the nose and ear are such that the examination is very easy.

Anatomy of the Ear

EMBRYOLOGY

In the early stages of fetal development, a series of six branchial (visceral/mesenchymal) arches develops on the lateral aspect of the head to produce serial ridges over the surface and projections within the pharynx, being separate from each other by furrows.

The outer one (ectodermal) is called the visceral cleft while the inner one (entodermal) is known as the pharyngeal pouch (Fig. 2.1).

Pinna   It is formed by fusion of six tubercles around the margin of the first visceral cleft, derived from the first and second branchial arches.

- **Double source of origin:** Hence, double nerve innervation.

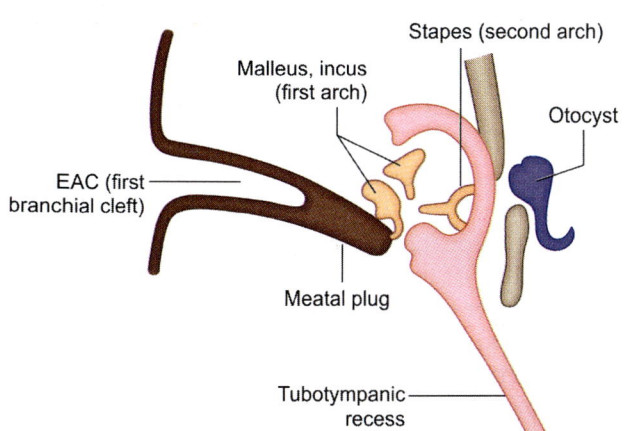

Fig. 2.1: Embryological development of the ear

- Greater auricular nerve
- Auriculotemporal nerve
- The site of fusion is at the interval between tragus and helix–common site of congenital preauricular sinus.

External auditory canal (EAC)
- The cartilagenous part is derived from the dorsal end of the ectoderm of the first branchial cleft.
- The bony part develops after birth from the tympanic ring.

Tympanic membrane   It is derived from the membrane separating first branchial cleft and the tubotympanic recess, which develops from first and second branchial pouches.

Origin of different layers of tympanic membrane:
- **Outer squamous layer:** Ectoderm of first branchial cleft
- **Intermediate fibrous layer:** Mesoderm between first branchial cleft and tubotympanic recess
- **Inner mucous layer:** Entoderm of the tubotympanic recess

Middle ear cleft   (Eustachian tube, middle ear, mastoid air cells) Derived from the tubotympanic recess (entodermal) between first and second visceral arches.
- Ossicles
  - *Malleus and incus:* Developed from dorsal end of mandibular (Meckel's) cartilage (first branchial arch)

- ♦ *Stapes suprastructure:* Derived from the dorsal end of the Reichert's cartilage (second branchial arch).
- ♦ *Stapes footplate:* Derived from otic capsule, which develops in the mesoderm surrounding the membranous labyrinth.

Inner ear It develops from the ectoderm in the hindbrain which gets invaginated to form the auditory pit which later forms the auditory vesicle (otocyst) which then develops into the membranous labyrinth.

Its cartilaginous otic capsule orginates from surrounding mesoderm which later ossifies into the bony labyrinth. (The inner ear and auricles reach adult size by fourth month of intrauterine life.)

- • Temporal bone: It is formed by fusion of morphological elements of tympanic ring sepama, styloid process (cranial end of cartilage of second branchial arch) and petromastoid bone.

ANATOMY

External ear It consists of pinna and external auditory canal (Fig. 2.2).

- • Pinna (Auricle): It comprises of a single sheet of yellow fibrocartilage 0.5–1 mm thick covered by perichondrium and skin.

  It is attached to the side of the head with three vestigeal muscles (auricularis anterior, posterior and superior) and fibrous ligaments.
  - ♦ *Lobule:* Fibro-fatty tissue without cartilage.
  - ♦ *Helix:* Outer rim of auricle, begins at concha and ends at lobule.

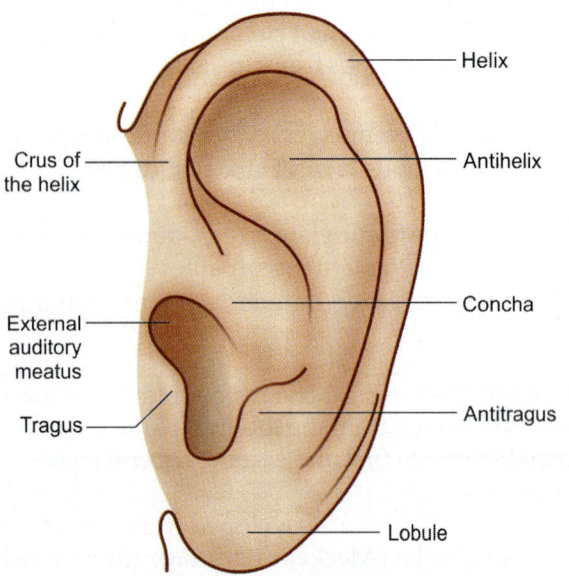

Crus of the helix

External auditory meatus

Tragus

Helix

Antihelix

Concha

Antitragus

Lobule

Fig. 2.2: Anatomy of the left pinna

- ♦ *Antihelix:* Prominence anterior to and parallel with the helix, which has two crura dividing to form a triangular fossa, 'scaphoid fossa'.
- ♦ *Concha:* It is a part of the auricular cartilage that lies anterior to the antihelix, anterosuperiorly, covered by the crus of the helix lies the cymba conchae.
- ♦ *Tragus:* A triangular small blunt prominence that overlays the concha anteriorly.
- ♦ *Antitragus:* It lies opposite to tragus at inferior limit of antihelix.
- ♦ *Gaps*
  - • Incisura terminalis — gap between tragus and helix.
  - • Intertragic notch — gap between tragus and antitragus.
- ♦ *Fissures of santorini:* These lie in the auricular cartilage to enable vessels and nerves to pass through from one surface to another
- ♦ *Arteries:* Anteriorly — superficial temporal artery. Posteriorly — posterior auricular artery
- ♦ *Veins:* Superficial temporal and posterior auricular veins
- ♦ *Lymphatics:* Preauricular, postauricular and superficial cervical lymph nodes
- ♦ *Nerves:*
  - • *Motor supply:* Facial nerve — extrinsic muscles.
  - • *Sensory supply*
    - ▪ Auriculotemporal (V3) — upper two-thirds on lateral side
    - ▪ Greater auricular (C2, C3) — lower one-third on both sides
    - ▪ Lesser occipital (C2) — upper two-thirds on medial side
    - ▪ Auricular branch of facial nerve

Clinical significance

- • If perichondrium is stripped by hemorrhage or suppuration, the entire auricular cartilage may necrose, as it is a single sheet.
- • Endaural incision, can be taken at incisura terminalis, as it does not cut through cartilage at this point.
- • Cymba conchae are related directly to suprameatal triangle of the temporal bone. These are site to check for mastoid tenderness in mastoiditis.
- • External auditory canal: It extends from the base of the concha to the tympanic membrane.
  - ♦ *Size* : 2.4 cm (1 inch) approximately
  - ♦ *Parts* : Outer one-third (cartilagenous)—8 mm
    Inner two-thirds (bony)—16 mm
  - ♦ *Shape* : 'S' shaped

Constrictions

- At the junction of cartilage and bone.
- At the isthmus, (narrowest) at 5 mm (0.2 inches) from the tympanic membrane and the isthmus, the floor of the external auditory canal dips steeply downwards and forwards forming the anterior recess.

Lining

- *Outer one-third (cartilagenous)*: The skin is adherent to the cartilage with hair follicles and ceruminous glands which secrete wax.
- *Inner two-thirds (bony)*: Skin is thin, lacks sebaceous and ceruminous glands.

Relations

- *Anteriorly* : Temporomandibular joint
- *Superiorly* : Middle cranial fossa
- *Posteriorly* : Mastoid air cells and antrum
- *Inferiorly* : Parotid gland

Arteies

- *Cartilagenous portion*
  - Auriculotemporal branch of superficial temporal artery.
  - Posterior auricular branch of external carotid artery.
- *Bony portion (including the outer surface of the tympanic membrane)*
  - Deep auricular branch of maxillary artery (first part).

Veins: Superficial temporal and posterior-auricular veins

Lymphatics: Preauricular, post-auricular and external jugular lymph nodes

Nerves

- Auriculotemporal branch of trigeminal nerve anterior half of the EAC
- Auricular branch of vagus nerve (Arnold's/Alderman's) posterior half of the EAC

Clinical significance

- *Shape*: In children, canal is short and straight without hair, thus eardrum is directly examined, pulling the pinna downwards and backwards, unlike adults where it has to be pulled upwards laterally and backwards.
- *Constriction*: At isthmus, the commonest site where foreign body is lodged.
- *Anterior recess*: It is site of accumulation of debris.
- *Lining*: It is outer cartilagenous portion. Skin is adherent, hence even a minimum subcutaneous

collection (e.g. furuncle) may stretch it to produce severe pain.

- *Fissures of santorini*: These lie in the anterior wall, are a pathway through which parotid abscess may drain via the external auditory meatus.
- *Arnold's nerve*: Innervation (posterior half), it triggers coughing and vasovagal syncope–on manipulation in this area for removal of foreign body or wax.

Tympanic membrane (Drum head, eardrum) The tympanic membrane is thin, pearly white in colour and lies in between the external and middle ears. It forms the lateral wall of the middle ear cavity (Fig. 2.3).

It is divided into two parts:

- Pars flaccida (Shrapnell's membrane): It is formed of three layers that is outer squamous, inner mucous and middle fibrous. It is situated above the lateral process of malleus between the notch of Rivinus and the anterior and posterior malleolar folds. It appears flaccid and is pinkish in colour.
- Pars tensa: It forms the larger part of the tympanic membrane. It has a thickened fibrocartilagenous ring at the margin called the annulus which fits into the bony tympanic sulcus (sulcus tympanicus).

The central part (most concave part of the tympanic membrane) is tented inwards at the level of the tip of the malleus and it is called the umbo.

The three layers of the pars tensa are:

- Outer epithelial layer: It is continuous with the meatal skin.
- Middle fibrous layer: It encloses the malleus handle and has radial and circular fibres.
- Inner mucosal layer: It is continuous with the mucosa of the middle ear.

Size, shape and position of the tympanic membrane

- *Size*: 9–10 mm vertical diameter and 8–9 mm horizontal diameter and approximately 0.1 mm thick.
- *Surface area*
  - 80 mm^2 with effective area (i.e. area of vibration) of 55 mm^2
  - Lateral surface is concave
  - Medial surface is convex
- *Shape*: Oval to elliptical
- *Position*: In adults, obliquely placed at an angle of 55° with floor of the deep part of the external auditory canal.
- The anterior and posterior malleolar folds have an attachment of the lateral process of malleus.

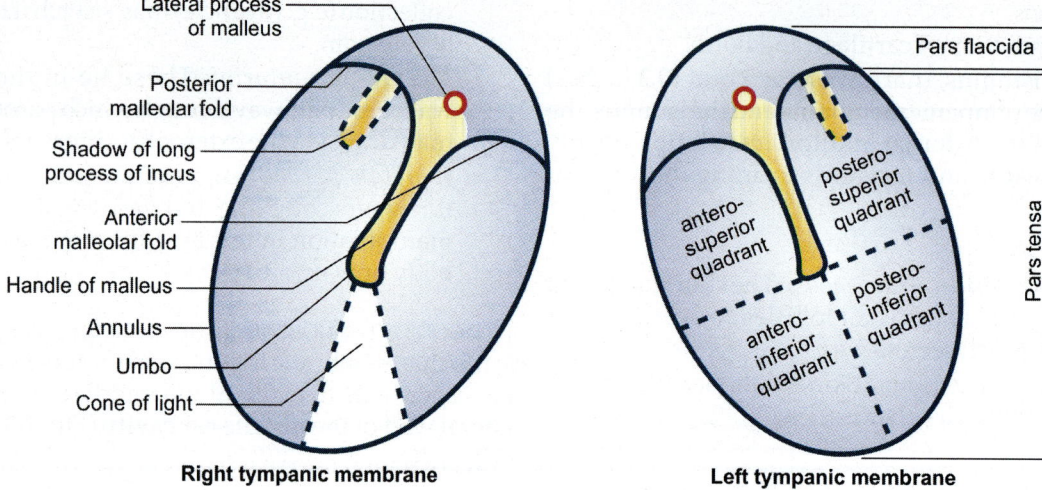

Right tympanic membrane   **Left tympanic membrane**

Fig. 2.3: Diagrammatic representation of tympanic membrane

- *Umbo*: Lies at the tip of the malleus handle. It is the most concave portion of the tympanic membrane.
- *Cone of light*: It is a conical reflection of light extending to the anteroinferior quadrant of the eardrum because that is the part where the light rays of the otoscope or Bull's eye lamp are reflected back at right angles to the observer's eye.
- *The long process of incus*: It lies posterior to the handle of malleus, and runs parallel to it midway between the posterior bony wall of the middle ear and malleus.
- *Pars flaccida* is the part of the eardrum above the malleolar folds.
- *Pars tensa* forms the rest of the tympanic membrane which is divided into four quadrants by drawing an imaginary line extending from the handle of malleus down and another imaginary line at right angles to the first line at the level of the umbo.

    The quadrants thus created are anteriosuperior, anterioinferior, posteroinferior and posterosuperior quadrants.

Arteries
- *Outer surface*: Deep auricular artery which is the branch of the maxillary artery (first part). (The artery encircles the membrane peripherally and sends branches towards the centre in a cart-wheel fashion).
- *Inner surface*
    - Anterior tympanic branch of maxillary artery (second part).
    - Posterior tympanic branch of stylomastoid artery (branch of posterior auricular artery).

- Inferior tympanic artery (branch of ascending pharyngeal artery).
- Arteria nutrica incudo-mallei (twig from middle meningeal artery).

Veins
- *Outer surface*: Drained by external jugular vein.
- *Inner surface*: Drained by the transverse sinus and venous plexus located around the Eustachian tube.

Nerve supply
- *Outer surface*: Same as that of the external auditory canal.
    - Anterior half—by auriculotemporal nerve
    - Posterior half—by auricular branch of vagus nerve
- *Inner surface*: By the tympanic plexus, which also supplies the middle ear.

Clinical Significance
- In newborn, tympanic membrane is horizontal but with development of tympanic portion of the temporal bone, it becomes oblique (adults).
- Pars flaccida is a common area for occurance of retraction and cholesteatoma formation due to laxity of the eardrum, as it does not have an annulus.
- During myringotomy, curved incision is preferred as straizght incision cuts the radial fibres and allows the circular fibres to appose and close the wound, thus preventing adequate drainage of the secretions in the middle ear.

Middle ear cleft   The middle ear together with the Eustachian tube, aditus, antrum and mastoid air cells is called the middle ear cleft which is lined by respiratory mucous membrane and filled with air (Fig. 2.4).

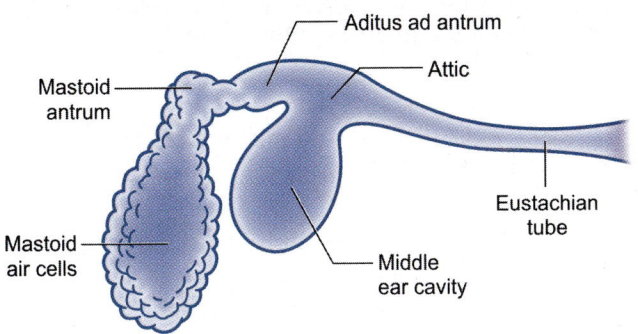

Fig. 2.4: Diagrammatic representation of the middle ear cleft

- Eustachian tube (pharyngotympanic tube): Valsalva gave the name 'Eustachian' to the auditory tube in honor of Bartholemus Eustachius, who had first described it.

  The Eustachian tube connects the middle ear cavity to the pharynx.

  - *Size and position:* 36 mm (adults) in length, the pharyngeal opening in the lateral wall of the naso-pharynx is situated 1.5 cm behind and at the level of the posterior end of inferior turbinate with a 45° inclination.

  It is divided into two parts:
  - Lateral one-third—bony (12 mm)
  - Medial two-thirds—cartilagenous (24 mm)

  Both portions meet at an angle called the isthmus, which is the narrowest part of the tube.

  - *Muscles attached to the Eustachian tube:*
  - Tensor tympani muscle
  - Tensor palati muscle
  - Levator palati muscle

Clinical Significance: In infants the tube is inclined at an angle of 30°, it is shorter and more horizontal, thus permits infections to travel easily from nasopharynx to the middle ear cleft. The milk may regurgitate into the middle ear, if the infant is not fed in a head-high position.

- Tympanic cavity (middle ear): The middle ear is a six-sided cavity, situated between the tympanic membrane laterally and inner ear medially (Figs 2.5 and 2.6).

  - *Size, shape and position:* The vertical and antero-posterior diameters are approximately 15 mm, while the transverse diameter is 6 mm at the upper part (epitympanum), 2 mm at the centre (mesotympanum) and 4 mm at the lower part (hypotympanum).

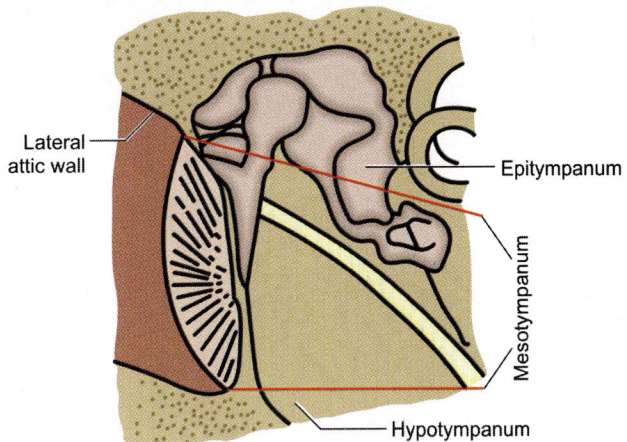

Fig. 2.5: The tympanic cavity

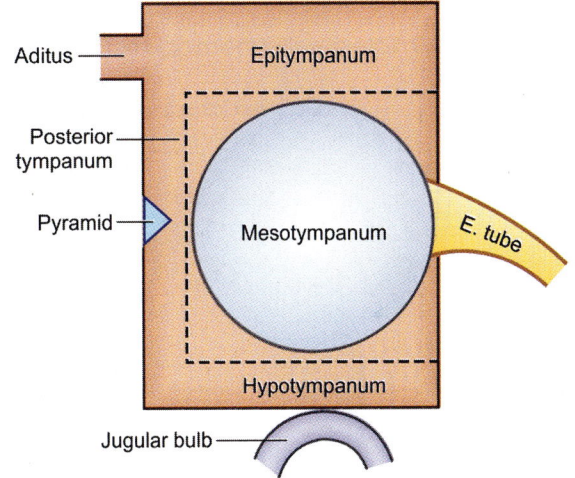

Fig. 2.6: Diagrammatic representation of the tympanic cavity

- *Boundaries*
  - *Lateral wall:* Tympanic cavity is divided into three parts (Fig. 2.7):
    - *Epitympanum (Attic):* It lies above the pars tensa but medial to the pars flaccida and bony lateral attic wall (scutum), extending above the tympanic membrane. It contains upper half of malleus and a large part of incus.
    - *Mesotympanum:* It lies medial to the pars tensa.
    - *Hypotympanum:* It lies medial to and below the level of pars tensa.
  - *Medial wall:* It is formed by the bony labyrinth and has the following structures (Fig. 2.8):
    - *Promontory:* It is a smooth, round projection of the basal turn of the cochlea containing the tympanic plexus of nerves on its surface.

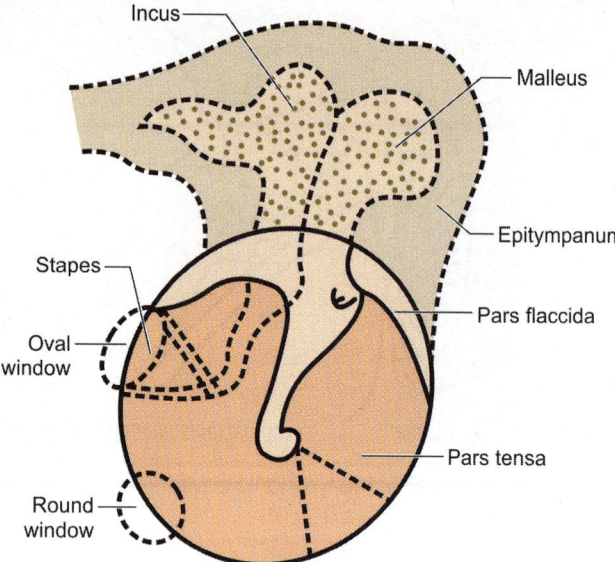

Fig. 2.7: Lateral wall of the middle ear

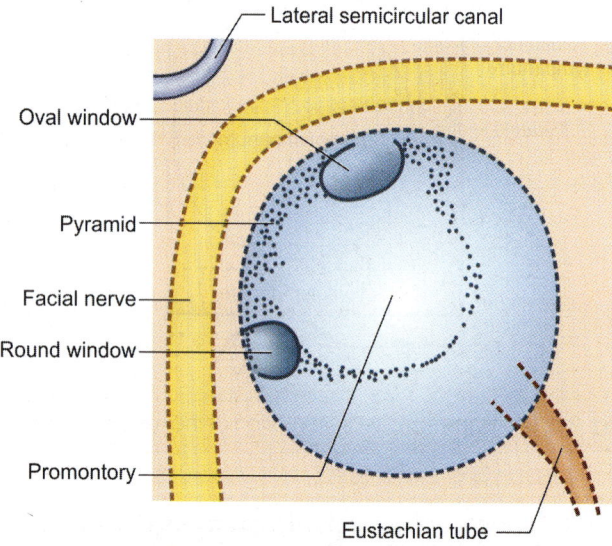

Fig. 2.8: Medial wall of the middle ear

- *Oval window (fenestera vestibuli)*
  - *Size:* 3.25 mm long and 1.75 mm wide.
  - *Shape:* Kidney-like.
  - *Position:* It lies behind and above (postero-superior) the promontory.

  It is covered by the stapes footplate which is surrounded by the annular ligament. It lies between the middle ear and the scala vestibuli of the cochlea.

Clinical significance
- The facial nerve lies above the oval window. Its bony covering may be congenitally dehiscent,

exposing, the nerve to infection and injuries.
- In otosclerosis, the annular ligament and footplate are affected, thus making them immobile and preventing conduction of sound into the inner ear.

- *Round window (fenestera cochlea)*
  - *Size:* Anterior—1.5 mm, superior—1.3 mm, posterior—1.6 mm
  - *Shape:* Spatulate
  - *Position:* It lies below and behind the promontory.

    It is sealed by the secondary tympanic membrane (round window membrane) which separates the middle ear from the scala tympani of the cochlea.

  Clinical significance: Posterior ampullary nerve (Singular nerve) lies in the inferior edge of the round window niche and it is resected here for treatment of benign paroxysmal positional vertigo (BPPV).

- *Sinus tympani* is a narrow space at the junction of posterior and medial walls (medial to the pyramidal process).

  Clinical significance: It is the area in which cholesteatoma or granulation tissue is not easily visible and difficult to clear. It is cleared by canal-wall-down mastoidectomy.

- *Processus cochleariformis:* It is a bony canal of the tensor tympani muscle appearing as a hook-like projection just anterior to the oval window.

  Clinical significance: Facial canal lies above the process cochleariformis, which forms a landmark for the facial nerve.

- *Anterior wall:* It has a thin plate of bone which separates the cavity from the internal carotid artery. It has the following openings:
  - Canal for chorda tympani nerve (canal of Hugier).
  - Canal for tensor tympani muscle.
  - Eustachian tube opening.

Clinical Significance
- Erosion of the anterior wall with the ICA lying covered by granulation or cholesteatoma is seen sometimes in extensive disease.
- Any trauma to anterior wall during ear surgery can injure the internal carotid artery causing torrential bleeding.

- *Posterior wall:* It lies close to the mastoid air cells, and includes:

- *Superiorly*: Aditus ad antrum which leads from epitympanum to the mastoid antrum.
- *Middle*: Small conical projection called the pyramidal process which contains the stapedius muscle.
- *Inferiorly*: Below the pyramidal process and lateral to it, is the opening for the chorda tympani nerve.

    Clinical significance: Facial nerve canal turns (second genu) and lies deep in the posterior wall of the middle ear, hence, it is a landmark for the vertical/mastoid part of the facial nerve.

- *Superior wall (roof, tegmental wall):* It is formed by a thin plate of bone called the 'tegmen tympani' which separates the middle ear from the middle cranial fossa and extends posteriorly to form the roof of the aditus ad antrum.

    Clinical significance
    - It is at times very thin and can become a potential route for infection from middle ear to spread to the middle cranial fossa.
    - In case of extensive cholesteatoma or granulations, it may be eroded by disease, and the bare meninges can be injured during surgery.
- *Inferior wall (floor, jugular wall):* This is formed by an irregular plate of bone that separates the middle ear from the bulb of the internal jugular vein.

    There is an opening at the junction of floor and medial wall of the cavity where the tympanic branch of the glossopharyngeal nerve enters into the middle ear from its origin below the base of the skull.

    Clinical significance: The floor may occasionally be dehiscent and covered by fibrous tissue and mucous membrane, allowing the jugular bulb to bulge into the middle ear cavity. If the surgeon is not careful, it may be damaged with resultant torrential haemorrhage.

Contents of the Middle Ear Cleft

The middle ear cleft contains three ossicles, two muscles, and two nerves (chorda tympani nerve and the tympanic plexus of nerves).
- Ossicles: Andreaus vesalius was first to describe the malleus and compared incus to a molar tooth.
    - *Malleus* (Fig. 2.9)
    - Largest ossicle
    - *Parts*

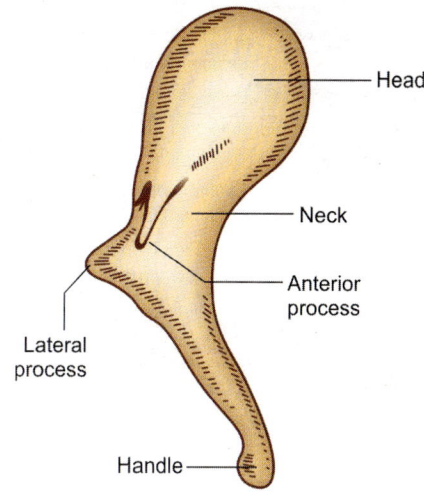

Fig. 2.9: Malleus

- Head lies in epitympanum.
- Neck constricted mid-portion.
- Two processes:
    - *Anterior process*: It is the process from which the slender anterior ligament arises.
    - *Lateral process*: It is the process which receives the anterior and posterior malleolar folds.
- *Handle*: It lies between the mucosal and fibrous layer of the tympanic membrane.
- *Size:* 7.5–9.0 mm
- *Shape:* Hammer-like
- *Incus* (Fig. 2.10)
- Second largest ossicle.
- *Parts:*
    - Body lies in epitympanum.
    - Short process (5 mm) lies in fossa incudis.

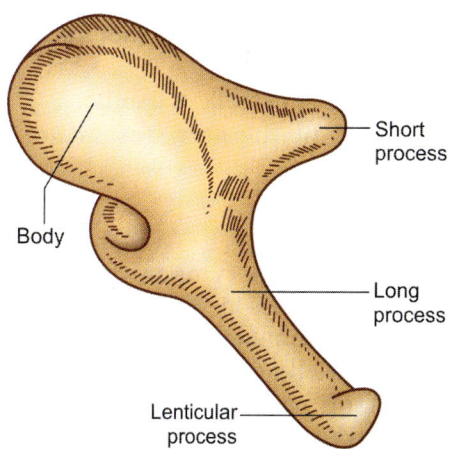

Fig. 2.10: Incus

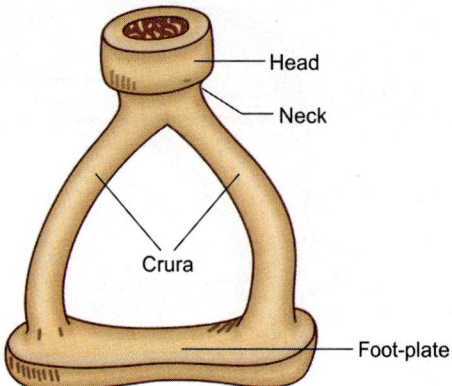

Fig. 2.11: Stapes

- Long process (7.7 mm) lies medial to handle of mallues with a lenticular process to articulate with the stapes head.
  - *Shape:* Anvil-like
- *Stapes* (Fig. 2.11)
  - Smallest ossicle
  - *Parts:*
    - Head articulates with the lenticular process of the incus
    - Neck has the insertion of the stapedius tendon
    - Two crura
    - Footplate which covers the oval window
  - *Shape:* Stirrup-like
- Muscles
  - *Stapedius muscle*
    - *Origin:* Pyramidal process.
    - *Insertion:* At the neck of the stapes.
    - *Nerve supply:* Branch of facial nerve.
  - *Tensor tympani muscle*
    - *Origin:* Bony canal above the Eustachian tube and partly from the cartilagenous portion of the Eustachian tube
    - *Insertion:* Into the malleus handle
    - *Nerve:* Mandibular nerve (branch of the fifth cranial nerve)
- Nerves
  - *Chorda tympani nerve:* It is a branch of the facial nerve. It enters the tympanic cavity from the posterior wall, runs medial to the upper portion of the handle of malleus and escapes out through the anterior wall.

    It contains parasympathetic fibres to supply the submandibular and sublingual salivary glands and taste fibres to the anterior two-thirds of the tongue.

- *Tympanic plexus:* It lies over the promontary. This is formed by:
  - Tympanic branch of the glossopharyngeal nerve (parasympathetic)
  - Caroticotympanic nerves arise from sympathetic plexus around the internal carotid artery.

  Branches of the tympanic plexus:
  - Nerve supply to mucous lining of tympanic cavity, Eustachian tube, and mastoid antrum.
  - Branch joining greater superficial petrosal nerve.
  - Lesser superficial petrosal nerve.
  - To twig of facial nerve.
- Mastoid
  - It is a part of the temporal bone, situated behind the ear.
  - It is not developed at birth, it develops gradually as the child grows.
  - It is formed from squamous and petrous bones. When the petrosquamous suture persists as a bony plate, it is called the 'Korner's septum', which separates the superficial squamosal cells from the deep petrosal cells. This creates a difficulty in location of the mastoid antrum, and incomplete removal of disease during the mastoidectomy operation.
  - It comprises of three parts:
    - *Aditus ad antrum*
      - It is an opening through which the attic communicates with the antrum.
      - At its floor, there lies the short process of the incus and the facial nerve canal.
      - At its medial wall there lies the lateral semicircular canal.
    - *Mastoid antrum:* It is the largest air cell in the mastoid process and communicates with the attic through the aditus.
      - *Boundaries*
        - *Roof:* Tegmen plate
        - *Anterior:* Aditus ad antrum
        - *Medial:* Horizontal (lateral) semicircular canal
        - *Lateral:* Mastoid bone cortex of 1.5 cm thickness
        - *Posteroinferiorly:* Numerous mastoid air cells.
    - *Mastoid air cells* (Fig. 2.12)
      - Depending upon the air cell development, the mastoid can be of following types:
        - *Cellullar:* Well-developed air cells with intervening thick bony septae.

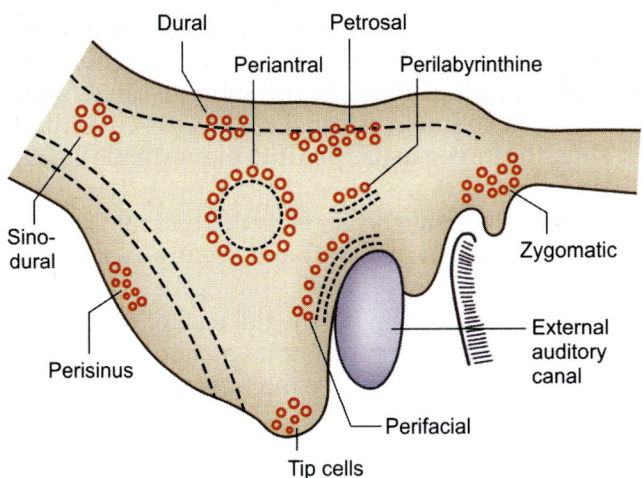

Fig. 2.12: Mastoid air cells

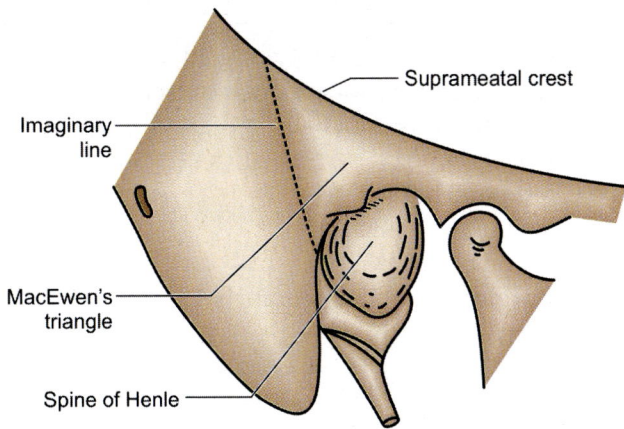

Fig. 2.13: MacEwen's triangle

- *Diploic*: These consist of marrow spaces with few air-cells.
- *Sclerotic or acellular*: No air cells or marrow spaces
- Depending upon their location the air cells are named as follows:
  - Zygomatic cells (in root of zygoma)
  - Tegmen cells (extend in tegmen tympani)
  - Perisinus cells (overlying sinus plate)
  - Perifacial and retrofacial cells (surround the facial nerve)
  - Perilabyrinthine cells (above, below, and behind the labyrinth)
  - Peritubal cells (around Eustachian tube)
  - Marginal cells (behind sinus plate and extend into occipital bone)
  - Tip cells (of the mastoid tip, i.e. medial and lateral to digastric ridge)
  - Squamous cells (squamous part of temporal bone).

MACEWEN'S TRIANGLE (SUPRAMEATAL TRIANGLE)

It is surgical landmark for the mastoid antrum (Fig. 2.13).
- Boundaries
  - *Superiorly*, suprameatal crest
  - *Anteriorly*, the posterosuperior margin of the external auditory canal
  - *Posteriorly*, a vertical tangential imaginary line from posterior meatal wall cutting the suprameatal crest.
- Mastoid antrum
  - It lies at a depth of approximately 1.5 cm (adults) from this surface landmark.

- In children, it is more superficial.
- Depth increases by 1 mm per year of age till the antrum is approximately 14–15 mm deep.

FACIAL NERVE

- Roots: It comprises of motor and sensory roots.
  - *Motor root*: Facial nucleus in pons.
  - *Sensory root*
    - Nervus intermedius of Wrisberg joins the facial nerve at the brainstem
    - Secretomotor parasympathetic fibres arise from the superior salivatory nucleus
- Parts: It has three parts:
  - *Intracranial part*: It extends from origin in the pons to the lateral end of internal auditory meatus.
  - *Intratemporal part*: The facial nerve in the facial canal (fallopian canal) is divided into three segments:
    - *Labyrinthine segment* extends from the internal acoustic meatus up to the geniculate ganglion by making a first turn (internal or first genu).
    - *Tympanic segment* extends from geniculate ganglion up to pyramidal process and again makes a second turn (external or second genu).
    - *Mastoid segment* extends from pyramidal process up to the stylomastoid foramen.
  - *Extra temporal part*: It extends beyond the stylo-mastoid foramen into the face and neck.
- Branches
  - *Geniculate ganglion*: Greater superficial petrosal nerve.
  - *Within the facial canal:*
    - Nerve to stapedius
    - Chorda tympani nerve
    - Sensory branch to external auditory canal

- **Branches in neck:**
  - Stylohyoid branch to stylohyoid muscles
  - Branch to posterior auricular muscles
  - Branch to posterior belly of digastic muscle
- **Terminal branches in the face:**
  - Temporal branch
  - Zygomatic branch
  - Buccal branch
  - Marginal mandibular branch
  - Cervical branch.

INNER EAR (THE LABYRINTH)

It is an organ of hearing and balance. It lies in the petrous part of the temporal bone (Fig. 2.14). It consists of two parts: (1) Bony labyrinth and (2) Vestibular labyrinth.

Bony labyrinth (capsule): It contains perilymph fluid and consists of: (a) vestibule, (b) semicircular canals (three) and (c) cochlea.

- **Vestibule:** It is the central chamber of labyrinth.
  - **Relations**
    - **Lateral wall**—oval window.
    - **Medial wall**
      - Spherical recess for saccule
      - Elliptical recess for utricle
    - Below the elliptical recess, there is the aqueduct of the vestibule through which endolymphatic duct passes.
    - Posterosuperiorly, the vestibule has five openings of the semicircular canals.

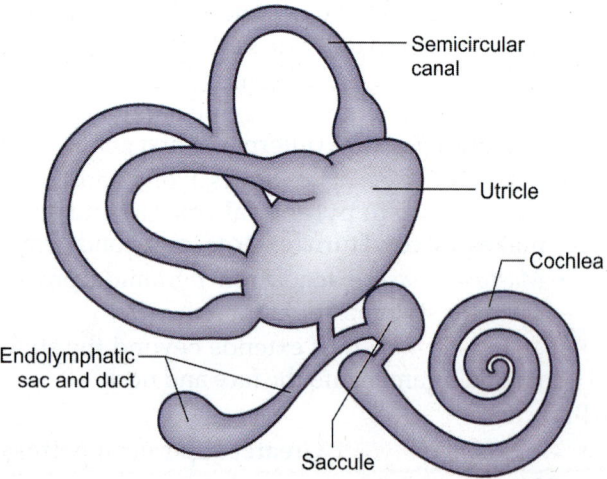

Fig. 2.14: The labyrinth

- **Semicircular canals:** They are three in number. The lateral (horizontal), posterior, and superior canals which lie in planes at right angles to one another. Each

canal has an ampullated end which opens into the vestibule and a non-ampullated end. The non-ampullated ends of posterior and superior canals unite to form a common channel called crus commune. Thus, the three canals open into the vestibule by five openings.

- **Cochlea:** The bony cochlea is a coiled tube making two and three-quarter turns around a central pyramid of bone called the 'modiolus'.

  The bony bulge in the medial wall of the middle ear—the promontory is due to basal coil of the cochlea. The bony cochlea contains three compartments:
  - Scala vestibuli
  - Scala tympani
  - Scala media or membraneous cochlea.

  The scala vestibuli and scala tympani are filled with perilymph and communicate with each other at the apex of the cochlea through an opening called 'Helicotrema'.

  The scala vestibuli is closed by the footplate of the stapes which separates it from the air-filled middle ear cavity. The scala tympani is closed by the secondary tympanic membrane; it is also connected with the subarachnoid space through the aqueduct of the cochlea.

Vestibular labyrinth (Fig. 2.14): It consists of: (1) cochlear duct, (2) utricle and saccule, (3) three semi-circular ducts and (4) endolymphatic duct and sac.

- **Cochlear duct (membranous cochlea / scala media):** It is a coiled tube. It appears triangular on cross-section and its walls are formed by:
  - **Basilar membrane**, which supports the organ of corti.
  - **Reisner's membrane**, which separates it from the scala vestibuli.
  - **Stria vascularis**, which contains vascular epithelium and is concerned with the secretion of endolymph. Cochlear duct is connected to the saccule by the ductus reuniens. The length of the basilar membrane increases from the basal coil to the apical coil of the cochlea.

  Organ of Corti: It is the end organ of the cochlea and forms the neuroepithelium. It consists of the tunnel of corti, which is formed of two rows of rods of Corti. It forms a triangle with the basilar membrane and contains corti-lymph. There are rows of inner and outer hair cells.

  The hair cells are supported within the organ of corti by:
  - Pillar cells

- Deitor's cells
- Hensen's cells.

The tectorial membrane over-hangs the organ of Corti. The terminal fibres of the cochlear division of the eight cranial nerve are in contact with the hair cells.

- *Utricle and saccule*: They lie in the vestibule of the bony labyrinth. The utricle lies in the posterior part of the bony vestibule while the saccule lies anterior to the utricle and medial to the stapes footplate.

  The sensory epithelium in both are called '*macula*', which responds to gravity and linear accleration.

- *Semicircular ducts*: They correspond to three bony canals. They open in the utricle. The ampulated end of each duct contains a thickened ridge of neuroepithelium called 'cristae ampullaris'.

- *Endolymphatic duct and sac*: The duct is formed by the union of two ducts, each from the saccule and utricle. Its terminal part is dilated to form the endolymphatic sac which lies between two dural layers in the petrous bone.

Significance: In Meniere's disease, the endolymphatic shunt operation is done to reduce the pressure in the distended endolymphatic sac.

Arteries of inner ear: Internal auditory (labyrinthine) artery (branch of anterior inferior cerebellar artery or sometimes of the basilar artery).

Veins draining inner ear:
- Internal auditory vein
- Vein of the cochlear aqueduct
- Vein of the vestibular aqueduct

Nerve supply of inner ear:
- Ampullary, utricular and sacular nerves joint to form the vestibular nerve
- Cochlear nerve and vestibular nerve join to form the VIIIth cranial nerve (vestibulo-cochlear nerve).

Physiology of the Hearing

Functionally, the ear is divided into two parts (Figs 3.1 and 3.2):

- Conductive apparatus
- Perceptive apparatus

The conductive apparatus comprises of the structures in the external and middle ears whereas the perceptive apparatus comprises of the inner ear and cortical fibres.

THE CONDUCTIVE MECHANISM OF HEARING

- The pinna helps to collect sound waves and direct them towards the external auditory canal (EAC).
- The external auditory canal transmits the physical sound waves to the tympanic membrane.
- The tympanic membrane is set into vibrations by the sound waves. This in turn, results in vibrations of the ossicular chain. These vibrations are transmitted to

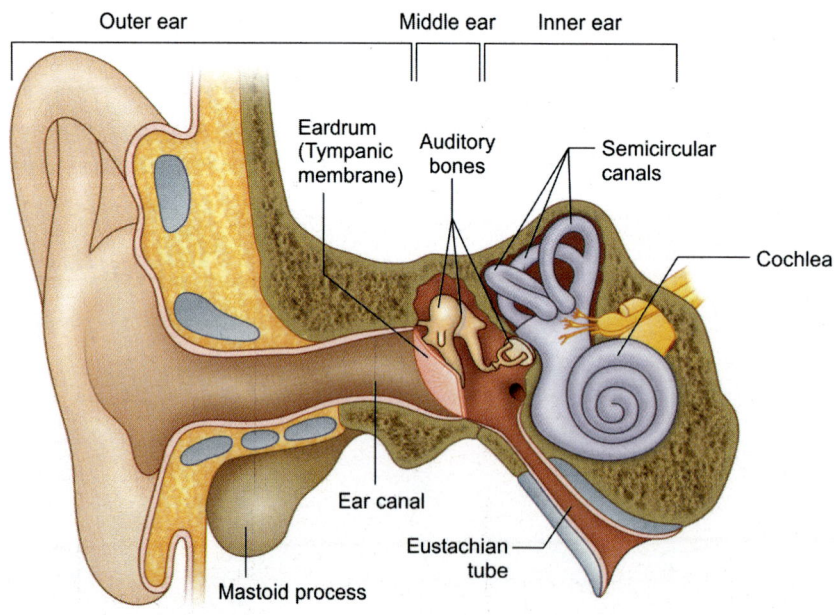

Fig. 3.1: Diagrammatic representation of the internal structure of ear

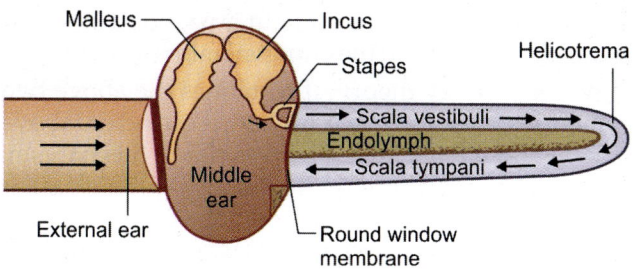

Fig. 3.2: Diagrammatic representation of the conductive and perceptive apparatus of hearing

the inner ear fluids by the stapes footplate via the oval window.

The vibrating surface area of the tympanic membrane is 17 times the area of the oval window, i.e. the areal or hydraulic ratio is 17. The ratio of the length of the malleus handle to that of the long process of incus is 1.3:1, i.e. the ossicular leverage ratio is 1.3. 17 1.3 = 22 approx. These fractions increase the force of sound by 22 times or 28 dB as it courses from the middle ear to inner ear. This is termed as the 'middle ear transformer action' (Fig. 3.3).

- Muscles of the middle ear play a role in protecting the inner ear from the effects of very loud sound. By contracting, they reduce the mobility of the ossicular chain and hence reduce the intensity of the sound reaching the inner ear.
- Bone conduction is also responsible for transmitting sound to the inner ear by vibrations through the skull bones which are transmitted to the inner ear fluids. There are three theories of bone conduction:
  - *Inertial theory*: The skull is set into vibration by the sound stimulus. The ossicles lag behind due

to inertia. Hence, the ossicles and the skull bones vibrate out of phase to each other resulting in a piston-like movement of the stapes footplate in the oval window.
  - *Compressional theory*: The skull bones including the bony labyrinth vibrate in response to the sound stimulus and set the inner ear fluids into vibration.
  - *Osseotympanic theory*: When the skull bones including the bony labyrinth vibrate, the mandible lags behind due to inertia. This sets the air in the EAC into vibration (since the mandible is closely related to the floor of the cartilagenous EAC) which in turn vibrates the tympanic membrane.

THE PERCEPTIVE MECHANISM OF HEARING

It includes the transmission of the auditory signals received by the perilymph in the cochlea to the organ of Corti and from there to the nerve endings. Thus, physical sound is converted into an electrical impulse which is transmitted via the VIIIth cranial nerve to the cerebral cortex. There exists a phase difference between the round and oval windows due to the presence of the tympanic membrane. This is essential for fluid displacement in the inner ear. The eardrum protects the round window and preferentially directs sound to the oval window via the ossicles (Figs 3.4 and 3.5).

THEORIES OF HEARING

There are various theories of hearing which explain the mechanism by which the cochlea perceives sound.
- **Rutherford's telephone theory:** It states that in response to a sound stimulus, the basilar membrane of the cochlea vibrates uniformly in all parts and the amplitude of vibration represents the intensity of

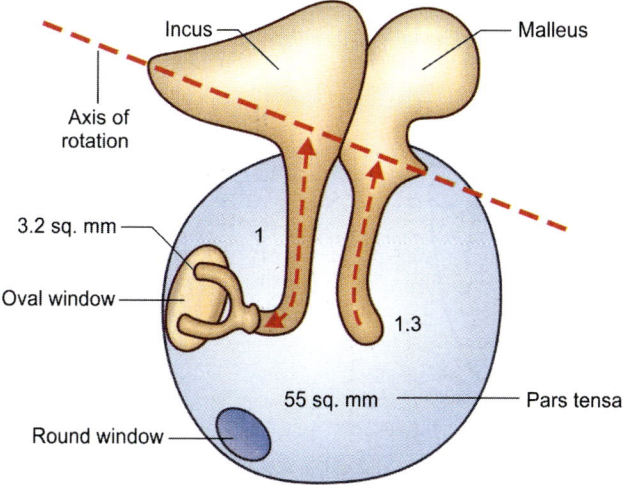

Fig. 3.3: The middle ear transformer

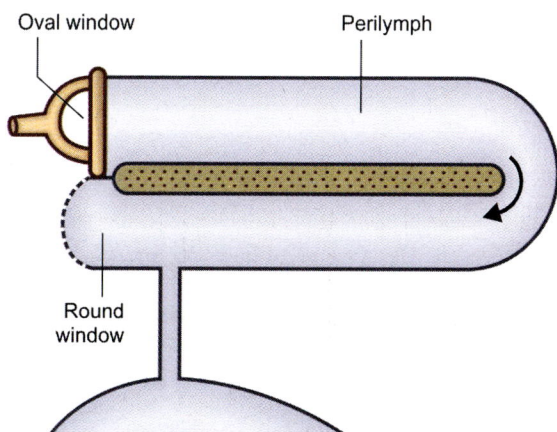

Fig. 3.4: Movement of perilymph in the cochlea

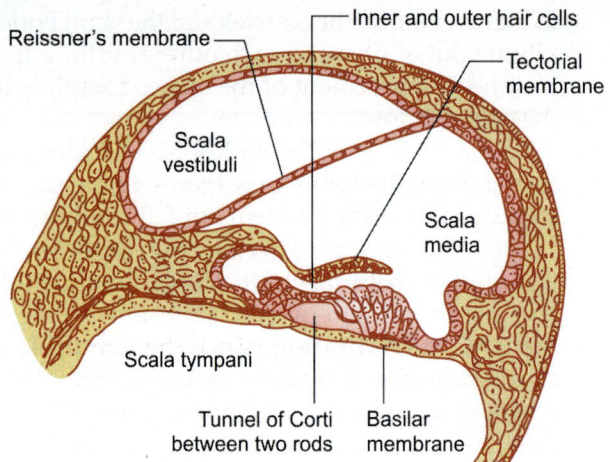

Fig. 3.5: Diagrammatic representation of the cochlea

sound. Also, the rate of firing of the auditory nerve fibres determine the frequency of sound.

- Helmholtz's place theory: It states that the cochlea detects the frequency of sound due to the fact that each pitch causes a vibration of its own particular 'place' on the basilar membrane, i.e. a particular pitch vibrated only a particular part of the basilar membrane and not the entire membrane.

- Wever's volley theory: It combines the above two theories by stating that higher frequencies (above 5000 Hz) are perceived by the 'place' mechanism, i.e. they vibrate only particular areas on the basilar membrane at the basal turn of the cochlea. Whereas, the low frequencies (below 400 Hz) are perceived by the 'Telephone mechanism,' i.e. they stimulate the entire basilar membrane according to their frequency. Frequencies between 400–5000 Hz are perceived by both mechanisms.

- Bekesy's travelling wave theory: This states that, in response to a sound stimulus at the oval window a wave-like vibration of the basilar membrane occurs, which starts from the basal turn and travels upwards to the apex of the cochlea. It increases in amplitude as it moves, until it reaches a maximum and then it dies off. The frequency of sound is determined by the point of maximum amplitude.

Final perception of sound occurs in the cerebral cortex (Fig. 3.6).

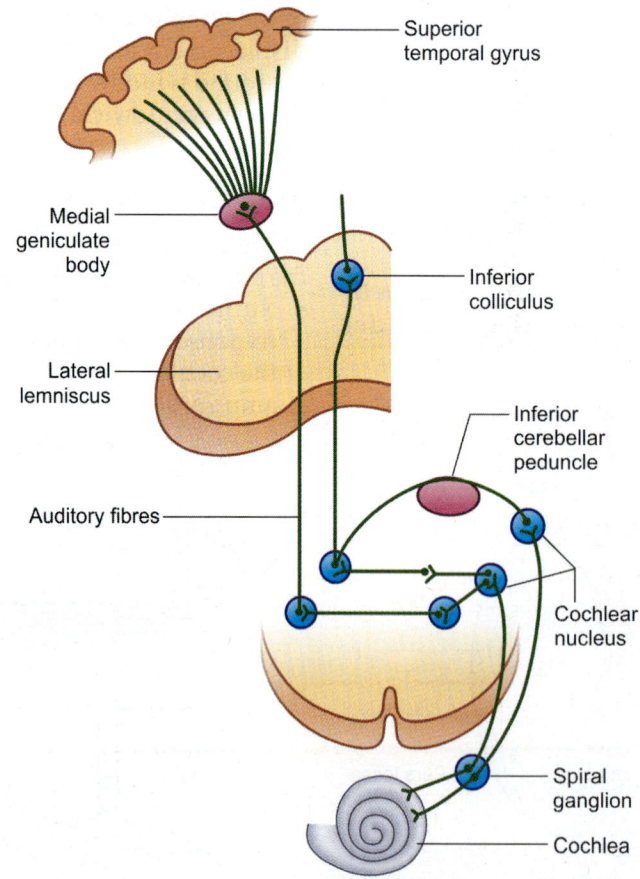

Fig. 3.6: Diagram of the final pathway of hearing

PHYSIOLOGY OF EQUILIBRIUM

The cerebrum and cerebellum are responsible for the perception of equilibrium (Fig. 3.7). The proprioceptive end-organs are the vestibule, tendons, muscles, joints, skin and eyes.

There are three pairs of semicircular canals:
* Two lateral/horizontal
* Two superior
* Two posterior

These are stimulated by angular acceleration which causes movement of the endolymph resulting in stimulation of the crista in the ampullae of the semicircular canals.

All the three semicircular canals of one side are situated at right angles to each other. Hence, both lateral (horizontal) canals lie in the same plane and the superior canal of one side lies in the same plane as the posterior canal of the opposite side.

The vestibule also contains the saccule and the utricle which play a role in maintainence of equilibrium. The saccule and utricle are stimulated by linear acceleration.

Proprioceptive reflexes produced by the end-organs are of two types:
* Static, which occur at rest and
* Kinetic, which occur during a movement.

These are responsible for maintainence of body posture.

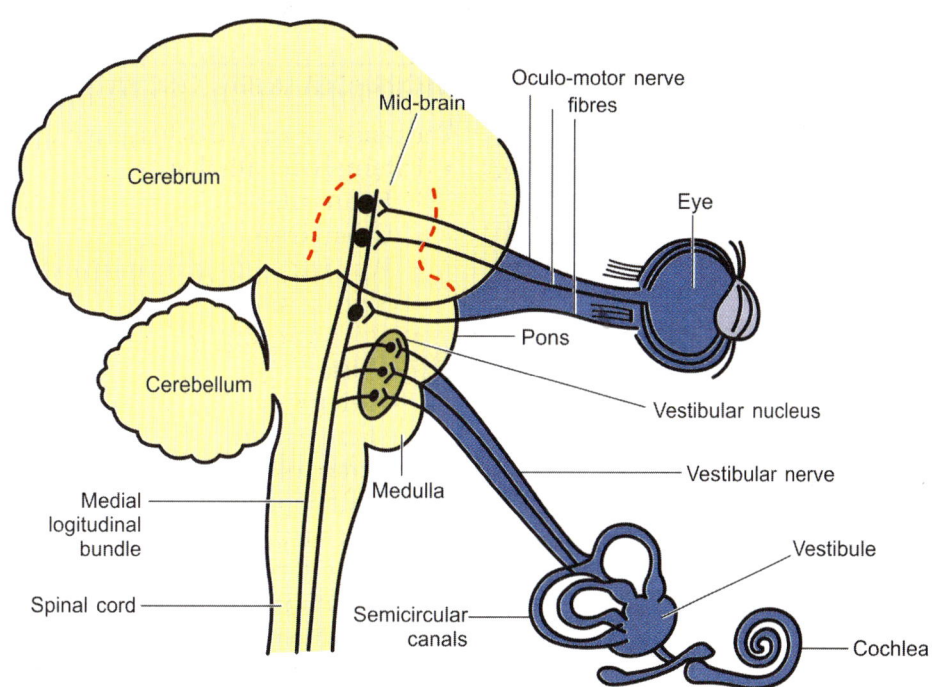

Fig. 3.7: Physiology of equilibrium

CHAPTER 4

Examination of the Ear

Just like any other branch of medicine, history-taking is a very important and preliminary part of otology. The common symptoms in otology may be broadly divided into two parts: (1) local symptoms and (2) generalised symptoms.

LOCAL SYMPTOMS

The cardinal local symptoms of ear disease include:
- Otalgia
- Aural discharge (otorrhoea)
- Disorders of auditory perception or deafness
- Tinnitus
- Vertigo

Whenever an enquiry is made about the local symptoms of the ear, the following points must be considered:
- Origin
- Duration
- Progress
- Severity
- Unilateral/bilateral disease
- Intermittent/continuous
- Aggravating and reliving factors.

Of the above mentioned local symptoms, otalgia, disorders of auditory function and vertigo have been dealt within detail in subsequent chapters. In this chapter, we would like to stress upon mainly two symptoms namely otorrhoea and tinnitus.

OTORRHOEA (AURAL DISCHARGE)

The causes of aural discharge include:
- External ear pathology
  - Furunculosis
  - Otomycosis
  - Wax with secondary otitis externa
  - Myringitis
  - *Otitis externa*
    - Viral
    - Seborrhoeic
    - Eczematous
  - Tumours of external auditory canal (EAC), e.g. ceruminoma.
- Middle ear pathology
  - Acute suppurative otitis media (ASOM)
  - Chronic suppurative otitis media (CSOM)
    - Safe type
    - Unsafe type
  - Tumours—carcinoma of the middle ear
  - Syphilitic otitis media
  - Tuberculous otitis media
- Other causes
  - Cerebrospinal fluid (CSF) rhinorrhoea
  - Rupture of a parotid or temporomandibular joint abscess in the EAC

Types of Discharge
- Watery
  - CSF rhinorrhoea

- ✦ Safe CSOM
- ✦ Otomycosis
- Serous
  - ✦ Safe CSOM
  - ✦ Secretory otitis media
  - ✦ Myringitis
  - ✦ Eczematous otitis externa
- Mucoid: Mucous-containing discharge is produced by secretory glands within the middle ear cleft. It passes into the external auditory meatus either through a perforated drum or open mastoid cavity.
- Purulent
  - ✦ Furunculosis
  - ✦ Suppurative stage of ASOM
  - ✦ CSOM
  - ✦ Parotid or temporomandibular joint abscess drains into the EAC
- Malodorous discharge
  - ✦ Long standing safe CSOM due to superadded infection with saprophytic organisms
  - ✦ Presence of cholesteatoma or granulations
  - ✦ Syphilitic otitis media (foul smelling painless discharge)
- Blood stained otorrhoea (serosanguinous)
  - ✦ Granulations in the ear
  - ✦ Carcinoma of the ear
  - ✦ Malignant otitis externa
- Frank blood
  - ✦ Trauma
  - ✦ Glomus tumour
  - ✦ Rare cases of vascular malformation in middle ear or external ear

A detailed history of otorrhoea should include the following features:

- Since when it started.
- Quantity: Scanty/Profuse.
- Quality:
  - ✦ Serous
  - ✦ Seromucinous
  - ✦ Serosanguinous
  - ✦ Mucopurulent
- Unilateral/Bilateral
- Odour present/Absent
- Continuous/Intermittent.
- Aggravating and relieving factors
- Any treatment taken for this. If history is present, details of drugs taken should be asked to the patient. Any surgery performed.

- Presence of associated symptoms, such as deafness, vertigo, tinnitus, otalgia, etc.

TINNITUS

Tinnitus is a frequent presentation of various diseases of the ear. It may be defined as noise within the ear or head, produced in absence of any external stimulus. Tinnitus may be classified into two types:
- Subjective tinnitus
- Objective tinnitus

Subjective Tinnitus: Sounds like ringing, whistling, etc., are heard by the patient only and not by the examiner. Subjective tinnitus differs from the 'auditory hallucination' in the fact that the latter name is reserved for conditions where the individual hears voice and sentences due to certain functional disturbances, when they actually do not exist.

Objective Tinnitus: It is heard by both, the examiner and the patient.

Causes of Tinnitus

- Subjective tinnitus
  - ✦ *Local causes*
    - Postoperative (following stapedectomy)
    - Acoustic neuroma
    - Meniere's disease
    - Ototoxic drugs, e.g. aspirin, quinine
  - ✦ *Systemic causes*
    - Anaemia
    - Cerebrovascular accidents
    - Cardiovascular disorders, e.g. hypertension and hypotension
    - Diabetes, mellitus
    - Thyroid disorders
    - Impacted wisdom tooth
    - Caried tooth
    - Anxiety
    - Depression
- Objective tinnitus
  - ✦ Impacted wax
  - ✦ Foreign body in external auditory canal
  - ✦ Secretory otitis media
  - ✦ Otosclerosis
  - ✦ Eustachian tube dysfunction
  - ✦ Glomus tumour
  - ✦ Vascular bruits

- Ateriovenous malformation in head and around EAC
- Hydrocephalus
- Palatal myoclonus
- Chronic contraction of tensor tympani and stapedius muscles
- Clicking of temporomandibular joint

Characteristics of Tinnitus

A dull and continuous tinnitus occurs in conductive hearing loss due to the fact that masking effect of environmental sounds is lost. The normal noise level now becomes obvious and the patient complains of tinnitus. Successful treatment of conductive hearing loss may sometimes cure such tinnitus.

Pulsatile tinnitus occurs in vascular tumours like glomus. Clicking tinnitus is seen in palatal myoclonus. Fluctuant tinnitus may be associated with Meniere's disease. Its intensity increases prior to the aura of Meniere's disease.

A high pitched whistling continuous tinnitus occurs in cochlear pathology (sensorineural hearing loss).

GENERAL SYMPTOMS

Various general symptoms are often associated with disease of the ear. Most of these symptoms arise as a result of intracranial extention of the disease. They may sometimes be the presenting symptom in case of complications. These include:

- Headache,
- Nausea,
- Fever with chills,
- Vomiting,
- Neck rigidity,
- Central nervous system depression.

History of Past Illness

- Careful history should be taken about recurrent upper respiratory tract infection (URTI), presence of cleft palate and acute tonsillitis. These may be the predisposing factors for CSOM.
- Swimming and probing of ears can lead to otitis externa.
- History of diabetes, syphilis, hypertension and prolonged use of ototoxic drugs is important.
- Family history becomes important in otosclerosis.
- Poor living conditions and poor hygiene predispose to ear diseases.

Local Examination

Preauricular region　Look for:
- Preauricular sinuses
- Scars of end-aural inscision
- Preauricular lymph node enlargement.

Postaural region　Look for fistula, abscess, tenderness over the mastoid and postaural scars. Retroauricular suclus may be obliterated in otitis externa and mastoid abscess.

Pinna　Various congenital and acquired defects may be seen.
- Congenital anomalies of pinna:
  - *Anotia* is the congenital absence of the auricle.
  - *Microtia* is the incomplete development of the auricle.
  - *Synotia* is the condition where the auricular tags lie behind and beneath the mandible and is associated with hypoplasia of the mandible, buccal cavity and tongue.
  - *Melotia* is the condition where ears are displaced caudoventrally. It is associated with hypoplasia of the mandible.
  - *Darwin's tubercle* is an elevation of the postero-superior part of the helix.
  - *Bat ear* is the commonest congenital deformity of the external ear and is characterised by abnormal ear protrusion, reduced or absent antihelix and is occasionally associated with congenital disorders of genitourinary tract.
  - *Lop ear* is a more severe variant of bat ear.
  - Trisomy 21 (Down's syndrome).
  - There is presence of rounded pinna with poorly developed lobule. The posterior-superior aspect of helix may be folded.
  - *Wrinkle's disease* (chondrodermatitis nodularis chronicus helices) is characterised by small painful nodular lesions occurring in the upper part of pinna brought about by low temperature resulting in local vasoconstriction.
- Acquired lesions
  - *Cauliflower ear* results due to fibrosis following hematoma formation in the pinna.
  - *Perichondritis of pinna* results in a deformed pinna.

External auditory canal　External auditory canal is examined using either a Bull's eyelamp with a head mirror and an aural speculum or an otoscope. The pinna is gently pulled in the upward, outward and backward direction in adults in order to align the cartilagenous

EAC with the bony EAC. In children the traction is given in the downward, backward and outward directions (Fig. 4.1).

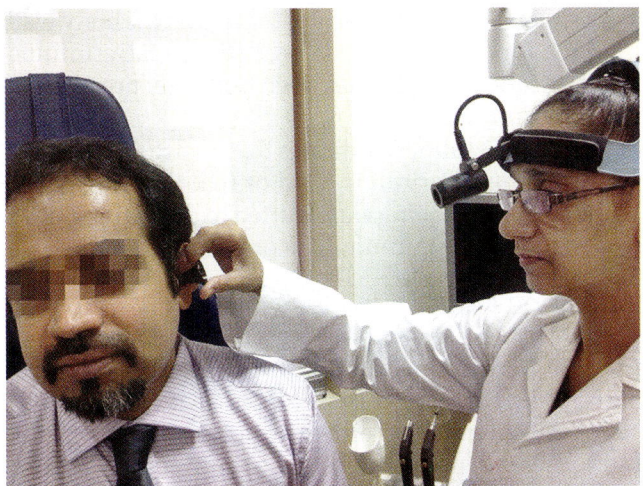

Fig. 4.1: Examination of ear using aural speculum

The various conditions which may be seen include:

- Wax, which may be removed using a wax hook or by an aural syringe.
- Canal stenosis may occur after ear surgery or chronic otitis externa.
- Foreign body in EAC
- Otitis externa which may be in the form of:
  - Furuncle,
  - Diffuse infective otitis externa,
  - Otomycosis,
  - Eczematous otitis externa,
  - Seborrhoeic otitis externa,
  - Granular myringitis,
  - Herpetic lesions like herpes simplex, bullous myringitis and herpes zoster,
  - Keratosis obturans.
- Polyp in the EAC.
- Sagging of the posterior-superior canal wall due to mastoiditis.
- Neoplasms of the external ear.

Tympanic membrane The method of visualising the tympanic membrane is similar to that described in examination of EAC (i.e. by gentle traction of pinna).

The entire tympanic membrane should be visualised. Besides noting the anatomy of the tympanic membrane, its mobility should also be seen. Mobility of tympanic membrane is seen either with Seigle's pneumatic speculum or by using a pneumatic bulb connected to an otoscope. Alternating positive and negative pressure in ear canal results in tympanic membrane moving inwards and outwards. Whenever there is a perforation in the tympanic membrane or there is fluid in the middle ear, the normal mobility of tympanic membrane is lost.

While looking at the tympanic membrane, the following should be noted:

- Congestion
- Granulation
- Perforation: If a perforation is seen then, the following details must be noted:
  - Whether it is in the pars tensa or the pars flaccida,
  - The condition of the ossicles seen through the perforation should be noted,
  - Condition of the middle ear mucosa through the perforation should be seen,
  - Edges of perforation, whether thin or thick.
- Pathology like granulation, polyps, and cholesteatoma are to be noted.
- Air fluid level/Air bubbles in the stagnant ear discharge.
- Retraction pocket, site and presence of adhesions with middle ear structures is noted.

Eustachian tube patency Presence of Eustachian tube patency does not necessarily indicate a normally functioning tube. The following tests are used to test Eustachian tube patency:

- **History:** Patient gives a history that when he/she instills eardrops, they enter the throat. This indicates that there is a perforated eardrum with a patent Eustachian tube.
- **Air bubbles:** Eardrops are put in the middle ear and the patient is asked to blow forcefully through the nose. Presence of air bubbles in the EAC indicates a patent Eustachian tube.
- **Valsalva's manoeuvre:** Patient is asked to attempt to blow out air with his mouth and nose closed. The examiner sees the movement of the tympanic membrane when the patient blows out, with an otoscope. Tympanic membrane bulges outwards (laterally) when patient blows. This indicates a patent Eustachian tube.
- **Toynbee's manoeuvre:** Patient is asked to swallow with nose and mouth closed. This creates a negative pressure in the middle ear and draws the tympanic membrane inwards, if the Eustachian tube is patent. This can be visualised with an otoscope. When the patient swallows with the nose patent, the Eustachian tube comes back to the normal position.
- **Frenzel manoeuvre:** This method was popularised by Frenzel who was a popular figure in German aviation medicine during the time of World War II.

In this method, the air in the nasopharynx is compressed by the muscles of the floor of mouth and tongue with the nose and the glottis closed.

The advantage of this procedure is that it can be performed without using a hand for closing the nostrils, once it is properly learnt. Secondly, it can be performed in any phase of respiration and it is independent of intrathoracic pressure.

- Politzerisation: The nozzle of the politzer bag is inserted into one of the nostrils. Both nostrils are pinched by the patient with his hand. Patient is asked to make swallowing movements and simultaneously at that time, the politzer bag is squeezed. Patient may feel air rushing into the ears and the examiner can see the tympanic membrane bulging outwards.

- Eustachian tube catheterisation: Eustachian catheter may be used for determining the patency of the Eustachian tube.

After spraying the nasal mucosa with 4% xylocaine the Eustachian catheter is introduced with its tip pointing downwards towards the floor of the nose up to the posterior pharyngeal wall, when the Eustachian catheter touches the posterior pharyngeal wall, it is rotated by 90° so that the tip points medially. The Eustachian catheter is then pulled outwards gently till it touches the posterior end of nasal septum.

At this stage, the Eustachian catheter is rotated by 180°, so that the tip faces laterally. By gently manipulation, it is made to enter into the Eustachian tube orifice which lies behind the posterior end of the inferior turbinate.

Politzer bag is attached to the proximal end of the catheter and the bulb is squeezed, thus raising the nasopharyngeal pressure.

Interpretation of results

- If the Eustachian tube is patent, then the sound of air entering the middle ear is heard by the patient.
- If the Eustachian tube is blocked, the sound of air entering the middle ear is not heard by the patient.
- In secretory otitis media, bubbling sounds may be heard by both the examiner and the patient.
- Impedence audiometry can give an idea of functioning of the Eustachian tube.

Fistula test

Positive fistula sign is present when nystagmus and vertigo result on increasing the pressure in the external auditory meatus. Pressure in the external auditory meatus may be increased by various ways:
- Compressing the tragus into the external auditory meatus with a finger.
- Pneumatic otoscope.

- Siegle's speculum.
- Impedence tympanometer.

Clinical Importance

- Positive fistula test indicates that either the bony wall of the inner ear has been eroded or a labyrinthine fenestration surgery has been done, i.e. presence of a labyrinthine fistula.
- Negative fistula test indicates that no fistula is present or that the labyrinth is dead or that the pressure in the EAC is not being transmitted to the fistula due to obstruction by granulations or cholesteatoma.

Hennebert's sign

This is the name given for the positive fistula sign with an intact tympanic membrane and with no evidence of middle ear disease. The exact pathophysiology of this sign is not known and it is believed to be due to either adhesions between the vestibule and stapes footplate or presence of a third window caused by osteitis. It is most commonly seen in congenital and late syphilis.

Auscultation of ear and temporal bone

It is useful in cases of glomus tumours and vascular anomalies where bruits may be heard.

Examination of eyes

- Ophthalmoscopic examination: This is a very important examination in ENT. Papilloedema may be seen in cases like cerebellopontine angle tumours, temporal lobe abscess and otitic hydrocephalus. Optic nerve atrophy is seen in demylinating diseases, which may also present with auditory or vestibular disturbances.

Nystagmus

Nystagmus is a condition in which there is failure of maintenance of posture of the eyes characterised by rhythmic, involuntary and occilatory movement of the eyes when fixed on an object.

To test for nystagmus the patient is asked to look straight ahead and the physician observes whether the eyes remain steady. The patient is then asked to look to the extreme right, extreme left, upwards and downwards. First degree nystagmus to the left is seen only on looking to the left. Second degree nystagmus to the left is seen on looking straight but increased on looking to left. Third degree nystagmus is seen on looking straight and to the left and to some extent on looking to the right.

Five or more jerks of eye movement characterise the presence of nystagmus. The finger of the examiner should never extend beyond the limit of binocular vision.

Positional nystagmus: Patient made to sit on a chair. Head is rotated to 30–40° to one side and it is also brought at an inclination of 30° below the horizontal. Then, look for nystagmus.

Visual fixation can be reduced either by using Frenzel's glasses or using a darkroom with an infrared viewer.

Nystagmus is broadly classified into two types:

- Pendular
- Jerk varieties
  - Horizontal
  - Vertical
  - Rotatary

Congenital nystagmus: It is characteristically pendular, whereas vestibular nystagmus may be horizontal or rotatory. It has two components a slow phase and a fast phase (corrective phase). The direction of nystagmus is conventionally labelled as the direction of the fast component. The first degree nystagmus is that where eyes show nystagmus when they are deviated in the direction of the fast phase.

Nystagmus may be labelled as direction changing nystagmus, if it changes direction with gaze. This type of nystagmus is seen in central lesions.

Benign paroxysmal positional vertigo (BPPV) presents with nystagmus in the direction of the undermost ear when the patient's head is tilted and is characterised by the presence of a latent period, the type is rotational or horizontal and it lasts for 20–30 seconds and is fatiguable. However, if the patient is found to have positional nystagmus but is not meeting the criteria for BPPV, then in such cases one should think of the presence of central lesions.

Examination of cranial nerves III to VI Examination of the III to VIth cranial nerves is important in cases of unsafe CSOM with Gradenigo's syndrome, where there is a triad of aural discharge, pain and sixth nerve palsy.

Pupillary reflexes In Argyll Robertson's pupils, accommodation reflex persists and light reflex is lost. This is seen in tertiary syphilis.

Visual field defects ENT causes of visual field defects include intracranial complications like papilloedema, cerebellopontine angle tumours, otitic hydrocephalus and temporal lobe abscess.

Corneal reflexes Loss of corneal reflexes is a late manifestation of acoustic neuroma.

Examination of facial nerve Examination of the facial nerve is important as facial palsy is encountered in various ENT diseases. One should clearly determine, if the facial palsy is of upper motor neurone type or lower motor neurone type. Also, it should be stated if there is a facial palsy or simply a paresis. Upper motor neurone type of facial palsy results in involvement of lower half of the face of the opposite side.

Somatic sensory component of facial nerve may be paralysed in acoustic neuroma, where the touch sensation on the external auditory meatus is lost (Hitselberger's positive sign).

Parasympathetic secromotor function is tested by noting the rate of tear production, i.e. lacrimation (Schirmer's test).

Special sensation of facial nerve is tested over tongue and by electrogustometry.

Cranial nerves IX to XII Glossopharyngeal nerve (IXth cranial nerve) is tested by noting the gag reflex.

Vagus nerve (Xth cranial nerve) can be tested on indirect laryngoscopy by noting the vocal cord movements. Hypoglossal nerve function (XIIth cranial nerve) is seen by asking the patient to protrude the tongue. Protrusion of tongue leads to deviation to the side of lesion.

Examination of nose and throat Rhinitis and sinusitis will affect Eustachian tube function.

When there is middle ear effusion without an obvious explanation, the postnasal space (nasopharynx) should be examined for any growth in the nasopharynx.

Examination of VIIIth cranial nerve Eighth cranial nerve examination consists of two parts, i.e. the auditory component and the vestibular component.

SYSTEMIC EXAMINATION

A brief systemic examination of the cardiovascular, respiratory, abdominal and central nervous system follows the local examination.

DIAGNOSIS

A diagnosis comprising of the following is to be prepared as follows:

- CSOM/SOM/ASOM
- Safe/Unsafe (in case of CSOM)
- Unilateral/Bilateral (specify side left/right if unilateral)
- Active/Inactive stage
- With mild/Moderate/Severe conductive/Sensorineural (SN)/Mixed deafness
- Without/With complications

INVESTIGATIONS

Specific investigations   These include:
- Confirmation of clinical findings using an operating microscope.
- Pus (if present) should be sent for culture of organisms and antibiotic sensitivity.
- Pure tone audiometry:
  - To confirm type (SN or conductive) and intensity (mild / moderate / severe) of hearing loss.
  - For documentation of findings.
- X-ray mastoid Schuller's view:
  - To see the anatomical variants in the mastoid
  - To see any pathology like sclerotic mastoid or erosion of bone.
- X-ray paranasal sinuses:
  - To see associated sinusitis especially in safe CSOM as this has to be treated first if present, prior to ear surgery.
  - CT scan of temporal bone if in an unsafe CSOM, intracranial complications are suspected.

Routine investigations These include:
- Complete haemogram
- Erythrocyte sedimentation rate (ESR) if tuberculosis is suspected as a cause of CSOM.
- Blood sugar, if patient is diabetic or on suspicious history.
- ECG, if patient has cardiac problems or for anaesthesia fitness.
- X-ray chest for fitness for general anaesthesia, fitness and to rule out tuberculosis, if suspected.

AUDIOLOGICAL TESTS

Test for hearing
- Voice test
  - *Conversational voice*: Normal range for hearing conversational voice (CV) in a quiet surrounding is up to 12 meters. Inability to hear normal conversation beyond 1–2 meters from the ear indicates moderate to severe deafness.
  - *Whispered voice*: Normal range for hearing whispered voice (WV) in a quiet surrounding is up to 4½ meters. If whispered voice is not heard but, patient can have normal conversation, he may have a mild deafness.
- Watch test: Not a standard test. Not usually carried out.
- Tuning fork tests: These include Rinne test, Weber test and absolute bone conduction (ABC) test [Figs 4.2(A, B) and 4.3].
  - *Rinne test*: Performed to detect type and degree of hearing loss (qualitative and quantitative tests). Always interpreted in association with Weber test.
    Three frequencies of tuning forks, i.e. 256 Hz, 512 Hz, and 1024 Hz are used.
  - *Principle:* It compares duration of air conduction (AC) with duration of bone conduction (BC) of the same ear.
  - *Procedure:* The entire procedure is first explained to the patient. The tuning fork is held by the stem and set into vibrations by striking it gently on a firm but yielding surface (rubber pad, elbow

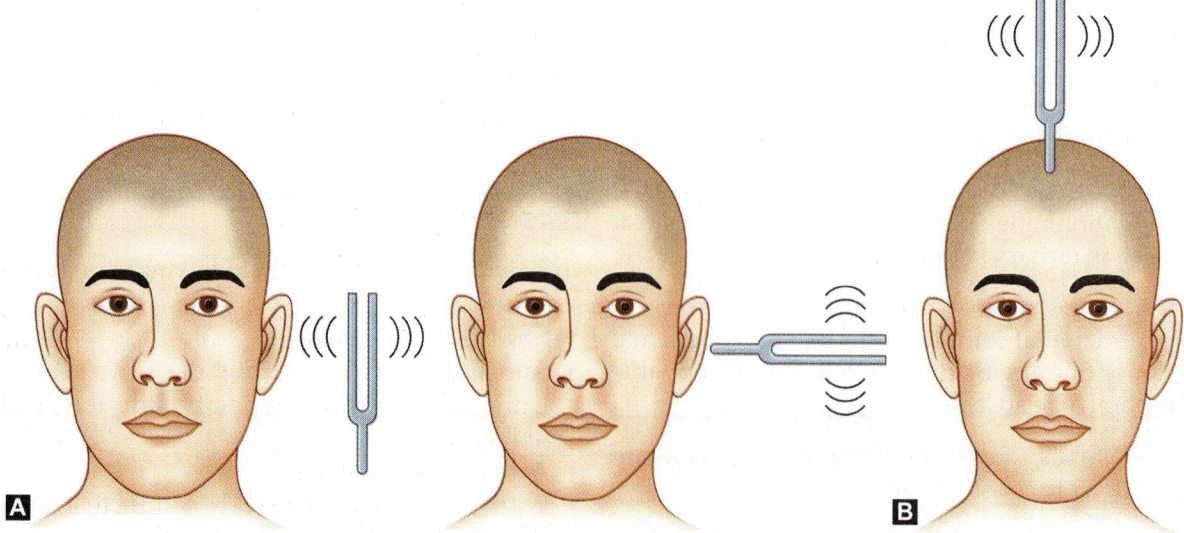

Fig. 4.2: (A) Rinne test, (B) Weber test

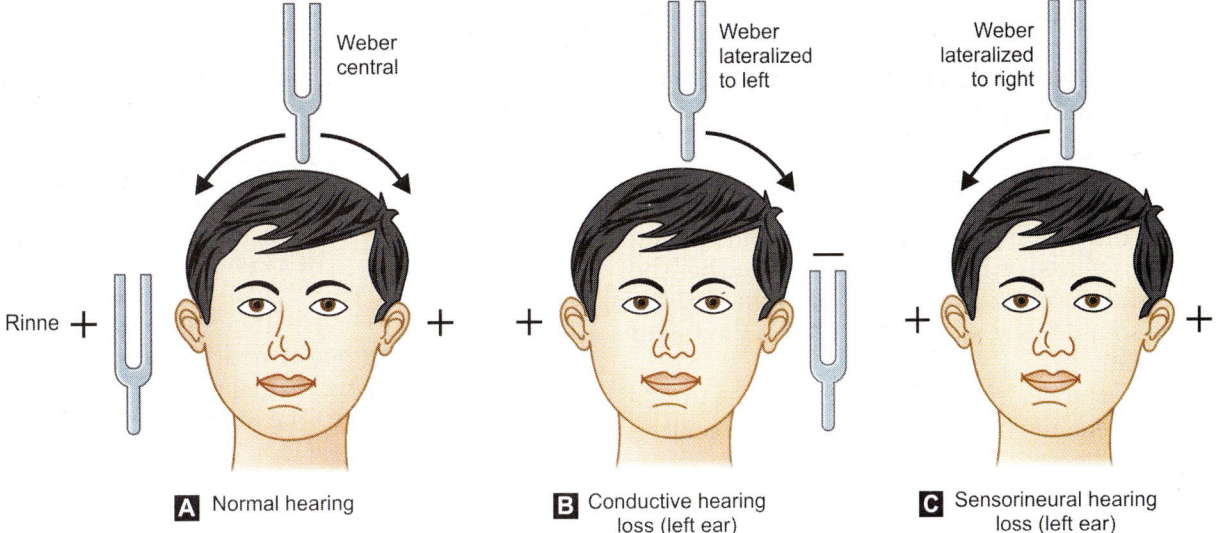

Fig. 4.3: Interpretation of tuning fork test

above the olecranon process, knee, or heel of hand). It is then held vertically 1 inch away from the EAC to be examined, so that the prongs are parallel to the EAC. By doing this, the acoustic axis is in line with the EAC. The patient is asked to indicate when he stops hearing the sound. When he says so, the base of the tuning fork is placed on the mastoid cortex and he is asked, if he can still hear the sound. If he says 'no', it indicates that AC > BC but, if he further continues to hear the sound after it ceases to be heard by air conduction, it indicates that BC > AC.

The procedure is performed with all the three tuning forks. (256 Hz, 512 Hz and 1024 Hz)

- *Inference*
  - AC > BC, then Rinne positive (+).
  - BC > AC, then Rinne negative (–).
- *Type of hearing loss* (Table 4.1)
  - *Rinne* + AC > BC: Normal hearing or sensorineural deafness
  - *Rinne* – BC > AC: Conductive deafness
  - *Rinne equivocal* AC = BC: Mild conductive hearing loss.

TABLE 4.1: Degree/Intensity of hearing loss

Tuning fork freq.	Rinne test	Degree of conductive deafness
256, 512, 1024	—, +, +	Mild
256, 512, 1024	—, —, +	Moderate
256, 512, 1024	—, —, —	Severe

- *False Rinne negative:* In unilateral severe sensorineural deafness, BC is apparently heard better than AC in the deaf ear. Hence, it is interpreted as Rinne negative. This is because, the BC is actually being heard by the normal ear when the tuning fork is placed on the mastoid cortex. However, Weber test will be lateralized to the normal ear indicating that this is a falsely negative Rinne result. It can further be confirmed by masking the normal ear and repeating the test, which will now reveal the positive Rinne result.

To accurately detect the type of hearing loss, Rinne's test has to be interpreted in association with Weber test.

- *Masking:* A continuous noise is presented to the normal ear to prevent crossing over of sound from the deaf ear to the normal ear during the Rinne test. This will help in preventing a false Rinne negative result in a case of severe unilateral SN deafness. It can be done by:
  - Rustling a piece of paper near the good ear,
  - Placing a ticking watch near the good ear,
  - Barany noise box near the good ear,
  - Masking can be done also by using the audiometer.
- *Weber test:* It is performed using only one tuning fork of 512 Hz frequency (Fig. 4.3). This tuning fork is chosen for the following reasons:
  - 512 Hz falls in the mid-speech frequency
  - Tuning fork of higher frequency has more overtones

- Tuning fork of lower frequency has more vibrations.
- Decay is faster in a tuning fork of higher frequency.
  The result is interpreted in association with Rinne's test.
- *Procedure:* The tuning fork of 512 Hz frequency is set into vibration by striking it gently against a firm but yielding surface. The base of the tuning fork is placed on the patient's vertex and he/she is asked to identify in which ear he/she can hear the sound better. (i.e. to which ear is the sound lateralised).
- *Interpretation:* In a normal patient the sound is heard equally in both ears or it may be central, i.e. not lateralised to any side.
  - *In conductive deafness:* The sound lateralises to the ear with poorer hearing.
  - *In sensorineural deafness:* The sound lateralises to the ear with better hearing.
    The tuning fork can also be placed on the nasion, mentum or the upper central inscisor teeth instead of the vertex.
- *Absolute bone conduction test:* Also known as modified Schwabach test. This test helps to detect presence of sensorineural deafness. It compares the absolute bone conduction (ABC) of the patient with that of the examiner assuming that the examiner's hearing is normal.
  - *Procedure:* A tuning fork of 512 Hz frequency is set into vibration by gently striking it against a firm but yielding surface. The base of the vibrating tuning fork is placed over the mastoid process of the patient after blocking the EAC of the same ear with a finger pressed lightly on the tragus. When the patient ceases to hear the sound, the same tuning fork is now placed on the same side ear of the examiner with the EAC blocked in a similar manner. The tuning fork is not set into vibrations again. If the examiner can hear the sound after the patient ceases to hear it, it indicates that the ABC of the patient is diminished. This test is done with the assumption that the examiner has normal hearing. It is repeated for the other ear.
  - *Interpretation*
    - *In normal ear or conductive deafness:* ABC of the patient is equal to that of examiner.
    - *In sensorineural hearing loss:* ABC of patient is diminished.
- *Schwabach test:* This test is similar to ABC test, only in this, the EAC is not occluded during the test. However, the ABC test is more reliable and hence this is not used nowadays.

- Audiometry: It is the graphic recording of hearing. It is both quantitative and qualitative. However, it is subjective and not an objective method of testing hearing (Figs 4.4 – 4.13).

Subjective	Objective
• Pure tone audiometry	• Impedence audiometry
• Bekesy audiometry	(tympanometry)
• Speech audiometry	• Evoked response audiometry (ERA)

- *Pure tone audiometry:* It is the commonest form of audiometry performed. It is a subjective test performed using an electronic device known as an audiometer. The audiometer is capable of presenting a single tone (pure tone) of sound in different frequencies to the ear at various intensities. This is heard by means of a headphone for air conduction and a vibrator for bone conduction. The graph of frequency in hertz on the X-axis with intensity in decibels (dB) on the Y-axis is called the audiogram.
  The audiometer has a frequency range from 125 Hz to 8 kHz (8000 Hz). The intensity is from 0 dB to 110 or 120 dB. It is performed in a sound-proof room.
  - *Applied importance*
    - Diagnosis of type and degree of deafness.
    - Documentation of hearing loss for
      - comparative study
      - medicolegal purposes.
    - Diagnosis of otosclerosis, presbyacusis or acoustic trauma as these have characteristic graph patterns on the audiogram.
    - For fitting of an appropriate hearing aid.
    - For masking.
    - Special tests can be performed using pure tone audiometry like:
      - Tests for recruitment
        - ☞ Alternate binaural loudness balance (ABLB) test
        - ☞ Short increment sensitivity index (SISI) test
        - ☞ Tone decay test
      - Tests for functional deafness
      - Free field audiometry used for testing hearing loss in children.
- *Bekesy audiometry:* The Bekesy audiometer is a self-recording automatic audiometer with which the patient himself records his/her hearing.
- *Speech audiometry:* Recorded test words are used to measure the intelligibility of spoken words in patients. It is closer to testing the natural hearing

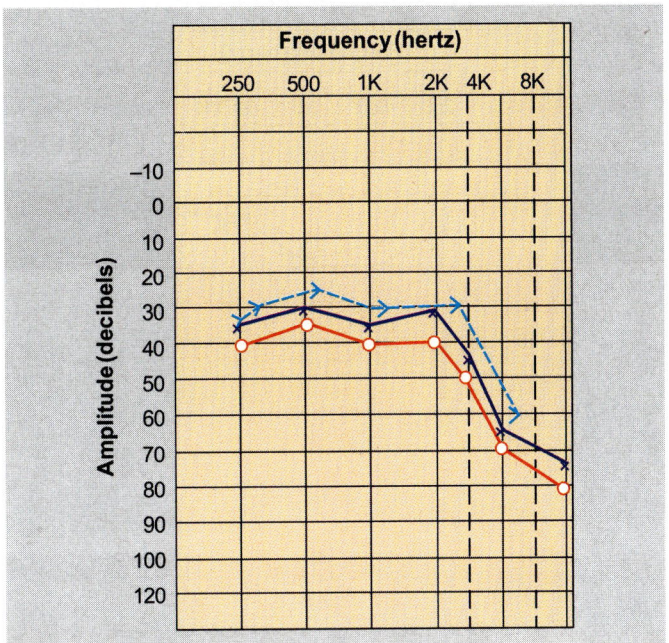

Fig. 4.4: Pure tone audiogram showing bilateral symmetrical hearing loss which is sensorineural in type, mild in the low frequencies and sloping to moderate-severe in the higher frequencies

Differential diagnosis: Sloping sensorineural hearing loss. 1. Ototoxicity 2. Presbycusis

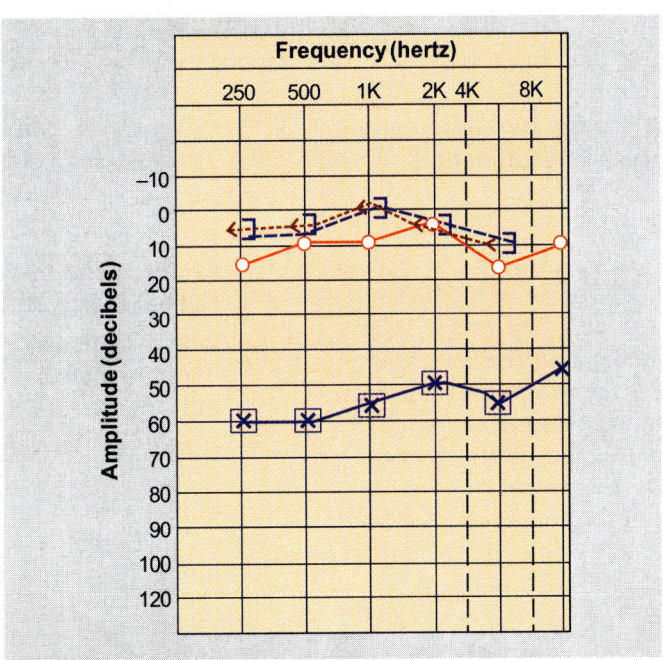

Fig. 4.5: Pure tone audiogram showing left sided conductive hearing loss which is moderately severe in intensity with an air-bone gap of about 55dB. The hearing in the right ear is within normal limits

Differential diagnosis: Unilateral conductive hearing loss.

1. Inflammatory—acute otitis media, chronic otitis media and otitis media with effusion.
2. Tympanic membrane perforation—traumatic or infective.
3. Ossicular chain discontinuity
4. Unilateral otosclerosis, tympanosclerosis.
5. Benign or malignant tumours of external auditory canal or middle ear.
6. Wax, foreign body in external auditory canal

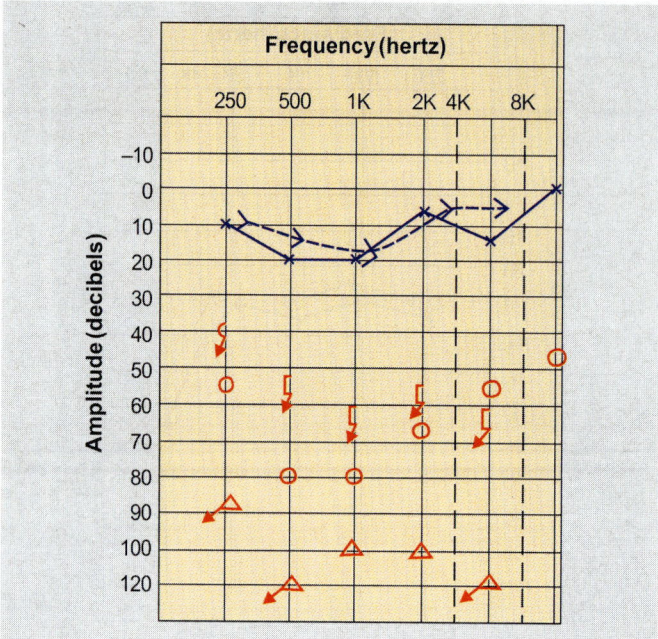

Fig. 4.6: Pure tone audiogram showing right sided sensorineural hearing loss which is profound in intensity. The hearing in the left ear is within normal limits

Differential diagnosis: Unilateral sensorineural hearing loss.

1. Infective labyrinthitis—bactrrial, spirochaetal and viral-mumps
2. Trauma
3. Endolymphatic hydrops.
4. Haematological embolism, coagulation disorders.
5. Vestibular schwannoma
6. Idiopathic.

but, not as standardised as pure tone audiometry.

- *In a normal ear,* the speech discrimination (SD) score is 95–100%.
- *In conductive deafness* SD score is 95–100% at higher intensity.
- *In SN deafness* SD score is low.
- *Impedence audiometry (tympanometry):* It is an objective method of measuring the resistance offered by the tympanic membrane and middle ear and their compliance to sound pressure transmission. A tympanogram is the graphic representation of middle ear pressure on the X-axis and compliance of the sound conducting apparatus on the Y-axis. **(Figs 4.14–4.17).**

The various types of graphs obtained are:

- *Type A* : Normal curve.
- *Type As* : Normal pressure with reduced compliance. It is seen in oto-sclerosis.
- *Type Ad* : Normal pressure with increased compliance. It is seen in ossicular discontinuity.
- *Type B* : Dome shaped or flat curve. It is seen in secretory otitis media.

- *Type C* : Maximum compliance at nega--tive pressure. It is seen in Eustachian tube dysfunction.

- *Applied importance*
  - Children and mentally handicapped patients can be objectively tested.
  - It helps to diagnose different types of pathology like otosclerosis, ossicular discontinuity, serous otitis medis (SOM), etc.
  - It is used for testing the stapedial reflex or acoustic reflex in facial palsy. It helps to detect site of lesion and presence of this reflex is the first sign of recovery of nerve function.

- *Brainstem evoked response audiometry (BERA):* It records the electric response to sound in the auditory system till the brainstem. It is useful for testing children, psychiatric patients and patients with psychogenic (functional) deafness. It is important to distinguish between cochlear deafness (Meniere's disease) and retrocochlear deafness (acoustic neuroma), i.e. it helps in the differential diagnosis of sensorineural deafness.

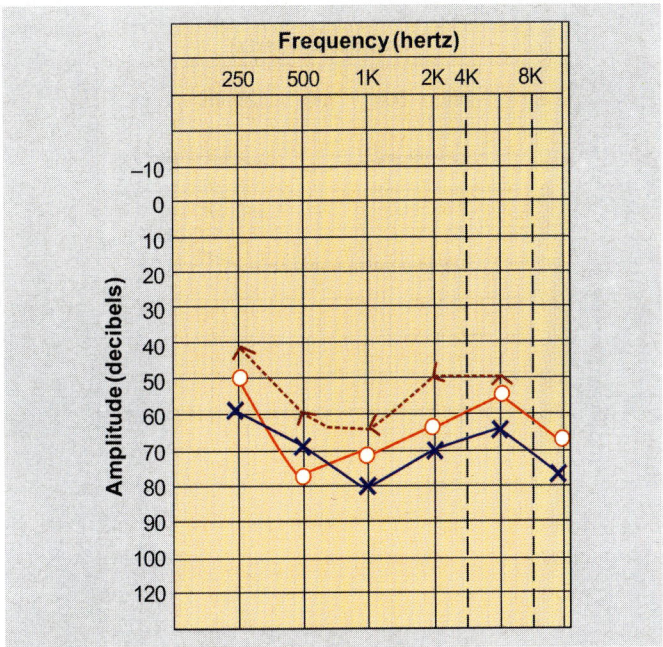

Fig. 4.7: Pure tone audiogram showing bilateral symmetrical hearing loss which is sensorineural in type, severe in intensity

Differential diagnosis: Bilateral sensorineural hearing loss.

1. Presbycusis
2. Acoustic trauma
3. Ototoxicity
4. Inflammatory/infective—typhoid, meningitis
5. Congenital
6. Systemic diseases–diabetes mellitus, hypertension
7. Auto immune diseases.

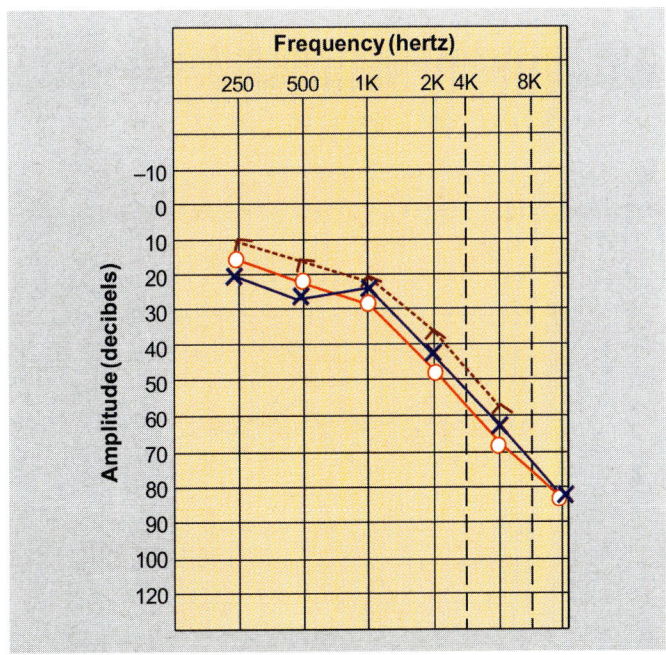

Fig. 4.8: Pure tone audiogram showing bilateral symmetrical hearing loss which is sensorineural in type, sloping from mild-severe in the higher intensities

Differential diagnosis:

1. Ototoxicity
2. Presbycusis

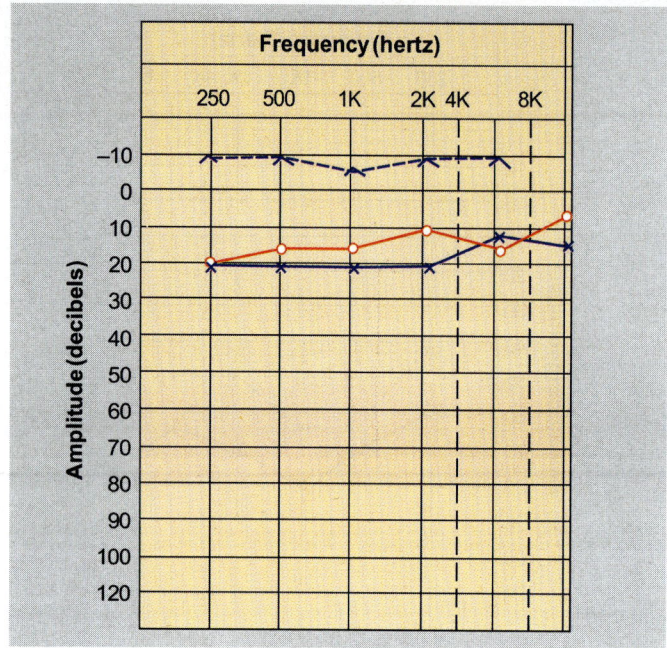

Fig. 4.9: Pure tone audiogram showing bilateral symmetrical hearing loss which is conductive in type and mild in intensity

Differential diagnosis: Bilateral conductive hearing loss.

1. Bilateral otosclerosis   3. Wax in both ears
2. Bilateral otitis media

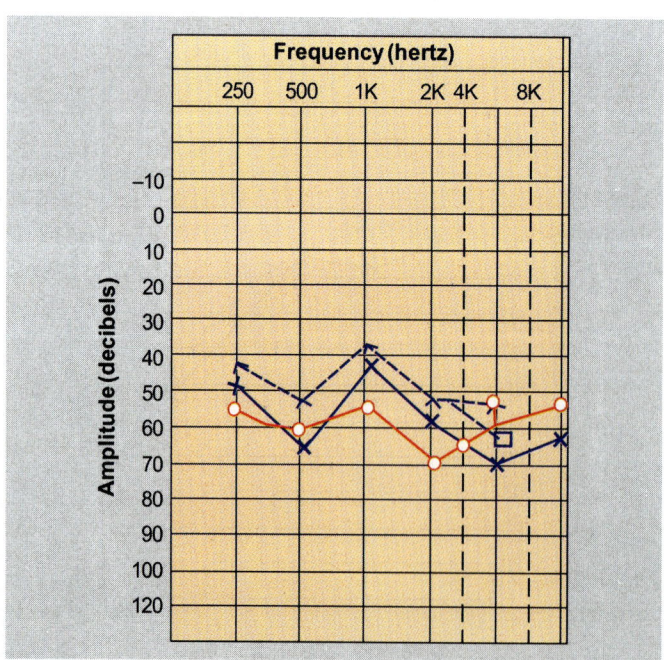

Fig. 4.10: Pure tone audiogram showing bilateral symmetrical hearing loss which is sensorineural in type, severe in intensity.

Differential diagnosis:

1. Congenital sensorineural hearing loss

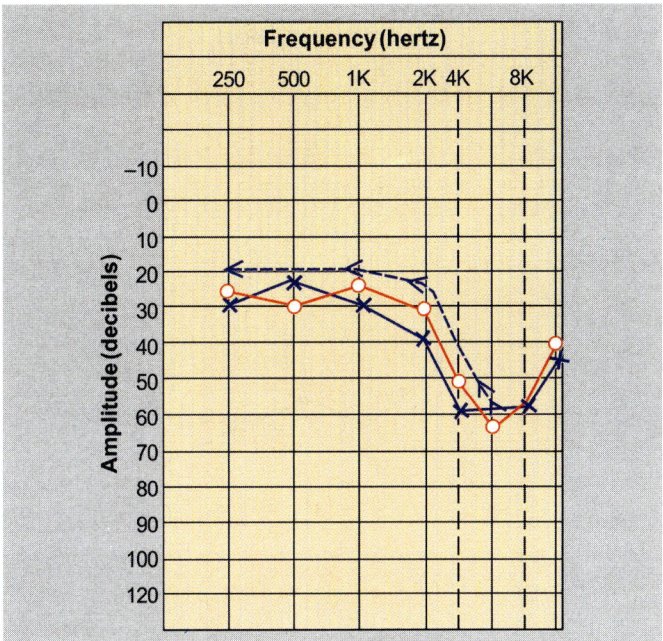

Fig. 4.11: Pure tone audiogram showing bilateral symmetrical hearing loss which is sensorineural in type/nature and mild in intensity with dip at 4 kH

Differential diagnosis:

1. Noise-induced hearing loss (acoustic brauma)

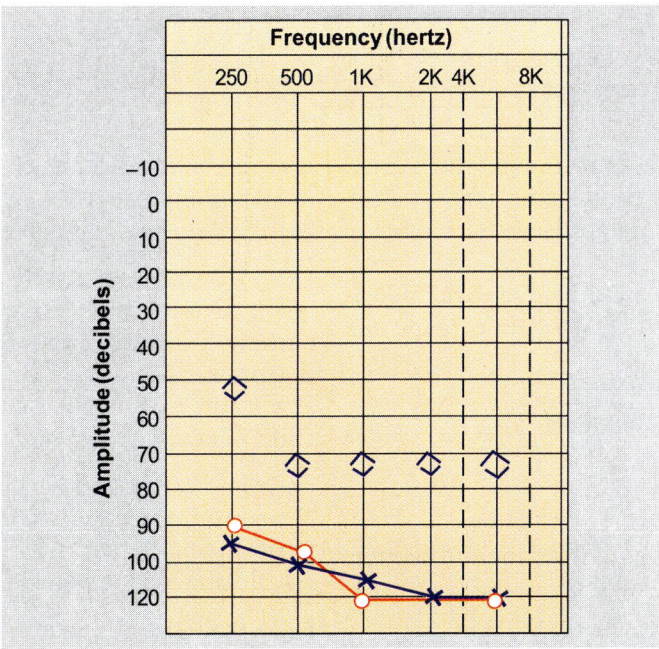

Fig. 4.12 : Pure tone audiogram showing bilateral symmetrical hearing loss which is sensorineural in type/ nature and profound in intensity

Differential diagnosis:

1. Congenital sensorineural hearing loss

2. Bilateral sensorineural hearing loss following exanthematous fevers/meningitis

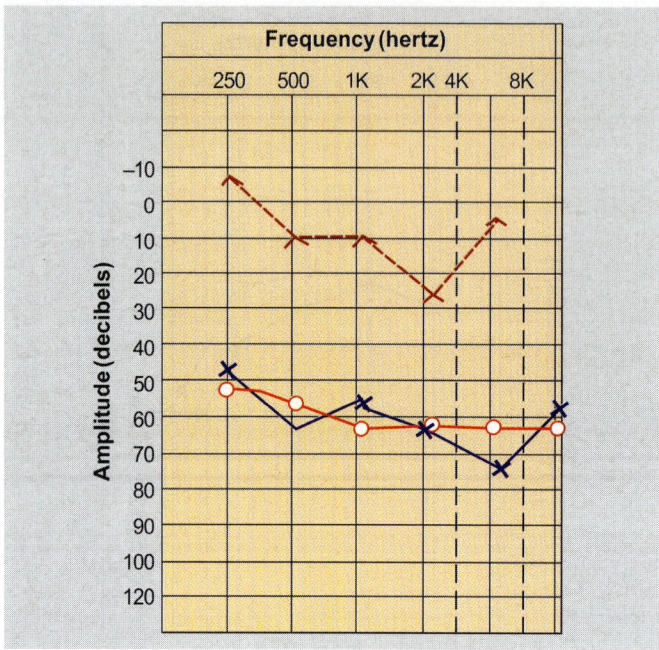

Fig. 4.13: Pure tone audiogram showing bilateral symmetrical hearing loss which is conductive type/ nature and moderate — severe in intensity with the bone conduction curve showing a 5 dB dip at 500 Hz, 5–10 dB dip at 1 khz, 10–15 dB dip at 2 kHz, 5–10 dB dip at 4 kHz. This is the characteristic Carhart's notch seen in ossicular chain fixation

Differential diagnosis: Conductive hearing loss with Carhart's notch

1. Otosclerosis
2. Congenital ossicular fixation
3. Tympanosclerosis
4. Persistent stapedial artery over stapes footplate
5. Facial nerve coursing over stapes footplate

A series of five peaks is recorded which arise from the cochlear nerve, cochlear nucleus, superior olivary nucleus, lateral lemniscus and inferior colliculus.

Other similar tests include electrocochleography (ECoG) and cortical evoked response audiometry (CERA).

HEARING TESTS USED FOR CHILDREN

Reflex tests
• Used for infants.
• Blinking or turning the eyes or head in the direction of sound, e.g. voice, clap, bells, etc.

Distraction tests
• Used for children between 1 and 2 years of age.
• Turning towards the sound, e.g. rattle, etc.

Behavioural observation audiometry   In behavioural observation audiometry (BOA) response of an infant to sound stimulus is observed.

Visual reinforcement audiometry   In visual reinforcement audiometry (VRA), the child is asked to look at an object when he/she is given a sound stimulus.

Conditioned audiometry   The child is given time to get accustomed to the earphones used for pure tone audiometry and a proper pure tone audiometry is then performed. Most children are afraid of the earphones and if this fear can be overcome by conditioning the child, this is the most preferred test.

Free field audiometry   It is performed only if conditioned audiometry is not possible. The child is taught to perform a particular task in response to sound stimulus, e.g. closing a door, placing a toy in a basket, etc.

BERA is the best objective test for testing hearing in children.

VESTIBULAR TESTS

Tests to assess the function of the vestibular apparatus are concerned with equilibrium.

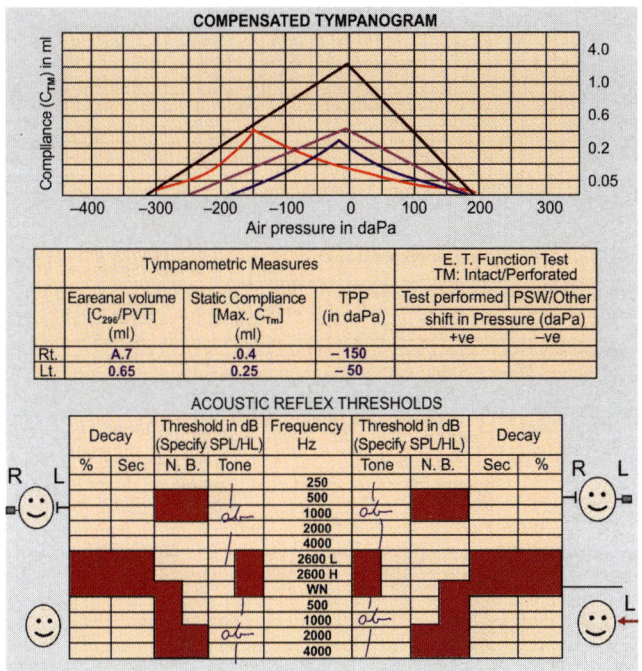

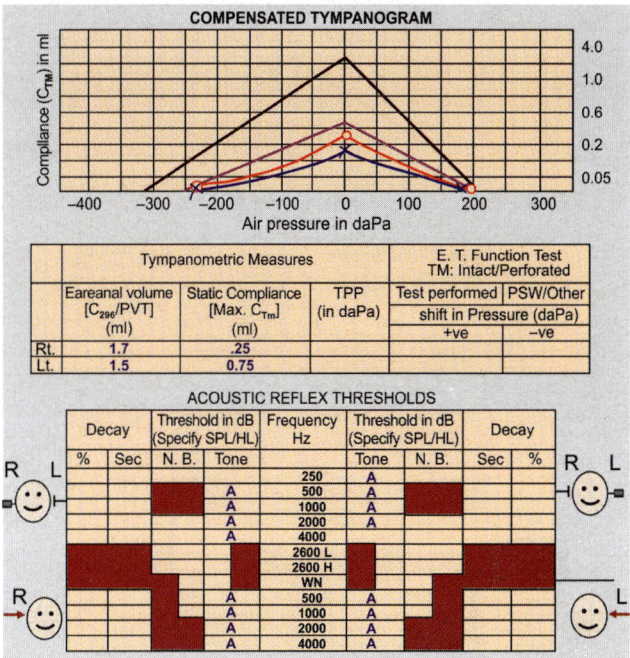

Fig. 4.14: Impedance audiogram showing in the right ear, the compliance is normal with a negative middle ear pressure, in the left ear, the compliance is reduced with normal middle ear pressure. In both ears, the stapedial/ acoustic reflexes are lost/ absent. This is type 'C' tympanogram for the right ear

Type C curve
1. Uncomplicated Eustachian tube obstruction
2. Eardrum abnormality super-imposed upon Eustachian tube obstruction(high compliance)

Symptoms and signs associated with vestibular dysfunction include:

Symptoms
- Vertigo
- Nausea and vomiting

Signs
- Nystagmus
- Loss of equilibrium
- Pastpointing

Nystagmus It is a rhythmic involuntary eye movement. It has two components, i.e. slow and fast. The slow component is caused due to vestibular dysfunction and the fast component is caused due to cerebral correction. The direction of the nystagmus is decided from the direction of its fast component since this is easily visible on examination of the patient's eyes. Vestibular nystagmus can be either:

Fig. 4.15: Impedance audiogram showing bilateral decrease in compliance with normal middle ear pressure and absence/ loss of stapedial/acoustic reflex in both ears. This is type 'As' tympanogram for both the ears

Type A – Normal ears, some cases of otosclerosis.
As type of curve
1. Otosclerosis
2. Thickened tympanic membarane
3. Tumours of the middle ear
4. Fixed malleus syndrome
5. Tympanosclerosis
6. Congenial fixation of stapes head
7. Paget's disease,osteogenesis and imperfect

- **Spontaneous:** It occurs in all positions and without any stimulus.
- **Positional:** It occurs only in a particular position of the patient.
- **Induced:** It occurs only on stimulation or induction using various tests like the caloric test and rotation test.

Nystagmus is classified into three degrees:
- *First degree* : Nystagmus occurs only when the patient looks in the direction of the fast component.
- *Second degree* : Nystagmus occurs when the patient looks straight ahead.
- *Third degree* : Nystagmus occurs when the patient looks in the direction of the slow component.

Third degree is the most severe type.

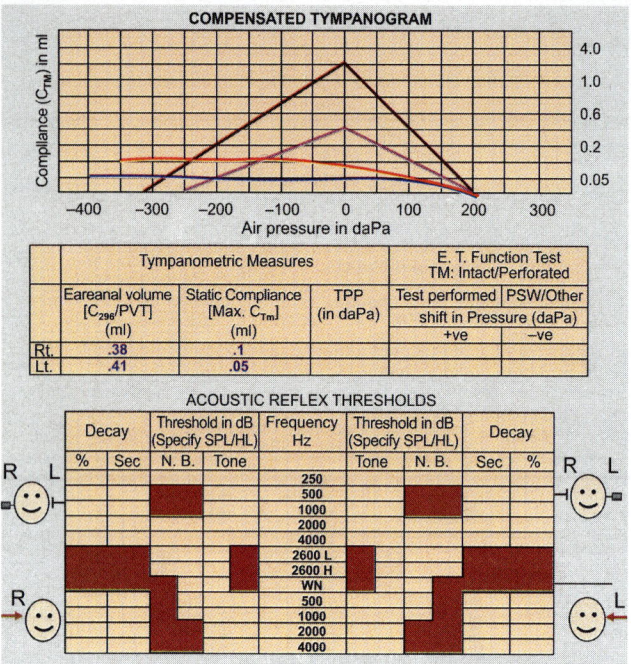

Fig. 4.16: Impedance audiogram showing bilateral very low compliance with low middle earpressure. This is a typical 'flat curve' tympanogram. This is type 'B' tympanogram for both

Type B curve
1. Otitis media with effusion
2. Adhesive otitis media
3. Tympanic membrane perforation, patent grommet
4. Artifact-blocked probe tip
5. Cerumen blocking external auditory canal

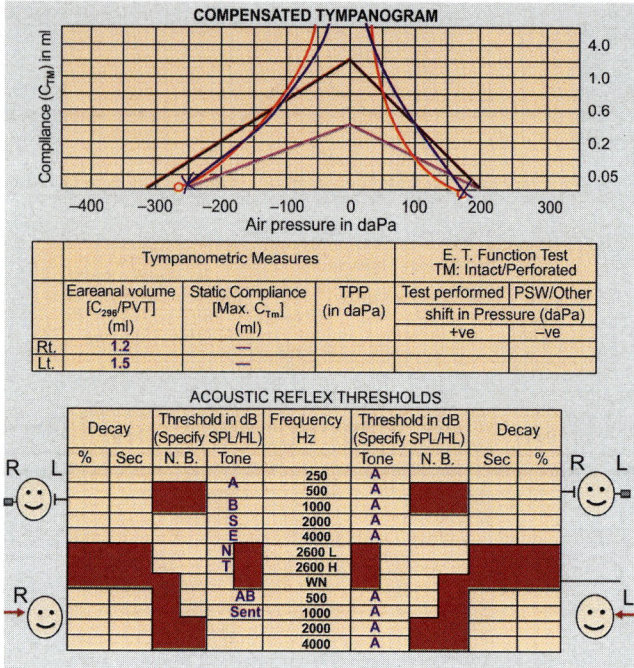

Fig. 4.17: Impedance audiogram showing bilateral very high compliance with normal middle earpressure and bilateral loss/absence of the stapedial/acoustic reflexes. This is type 'Ad' tympanogram for both the ears

Ad type of curve
1. Ossicular chain discontinuity
2. Hypermobile tympanic membrane
3. Large tympanic membrane (rare)

Loss of equilibrium   The patient tends to fall to one side, since he has a hallucination of movement and tries to correct it.

Pastpointing   The patient tends to reach beyond an object while attempting to touch it. This occurs as he/she feels that the object is moving away and hence he/she tries to compensate for this.

The various tests for assessment of vestibular function include:
- Caloric test (Hallpike test).
- Position test.
- Cold caloric test.
- Cold air caloric test.
- Rotation test.
- Electronystagmography (ENG).
- Fistula test.
- Rhomberg's test.

Caloric test (Hallpike test)

Principle: The vestibular labyrinth is stimulated using saline/water of different temperatures and the response is noted. The essential prerequisite is that the eardrums should be intact.

Procedure: Patient is placed supine with 30° head high (this position brings the horizontal semicircular canals in the vertical position). Water or saline is gently passed into the EAC of the patient using a soft rubber tubing and the returning water is collected into a kidney-tray. 200–300 cc of water is passed over a period of 40 seconds, using an enema can. The temperature of water used is 7°C above and below normal body temperature i.e. 30°C and 44°C. Each ear has two readings.

The response is noted in the form of a nystagmus and the duration from onset of the test to disappearance of nystagmus is measured. Cold water produces nystagmus to the opposite side and hot water produces nystagmus to the same side (COHS).

In a normal person, the duration ranges from 1 minute 20 seconds to 2 minutes.

Inferences

- *Normal:* All the four readings are almost equal.
- *Canal paresis:* The duration of nystagmus is shortened for both, hot and cold water in one ear. It is seen commonly in Meniere's disease or acoustic neuroma.
- *Canal palsy:* No response to both, hot and cold water in one ear.
- *Directional preponderance:* Nystagmus shows a preponderance to one side, i.e. either right or left side.

Contraindications

- *Presence of tympanic membrane perforation:* Test is performed using cold air instead of water.
- *Severe vertigo:* It is controlled first.
- *Patient on labyrinthine sedatives:* Patient is asked not to take them for at least 48 hours prior to the test.

Position test: Preferred in patients of positional vertigo. Positional nystagmus is seen on turning the head. The nystagmus shows fatigue on repetition whereas neurological (central) nystagmus does not show fatigue.

Cold caloric test: A small quantity of ice cold water is flushed in the external auditory canal and nystagmus is noted. It is a rough method of testing.

Cold air caloric test: In the presence of tympanic membrane perforation air is used instead of water to induce nystagmus as water may cause infection. The Dundas Grant apparatus is used for supplying air.

Rotation test: Patient is rotated and nystagmus is observed.

Electronystagmography (ENG): It is an electrical recording of nystagmus in the form of a graph and it is capable of detecting even minute nystagmus or nystagmus with eyes closed or in darkness. Both spontaneous and positional nystagmus are recorded. Induction of this nystagmus is by the caloric test.

Fistula test: It is used for the diagnosis of a labyrinthine fistula, i.e. an abnormal communication between the inner ear and the middle ear.

Procedure: The pressure in the external auditory canal is raised. This is transmitted to the inner ear from the middle ear via this fistula and results in labyrinthine stimulation which is manifested as vertigo, nausea, vomiting and nystagmus. Pressure in the EAC is raised by gently pressing the tragus against the external auditory meatus or using a Siegle's pneumatic speculum or an otoscope with attached pneumatic bulb or an impedence bridge.

The commonest site of fistula is the lateral semicircular canal.

- A positive test indicates the presence of labyrinthine fistula.
- A false positive test in presence of intact tympanic membrane is known as a positive '*Hennebert's sign*' and seen in syphilis and Meniere's disease at times.
- A false negative test can be due to a fistula being covered by granulation or cholesteatoma, or a dead labyrinth or an improperly performed test.

Rhomberg's test: The patient is made to stand with both feet together and hands by his side with eyes closed. Normally, he should not sway or fall.

- Vestibular paralysis: Patient sways towards the side of the lesion.
- Central disorder: Patient sways in different directions.
- Hysteria: Patient falls backwards.

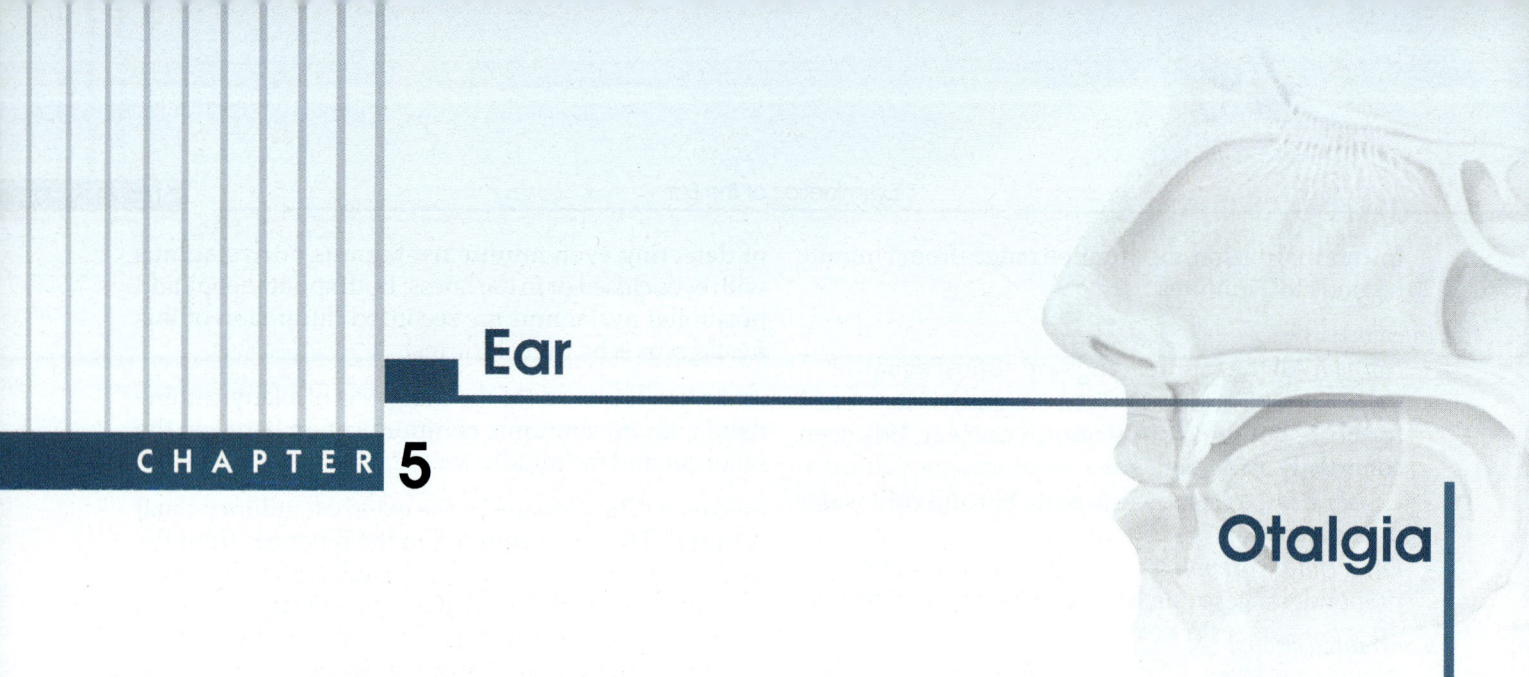

Ear

CHAPTER 5

Otalgia

LOCAL CAUSES OF OTALGIA (Flowchart 5.1)

Conditions affecting the external ear
• Wax
• Otitis externa
• Furuncle of the external ear
• Otomycosis
• Perichondritis
• Trauma
• Foreign body
• Viral infections such as herpes
• Myringitis
• Malignant otitis externa
• Maggots.

Flowchart 5.1: Causes of otalgia

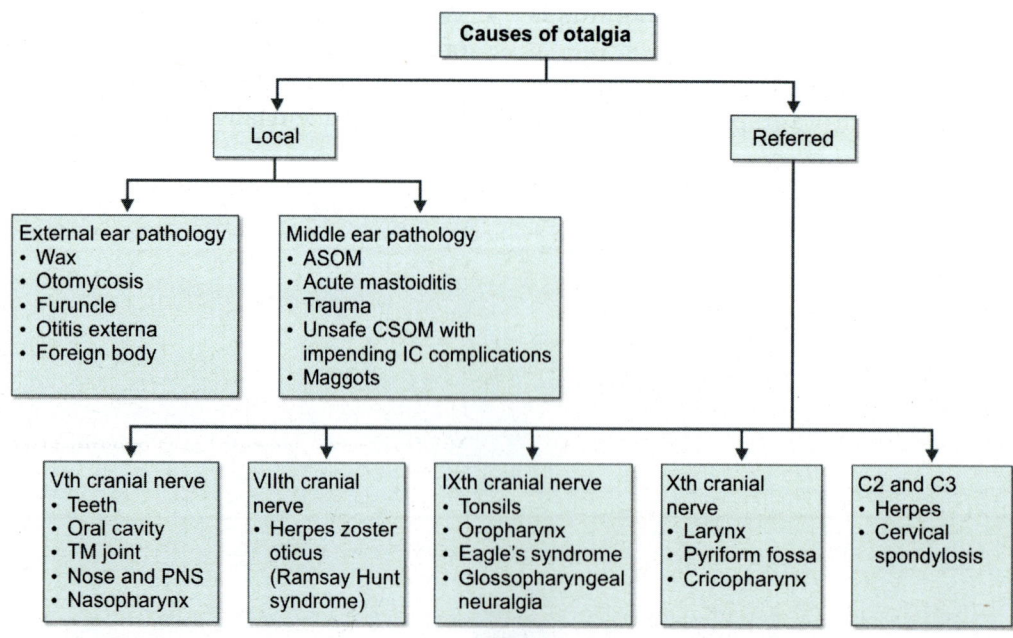

Conditions affecting the middle ear

- Acute suppurative otitis media (ASOM)
- Eustachain tube catarrh
- Acute mastoiditis
- Traumatic perforation of tympanic membrane
- Haemotympanum following trauma
- Barotrauma
- Unsafe suppurative otitis media—CSOM with impending intracranial complications
- Tumours
- Maggots.

REFERRED CAUSES OF OTALGIA

Through Vth cranial nerve (trigeminal nerve) This is via the auriculotemporal branch of the mandibular division of the Vth cranial nerve which supplies the external ear:

- Teeth
  - Dental caries
  - Dental abscess
  - Impacted third molar tooth
  - Malocclusion of jaws (Costen's syndrome).
- Oral cavity: Conditions involving the palate, cheek, tongue, floor of mouth, lips and salivary glands such as:
  - Infection
  - Abscess, e.g. Ludwig's angina
  - Ulcers
  - Malignancy
  - Salivary calculus
  - Sialadenitis.
- Temporomandibular joint
  - Arthritis
- Nose and paranasal sinuses
  - Tumours
  - Impacted DNS
  - Sinusitis.
- Nasopharynx
  - Infection
  - Adenoiditis
  - Post-adenoidectomy
  - Tumours.
- Trigeminal neuralgia

Through the VIIth cranial nerve (facial nerve) Via the sensory branch of the facial nerve which supplies the deep part of the posterior wall of the EAC.

- Herpes zoster oticus (Ramsay Hunt syndrome)

Through the IXth cranial nerve (glossopharyngeal nerve) Via the tympanic branch of the glossopharyngeal nerve which supplies the middle ear.

- Tonsils
  - Tonsillitis
  - Peritonsillitis and peritonsillar abscess
  - Post-tonsillectomy
  - Malignancy.
- Oropharynx: Conditions affecting the posterior pharyngeal wall, posterior one-third of tongue and soft palate such as:
  - Infection
  - Retropharyngeal abscess
  - Parapharyngeal abscess
  - Ulcers
  - Trauma
  - Malignancy
- Eagle's syndrome/stylalgia:
  - Due to elongated styloid process
- Glossopharyngeal neuralgia.

Through the vagus nerve (Xth cranial nerve) Via the auricular branch of the vagus nerve (Arnold's nerve) which supplies the external auditory canal and tympanic membrane.

- Larynx
  - Malignancy
  - Tuberculosis
  - Infections
  - Trauma.
- Pyriform fossa
  - Malignancy
  - Tuberculosis
  - Infections
  - Trauma.
- Cricopharynx
  - Malignancy
  - Trauma
  - Infections
  - Foreign body.

Through second and third cervical nerves (C2 and C3)

- Via the lesser occipital and greater auricular nerves which supply the external ear:
  - Herpes
  - Cervical spondylosis.

The common causes of referred otalgia in clinical practice: These include:

- Quinsy

- Dental causes
- Following tonsillectomy
- Temporomandibular joint arthritis
- Malignancy of the oral cavity, oropharynx and larynx
- Cervical spondylosis.

DIAGNOSIS

Diagnosis for the cause of otalgia should include a complete examination of the ear and examination of other structures which could be the cause of referred otalgia such as oral cavity, oropharynx, nose, nasopharynx, larynx, neck, and temporomandibular joint.

INVESTIGATIONS

Specific investigations should be aimed to find the cause of otalgia. These include:

- X-ray of cervical spine to rule out spondylosis
- X-ray of temporomandibular joint to rule out ankylosis
- X-ray of molars to rule out impacted third molar, (orthopantomogram)
- X-ray of chest to rule out tuberculosis which may have also infected the larynx
- Routine examination of ear, nose, throat and neck to rule out cause of otalgia
- Endoscopy to examine nose, nasopharynx, oropharynx, hypopharynx and larynx.

TREATMENT

- Treatment of the cause
- Systemic—Analgesics
- Systemic—Antibiotics
- Occasionally, analgesic or antibiotic or steroid eardrops or antimycotic eardrops, depending on the cause.

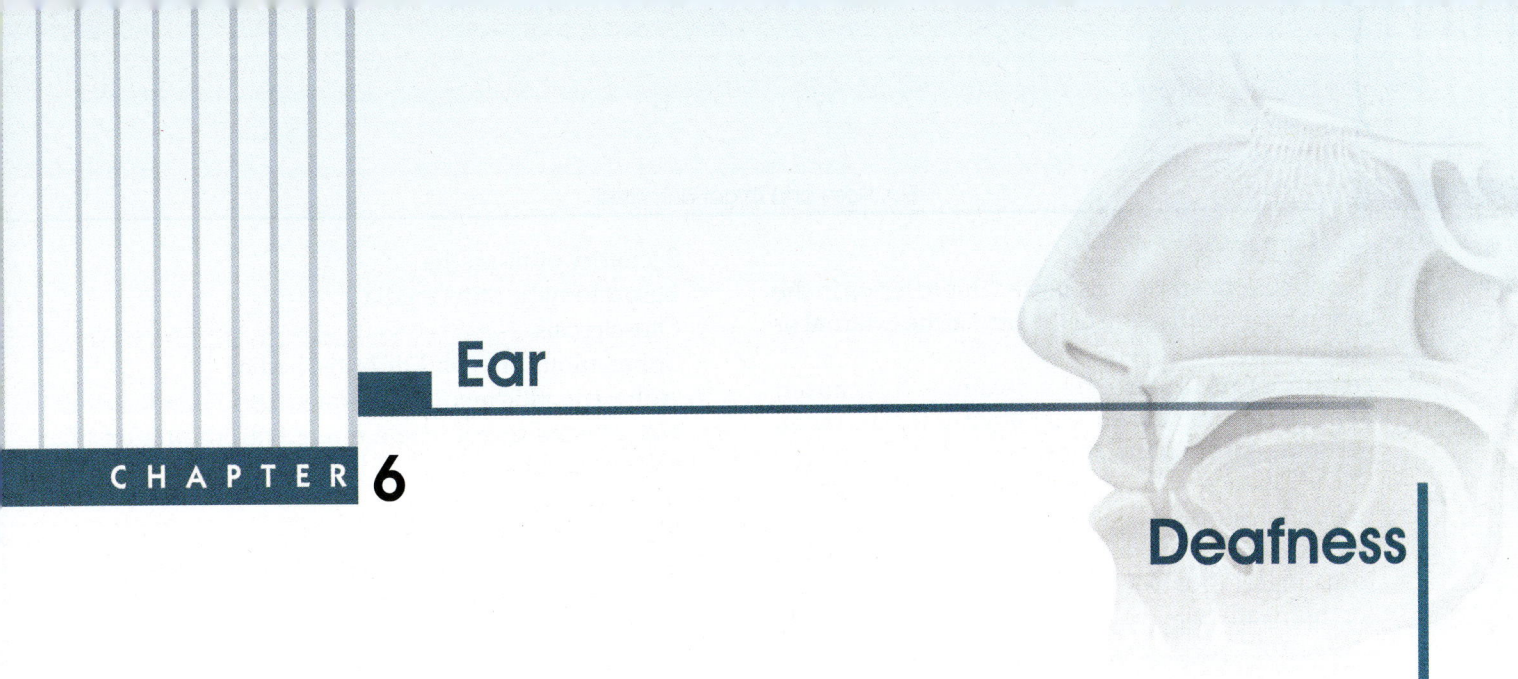

DEFINITION

Deafness is defined as impairment of hearing.

CLASSIFICATION

Classification of deafness include following types (Fig. 6.1):

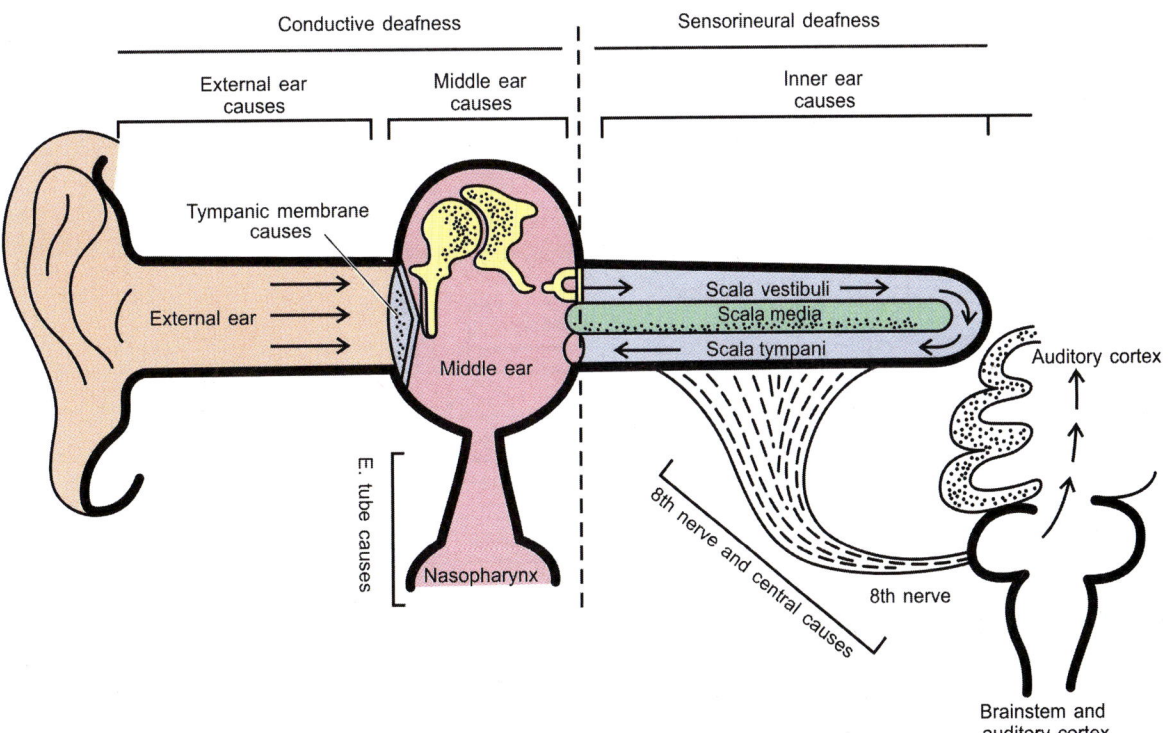

Fig. 6.1: Classification of causes of deafness

Types of deafness

- **Conductive deafness:** It is caused due to lesion in the conducting mechanism of the ear, i.e. the external or middle ear.
- **Sensorineural or perceptive deafness:** It is caused due to lesion in the inner ear (labyrinth), 8th cranial nerve or central connections.
- **Mixed deafness:** This is conductive as well as sensorineural deafness.
- **Psychogenic or functional deafness:** It is caused due to malingering or hysteria. There is no organic cause for this deafness.

AETIOLOGY (Flowchart 6.1)

Conductive deafness

- **External ear**
  - Wax or cerumen
  - Fungus (otomycosis)
  - Impacted foreign body
  - Otitis externa
  - Aural polyp
  - Neoplasm–benign or malignant
  - Congenital causes like stenosis or atresia.
- **Middle ear**
  - Bullous myringitis
  - Traumatic rupture of eardrum
  - Ossicular deformity due to congenital or traumatic causes
  - Chronic suppurative otitis media (CSOM)
  - Acute suppurative otitis media (ASOM)
  - Secretory otitis media
  - Barotraumatic otitis media
  - Otosclerosis
  - Tuberculous or syphilitic otitis media
  - Adhesive otitis media
  - Neoplasms of middle ear, e.g. carcinoma or glomus jugulare.
- **Eustachian tube**
  - Eustachian tube catarrh
  - Eustachian tube dysfunction due to diseases in nose, paranasal sinuses and nasopharynx
  - Barotrauma.

Sensorineural deafness

- **Causes in the inner ear or cochlea**
  - *Congenital:* Maldevelopment of inner ear structures
  - *Infective:* Labyrinthitis due to bacterial infections, measles, mumps, influenza, etc.
  - *Traumatic:* Fracture of bony labyrinth due to head injury or operative trauma during ear surgery
  - Meniere's disease
  - Ototoxic drugs, e.g. streptomycin, gentamycin, frusemide, salicylates
  - Tumours like acoustic neuroma
  - Senile deafness (presbyacusis)
  - Noise induced trauma to inner ear.
- **Systemic disorders**
  - Diabetes mellitus
  - Hypertension
  - Hypothyroidism

Flowchart 6.1: Aetiology of deafness

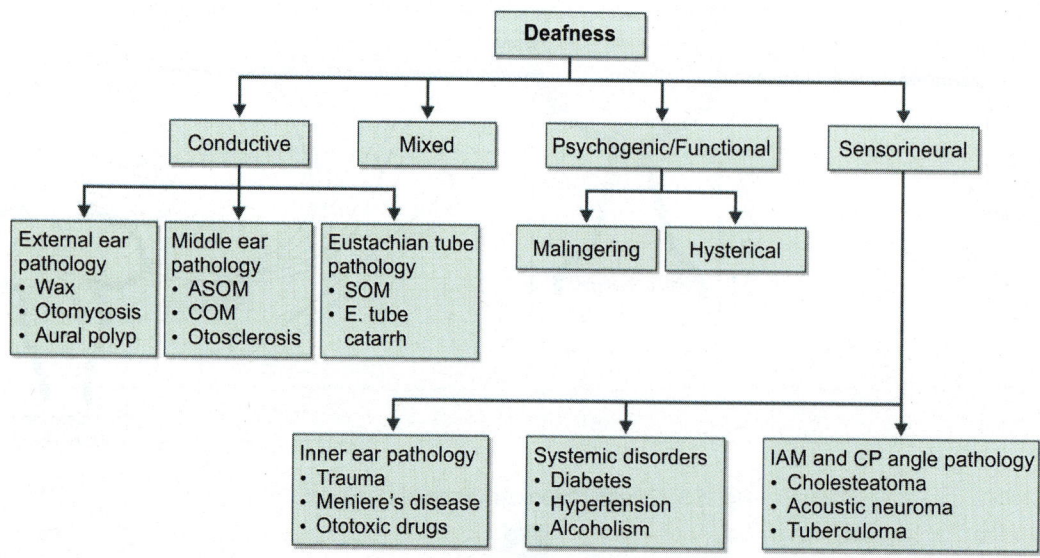

- Vitamin deficiency
- Smoking
- Alcoholism
- Cerebrovascular insufficiency
- Atherosclerosis.
- Causes in the internal auditory meatus (IAM) and cerebellopontine (CP) angle
  - Acoustic neuroma
  - Meningioma
  - Tuberculoma
  - Cholesteatoma
  - Arachnoid cyst.

Mixed deafness
- It causes where both, the conductive apparatus and end-organ are affected:
  - CSOM—Cholesteatoma resulting in damage to ossicles and inner ear. Usually unsafe ear disease causes mixed deafness.
  - Otosclerosis in the advanced stage
  - Senile deafness superimposed on conductive deafness
  - Trauma—Acoustic trauma
    - Blast injury
    - Head injury.

Psychogenic deafness
It is caused where there is no organic cause for the hearing loss. It is of two types:
- Malingering: If the patient purposely pretends not to hear. He is aware of the deception.
- Hysterical: If the patient stops listening and hence fails to hear. It is outside conscious control.
  This is usually seen in females following some emotional shock.

Causes of Sudden Sensorineural Deafness
- Vascular: Spasm, embolism or hemorrhage
- Infection: Viral labyrinthitis, influenza, mumps
- Traumatic: Acoustic trauma, head injury, round window rupture or oval window fistula
- Ototoxicity
- Meniere's disease
- Meningitis, encephalitis
- Acoustic neuroma
- Functional.

INVESTIGATIONS

Clinical examination of ears
- Tests of hearing
  - Voice test
    - Tuning fork tests
    - Pure tone audiometry.
- Caloric test
- BERA (Brainstem evoked response audiometry)
- Venereal disease research laboratory (VDRL)
- Haematological tests
- Blood sugar
- Serum lipid profile
- Blood pressure
- X-ray and CT scan of temporal bone and cerebellopontine (CP) angle
- Neurological examination.

TREATMENT

Conductive deafness
- Treat the cause, e.g. tuberculosis, etc.
- Surgical management—tympanoplasty, ossiculoplasty mastoidectomy, stapedectomy or endolymphatic sac decompression
- Hearing aid—if patient refuses or is unfit for surgery.

Sensorineural deafness
- Treat the cause, e.g. syphillis, diabetes, etc.
- Vasodilators: Nicotinic acid derivatives parenterally or orally—help by improving blood flow to cochlea.
- Steroids: Parenterally or orally.
- Vitamin B1, B6, B12: To help nerve tissue regeneration.
- Vitamin A, C and E: As they are antiatherosclerotic.
- Labyrinthine sedatives and tranquillisers
- Hearing aids
- Auditory training and lip reading.

Tests for Malingering
- General observation of behavioural changes in patient without his knowledge.
- Stenger's test: When two identical tones are simultaneously presented in both the ears, the sound is heard only by the ear nearer to the tone.
- Chimani Moos' test: Tuning fork is placed on the forehead (vertex) of the malingerer and the patient will claim to hear only with the good ear. If the EAC of the good ear is occluded, he will deny to hear the sound whereas in a truly deaf patient, he will continue to hear sound even after the EAC of the good ear is occluded.
- Lombard's test: Barany's noise box is placed on the good ear and patient is asked to read aloud. A deaf patient starts reading very loudly but a malingerer's voice will not be raised.
- Objective test like BERA.

CHAPTER 7

Vertigo and Tinnitus

VERTIGO

DEFINITION

Vertigo is a hallucination of movement due to a disturbance of the sense of equilibrium

In this the person feels that his surroundings are going around him or he himself is rotating. It may be accompanied by nausea, vomiting, sweating, and diarrhoea due to stimulation of the vagus.

PHYSIOLOGY OF EQUILIBRIUM

The labyrinth has two parts, the cochlea which is concerned with hearing and the vestibule which maintains equilibrium. Equilibrium is maintained by the vestibule in coordination with visual and proprioceptive senses. The higher centres for maintenance of equilibrium lie in the cerebellum and cerebrum.

If there is any disturbance in the coordination of this mechanism, vertigo is experienced.

AETIOLOGY

- Pathological vertigo
- Nonpathological vertigo
- Functional vertigo

Pathological vertigo
- Central cause: Vertigo is caused due to cerebellar and cerebral disease.

- Peripheral cause
  - *Local causes* (Causes in the ear)
    - *Inner ear diseases*
      - Motion sickness
      - Meniere's disease
      - Acoustic neuroma
      - *Infections*
        - Viral labyrithitis due to mumps, measles, etc.
        - Labyrinthitis as a complication of chronic suppurative otitis media (CSOM) or acute suppurative atitic media (ASOM).
        - Syphillitic labyrinthitis.
      - *Traumatic*
        - Head injury
        - Postoperative trauma to inner ear
        - Perilymph fistula
        - Acoustic trauma. Very loud sound may cause vertigo in some individuals (Tullio phenomenon).
        - Ototoxic drugs, e.g. streptomycin.
    - *Middle ear diseases*
      - ASOM
      - Unsafe CSOM
      - Eustachian catarrh
    - *External ear causes*
      - Impacted wax
      - Furuncle in external auditory canal

- ◆ *Systemic causes*
  - *Cervical spondylosis:* Osteophytes reduce the blood supply to the labyrinth by compression of the vertebral arteries
  - *Visual disorders:* Refractory errors and glaucoma
  - *Cardiovascular diseases*
    - Hypertension
    - Hypotension
    - Atherosclerosis
      These reduce the blood supply to the labyrinth and brain resulting in vertigo.
  - *Neurological diseases*
    - Cerebellar tumours or abscess
    - Vertebrobasilar artery syndrome
    - Raised intracranial tension
    - Disseminated sclerosis
  - *Anaemia*, which results in diminished oxygen supply to the labyrinth.
  - *Metabolic disorders*
    - Diabetes mellitus resulting in VIII cranial nerve neuritis
    - Hypoglycaemia resulting in reduced nutrition to vital centres.

Non-pathological vertigo
- Vertigo due to lights
- Vertigo after rotation or motion sickness
- Vertigo due to sudden change in floor-texture

Functional vertigo   This is quite common and seen due to hysteria, usually in females.

INVESTIGATIONS

The primary aim of treatment is to achieve symptomatic relief and then investigate the cause :
- A detailed history and clinical examination is a must for ascertaining the diagnosis.
- Tuning fork tests, audiometry, brainstem evoked response audiometry (BERA).
- Vestibular function tests: Electronystagmography (ENG), caloric test, videonystagmography (VNG)
- X-ray of the mastoid and cervical spine
- CT scan of head and temporal bone
- Haematological investigations:
  - ◆ Complete blood count
  - ◆ Blood sugar
  - ◆ Serum cholesterol
  - ◆ VDRL.

- ECG
- Neurological investigations if required.

TREATMENT
- Reassurance to the patient
- Treatment of cause
- General treatment is same as for Meniere's disease.
  Vasodialators are contraindicated in cases of head injury or cardiovascular diseases and should be used with caution.

TINNITUS

DEFINITION

Tinnitus is the perception of sound in the absence of any external auditory stimulus.

Synonym   Tinnitus aurium

CLASSIFICATION

- Unilateral: Heard in only one ear
- Bilateral: Heard in both ears
- Subjective: Heard only by the patient
- Objective: Heard by the patient and the examiner
- Continuous
  Intermittent
- High pitched
  Low pitched.

AETIOLOGY

- Subjective tinnitus
  - ◆ *Tinnitus with deafness:*
    - *Due to local cause in the ear:* Any pathology causing deafness can also cause tinnitus, e.g. ASOM, glomus tumour, otosclerosis, serous otitis media (SOM), etc.
    - *Systemic causes,* which cause deafness, can also cause tinnitus
  - ◆ *Tinnitus without deafness:* It occurs in:
    - Anaemia
    - Aortic incompetence
    - Hypertension
    - Hypotension
  - ◆ *Functional tinnitus:* It is rare and occurs due to emotional factors. However, usually tinnitus is responsible for emotional disturbances.
  - ◆ *Idiopathic:* The cause for tinnitus is not known.

- Objective tinnitus:
  - Patulous Eustachian tube
  - Clonic contractions of palatal muscles or muscles of middle ear
  - Clicking temporomandibular joint
  - Aneurysm in the ear or around the ear
  - Arteriovenous shunt around the ear
  - Intracranial vascular tumours
  - Live insect in the ear or maggots.

INVESTIGATIONS

Similar to investigations for deafness and specific investigations to find the cause.

Detailed history and examination to search for systemic causes.

TREATMENT

- Treatment of cause
- Mild sedatives and anxiolytics
- Vasodilators
- Carbamazepine
- Tinnitus maskers: These are devices used to mask the tinnitus in a quiet atmosphere, e.g. alarm clock, bed-side radio, Barany noise box, etc.
- Hyperbaric oxygen
- Surgical treatment is not very much useful and results in deafness, e.g. sectioning of cochlear nerve or ultrasonic destruction of cochlea. It can be used in a patient of tinnitus with profound sensorineural hearing loss in the same ear.

CHAPTER 8

Conditions of the External Ear

CONGENITAL MALFORMATIONS

Variations in shapes of the pinna
- Bat ear/Lop ear: Abnormal protrusion of pinna outwards
- Microtia: Small-sized pinna
- Macrotia: Large-sized pinna

Accessory auricles   Small skin tags seen anterior to the auricle. These are rudimentary.

Congenital atresia of the external auditory canal
It can be partial or total.

Treatment of the above three types of defects:
- Plastic surgery
- To adopt a hair style to camouflage the defect

Congenital absence of pinna   Commonly associated with atresia of external auditory canal.
- Treatment: Surgical reconstruction of external auditory canal (EAC) with use of prosthesis for the pinna.

Preauricular sinus
- Aetiology: Improper fusion of the auricular tubercles which develop from the first and second branchial arches.
- Treatment: If it is infected recurrently, excision should be done after adequate antibiotics. Recurrence is rare if the entire tract is excised.

Treacher–Collin's syndrome   This is a syndrome comprising of hypoplasia of the external and middle ear, eyes, maxilla and mandible. It is unilateral or bilateral.
- Treatment is by plastic surgery.

INFECTIONS OR INFLAMMATORY CONDITIONS

- Perichondritis of pinna
- Otitis externa

PERICHONDRITIS OF THE PINNA

Definition   Infection and inflammation of the perichondrium and cartilage of the pinna.

Aetiology
- After trauma to pinna
- Following haematoma
- Iatrogenic, rarely after ear surgery

Causative organisms
- *Staphylococcus aureus*
- *Bacillus pyocyaneus*

Clinical features
- Symptoms
  - Severe pain over pinna causing loss of sleep at times
  - Swelling and redness over pinna
  - Headache, fever and malaise.
- Signs
  - Tenderness and local rise in temperature over pinna

- ◆ Redness over pinna and swelling
- ◆ Deformity of pinna due to necrosis of cartilage
- ◆ Cauliflower ear is the end-result of perichondritis of pinna due to necrosis of the supporting cartilage. It is also commonly seen in wrestlers and boxers due to injury caused during fights.
- • Treatment
  - ◆ Intravenous antibiotics
  - ◆ If haematoma/pus is present incision and drainage with aseptic precautions is performed followed by regular dressings
  - ◆ Plastic surgical repair of pinna at a later date.

OTITIS EXTERNA

Definition   It is the inflammation of the external ear.

Classification
- • Acute or chronic: Acute can be either localized or generalised.
- • Primary or secondary: Primary is due to a cause in the external ear and secondary is due to spread of infection from cheek, etc.

Aetiology
- • Infectious causes (Table 8.1)

TABLE 8.1: Various types of infections

Bacterial	Viral	Fungal

• Acute otitis externa
  ◆ Localized (furuncle)
  ◆ Generalized
• Erysipelas
• Lupus vulgaris
	• Herpes simplex
	• Herpes zoster
	• Bullous myringitis
		• Otomy-cosis

- • Miscellaneous
  - ◆ Malignant otitis externa
  - ◆ Myringitis
  - ◆ Eczematous otitis externa
  - ◆ Seborrhoeic otitis externa
  - ◆ Neurodermatitis.

Acute otitis externa

Definition: Acute otitis externa (AOE) is the acute inflammation of the external ear.

Classification
- • Localized: It presents as a furuncle in the external auditory canal.
- • Generalized: It presents as thickening or desquamation of the EAC skin.

Aetiology
- • Diabetes: Diabetic individuals are more prone to furunculosis of the external auditory canal. If untreated or if inadequately treated, it may lead to malignant otitis externa.
- • Scratching the ear with dirty nails or cleaning the ear with pencil, hair-pin, etc.
- • Humid climate predisposes to AOE.
- • Bathing and swimming with water entering the ear predisposes to AOE.
- • In a case of chronic suppurative otitis media (CSOM), recurrent discharge from the middle ear acts as a source of constant irritation to the EAC with resultant secondary infection and AOE.
- • Allergy may also predispose to AOE.

Clinical features
- • Symptoms
  - ◆ *Pain:* Acute and severe pain which is aggravated by movement of the jaw.
  - ◆ *Deafness:* Usually a sensation of blocking of the ear is present, if the lumen of the EAC is occluded due to oedema, furuncle or accumulation of debris.
  - ◆ *Itching*
  - ◆ *Otorrhoea:* If furuncle ruptures, otorrhoea is followed by relief from pain. The discharge is purulent and occasionally blood stained. In generalized otitis externa, the discharge is usually serous.
  - ◆ *Trismus:* The anterior wall of the EAC is in close proximity to the temporomandibular joint. Any jaw movement causes aggravation of pain, therefore the patient restricts opening of the mouth to the minimum.

- • Signs
  - ◆ Tenderness over pinna
  - ◆ Local rise of temperature
  - ◆ Oedema of EAC with congestion or furuncle may be seen pointing in the EAC
  - ◆ Cellulitis of pinna extending to the mastoid region with obliteration of the postauricular sulcus
  - ◆ Aggravation of pain when tragus is pressed lightly over the external auditory meatus
  - ◆ Trismus
  - ◆ Discharge in the EAC
  - ◆ Tympanic membrane may not be seen due to tenderness of the pinna or occlusion of EAC due to oedema. If seen, it is usually normal.
  - ◆ Tuning fork tests reveal normal hearing.
  - ◆ Localized lymphadenitis is present occasionally.

Causative organisms

- Furunculosis is due to infection by *Staphylococcus aureus*.
- Generalized otitis externa is due to staphylococcus, streptococcus or gram negative bacilli.

Differential diagnosis

- Acute suppurative otitis media (ASOM) with acute mastoiditis (AM) (Table 8.2).
- Wax: Brownish or Blackish mass is seen filling the entire EAC.
- Otomycosis: It is characterized by itchness in ear. Cotton-like growth or wet newspaper-like mass is seen in the EAC.
- Keratosis obturans: Blackish mass with debris and granulations is seen in the EAC with very intense pain. Tympanic membrane is normal. Associated usually with chronic sinusitis and bronchiectasis.
- Referred causes of otalgia: External ear is normal in this condition.

Management

- Curative treatment
  - *Local treatment*
    - 10% glycerine ichthammol eardrops over a light ear-pack (wick) dipped in the same solution and placed in the EAC. Glycerine is hygroscopic and hence reduces oedema. Ichthammol is antiseptic. A wick helps to keep the solution in contact with the affected part continuously and splints the cartilagenous EAC. Also, in case of furuncle, the oedema and pain subside due to softening and rupture of the furuncle.
    - Magnesium sulphate and glycerine dipped ear-packs may also be used in severe cases for their hygroscopic property.

- Magnesium sulphate soaked gauze pieces are placed over the pinna for rapid relief from oedema and pain.
- Antibiotic eardrops may be used. Use of steroids in the form of eardrops should be done with caution and only under cover of systemic antibiotics provided the patient is not diabetic. Usually, response to antibiotic eardrops is good.
- All secretions and debris in the EAC are removed.
- If furuncle is present, careful incision and drainage is done under strict aseptic conditions taking care not to damage the underlying cartilage as this can result in perichondritis.
- *Systemic treatment*
  - *Antibiotics:* Oral or intravenous antibiotics are used depending on the severity. Injection ampicillin (250 mg) IV six hourly with injection cloxacillin (250 mg) IV six hourly in severe cases. If discharge is present it may be sent for culture and antibiotic sensitivity.
  - *Anti-inflammatory analgesics:* Anti-inflammatory analgesics are given to relieve pain and oedema.
  - If diabetes is present, the patient's blood sugar is kept within normal range using insulin subcutaneously.
- Preventive management
  - *Regular aural toilet:* Ear should be kept dry at all times.
  - *Prompt drying of ears:* If water has entered into the ears accidentally, e.g. while bathing or swimming.
  - Bathing with cotton plugs in EAC
  - Swimming with ear plugs
  - Avoid putting hair-pin or pencils into the ear for scratching

TABLE 8.2: Difference between acute otitis externa and acute suppurative otitis media with acute mastoiditis

	AOE	ASOM with AM
• History	Scratching, trauma, swimming	Upper respiratory tract infection (URTI)
• Otalgia	More severe	Less severe
• Deafness	Absent or mild blocking sensation	Present
• Otorrhoea	Scanty — if present, serous or purulent	Profuse if present seromucinous
• Tinnitus	Absent	Present (bubbling sound)
• Tenderness	Over the pinna and tragus. Aggravated on pressing tragus lightly over EAM	Over mastoid antrum. Absent on movement of tragus/pinna
• Displacent of pinna	Forwards	Downwards, outwards, and forwards
• Postauricular groove	May be obliterated	Deepened
• External auditory canal	Oedematous and congested in entire extent	Normal or oedema in deep bony portion
• Postaural lymphadenitis	May be present	Absent
• X-ray mastoid-Schuller's view	Normal	Haziness or destruction of mastoid air cells in acute mastoiditis

♦ Keep nails clean and avoid scratching ears.

♦ Keeping diabetes under control, if patient is diabetic.

Erysipelas: It usually occurs following a scratch. It is an acute streptococcal infection characterised by lymphangitis and dermatitis. It spreads rapidly.

• Treatment: It responds to the same systemic and local therapy given in acute otitis externa.

Otomycosis: It is the fungal infection of the external ear accompanied by itching and pain.

Aetiology

• **Humidity and moisture:** Water entering the ear during bathing or swimming may carry the fungus into the ear. Also, this infection is seen to occur commonly in the rainy seasons. The fungus grows on the skin of the EAC (sometimes under the epidermis).

• Prolonged use of antibiotic eardrops predisposes to fungal infection.

• Common in diabetics.

• Common in immunocompromised individuals due to immunodeficiency as a result of either disease or poor socioeconomic status.

Causative organisms

• *Aspergillus niger:* The commonest organism in tropical countries.

• *Candida albicans:* It is common in western countries.

• Monilial and other fungal infections are rare.

Clinical features

• Symptoms

♦ *Irritation and itchness* in the EAC initially.

♦ *Pain:* Usually very severe and unbearable.

♦ *Blocking* of the ear.

♦ *Otorrhoea:* Brownish or blackish scanty discharge.

♦ *Tinnitus* may be present.

♦ *Trismus:* Since the pain is aggravated on jaw movement.

• Signs

♦ Tenderness on lightly pressing the tragus over the external auditory meatus.

♦ Cotton-like whitish growth with black spots (sporangia) or wet-newspaper-like mass is seen in the EAC. Sometimes, completely blocking it.

♦ If secondary infection has occurred, there will be associated fever and malaise.

Treatment: (1) Local and (2) systemic treatment

• Local treatment

♦ *Aural toilet:* Removal of the fungal mass from the EAC by aural suction under microscope followed by application of boric spirit locally.

• 2% salicylic acid[†] in alcohol eardrops 3–4 times daily for 7 days.

• 1% clotrimazole[‡] and tolnaflate eardrops.

• 2% acetic acid eardrops.

• Amphoterecin B eardrops.

• 3% gentian violet eardrops.

• Nystatin eardrops.

• Neomycin and bacitracin eardrops.

• Systemic treatment

♦ *Antibiotics:* To control secondary infection.

♦ *Anti-inflammatory analgesics:* To relieve the pain and inflammation.

♦ *Antihistaminics:* To relieve the itching.

Herpes simplex: Similar to herpes simplex infections elsewhere in the body.

Herpes zoster: It is characterized by serous-fluid filled vesicles in the EAC associated with pain, facial nerve paralysis or involvement of other cranial nerves (the Ramsay-Hunt syndrome, affection of the geniculate ganglion by *Herpes zoster* virus).

Bullous myringitis: Usually followed by influenza and is characterised by severe otalgia and haemorrhagic (bluish) vesicles on the external surface of the eardrum. There is mild conductive deafness and serosanguinous otorrhoea.

Treatment for herpes simplex, herpes zoster and bullous myringitis, which are all caused by a neurotropic virus is as follows:

• Analgesics: To relieve the pain.

• Antibiotics: To control secondary infection.

• Vit. $B_1 B_6 B_{12}$.

• Antiviral agents like acyclovir.

Eczematous otitis externa: It is the sensitization of the skin to a local irritant. It is a form of allergic dermatitis.

Aetiology

• Misuse of local antibiotic eardrops like neomycin, etc.

• Secondary to spread of eczema from cheek.

Clinical features

• Itchiness and irritation of EAC.

---

[*]Aural toilet regularly is of utmost importance in prevention of a recurrence.

[†]2% salicylic acid eardrops are used most commonly. They help by killing the fungus and causing desquamation of the superficial layer of the skin, hence enabling the drops to reach the deep layer of the skin, which harbours the fungus.

[‡]Clotrimazole is a broad spectrum antimycotic and gives good results.

- Oedema, redness, weeping eczema and crusting in the EAC.
- Secondary infection.
- Scaling and fissuring of the external auditory meatus.
- Fibrosis and stenosis of the EAC.

Treatment
- The irritant should be removed.
- Antibiotic cream with steroid is applied locally, 2–3 times a day.
- Antihistaminics orally.
- 10% silver nitrate may be applied.
- Calamine lotion locally.

Seborrhoeic otitis externa: It is a condition characterised by scaling and crusting of the skin of the external auditory canal.

Usually associated with seborrhoeic dermatitis of the scalp.

Clinical features
- Itchiness and irritation in the external auditory canal.
- Greasy, scaly skin with crusting in the external auditory canal.
- Secondary infection usually follows.

Treatment
- **Aural toilet:** Regular cleaning of the EAC with removal of crusts.
- Steroid with antibiotic ointment or eardrops 3–4 times a day for 7 days.
- A wick impregnated with sulphur salicylic ointment in the ear.
- Care of the scalp by regular shampooing twice or thrice a week with an antidandruff shampoo.
- Vit. B_1 B_6 and B_{12} orally.

Malignant otitis externa: It is a fulminant necrotising infection of the external ear which progresses to involve the entire temporal bone, base skull and cranial nerves.

The name 'malignant' is a misnomer, as it is not a neoplasm. However, this term has been used to describe the basic fulminant nature of this infection.

Aetiology: It is commonly seen in elderly diabetics.

Causative organism: Bacillus pyocyaneous

Clinical features
- Pain
- Otorrhoea—blood stained
- Deafness—progressive
- External ear is full of granulation tissue, which shows evidence of necrosis and slough with foul smell.

- Involvement of facial, glossopharyngeal, vagus and hypoglossal cranial nerves may occur.
- Headache
- Vertigo
- Intracranial complications like meningitis, cerebral abscess, etc.
- The course of this disease is rapidly progressive and may be fatal.

Treatment
- Control of diabetes with injection insulin.
- Wide debridement of all necrotic and granulation tissue.
- Local application of gentamicin or any antibiotic eardrops.
- Systemic antibiotics based on sensitivity of organisms as detected from biopsy of the granulation tissue.

Neurodermatitis: It is common in individuals suffering from psychological disorders caused by compulsive scratching of the EAC with finger-nails, hair pins, etc. Itching is the predominant symptom. There may be a secondary infection. Treatment comprises of psychotherapy and antibiotics for secondary infection. Sometimes, a ear bandage is given to prevent compulsive scratching.

TRAUMATIC CONDITIONS

Trauma to the external ear may involve either the pinna or EAC or both.

Minor accidental trauma such as cuts or lacerations of the pinna are treated with cleaning the wound using sterile water or saline on sterile cotton under strict aseptic conditions as infection of the exposed cartilage can cause severe deformity. Skin edges are approximated and sutured over exposed cartilage taking care not to go through cartilage.

In case of severe trauma, such as vehicular accidents, etc., a CT scan is mandatory to rule out injury to skull bones or brain tissue. These, if present, are treated on a priority basis. Associated tear of pinna is sutured after careful cleaning of wound. Lacerations in the EAC are allowed to heal by secondary intention and a wick soaked in antibiotic ointment is placed in the EAC, which is changed every 2–3 days. Associated fractures of the temporal bone with facial nerve palsy are treated by decompression of the nerve during a mastoidectomy. CSF leaks too are sealed with muscle or connective tissue by a mastoidectomy.

NEOPLASTIC CONDITIONS

Neoplasms rarely affect the external ear. A broad classification is presented in Flowchart 8.1.

Exostosis
- Synonym: Osseous external canal tumours.
- Definition: It is a benign bony outgrowth from the EAC projecting into the lumen and covered by skin. It arises only from the bony EAC.
- Aetiology: Not known, but seen commonly in swimmers or surfers or in those bathing in cold water.
- Classification
  - Single (osteoma) or multiple (exostosis).
  - Sessile (usually multiple) or pedunculated (solitary osteoma).
- Clinical features
  - Usually asymptomatic.
  - If very large, it may cause mild deafness and accumulation of wax in the EAC.
- Treatment
  - If asymptomatic, no treatment is required.
  - If symptomatic, surgical removal using an electric drill is required, taking care not to damage the facial nerve.

Sebaceous adenoma
- It is a benign tumour of the sebaceous glands of the skin, lining the EAC.
- It is a smooth painless swelling covered by skin.
- Treatment: Local excision surgically.

Ceruminoma (Hydradenoma)
- It is a benign tumour of the ceruminous glands of the skin, lining the EAC. It is firm, smooth, and painless and covered by skin. It may undergo malignant change.
- Treatment: Wide excision, as it has a tendency to recur and undergo malignant change.

Squamous cell carcinoma
- It can occur on the pinna or EAC, but it is more commonly seen to affect the EAC primarily.
- It is commonly seen in ears with long-standing chronic otorrhoea.
- It spreads rapidly to involve the middle ear, temporal bone, base skull, and cranial nerves.
- Clinical features
  - Elderly patient with blood stained, foul smelling otorrhoea.
  - Severe otalgia.
  - Headache.
  - Bleeding polyp or granulation tissue in the EAC.
  - Deafness.
  - Regional lymphnode enlargement.
  - Facial nerve palsy.
  - *Treatment*: Wide excision with postoperative radiotherapy.

MISCELLANEOUS CONDITIONS

Keratosis obturans
- Definition: It is a condition in which the EAC is filled up with a firm mass consisting of desquamated keratinised epithelium, wax and cholesterol. This can cause erosion and widening of the bony canal.
- Aetiology: Exact cause is unknown, but could be due to improper movement of wax in the EAC.

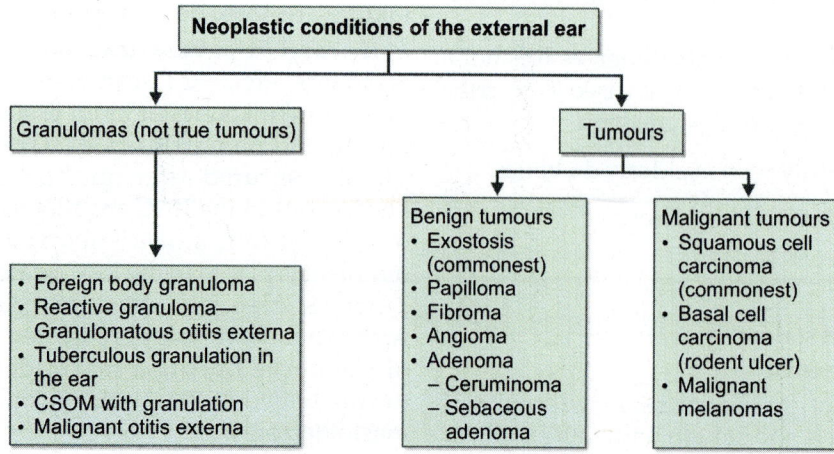

Flowchart 8.1: Neoplastic conditions of the external ear

- **Clinical features**
  - Pain
  - Deafness
  - Granulation tissue may be seen occluding the EAC
  - Chronic sinusitis and bronchiaetesis are associated features in some cases.
- **Treatment**
  - Removal of the mass under general anaesthesia as it is very painful.
  - Regular wax clearance to prevent recurrence.

Wax (Cerumen) Wax is the natural secretion of cerumenous and pilosebaceous glands situated in the skin of the cartilagenous part of the EAC. The relative proportion of their secretions determines the consistency of the wax. Wax is brown in colour, which is due to the oxidative process affecting it. The wax is expelled out by the movement of the jaw while eating and talking. The functions of wax are:

- Antibacterial action
- Self-cleansing action thereby cleaning the dust and debris present in EAC.

The secretions of ceruminous and sebaceous glands get mixed with desquamated epithelium (debris) of the EAC and may solidify to become hard and impacted.

Causes of excessive wax accumulation (impaction)
- Excessive formation of wax or desquamation of surface epithelium in the EAC
- Less oily secretion
- Stiff hairs in the EAC
- Exostosis or stenosis of EAC

- Dusty occupation–miners, etc
- Dry hot climate.

Clinical features
- Blocking of the ear with itching.
- Impacted wax leads to mild deafness (conductive type) and earache, which may be associated with tinnitus.
- On examination of ear, brownish mass filling the EAC is seen.

Treatment
- Removal of wax by wax hook or syringing
- If the wax is hard, wax softening agents are given.
- 5% sodium-bicarbonate eardrops.
- Oil, which is heated and cooled to sterilise.

For maximum action of wax softening agent, space is created between wax and EAC by a wax hook and after putting wax softening agents, the ear is kept up for 3–4 minutes. The ear is syringed after putting them 3–4 times per day for 3–4 days.

Syringing: Patient is in sitting position with head turned to opposite side, a towel is kept on the shoulder of the patient and an attendant holds a kidney tray below the ear (Fig. 8.1).
- The aural syringe is filled with boiled water which is cooled to room temperature, so that the labyrinth does not get stimulated leading to giddiness. There should be no air in the aural syringe.
- The nossel of the aural syringe is introduced in the EAC directed towards the posterosuperior canal wall. Constant and moderate force is used for syringing. The returning water and wax is collected in the kidney tray.

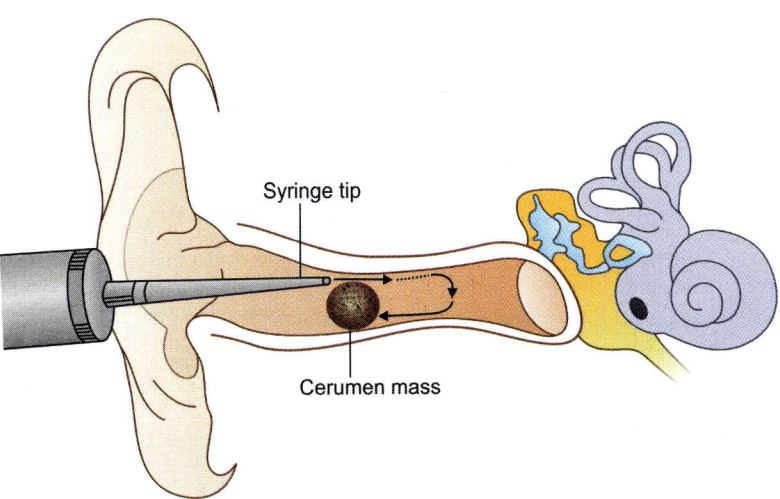

Fig. 8.1: Diagram showing aural syringing

- The ear is cleaned first with a dry cotton swab and then boric spirit is applied in the EAC. Patient is given 2% boric spirit eardrops to clean the external auditory canal and antibiotics if the tympanic membrane is congested. This prevents fungal infection due to moisture in the EAC.

Foreign bodies in the external auditory canal Foreign bodies in the external auditory canal commonly occur in children.

Flowchart 8.2: Classification of foreign bodies

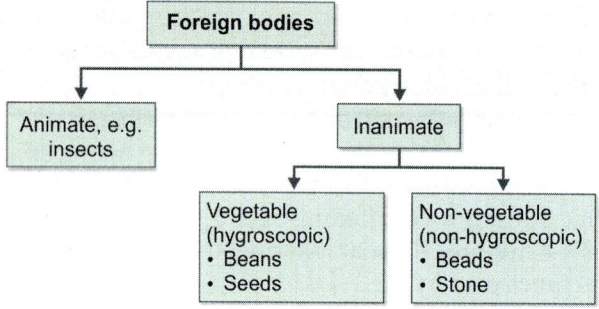

- **Classification**
  - *Animate:* Insects, flies, maggots, etc.
  - *Inanimate*
    - *Vegetable (Hygroscopic):* Beans, seeds, nuts, etc.
    - *Non-vegetable (Non-hygroscopic):* Beads, stones, pebbles, rubber, metallic, etc.
  - *Clinical features*
    - History of foreign body entering the ear.
    - Pain and deafness: The vegetable foreign body may swell up leading to earache and impaction.
    - Tinnitus: In case of animate, foreign-bodies due to their movement.
  - *Treatment*
    - Inanimate foreign bodies are removed by using a foreign body hook or vectis. It is passed gently behind the foreign body in the superior aspect of EAC and the foreign body is pulled out under vision to prevent tympanic membrane perforation (Fig. 8.2).
    - Non-vegetable foreign bodies are removed by syringing.

- In uncooperative children, it is preferable to remove foreign bodies under general anaesthesia to prevent damage to the ear.
- In case of animate foreign bodies, the insect is first killed by instilling sodium bicarbonate eardrops or warm oil and then removed.
- The EAC is cleaned with spirit and antibiotics are given if required.
- Vegetable or hygroscopic foreign bodies are *never* syringed as they tend to absorb water, swell and become impacted. They are removed with a vectis or wax-hook.
- *Complications*
  - Otitis externa
  - Perforation of tympanic membrane due to instrumentation
  - Foreign body may go into the middle ear leading to deafness and otitis media
  - Foreign body granuloma
  - Tetanus

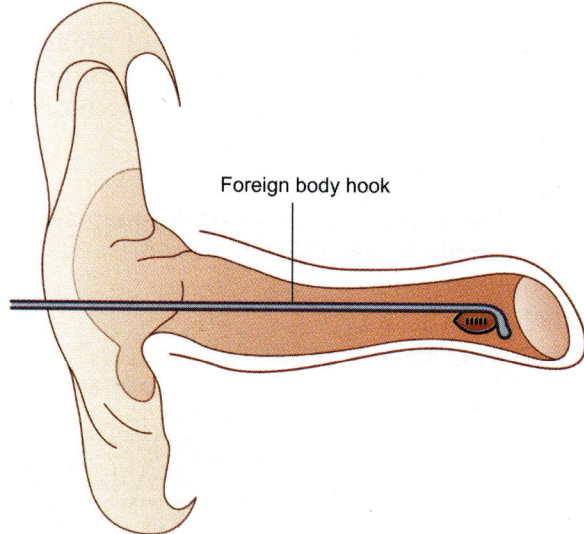

Fig. 8.2: Diagram showing the use of a foreign body hook for removal of aural foreign body

Ear

CHAPTER 9

Acute Suppurative Otitis Media and Mastoiditis

ACUTE SUPPURATIVE OTITIS MEDIA (ASOM)

DEFINITION

It is the acute infection of the mucosa of the middle ear cleft by pyogenic organisms.

AETIOLOGY

- **Age:** More common in children because the Eustachian tube is shorter, wider and more horizontal.
- **Commonly bilateral**, can be unilateral occasionally.
- **Sex:** Male : Female = 1 : 1.
- **Adenoids** blocking the Eustachian tube opening.
- Obstruction to Eustachian tube opening by nasopharyngeal tumours, e.g. carcinoma.
- Cleft palate.
- Rhinitis, sinusitis and pharyngitis.
- Forceful blowing of nose or performing the valsalva manoeuvre in presence of rhinitis may force infection into Eustachian tube.
- Swimming
- Deep sea diving may cause barotrauma and ASOM.
- Flying in an unpressurised aircraft or flying in the presence of rhinitis can cause ASOM.
- Infants fed in supine position, may develop ASOM due to milk entering the Eustachian tube as, in them the Eustachian tube is horizontal, wider and shorter. (More common in bottle fed infants).
- Iatrogenic scarring of Eustachian tube orifice after operations on the nasopharynx like adenoidectomy

or removal of angiofibroma during which Eustachian tube orifice is damaged. If a patient is asked to perform the valsalva manoeuvre in presence of rhinitis, pharyngitis or tonsillitis infection may go into the Eustachian tube from the nasopharynx. Hence, valsalva should never be performed in presence of infection.

Causative organisms
- *Haemophilus influenzae*
- *Staphylococcus aureus*
- *Streptococcus haemolyticus*
- *Pneumococcus*

STAGES

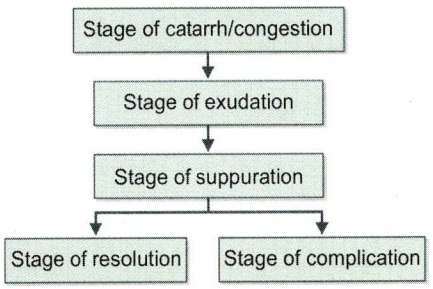

Stage of catarrh/congestion
↓
Stage of exudation
↓
Stage of suppuration
↓ ↓
Stage of resolution   Stage of complication

Stage of congestion/catarrh Obstruction of Eustachian tube → absorption of oxygen in middle ear cleft, increase in CO_2 content → irritation of middle ear mucosa → congestion in the middle ear.

55

Stage of exudation If occlusion persists, it will lead to exudation from capillaries in the middle ear (ME) due to congestion of the mucosa → collection of seromucinous exudate in middle ear eardrum budges laterally.

Stage of suppuration Seromucinous exudate accumulates in the ME and becomes mucopurulent. Tension in the ME increases and the eardrum perforates due to pressure necrosis. The exudate under pressure escapes into the EAC.

Stage of resolution/healing Infection starts resolving depending on:
- Immunity of host
- Virulence of organisms
- Efficacy of antibiotics. Usually there are no sequelae.

Stage of complications Infection from the ME, if untreated or if immunity of host is low or virulence of organism is high, spreads to the mastoid antrum, acute / catarrhal mastoiditis coalescent mastoiditis (empyma of the mastoid). Incidence and severity of complications are higher in pneumatized mastoids as compared to sclerotic mastoid.

CLINICAL FEATURES

Stage of congestion/catarrhal stage See Table 9.1 and Figs 9.1 and 9.2.

TABLE 9.1: Symptoms and signs in the stage of congestion/catarrhal stage	
Symptoms	*Signs*
• Blocking of ear/fullness of ear.	• Congestion of eardrum ('cart-wheel' appearance)
• Pain—severe and continous, more during sleep due to venous congestion in recumbent position	• Loss of light reflex
• Tinnitus—bubbling sounds are heard.	• Retraction of eardrum
• Deafness may not be noticed by patient due to the pain, but it progressively increases	
• Autophony—patient's words echo in his own ears	
• Fever and malaise	

Stage of exudation See Table 9.2 and Fig. 9.3.

TABLE 9.2: Symptoms and signs in the stage of exudation	
Symptoms	*Signs*
• Pain–worsens	• Congestion of eardrum
• Severe blocking of ear	• Bulging of eardrum
• Tinnitus is present	• Pressure point is seen as a yellow nipple at one spot on the eardrum
• Deafness progresses	• Tenderness of the suprameatal triangle (mastoidism)
• Fever and malaise (symptoms of toxaemia)	

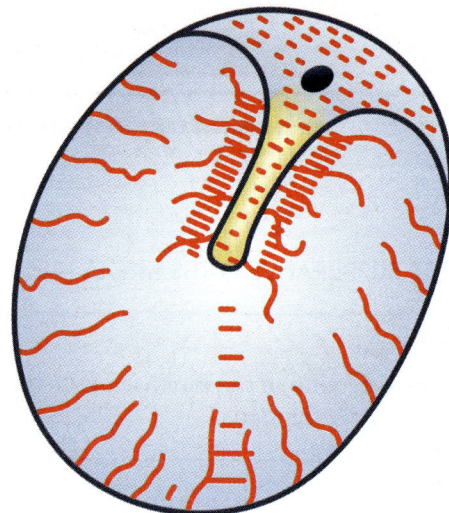

Fig. 9.1: ASOM in the catarrhal stage showing the characteristic 'cart-wheel' appearance due to congested blood vessels running radially

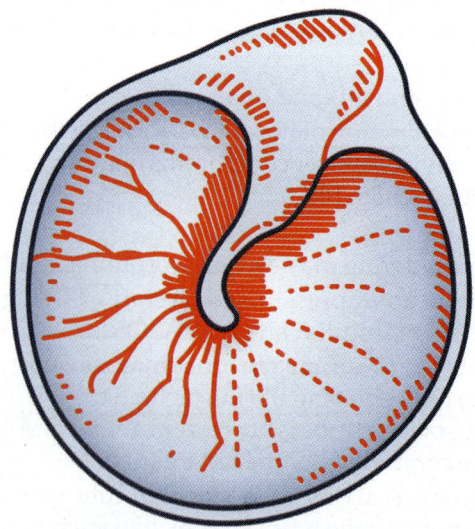

Fig. 9.2: Stage of congestion

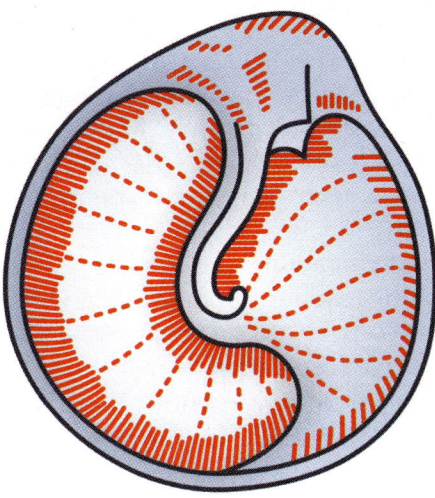

Fig. 9.3: Stage of exudation

Stage of suppuration   *See* Table 9.3 and Fig. 9.4.

TABLE 9.3: Symptoms and signs in the stage of suppuration	
Symptoms	*Signs*
• Otorrhoea: Mucopuru-lent and occasionally bloodstained	• Small perforation in antero-inferior quadrant of eardrum with pulsatile discharge which is mucopurulent (Lighthouse sign)
• Pain reduces	• Congestion of eardrum
• Fever and malaise reduce	• Mild conductive hearing loss
• Deafness	
• Tinnitus	

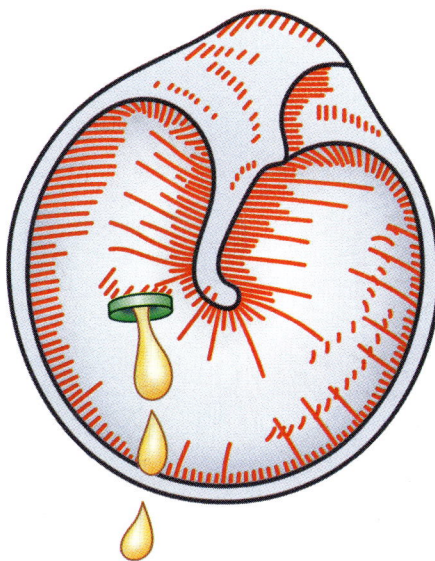

Fig. 9.4: Stage of suppuration

Stage of resolution/healing   Healing can begin after any stage. If it occurs after suppuration, a small scar may be seen in the anteroinferior quadrant of the eardrum.

Stage of complications   Extracranial and intracranial complications are shown in Table 9.4.

TABLE 9.4: Extracranial and Intracranial complications	
Extracranial	*Intracranial*
• Mastoiditis	• Meningitis
• Subperiosteal mastoid abscess	• Extradural abscess
• Subcutaneous mastoid abscess	• Subdural abscess
• Mastoid fistula	• Brain abscess
• Bezold's abscess	• Sigmoid sinus thrombosis
• Luc's abscess	• Otitic hydrocephalus
• Zygomatic abscess	
• Citelli's abscess	
• Petrositis	
• Facial nerve palsy	
• Labyrinthitis	

DIFFERENTIAL DIAGNOSIS

- Acute otitis externa.
- All causes of otalgia.
- Excessive crying in children can result in congestion of eardrum but as there is absence of oedema, light reflex is present.

INVESTIGATIONS

- Tuning fork tests show mild conductive hearing loss.
- Pure tone audiometry is usually not possible due to severe pain, but, if pain is less severe, it will reveal mild conductive hearing loss unless labyrinthitis has occurred, when it will show sensorineural hearing loss.
- X-ray mastoid Schuller's view is normal unless a complication such as mastoiditis has occurred, when the mastoid air cells show a haziness or ground-glass appearance or even absence of intercellular septae (coalescent mastoiditis).
- Culture and antibiotic sensitivity of the ear discharge is done.

TREATMENT

Aims of treatment

- To give symptomatic relief.
- To control and eradicate middle ear infection.
- To ensure Eustachian tube patency for ventilation of middle ear cleft.

Flowchart 9.1: Treatment of ASOM

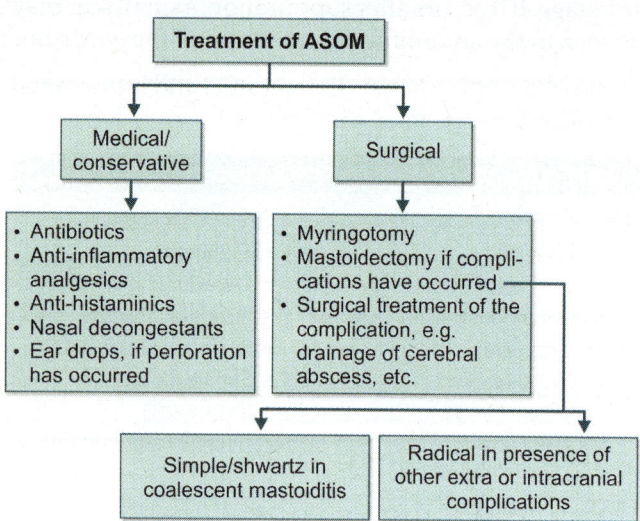

- To ensure drainage of middle ear cleft and return of auditory function.

Medical treatment
- Systemic antibiotics.
- Systemic antihistaminics.
- Antiinflammatory analgesics.
- Nasal decongestants.
- Local antibiotic eardrops in the presence of perforation.

Surgical treatment
- **Myringotomy:** An incision is made on the tympanic membrane to enable drainage and ventilation of the middle ear cleft (Fig. 9.5a, b, c).

- **Indications**
  - Stage of exudation in ASOM.
  - ASOM with a very small perforation in the stage of suppuration, where the ME discharge is not adequately draining.
  - ASOM with impending intracranial complications.
  - Haemotympanum
  - SOM, this requires a grommet along with myringotomy, if conservative management fails.
- **Preoperative preparation**
  - Written informed consent.
  - Injection atropine 0.6 mg intramuscular (IM) half hour pre-operatively.
  - Injection TT 0.5 cc IM preoperatively.
- **Anaesthesia:** In this condition, local anaesthesia does not act, as it is an acute inflammation. Hence, myringotomy in ASOM in always performed under general anaesthesia. In SOM, it can be performed under local anaesthesia if the patient is cooperative.
- **Procedure:** Patient lies supine with head turned to the opposite side. The surgeon operates using an operating microscope. Using an aural speculum, to visualise the eardrum a 'J' shaped incision is made in the posteroinferior quadrant of the eardrum, midway between the annulus and umbo using a microsurgery sickle knife. This 'J' shaped incision cuts the radial fibres of the eardrum and hence, heals slowly. This helps in adequate drainage.

  In SOM, a radial inscision is made in the antero-inferior quadrant of the eardrum and a grommet

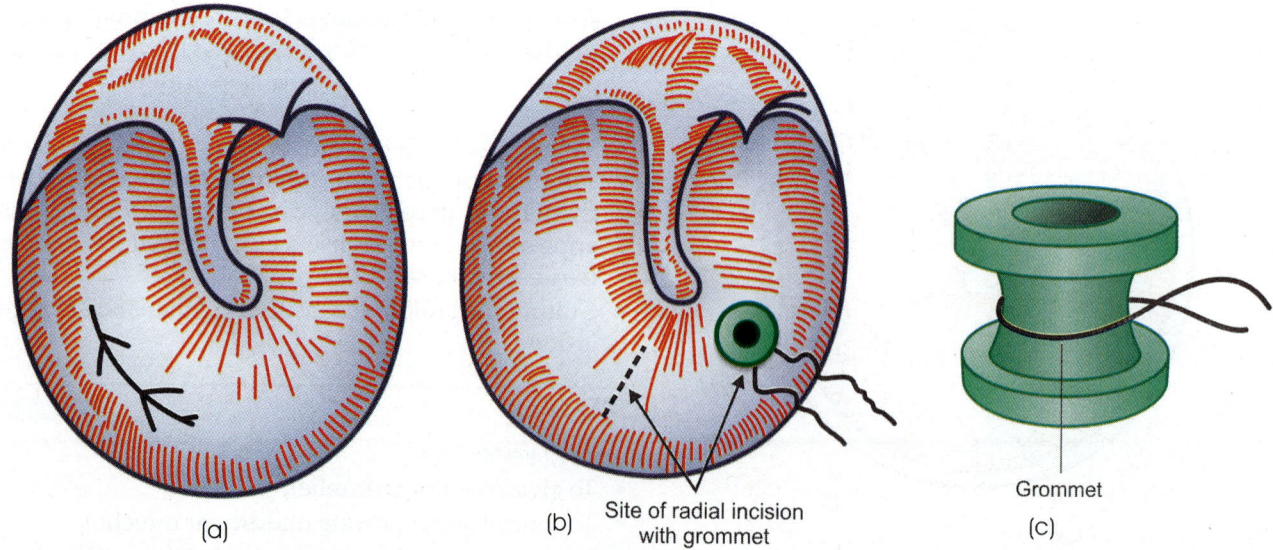

Fig. 9.5: Myringotomy—(a) site of J-shaped incision in ASOM; (b) site of radial incision with grommet in SOM; (c) grommet

(ventilation tube) is inserted as prolonged drainage is required.

- Postoperative care
  - A sterile cottonplug is placed in the EAC at all times
  - Antibiotics–systemic and local
  - Anti-inflammatory analgesics
  - Nasal decongestants.

SEQUELAE OF ASOM

- Deafness: Conductive deafness may persist due to failure of resolution of effusion.
  Sensorineural deafness may occur due to damage to the inner ear by toxins in the effusion fluid, which may permeate through the round window membrane.
- Perforation: The perforation from the stage of suppuration may persist due to Eustachian tube pathology.
- Persistence of Eustachian tube pathology and inadequate treatment may result in atelectasis at a later date.
- Healing of the perforation may occur with scarring of the eardrum or tympanosclerosis resulting in a conductive hearing loss.

COMPLICATIONS OF ASOM

- Acute mastoiditis due to spread of infection to the mastoid air cell system.
- Sensorineural hearing loss due to inner ear damage.
- Facial nerve paralysis.
- Intracranial complications like meningitis or brain abscess.
- Coalescent mastoiditis.
- Perisinus abscess and lateral sinus thrombosis.

MASTOIDITIS

Definition   Infection of the mucoperiosteal lining of the mastoid air cell system.

Classification

1. • Acute/Catarrhal   2. • Coalescent
   • Chronic   • Masked

Aetiology

- Acute mastoiditis occurs as a sequel to acute suppurative otitis media, if:
  - Organisms causing ASOM are very virulent.
  - Resistance of the individual is lowered.
  - Improper or inadequate antibiotics are administered for ASOM.

- The mastoid is very cellular in a case of ASOM.
- Drainage of the exudate in ASOM through the perforation is poor.
- Infection affects mastoid air cell system before the tympanic membrane perforates.

- Chronic mastoititis is seen in CSOM, where the mastoid process is sclerotic. Seen commonly in unsafe CSOM, where cholesteatoma or granulations erode the bone and the mastoid is filled with cholesteatoma and granulations. Sometimes, safe CSOM may give rise to granulations in the mastoid and chronic mastoiditis.

- Coalescent mastoiditis occurs as a sequel of acute mastoiditis, when granulations and oedema block the aditus to the antrum and pus collects in the mastoid air cells under pressure resulting in breakdown of the septae between the air cells. The entire mastoid is filled with pus as the air cells coalesce (empyma of the mastoid).

- Masked mastoiditis occurs, if inadequate or improper antibiotics are used in a case of acute mastoiditis. Here, the classical acute signs and symptoms are not seen (masked) and the patient develops complications which is the presenting feature.

Clinical features

- Acute mastoiditis: The symptoms and signs in acute mastoditis are shown in Table 9.5.

TABLE 9.5:	Symptoms and signs in acute mastoiditis
Symptoms	Signs
• Pain in the region of the ear	• Tenderness over the mastoid.
• Fever	• Febrile patient.
• Malaise	• Redness and increase in local temperature over the mastoid.
• Otorrhoea	• X-ray mastoid shows haziness but intact air cells.
• Deafness	

- Chronic mastoiditis: The symptoms and signs in chronic mastoiditis are shown in Table 9.6.

TABLE 9.6:	Symptoms and signs in chronic mastoiditis
Symptoms	Signs
• Otorrhoea	• Radiological examination of the mastoid shows a sclerotic mastoid which may show a radiolucent area due to bone erosion by granulations/cholestealoma.
• Deafness	
• No fever/pain	

- **Coalescent mastoiditis:** The symptoms and signs in coalescent mastoiditis are as given in Table 9.7 and represented in Fig. 9.6.
- **Masked mastoiditis:** This is a retrospective diagnosis, as the patient presents with serious complications and history of otalgia or headache for which inadequate treatment was taken in the recent past, is elicited.

Complications   Mastoiditis can result in any of the intracranial or extracranial complications of otitis media.

Management
- Diagnosis is based on history, clinical features, and radiological investigations.

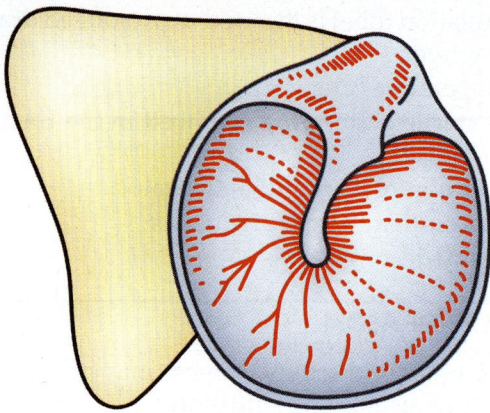

Fig. 9.6: Coalescent mastoiditis

TABLE 9.7:	Symptoms and signs occurred in chronic mastoiditis
Symptoms	*Signs*
• Severe throbbing continuous pain	• Mastoid tenderness.
• Otorrhoea	• Local increase in temperature.
• Deafness	• 'Reservoir sign' positive. i.e. the EAC continues to fill with discharge immediately on cleaning. This is due to collection of pus in the mastoid antrum, which overflows into the EAC.
	• Oedema of EAC with sagging of posterosuperior wall.
	• X-ray of mastoid shows ground-glass haziness with absence of intercellular septae.

- Management in the absence of complications is conservative followed by a mastoidectomy to treat the cause.
  - Antibiotics–orally or intravenously
  - Anti-inflammatory analgesics
  - Antipyretics
  - Antibiotic eardrops if there is perforation, discharge.
- Acute mastoiditis or coalescent mastoiditis following ASOM is treated by a simple/schwartz/cortical mastoidectomy.
- Chronic mastoiditis will require a radical mastoidectomy.
- Masked mastoiditis will require management of the complication with a radical mastoidectomy to treat the cause.

Chronic Suppurative Otitis Media

DEFINITION

Chronic suppurative otitis media (CSOM) is defined as the chronic infection of the middle ear cleft by suppurative organisms (Fig. 10.1).

Flowchart 10.1: Classification of chronic otitis media

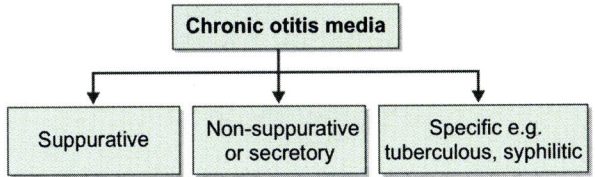

CLASSIFICATION

Based on aetiology
- Atticoantral (unsafe/dangerous)
- Tubotympanic (safe/benign)

Based on stage
- Active: Actively discharging ear.
- Inactive: Ear is dry for more than 6 months.
- Quiescent: Ear remains dry for a period upto 6 months.

AETIOLOGY

Safe CSOM   This includes central perforation in the pars tensa (Figs 10.2 and 10.3).

- Failure of complete resolution of acute suppurative otitis media (ASOM).
- Failure of traumatic perforation to heal.
- As a sequel of acute necrotizing otitis media.

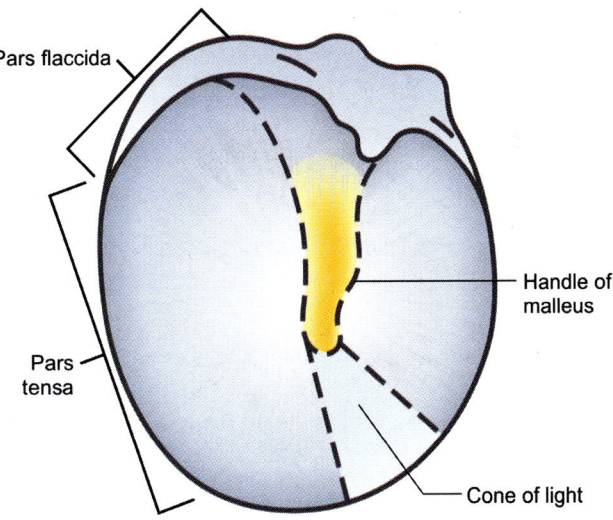

Fig. 10.1: Diagrammatic representation of a normal right tympanic membrane

Unsafe CSOM   This includes:
- Cholesteatoma (Fig. 10.4)
- Granulations
- Marginal/attic perforations (Figs 10.5 and 10.6)

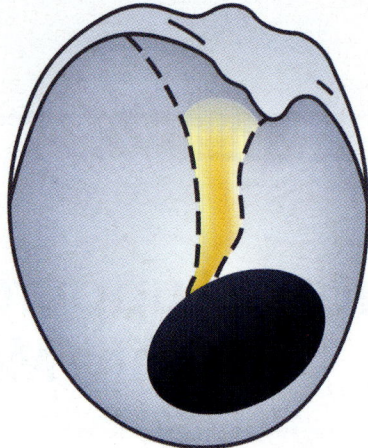

Fig. 10.2: Central perforation

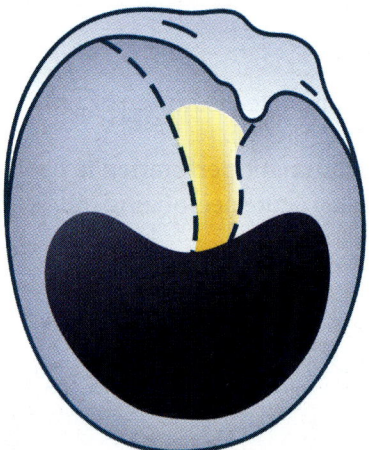

Fig. 10.3: Central perforation

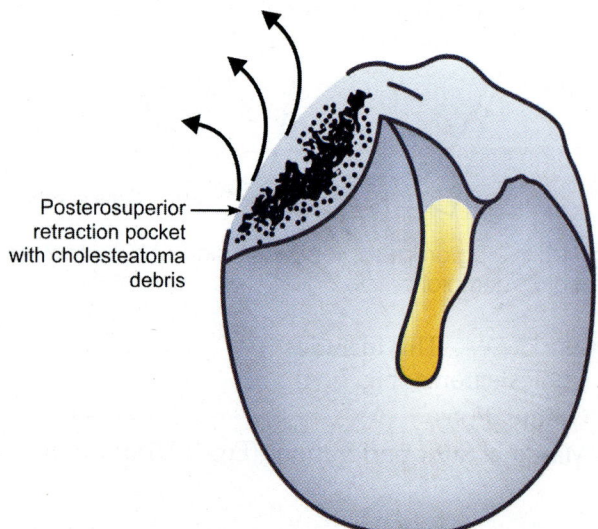

Posterosuperior retraction pocket with cholesteatoma debris

Fig. 10.4: Cholesteatoma

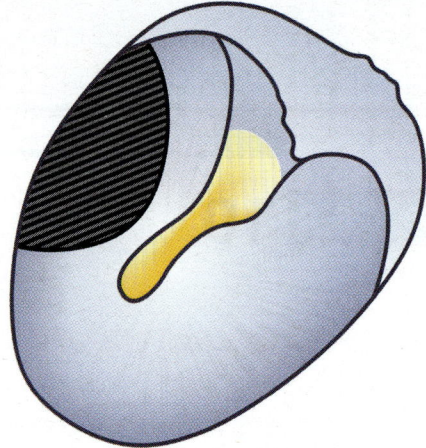

Fig. 10.5: Marginal perforation

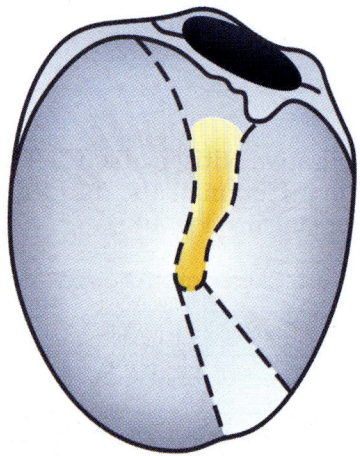

Fig. 10.6: Attic perforation

- **Cholesteatoma**

Flowchart 10.2: Classification of cholesteatoma

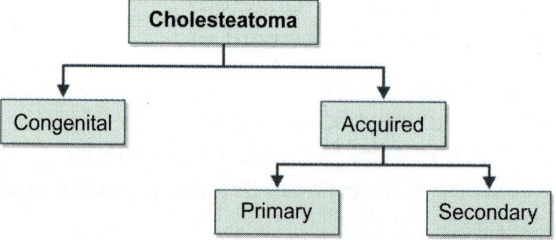

- *Congenital:* It occurs due to a sudden unexplained proliferation of dormant epithelial cell rests, caught in the suture lines of the temporal bone during embryological development.
- *Acquired*
  - *Primary:* Eustachian tube malfunction and poor aeration of middle ear by mastoid air cell system

(Fig. 10. 7) → retraction pocket formation in the pars flacidda (attic) or posterosuperior quadrant → inadequate clearance of desquamated epithelial debris → collection of debris and deepening of the pocket to form a sac with a broad fundus and narrow neck (Fig. 10.8).

- *Secondary:* There are two theories for secondary aquired cholesteratoma.
  - *Theory of immigration:* The outer layer of the eardrum, which is formed of stratified squamous epithelium migrates into the middle ear to form cholesteatoma. In the attic/pars flaccida, the irregular arrangement of the fibrous middle layer makes it more prone to formation of retraction pockets and cholesteatoma. In case of destruction of the fibrous annulus in the posterosuperior quadrant of the pars tensa due to disease or prior surgery, a cholesteatoma forms due to migration of squamous epithelium into the middle ear (Fig. 10.9).
  - *Theory of metaplasia:* Due to chronic infection of the middle ear, there is irritation to the mucosa, which may undergo a metaplastic change to squamous epithelium → formation of cholesteatoma (Fig. 10.10).

Organisms: Streptococci, staphylococci, pneumococci, *Esherichia coli*, B. proteus and anaerobes.

Pathogenesis of cholesteatoma: It is shown in Flowchart 10.3.

Black cholesteatoma—rarely seen: It is the black discolouration of cholesteatoma due to old haemorrhages within the sac.

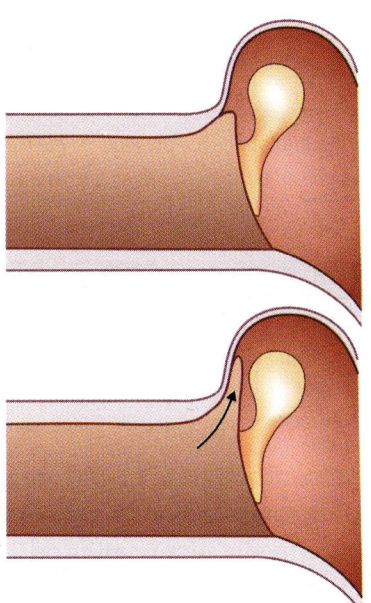

Fig. 10.7: Primary retraction pocket

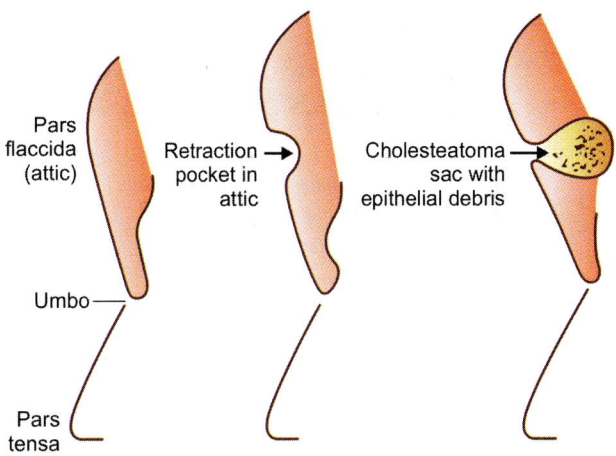

Fig. 10.8: Retraction pocket formation and epithelial debris

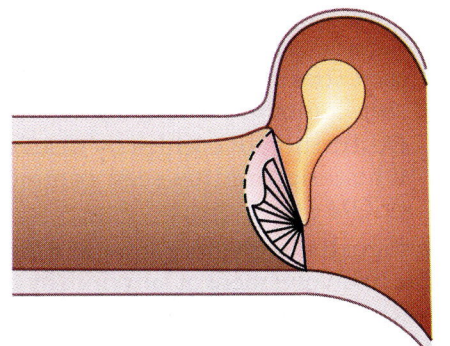
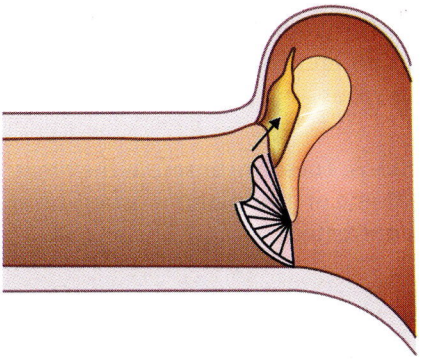

Fig. 10.9: Immigration of squamous epithelium

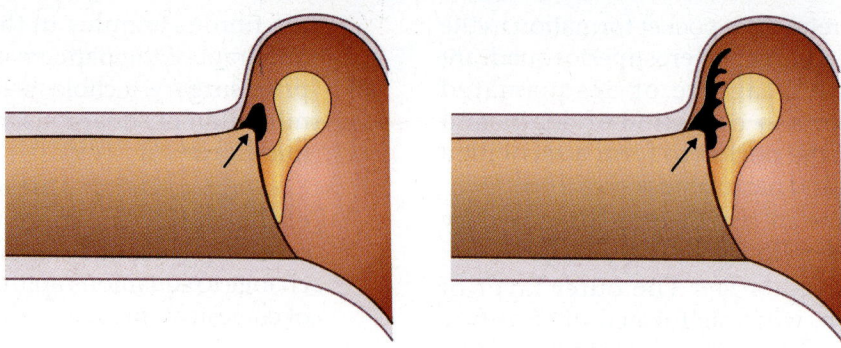

Fig. 10.10: Squamous metaplasia

Flowchart 10.3: Pathogenesis of cholesteatoma

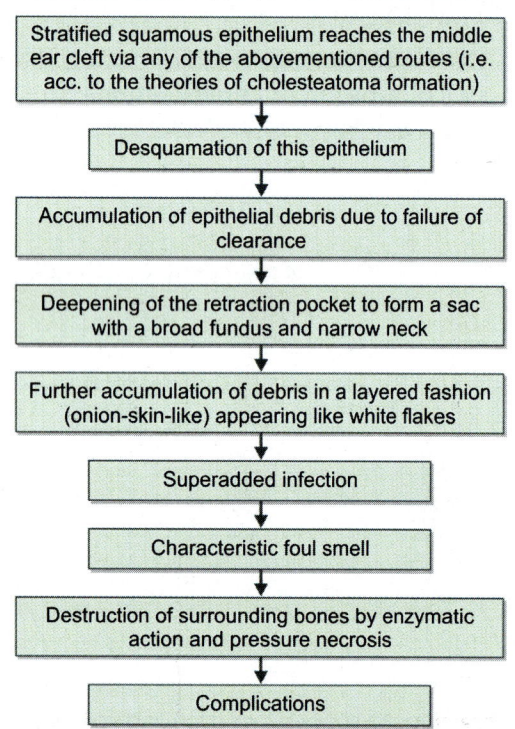

| | Stratified squamous epithelium reaches the middle ear cleft via any of the abovementioned routes (i.e. acc. to the theories of cholesteatoma formation) |
| Desquamation of this epithelium |
| Accumulation of epithelial debris due to failure of clearance |
| Deepening of the retraction pocket to form a sac with a broad fundus and narrow neck |
| Further accumulation of debris in a layered fashion (onion-skin-like) appearing like white flakes |
| Superadded infection |
| Characteristic foul smell |
| Destruction of surrounding bones by enzymatic action and pressure necrosis |
| Complications |

- **Granulations:** These occur in the mucosa of the middle ear cleft and are commonly associated with marginal perforations and chronic infection. These also destroy the surrounding bone and may result in complications.
- **Marginal perforations:** These are unsafe as they may result in cholesteatoma or granulation formation at a later date, if left untreated.

CLINICAL FEATURES

Symptoms
- Otorrhoea: *See* Table 10.1.

TABLE 10.1: Otorrhoea

Unsafe CSOM	*Safe CSOM*
• Scanty	• Profuse
• Foul smelling	• No foul smell
• Continuous	• Intermittent
• Purulent	• Mucopurulent
• Yellowish/brownish/greenish	• Yellowish/white
• Blood tinged if granulations are present	• Never blood tinged
• No change with URTI	• Increases with URTI

- **Deafness:** *See* Table 10.2

TABLE 10.2: Deafness

	Unsafe CSOM	*Safe CSOM*
Degree	Moderate to severe	Moderate
Type	Mixed or sensorineural common	Usually conductive Occasionally mixed

- **Otalgia:** Cause of otalgia in CSOM are as follows:
  - Impending complication in case of unsafe ear
  - Acute otitis media supervening on CSOM
  - Acute otitis externa
  - Malignant disease of ear
  - Malignant otitis externa.
- **Tinnitus:** It is caused due to:
  - Air from patent Eustachian tube bubbling through secretions in the hypotympanum bubbling tinnitus seen commonly in safe CSOM.
  - Destruction of cochlea by disease high pitched whistling tinnitus seen commonly in unsafe CSOM.
- **Vertigo:** It is seen more commonly in unsafe CSOM due to involvement of labyrinth by the disease.
  Rarely seen in safe CSOM, unless the round/oval windows are injured through the central perforation during cleaning of the ear or trauma to the ear, e.g. slap/fall on ear.

- **Postaural swelling:** It is common in unsafe CSOM due to abscess formation. Pinna is pushed outwards forwards and downwards.
- **Itchiness** in the ear due to chronic irritation of the EAC by the discharge or a superadded otomycosis.

Signs
- **Examination of the ear:** For the examination of ears in CSOM see Table 10.3.
- **Examination of the nose**
  - Rhinitis may be a feature in case of safe CSOM.
  - Deviated nasal septum may be present → ET dysfunction → CSOM (safe/unsafe).
- **Examination of the throat:** Children with CSOM usually have chronic tonsillitis, which may be the cause of repeated infections leading to the CSOM.

INVESTIGATIONS

Routine (for purpose of anaesthesia and to know general condition of the patient).
- Complete blood count.
- X-ray chest PA view.
- ECG and Blood sugar in all patients more than 35 years of age.

Specific
- **Otomicroscopy:** Examination of the ear under the magnification of a microscope with simultaneous cleaning using a suction to confirm the findings of clinical examination.
- **Pure tone audiometry:** To detect the exact degree and type of hearing loss.
  For purpose of documentation in case of mediolegal problem or for comparison of pre and postoperative improvement.
- **Swab of ear discharge** to be sent for culture of organisms and antibiotic sensitivity.
- **X-ray mastoids Schuller's view** to see
  - Whether mastoid is pneumatic/sclerotic.
  - Sinus plate, dural plate and sinodural angle.
  - Evidence of erosion of bone.
- **Eustachian tube patency:** It may be tested in a safe CSOM only in the absence of nose/throat infection by the valsalva manoeuvre in which the patient closes both nostrils and mouth with his fingers pinching the nose and gently attempts to breath out without opening nostrils and mouth. Air under pressure is pushed into the Eustachian tubes if they are patent and into the middle ear movement of the intact eardrum or the edges of perforation may show

TABLE 10.3: Examination of the ear in CSOM

	Unsafe	Safe
Postaural region	May show swelling	Normal
Preauricular region	May show swelling	Normal
Pinna	May be pushed outwards, forwards, and downwards	Normal
Mastoid tenderness	May be present	Absent
External auditory canal	May show eczematous changes due to constant irritation by the discharge	Discharge may be present in EAC
Tympanic membrane	• Marginal/Attic perforation • Cholesteatoma • Granulations with foul smell	Central perforation with discharge
Rinne test	Negative or Positive	Negative
Weber test	Lateralized to normal ear	Affected ear
ABC test	ABC decreased ⬇ Indicating Moderate to severe CHL or Mixed HL or SNHL	ABC normal ⬇ Indicating Mild to moderate CHL
Facial palsy	Infranuclear VIIth cranial nerve palsy may be present if disease has involved the facial nerve	Absent
Clinical stage	Always active	Active, inactive or quiescent

some movement or air is heard whistling out or air bubbles are seen through secretions collected in the hypotympanum,
- Fistula sign and examination of CNS: If complications are suspected.

DIFFERENTIAL DIAGNOSIS

ASOM
- Passes through various stages.
- Perforation is small, in anteroinferior quadrant, and usually with pulsatile discharge.

Acute necrotizing otitis media
- Common in children.
- History of acute exanthematous fever present.
- Subtotal/Total perforation.

Tuberculous otitis media
- Commonly present with complications.
- Characteristic tuberculous granulations present.
- Histopathological examination of granulation tissue is diagnostic.
- Sequestration of bone present.

Traumatic perforation
- History of trauma present.
- Dry perforation.
- Otalgia present.
- Ragged edges of perforation.
- Congestion of eardrum present at the site of perforation.

Otitis externa   Cleaning of the discharge and debris from the external auditory canal will reveal a normal and intact eardrum.

TREATMENT

- Medical: Only for safe CSOM
- Surgical: For safe and unsafe CSOM

Medical/Conservative
- Indications
  - Small or moderate central perforations.
  - Active stage of safe CSOM.
  - Traumatic perforation
    - *Antibiotics:* Systemic and local (eardrops)
    - *Aural toilet*
      - Keep ear dry
      - Clean with sterile swabs
      - Cotton plugs in EAM
      - No swimming
  - *Anti-inflammatory analgesics:* To reduce the inflammatory changes due to infection.

- *Multivitamins and B-complex orally:* To improve the immunity and general condition of the patient.
- *Chemical cauterization:* Done only in case of small central perforations, which are dry and have thin edges. The hearing loss should be mild and of the conductive type. Done every 4–5 days. Agents used: 50% trichloroacetic acid or 25% silver nitrate. Improvement is assessed after three turns.

Surgical (Flowchart 10.4)
- Indications
  - *Unsafe CSOM*
    - Cholesteatoma
    - Granulations and polyps
    - Marginal perforations
  - *Complications of CSOM*
    - Intracranial
    - Extracranial
  - *Failure of medical line of management in safe CSOM.*

Flowchart 10.4: Surgical treatment

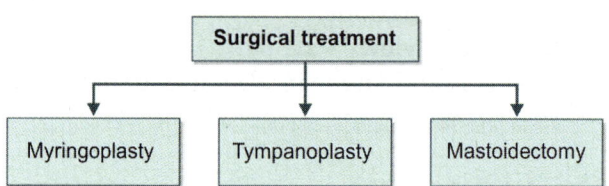

- **Myringoplasty** is defined as the reconstruction of the tympanic membrane without inspection of the ossicular chain or middle ear. This is indicated only in safe csom with normal hearing and normal middle ear mucosa.
- **Tympanoplasty**
  - *Definition*: Reconstruction of the tympanic membrane and/or the ossicular chain after complete eradication of the disease from the middle ear cleft.
  - *Aim*
    - To make the ear dry.
    - To restore hearing.
  - *Indications*
    - Safe CSOM with dry ear, i.e. inactive or quiescent stage, and not responding to 6 weeks of medical line of treatment.
    - Safe CSOM with large/subtotal central perforation.
    - Failure of small dry central perforation to heal after three turns of chemical cauterization.
    - Failure of traumatic perforation to heal with medical line of treatment.

- Safe CSOM with moderate to severe degree of conductive hearing loss, even if perforation is small, cauterization is not to be done as the ossicular chain needs to be checked.
- For better performance of a hearing aid because discharge from a perforation will spoil the hearing aid.

♦ *Contraindications*
- Age less than 12 years, i.e. once the immune system of the child is functioning well in order to safeguard against recurrent URTI, surgery can be performed.
- Elderly patient who is medically unfit due to hypertension/diabetes. This is a relative contraindication.

- Actively discharging central perforation, relative contraindication.
- Unsafe CSOM
- Presence of septic foci in nose, nasopharynx, paranasal sinuses and throat, these should be treated adequately prior to ear surgery.
- Eustachian tube dysfunction, this can result in failure of surgery.
- Fixed stapes footplate is a contraindication to ossicular repair.

♦ *Types of tympanoplasty*
- *Type I:* Only tympanic membrane repair with inspection of ossicular chain but, no reconstruction as chain is intact and functioning normally (Fig. 10.11).

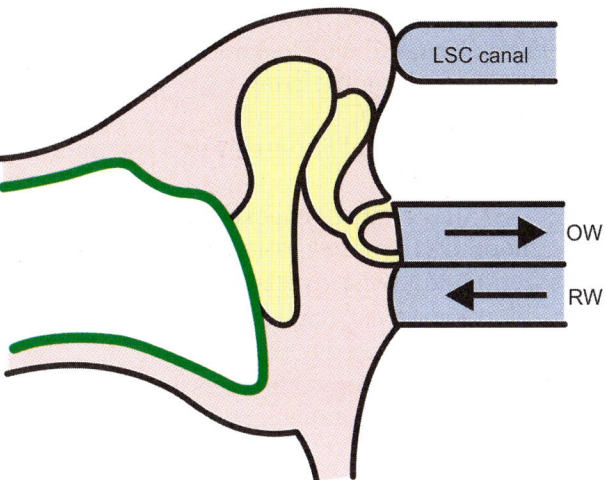

Fig. 10.11: Type I tympanoplasty

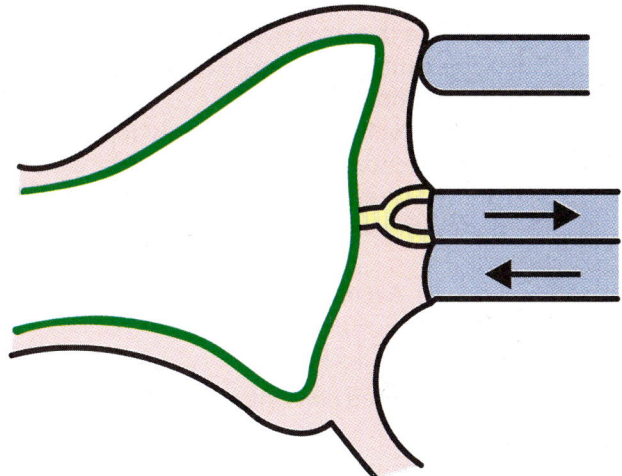

Fig. 10.13: Type III tympanoplasty (columella effect)

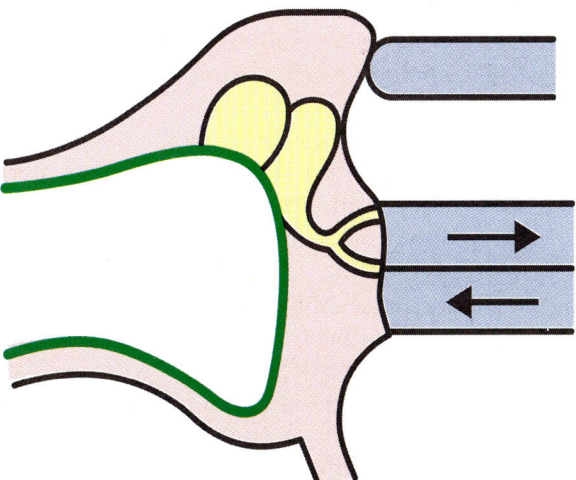

Fig. 10.12: Type II tympanoplasty

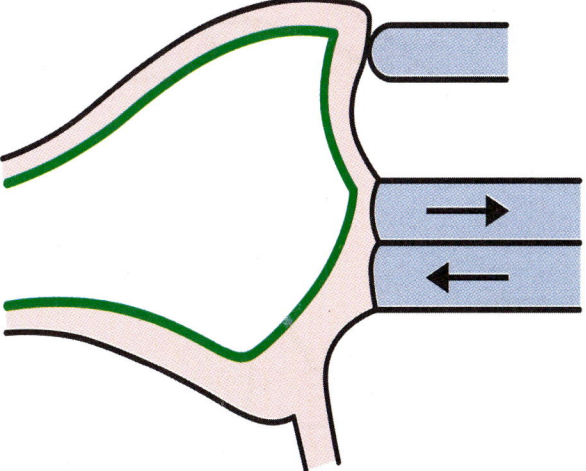

Fig. 10.14: Type IV tympanoplasty (Baffle effect)

- *Type II:* Necrosis of incus or malleus which is corrected by ossicular grafting, which results in a deformed but functioning ossicular chain (Fig. 10.12).
- *Type III:* Necrosis of incus and malleus is seen and the grafted eardrum is placed in contact with the stapes head (columella effect) (Fig. 10.13).
- *Type IV:* If stapes suprastructure is absent, oval window may be exposed to exterior and round window and Eustachian tube opening are covered by the grafted eardrum (Baffle effect) (Fig. 10.14).
- *Type V:* If stapes footplate is fixed, a fenestra is made in the lateral semicircular canal for facilitating hearing (fenestration operation) (Fig. 10.15).
- *Sonoinversion of Garcia (type VI):* The round window is exteriorized, and oval window and Eustachian tube opening are covered by grafted eardrum (sonoinversion).
- *Myringoplasty*: It comprises of only repair of the tympanic membrane where the middle ear and ossicular chain are not inspected. Indicated when the perforation is central, small and hearing loss is mild.

- *Anaesthesia*: LA or GA
- *Preoperative preparation*
  - Nil by mouth for 8 hours
  - Written informed consent
  - Injection TT 0.5 cc intramuscular (IM)
  - Injectiion atropine 0.6 mg IM, half hour before operation
  - Minimal shaving of postauricular hair

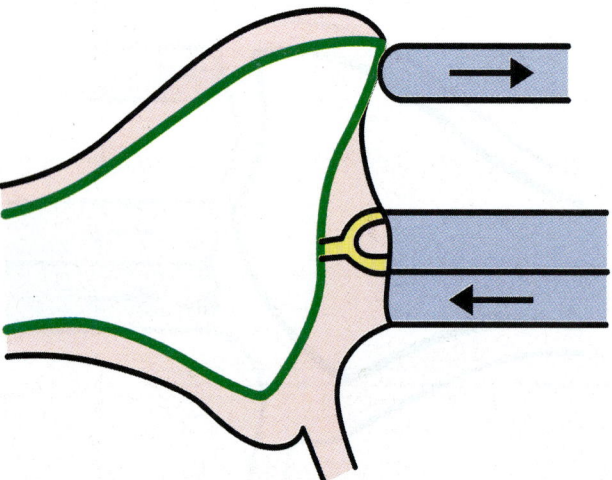

Fig. 10.15: Type V tympanoplasty (fenestration operation)

- Wash hair and do not apply oil on night prior to surgery.
- *Procedure*
  - *Position:* Supine with ear to be operated uppermost, i.e. head turned to opposite side.
  - *Postauricular:* Incision of Wilde, 0.5 cm behind the retroauricular sulus.
  - *Graft material:* Temporalis fascia graft approximately 2 × 2 cm is harvested (removed) and spread over a glass slide.
  - *Horizontal incision:* It is taken on the posterior meatal wall skin just deep to the spine of Henle.
  - Two Mollison's mastoid retractors are applied at right angles to each other for exposure and haemostasis.
  - Edges and under surface of central perforation are freshened with a sickle knife.
  - 12 o'clock and 6 o'clock incisions are taken on the skin lining the bony EAC, i.e. on the floor and roof of EAC.
  - Tympanomeatal flap is elevated and middle ear is visualized.
  - Ossicular chain is checked for continuity and mobility. If required, ossiculoplasty is performed.
  - Temporalis facia graft is placed underlay.
  - Tympanomeatal flap is replaced.
  - Gelfoam is placed in EAC.
  - Closure is performed in layers using 3–0 chromic catgut for subcutaneous tissue and 3–0 silk for skin.
- *Postoperative care*
  - Antibiotics for 7 days
  - Analgesics for 7 days
  - Sutures removed on 7th day
- *Methods of placement of graft*: There are two methods of placement of graft, i.e. underlay and overlay (Fig. 10.16).
  - The graft stays in position by the mechanism of surface tension due to the raw surface created by freshening of undersurface of the perforation.
  - Edges and undersurface of central perforation are freshened to:
    - Create a raw area on the undersurface of the remnant of the tympanic membrane to enable the graft to stay in position by surface tension.
    - Remove all squamous epithelium, which may have grown into the middle ear over the edge of the perforation.
    - In case of long standing perforations, the squamous layer and mucosal layer of the

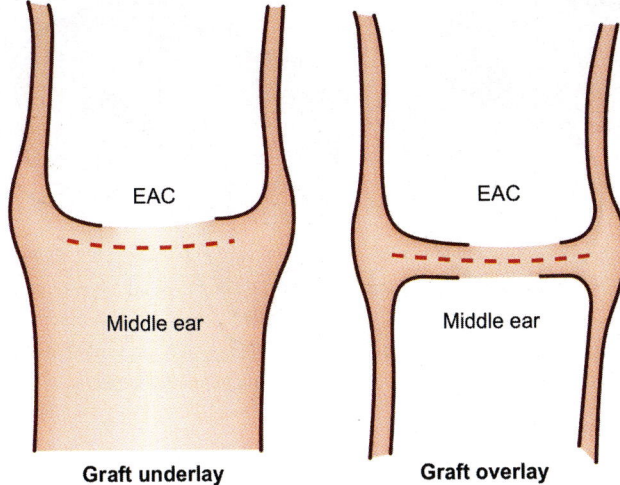

Fig. 10.16: Methods of placement of graft

eardrum tend to grow towards each other across the edge of the perforation and fuse. Thus, preventing further healing of the perforation. If the edge is removed, the layers grow towards each other along the graft and healing takes place.

- *Graft materials used in tympanoplasty*
  - For the tympanic membrane (Table 10.4)
  - For ossiculoplasty (Table 10.5)

TABLE 10.4: Grafts for tympanic membrane

Autografts	Homografts
• Temporalis fascia	• Lyophilised dura
• Tragal perichondrium	• Perichondrium
• Vein graft	• Cadaveric tympanic membrane
• Split-thickness skin	
• Conchal perichondrium	
• Facia lata	

TABLE 10.5: Ossicular graft materials

Autografts (From same person)	Homografts (From same species)	Implants (Biomaterials)
• Malleus head	• Malleus head	• Teflon
• Incus	• Incus	• Ceramics
• Tragal cartilage	• Tragal cartilage	• Gold
• Conchal cartilage	• Conchal cartilage	• Polyethylene
• Spine of Henle	• Tooth	• Plastipore

- *Implants*
  - *Partial ossicular replacement prosthesis (PORP):* PORP is used for ossicular reconstruction from eardrum to head of stapes
  - *Total ossicular replacement prosthesis (TORP):* TORP is used for reconstruction from eardrum to footplate of stapes.
- *Complications*
  - *Immediate*
    - Complications of anaesthesia.
    - Haemorrhage.
    - Sensorineural (SN) hearing loss if oval window or round window is damaged.
    - Injury to facial nerve.
  - *Delayed*
    - Perichondritis of the pinna → Cauliflower ear
    - Sensorineural hearing loss.
    - Facial palsy.
    - Failure of tympanic membrane graft to heal or failure of ossiculoplasty.
- Mastoidectomy
  - *Classification*
    - Simple / Cortical mastoidectomy (Fig. 10.17)
    - Modified radical mastoidectomy
    - Radical mastoidectomy

TABLE 10.6: Indications of mastoidectomy

Simple / Schwartz/ Conservative/Cortical	Modified radical	Radical
• Coalescent mastoiditis	• Unsafe CSOM with cholesteatoma	• Unsafe CSOM with intra or extracranial complications.
• With a tympanoplasty in the presence of glue in the middle ear	• Fenestration operation	• Extensive cholesteatoma involving anterior attic and tip of mastoid.
• As an approach for:		• Unsafe CSOM in children.
◆ Endolymphatic sac decompression		• Malignant otitis externa.
◆ Facial nerve decompression		• Malignant or benign tumours of mastoid and middle ear.
◆ Cochlear implant		
◆ Vestibular neurectomy		
◆ Labyrinthectomy		
◆ Acoustic neuroma removal		

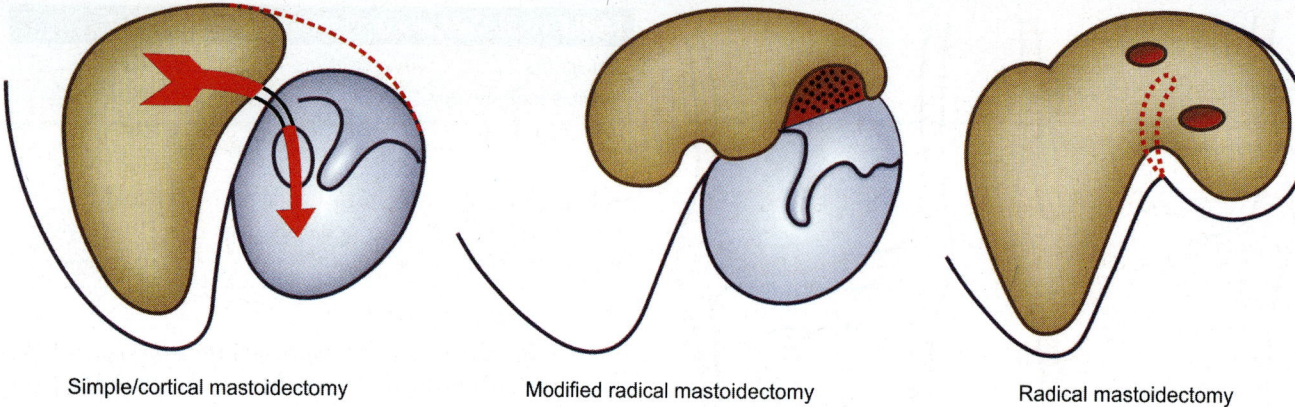

Simple/cortical mastoidectomy   Modified radical mastoidectomy   Radical mastoidectomy

Fig. 10.17: Simple/Cortical mastoidectomy

- *Indications*: For indications see Table 10.6.
- *Aims*
  - To make the ear safe and prevent complications.
  - To make the ear dry.
  - To restore hearing.
- *Preoperative preparation*: (Same as for Tympanoplasty).
- *Anaesthesia*: General anaesthesia (GA) preferred.
- *Procedure*
  - *Position*—supine with ear to be operated uppermost.
  - *Postauricular incision of Wilde*—0.5 cm behind retroauricular sulcus.
  - *Graft material*—Temporalis fascia graft is harvested.
  - *Horizontal incision* is taken on the posterior meatal wall skin deep to the spine of Henle.
  - *Soft tissues* on the mastoid cortex are incised and elevated off the cortex bone with a periosteal elevator.
  - Two self-retaining, haemostatic, mastoid retractors (Mollison's) are applied at right angles to each other for exposure of the mastoid cortex and haemostasis.
  - Using an electric drill with burr, the mastoid air cells are exenterated and whole disease is removed from the mastoid and middle ear.
    - The bony landmarks/limits of a cortical mastoidectomy are the tegmen plate superiorly, mastoid tip inferiorly, sinus plate posteriorly, bony EAC anteriorly, and lateral semicircular canal medially.
    - In a radical mastoidectomy, whole disease is removed from the middle ear and mastoid with removal of remnants of incus, malleus, and eardrum; with removal of bridge and lowering

of ridge, so that the mastoid, middle ear, and EAC are converted into a single cavity. The stapes is not removed.
  - In a modified radical mastoidectomy, whole disease is removed from middle ear and mastoid cavity with lowering of the ridge and removing of the bridge and only necrosed ossicles are removed. It is a much more conservative operation.
  - A reconstructive operation can be performed at the same time, such as tympanoplasty and/or ossiculoplasty. This helps to improve hearing as now disease is completely removed.
  - *Meatoplasty*–Widening of the external auditory meatus. Done in case of a radical or modified radical mastoidectomy only, to enable the new cavity to drain well and heal fast. It is done only if ridge is lowered and bridge is removed.
  - Soft tissues are sutured with 3–0 chromic catgut
  - EAC is filled with gelfoam and packed lightly with ribbon gauze impregnated with neosporin ointment. The gauze is brought out of the EAC.
  - Skin is sutured with 3–0 black silk.
  - A pressure dressing is given using a mastoid bandage.
- *Postoperative care*
  - Antibiotics for 7–10 days
  - Analgesics for 7 days
  - Skin sutures removed on 7th day
  - Earpack removed on 5th day.
- *Complications*
  - *Immediate*
    - Complications of anaesthesia
    - Haemorrhage
    - Damage to dura, sigmoid sinus, facial nerve, labyrinth, stapes and incus.

- *Delayed*
  - Infection of wound
  - Sigmoid sinus thrombophlebitis
  - Facial nerve palsy
  - SN hearing loss due to damage to labyrinth
  - Vertigo due to damage to labyrinth
  - Conductive deafness if incus is dislocated in a simple mastoidectomy
  - Stenosis of EAC
  - Residual or recurrence of cholesteatoma may occur.

DEFINITIONS

Cortical/Simple mastoidectomy Complete exenteration of the disease process from all the mastoid air cells. The boundaries of the cavity formed are: EAC anteriorly, sinus plate posteriorly, tegmen plate superiorly, mastoid tip inferiorly and lateral semicircular canal medially.

Radical mastoidectomy Complete exenteration of the disease from the middle ear, attic and mastoid air cells with removal of the diseased incus and malleus thus converting the mastoid and middle ear into a single cavity which drains into the EAC.

Modified radical mastoidectomy Complete exenteration of the disease from the attic and mastoid air cells converting the attic, mastoid, and EAC into a single cavity. The mesotympanium is not touched. Thus, it is radical as far as the disease is concerned and conservative as far as hearing is concerned.

Bridge This is the portion of the bony EAC, which lies lateral to the aditus ad antrum and short process of the incus. As it does not contain the facial nerve, it is removed completely during radical/modified radical mastoidectomy.

Ridge This is the portion of the bony EAC, which lies lateral to the facial canal (Fallopian canal). Deep/Medial to this runs the facial nerve in its canal and hence during a radical mastoidectomy, the ridge is lowered to the level of the facial canal.

Bridge is removed and ridge is lowered during radical mastoidectomy.

CHAPTER 11

Non-Suppurative Otitis Media

SYNONYMS

- Secretory otitis media (SOM)
- Serous otitis media
- Glue ear
- Catarrhal otitis media
- Otitis media with effusion
- Tubotympanic catarrh.

DEFINITION

Non-suppurative otitis media is a disease of the middle ear cleft characterised by the presence of non-purulent serous or mucoid effusion in the middle ear and a resultant conductive hearing loss.

AETIOLOGY

- Age: Common in children. Especially below 10 years of age.
- Climate: Common in winter.
- Eustachian tube dysfunction, e.g. due to repeated attacks of upper respiratory tract infection (URTI), patulous Eustachian tube.
- Eustachian tube obstruction, e.g. enlarged adenoids or following scarring due to surgery in the nasopharynx such as adenoidectomy, removal of nasopharyngeal angiofibroma, etc.
- Barotrauma: Sudden change in atmospheric pressure (e.g. flying in an unpressurised aircraft or scuba diving) may result in serous effusion in the middle ear.

- Cleft palate: It is commonly associated with adenoid hypertrophy and poor Eustachian tube function.
- Viral
- Allergy
- Tumours of nasopharynx causing obstruction to the Eustachian tube, e.g. nasopharyngeal angiofibroma, rhinosporidiosis, etc.
- Craniofacial anomalies: These affect Eustachian tube function.
- Disturbance of mucociliary clearance of the middle ear cleft, e.g. Young's syndrome, Kartagener's syndrome.
- Immunological disorders, e.g. hypogammaglobu-linemia.
- Radiotherapy of nasopharynx can result in scarring and stenosis of Eustachian tube opening.
- Inadequate treatment of ASOM: It may result in persistance of fluid in the middle ear cleft.
- Idiopathic.

CLINICAL FEATURES

Symptoms
- Deafness: It can be mild, conductive, and inter-mittent, usually bilateral and insidious in onset. Occasionally, sensorineural deafness may occur due to toxins affecting the inner ear.
- Tinnitus: It may be present and is usually of the 'bubbling' variety or of the 'whistling' type indicating inner ear affection.

Signs Tympanic membrane is intact but dull. Cone of light is absent. The eardrum may be bulging but unlike ASOM, there is no congestion. Fluid level or air bubbles may be seen occasionally (Figs 11.1 and 11.2) and the fluid level moves on sieglisation.

- Tuning fork tests: These usually show a mild conductive hearing loss.

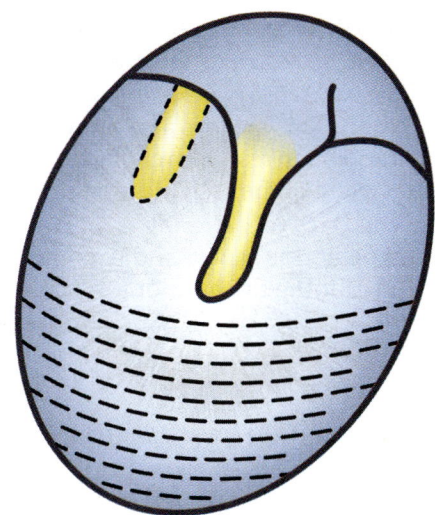

Fig. 11.1: Air-fluid level seen behind an intact eardrum in SOM

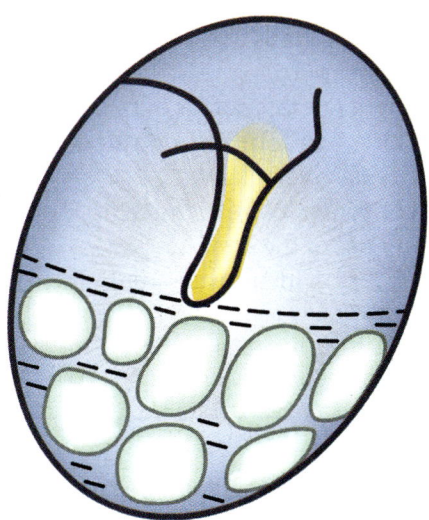

Fig. 11.2: Air-bubbles seen behind an intact eardrum in SOM

SEQUELAE

Long standing and inadequately treated cases can result in:

- Atelectasis
- Tympanosclerosis
- Sensorineural hearing loss
- Retraction pocket formation
- Cholesterol granuloma formation
- Cholesteatoma formation.

INVESTIGATIONS

- Pure tone audiometry: It will show mild to moderate conductive hearing loss.
- Impedence audiometry (tympanometry): It shows a flat 'type B' curve which is characteristic of secretory otitis media.

TREATMENT

Flowchart 11.1: Treatment of NSOM

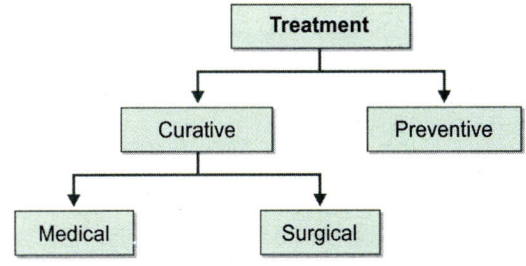

Treatment of the Cause

Medical
- Local nasal decongestants
  - 1% ephidrine nose drops.
  - 1% oxymetazoline hydrochloride or
  - 1% xylometazoline hydrochloride, nose drops.
    These help by reducing the congestion in the nose and around the opening of the Eustachian tube, thus, helping in spontaneous drainage of the effusion through the Eustachian tube.
- Systemic antihistaminics: If there is evidence of allergic rhinitis.
- Valsalva manoeuvre, politzerization or Eustachian catheterization may be useful in a few cases, as it helps in insufflation of the middle ear.
- Steroids: Systemic and topical steroids have given good results.

Surgical
- The commonest cause of SOM in children is enlarged adenoids and hence an adenoidectomy is useful in most cases.
- Myringotomy with grommet (ventilation tube): Radial incision is made in the anteroinferior quadrant of the pars tensa and the middle ear fluid

(seromucinous effusion) is aspirated. Following this, a grommet is put in position. A grommet (ventilation tube) helps in the following manner:

- It helps in drainage of the effusion.
- It ventilates the middle ear.
- It improves hearing.
- It helps the epithelium to revert back to normal.

   Sometimes, chymotrypsin instillation into the middle ear cavity through the myringotomy incision may help to liquefy the secretions and hence facilitate drainage.

- In some cases, a grommet too may fail to help and such patients benefit from a cortical mastoidectomy.
- In the presence of sequelae, the treatment is aimed at curing the disease, e.g. a tympanoplasty or a mastoidectomy.

Types of grommets used commonly
- Shah grommet
- Shepard grommet
- Silicone T tube

Preventive/Prophylaxis: All children who seem inattentive should be investigated for middle ear effusion :
- Cold should be treated immediately.
- Underlying sinusitis should be treated.
- Immunological disorder, if any, should be corrected.

ATELECTASIS

DEFINITION

This is a condition characterised by medial retraction of the pars tensa as a result of chronic non-suppurative otitis media.

AETIOPATHOGENESIS

If serous otitis media (SOM) persists due to inadequate treatment or lack of treatment, the middle ear effusion gets thickened and resorbed and in the presence of a persistent obstruction to the Eustachian tube, the pars tensa tends to retract towards the medial wall of the middle ear (promontory). This retraction is most pronounced in the posterosuperior quadrant of the tympanic membrane (as this region has less aeration due to presence of ossicles).

STAGES

- **Stage I:** The pars tensa is retracted medially, but does not touch the incudostapedial joint. It is characterised by prominence of anterior and posterior malleolar folds, absence of cone of light, dull lusture of the eardrum, prominence of the lateral process of the malleus, prominence of the annulus and foreshortening and retraction of handle of malleus.
- **Stage II:** The pars tensa is medially retracted and lies over the incudostapedial joint.
- **Stage III:** The pars tensa lies over the promontory but there are no adhesions between the promontory and the pars tensa (tested by sieglisation).
- **Stage IV:** The pars tensa is adherent to the promontory and lies over it. This stage is also known as *adhesive otitis media* and often results in cholesteatoma formation with erosion of the ossicular chain.
- **Stage V:** The pars tensa tends to perforate in the anterior or posterior aspect and squamous epithelium is seen draping the promontory.

CLINICAL FEATURES

Symptoms
- **Deafness:** Moderate to severe degree of conductive hearing loss.
- **Tinnitus:** It may be present.
- **Otalgia:** It may be present.
- **Otorrhoea:** It is characteristically absent.

Signs
- Features of retraction will be present, such as:
  - Prominent anterior and posterior malleolar folds
  - Prominent lateral process of malleus
  - Foreshortening and retraction of handle of malleus
  - Absence of cone of light
  - Loss of normal lustre of the tympanic membrane
  - Prominence of the annulus
  - Prominence of incudostapedial joint in stage II, III or IV atelectasis
- Tuning fork tests reveal a moderate to severe degree of conductive hearing loss.

INVESTIGATIONS

- Pure tone audiometry will show a moderate to severe degree of conductive hearing loss.
- Impedence audiometry will show a 'type B' flat curve characteristic of atelectasis in stages I to IV. However, this investigation needs an intact eardrum and hence is not possible in stage V atelectasis.

TREATMENT

- In stages I to III, myringotomy with grommet usually helps to equalize the pressure in the middle ear and hence improve hearing. Medical line of treatment is similar to SOM.

- If the hearing loss is more and indicates ossicular necrosis, a tympanomastoidectomy and ossiculoplasty are performed.
- In stages IV and V, a mastoidectomy is required.
- If sequelae have occurred, such as cholesteatoma, etc., a mastoidectomy is required.
- Tympanomastoidectomy using a silastic sheet in the middle ear is used recently to prevent adhesions in stages IV and V.
- In the absence of any sequelae, a hearing aid is most effective.

TYMPANOSCLEROSIS

DEFINITION

This is a condition characterised by subepithelial deposition of chalky calcarious plaques in the middle ear or in the tympanic membrane.

There is a hyaline degeneration of the fibrous layer of the middle ear mucosa followed by calcifications which appear like chalky patches in the eardrum or around the ossicular chain. It is the end-stage of chronic inflammatory ear disease.

SITES AFFECTED

- Tympanic membrane
- Incudostapedial joint
- Promontory
- Oval window and stapes footplate
- Round window

CLINICAL FEATURES

Symptoms

- It may be asymptomatic if it involves the anterior half of the tympanic membrane or if it is a small plaque involving promontory.

- Deafness usually conductive. It occurs if the plaque involves either the posterosuperior quadrant of the eardrum or the ossicular chain or oval window or round window, thus interfering with sound conduction. Rarely, it may result in sensorineural hearing loss, if the inner ear is involved either through the round or oval windows.
- Tinnitus and vertigo: These occur only if inner ear is involved.

Signs

- Chalky white plaques are seen in the tympanic membrane.
- If only middle ear is involved, the tympanic membrane may appear intact and normal and the condition may be discovered only on exploratory tympanotomy to find out the cause of the hearing loss.
- Tuning fork tests will show conductive hearing loss.

INVESTIGATIONS

- Pure tone audiometry reveals a conductive hearing loss.
- Impedence may show a low peaked curve if tympanic membrane is involved or a 'type As' curve, if the ossicular chain is fixed due to involvement. If ossicular necrosis has occurred a 'type Ad' curve is seen.

TREATMENT

- If asymptomatic, no treatment is required.
- If there is a conductive hearing loss, an exploratory tympanotomy is performed and the plaque is removed from the tympanic membrane and/or middle ear followed by a tympanoplasty and/or ossiculoplasty.
- If the oval window or round window are involved or if surgery fails, a hearing aid gives good results.

CHAPTER 12

Complications of Otitis Media

The middle ear is closely related to various important structures, such as the facial nerve, labyrinth, meninges, brain, venous sinuses, etc., and hence spread of infection beyond the middle ear can result in serious complications. Following the advent of antibiotics, however, the incidence of complications has greatly reduced. Also, advanced diagnostic techniques have helped to reduce the mortality rate. Complications can occur in acute as well as chronic otitis media.

CLASSIFICATION

Complications of otitis media (Fig. 12.1)
- Extracranial
  - Mastoiditis
    - Acute
      - Catarrhal
      - Coalescent
    - Chronic

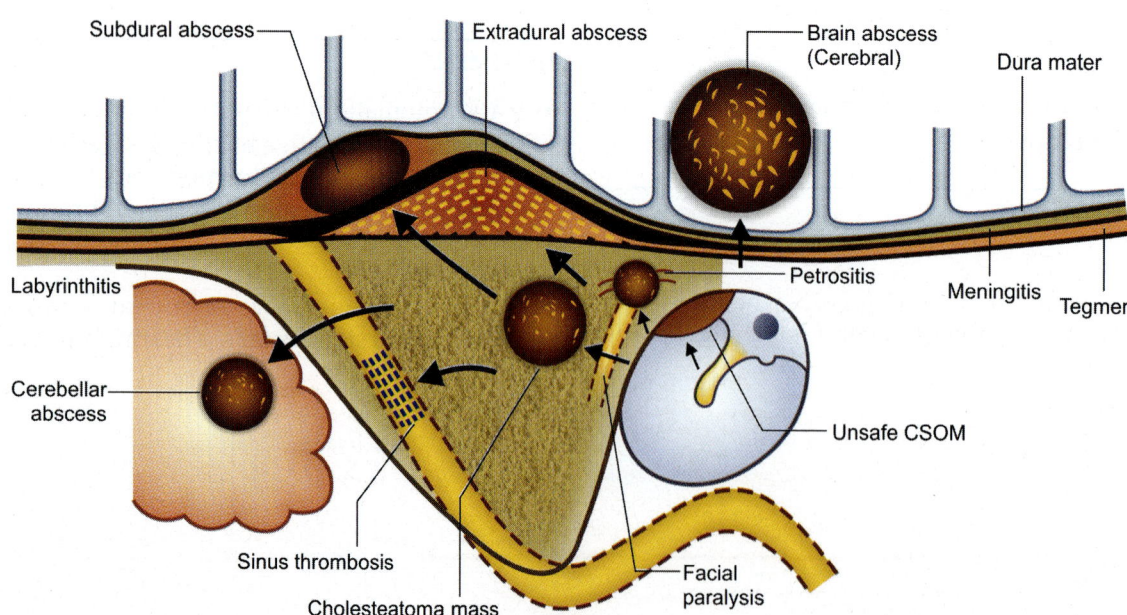

Fig. 12.1: Diagrammatic representation of the complications of CSOM

- Mastoid abscess
  - Subperiosteal mastoid abscess (Fig. 12.2A)
  - Subcutaneous mastoid abscess (Fig. 12.2B)
- Luc's abscess
- Bezold's abscess
- Citelli's abscess
- Zygomatic abscess
- Labrinthitis
  - Serous
  - Suppurative
- Petrositis and Gradenigo's syndrome
- Facial nerve paralysis.
- Intracranial
  - Extradural abscess
  - Subdural abscess
  - Meningitis

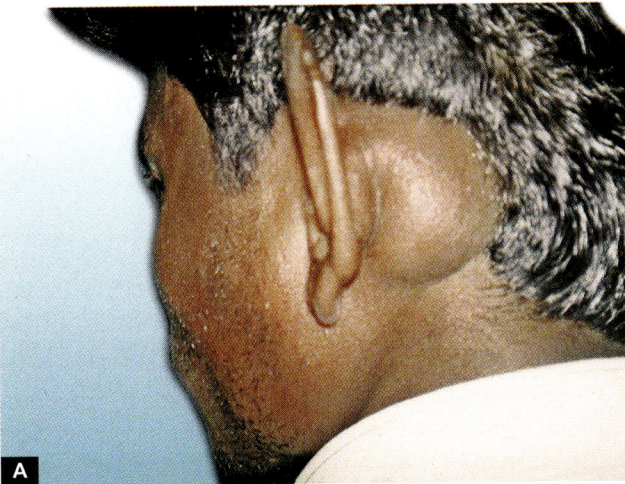

Fig. 12.2A: Subcutaneous mastoid abscess

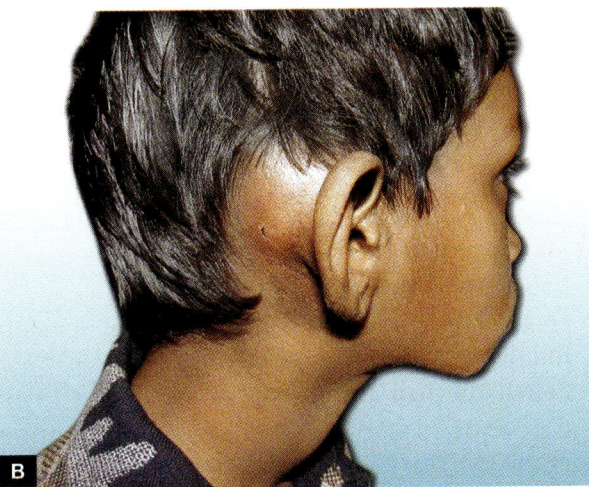

Fig. 12.2B: Subperiosteal mastoid abscess

- Sigmoid sinus thrombosis
- Otitic hydrocephalus
- Encephalitis
- Brain abscess:
  - Cerebral abscess
  - Cerebellar abscess

Rarely, one may encounter life-threatening complications like otogenic abscess, septicaemia and pyaemia.

MODE OF SPREAD OF INFECTION

- **Spread in continuity:** Infection of the middle ear mucosa can spread to the mastoid and result in mastoiditis.
- Direct spread through bone by erosion or osteitis as in CSOM or ASOM respectively.
- Venous spread by retrograde thrombophlebitis to the meninges, venous sinuses and brain.
- Spread via natural preformed pathways and developmental dehiscences like:
  - Congenital dehiscences of tegmen plate or facial canal,
  - Un-united suture lines such as petrosquamous suture,
  - Round window or oval window.
- Spread via perivascular spaces of Virchow-Robin intracranially.
- Occasionally, spread may occur in cases of recurrent CSOM postoperatively due to iatrogenic pathways created by the surgeon like labyrinthine fistula or destruction of dural or sinus plates during surgery.

The diagnosis of these complications is based on history, clinical features and CT scan of the temporal bone.

INTRACRANIAL COMPLICATIONS

Extradural abscess

- **Definition:** It is the localised accumulation of pus in the extradural space.
- **Aetiology:** It occurs as a complication of unsafe chronic suppurative otitis media when the infection spreads to the extradural space usually by erosion of the tegmen tympani. If this abscess goes around the sigmoid sinus, it is known as perisinus abscess.
- **Clinical features:** The features are similar to those of mastoid abscess but more severe. Occasionally, it may be asymptomatic.
- **Treatment:** Radical mastoidectomy with drainage of the abscess through the mastoidectomy.

Intravenous antibiotics for 7 days with anti-inflammatory analgesics.

Subdural abscess

- **Definition:** It is the collection of pus in the subdural space.
- **Aetiology:** It occurs as a complication of unsafe CSOM through the various modes of spread of infection described previously.
- **Clinical features**
  - Severe dull continuous headache
  - Fever
  - Malaise
  - Focal neurological symptoms may be present, e.g. epilepsy or paralysis.
  - Drowsiness
  - Coma, if untreated or undiagnosed.
- **Treatment:** Neurosurgical drainage of the abscess through a burr hole under intravenous antibiotic cover followed by a radical mastoidectomy.

OR

Radical mastoidectomy under intravenous antibiotic cover with drainage of the abscess through the mastoidectomy.

Meningitis

- **Definition:** It is defined as the inflammation of the meninges and it is one of the commonest intracranial complications of unsafe CSOM.
- **Aetiology:** Occurs as a complication of unsafe CSOM usually by erosion of the tegmen plate or sinus plate or spread through the labyrinth or petrous part of the temporal bone.
- **Clinical features**
  - High grade fever with rigors (Fig. 12.3).
  - Severe continuous headache
  - Projectile vomiting
  - Neck rigidity
  - Kernig's sign positive
  - Drowsiness and delerium may occur
  - Coma if untreated
  - Investigations of CSF reveal features of pyogenic meningitis–raised CSF pressure, turbid character of CSF, increased cell count, increased proteins and decreased glucose and chloride.
  - Blood count will show leucocytosis.
- **Treatment:** The meningitis is controlled first by conservative line (medical) of management and only when the patient is stable, surgical treatment of the cause by a radical mastoidectomy is carried out at the earliest.

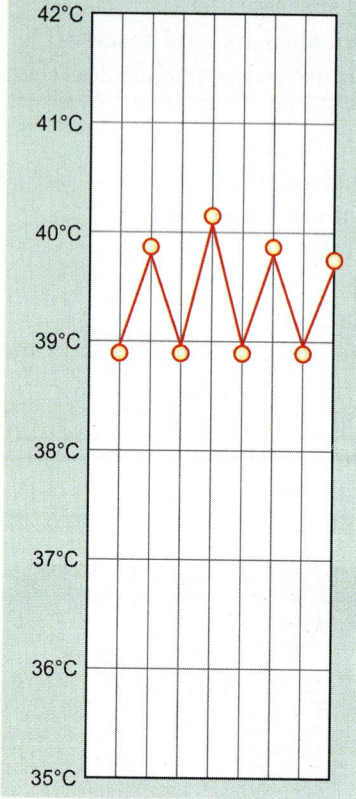

Fig. 12.3: High grade fever of meningitis

Sigmoid/Lateral sinus thrombosis

- **Definition:** It is a condition characterised by infection of the sigmoid sinus (thrombophlebitis) followed by thrombosis of the sinus.
- **Aetiology:** Occurs in unsafe CSOM due to erosion of the sinus plate following a perisinus abscess or due to retrograde venous thrombophlebitis.
- **Clinical features:**
  - Hectic rise of temperature associated with rigors (Fig. 12.4).
  - This is the classical fever of sigmoid sinus thrombosis. During rigors the temperature may shoot up to 104–105°F and patient looks ill but he may appear normal in between rigors.
  - Malaise and weakness.
  - Headache due to raised intracranial tension following blocking of the lateral sinus.
  - Pain in the post-aural area with swelling.
  - Griesinger's sign occurs due to inflammation of the emissary vein and is characterised by an indurated tender area over the occipital bone and mastoid region on palpation.

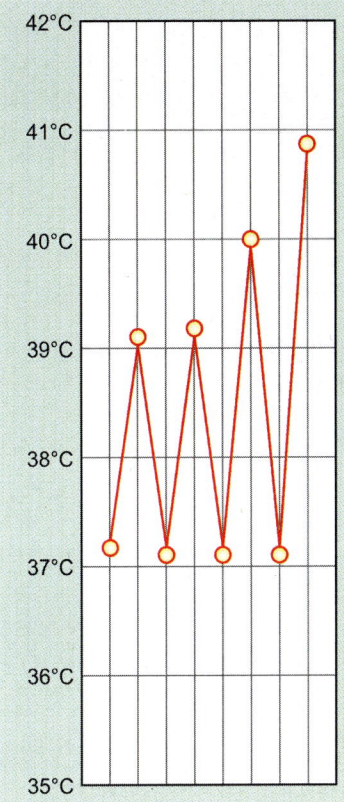

Fig. 12.4: Hectic fever of signoid sinus thrombosis

- ◆ Torticollis and pain over the upper part of the internal jugular vein may occur due to spread of infection into the internal jugular vein.
- ◆ Septicaemia, pyaemia and toxaemia are late features.
- ◆ Blurring of vision is indicative of cavernous sinus or superior sagittal sinus involvement.
- Investigations:
  - ◆ Blood count—polymorphonuclear leucocytosis is present.
  - ◆ Blood culture may be positive for bacteremia especially if collected in the febrile phase.
  - ◆ CT scan shows erosion of the sinus plate and presence of perisinus abscess with clot in the sinus.
  - ◆ CSF pressure may be raised.
  - ◆ Fundoscopy may show papilloedema.
  - ◆ Queckensted's test or Toby–Ayer test will show obstruction of the internal jugular vein on the affected side.
- Sequelae:
  - ◆ The thrombus may completely occlude the lumen of the sinus.
  - ◆ Emboli may be thrown off and may result in pulmonary embolism with instant death.

- ◆ Infection may spread deeper to result in meningitis, subdural abscess or brain abscess.
- ◆ Microemboli may result in septicaemia and pyaemia followed by death due to toxaemia.
- ◆ Thrombus may spread proximally to the transverse sinus.
- ◆ Distal spread of thrombus into the internal jugular vein may occur.
- ◆ Infection may spread through the mastoid emissary vein.
- ◆ Cavernous sinus thrombosis may rarely occur and is usually fatal.
- Treatment: Radical mastoidectomy with drainage of the perisinus abscess and removal of infected clot or pus from the sinus through the mastoidectomy under cover of intravenous antibiotics.

Otitic hydrocephalus
- Definition: Hydrocephalus occurring due to lateral sinus thrombosis following unsafe CSOM is termed as otitic hydrocyphalus.
- Aetiopathogenesis: Spread of thrombus from sigmoid sinus to the longitudinal sinus results in raised intracranial pressure due to blockage of arachnoid villi and brain oedema.
- Clinical features:
  - ◆ Frontal headache—dull and continuous.
  - ◆ Projectile vomiting
  - ◆ Malaise
  - ◆ Papilloedema—bilateral
  - ◆ Focal cerebral symptoms such as epilepsy or paralysis.
- Treatment:
  - ◆ Intravenous antibiotics
  - ◆ Steroids
  - ◆ To reduce intracranial pressure:
    - • Diuretics
    - • Hyperosmolar dehydrating agents
    - • Repeated lumbar puncture
  - ◆ Radical mastoidectomy with removal of pus and infected clot from the sigmoid sinus (which is the cause of this pathology) should be performed at the earliest.
  - ◆ If visual acuity worsens, a subtemporal decompression or a ventriculoperitoneal shunt may be required.

Brain abscess   A brain abscess due to unsafe CSOM occurs either in the temporal lobe of the cerebrum or in the cerebellum (Fig. 12.5).

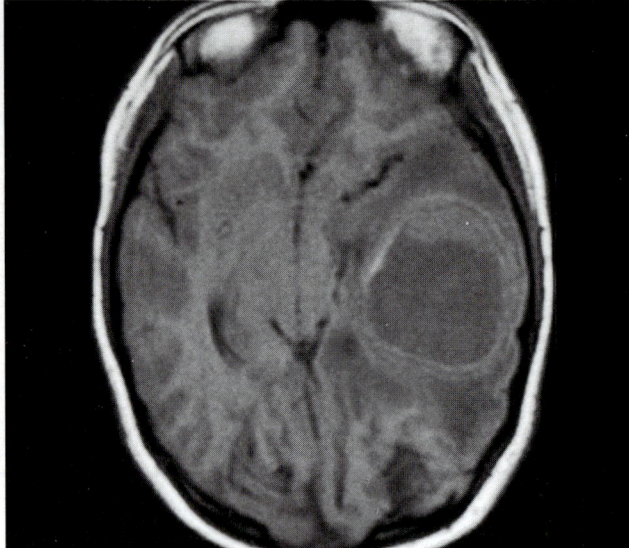

Fig. 12.5: Brain abscess

- The clinical features are due to:
  - Increased intracranial tension,
  - Pressure to surrounding areas due to a space occupying lesion,
  - Presence of infection.
- Pathology: The stages through which the abscess passes include:
  - Stage of encephalitis–inflammation of brain tissue,
  - Latent stage—this is a symptom free stage lasting for several days to several weeks. During this time, the abscess is localised due to capsule formation,
  - Stage of manifestation—when symptoms start occurring and signs are seen,
  - Terminal stage—when the abscess ruptures and purulent encephalitis or coning occurs resulting in death.
- Clinical features
  - General clinical features due to increased intra-cranial tension.
  - Localising signs due to pressure on surrounding brain tissue.

General signs and symptoms
  - Disorientation, malaise and anorexia.
  - Slow cerebration i.e. patient replies to questions after a latent waiting period
  - Bradycardia
  - Headache
  - Nausea and projectile vomiting
  - Subnormal body temperature may be present (Fig. 12.6).

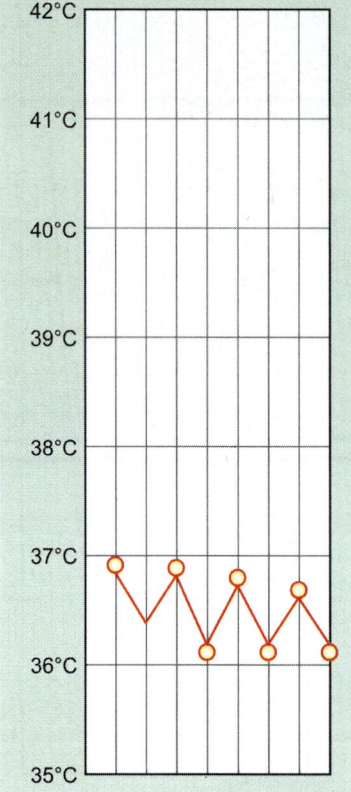

Fig. 12.6: Subnormal body temperature in brain abscess

Localising signs
  - *Temporal lobe abscess:*
    - Convulsions,
    - Dysphasia or aphasia if speech area is affected,
    - Homonymous hemianopia if optic radiations are involved,
    - VIth cranial nerve palsy,
    - Auditory or visual hallucinations may occur.
  - *Cerebellar abscess* (Fig. 12.7)
    - Ataxia—patient tends to fall to the side of lesion,
    - Incoordination or dysdiadokokinesia,
    - Nystagmus,
    - Romberg's test positive on the side of the lesion,
    - Slurred speech,
    - If pressure is on the medulla and pons in case of large abscess, cardiovascular and/or respiratory irregularities may occur.
- Investigations:
  - CSF—raised pressure and raised cell count.
  - Fundoscopy—papilloedema.
  - CT scan—plain and contrast of brain is the most important single investigation for definitive diagnosis.

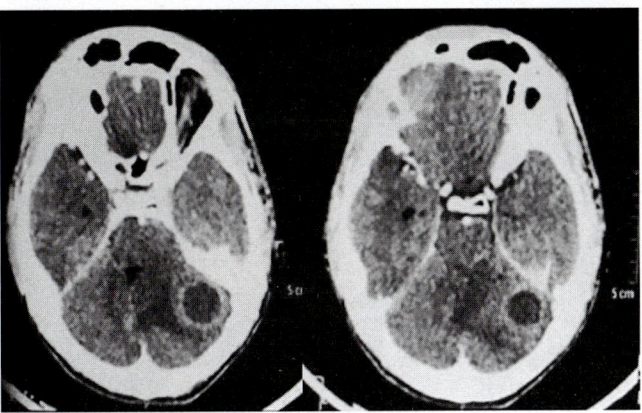

Fig. 12.7: Cerebellar abscess

- ◆ Carotid angiography
- ◆ Ventriculography
- ◆ X-ray skull
- ◆ Lumbar puncture is best avoided as in this condition, it can result in death due to coning of brainstem.
- ◆ EEG shows abnormal wave pattern.
- Treatment: Treatment is on a priority basis as this is a potentially life-threatening condition. The brain abscess is treated first by a neurosurgeon either by :
  - ◆ Drainage via a burrhole,
  - ◆ Excision of the abscess via a craniotomy.
    This is followed by a radical mastoidectomy by an ENT surgeon to eradicate the cause.
    Also antibiotics which cross the blood brain barrier are given along with metronidazole. The intracranial tension is controlled with mannitol and steroids.

EXTRACRANIAL COMPLICATIONS

Mastoiditis   *Refer* to Chapter 9.

Mastoid abscess:
- Subperiosteal abscess:
  - ◆ *Definition:* It is the collection of pus deep to the periosteum covering the lateral wall of the mastoid antrum after erosion of the bone.
  - ◆ *Clinical features:*
    - • *Symptoms:*
      - ▪ Severe pain over the mastoid region (post-auricular area).
      - ▪ Redness and swelling over the mastoid region.
      - ▪ Fever, malaise.
    - • *Signs:*
      - ▪ Inflammation and oedema in postauricular area.

- ▪ Raised local temperature and tenderness in postauricular area.
- ▪ Postauricular groove is deepened.
- Subcutaneous abscess:
  - ◆ *Definition:* It is the collection of pus in the subcutaneous postauricular region after destruction of the periosteum and bone covering the lateral cortical wall of the mastoid .
  - ◆ *Clinical features:*
    - • *Symptoms:*
      - ▪ Pain in the postauricular region reduces in severity.
      - ▪ Postauricular swelling increases.
      - ▪ Fever, malaise.
      - ▪ Pinna is prominent.
    - • *Signs:*
      - ▪ Inflammation and oedema in the post-auricular region.
      - ▪ Obliteration of postauricular grove by oedema and abscess.
      - ▪ Pinna is pushed outwards, downwards and forwards.
  - ◆ *Treatment:*
    - • Intravenous antibiotics.
    - • Anti-inflammatory analgesics.
    - • Urgent inscision and drainage of the post-auricular abscess with regular antibiotic dressings using strict aseptic measures.
    - • Mastoidectomy at a later date after infection and inflammation subsides (approximately 7–10 days).
- Luc's abscess: It occurs when the mastoid abscess erodes the postero-superior wall of the bony EAC to result in sagging of the roof of the EAC.
- Bezold's abscess: It occurs when the mastoid abscess erodes the tip of the mastoid to track along the sternomastoid muscle in the neck.
    The patient develops swelling in the upper portion of the neck with Bezold's Abscess (Fig. 12.8).
- Citelli's abscess: It occurs when the mastoid abscess erodes the bone of the digastric triangle to track along the posterior belly of the digastric muscle in the neck.
- Zygomatic abscess: It occurs when the mastoid abscess tracks along the zygomatic process to produce a swelling above and in front of the EAC.
- Labyrinthitis: This occurs when the infection reaches the inner ear either through the round or oval windows or through a fistula formation in the promontory or bony labyrinth.
    It is of two types—serous, which is reversible and if untreated, it becomes suppurative, which is irreversible.

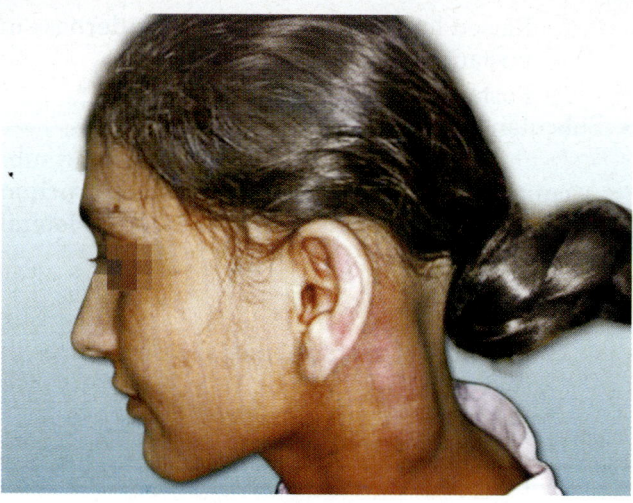

Fig. 12.8: Bezolds abscess

- *Clinical features:*
  - Sensorineural deafness
  - Vertigo
  - Tinnitus
  - Nausea and vomiting
  - Nystagmus
  - Positive fistula test
- *Treatment:*
  - Radical mastoidectomy in case of a fistula or serous labyrinthitis. In case of severe disabling vertigo (suppurative labyrinthitis), a labyrinthectomy is required.
  - Systemic antibiotics.
- Petrositis and Gradenigo's syndrome: This occurs when the cells of the petrous apex are involved due to spread of infection from the middle ear. The cells may coalesce to form an abscess. Localised meningitis may occur or an extradural abscess may occur. The VIth cranial nerve which supplies the ipsilateral lateral rectus muscle of the eye is involved in infection as it passes near the petrous apex and this results in the Gradenigo's syndrome (Fig. 12.9).
  - *Clinical features:* The Gradenigo's syndrome is a triad of symptoms comprising of:
    - Otorrhoea and mastoiditis,
    - Retro-orbital pain and deep temporal headache,
    - Paralysis of sixth cranial nerve and diplopia.
  - *Treatment:*
    - Radical mastoidectomy with drainage of the abscess from the petrous portion of the temporal bone.
    - Systemic antibiotics.

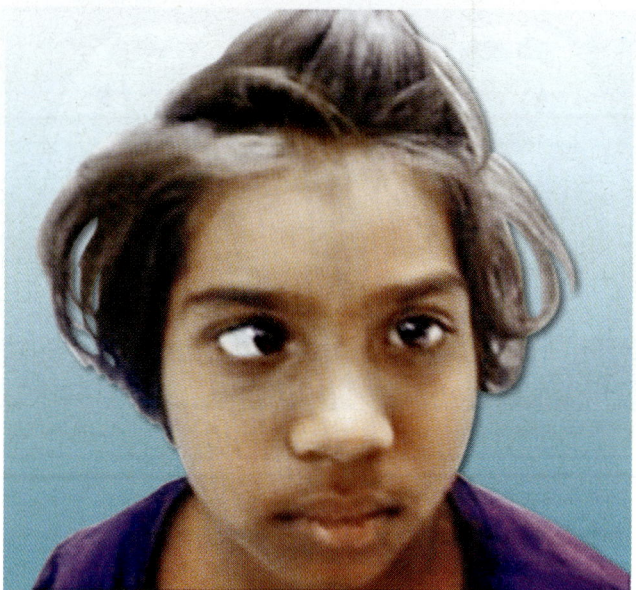

Fig. 12.9: Gradenigo's syndrome

- Facial nerve paralysis: Can occur due to (Fig. 12.10):
  - Direct involvement of the facial nerve in the middle ear or mastoid region either if the nerve is dehiscent or due to erosion of the facial canal. This is the common mode of involvement of the nerve, and results in ipsilateral infranuclear palsy.
  - Involvement of higher centres in case of a temporal lobe abscess. This is not very common and when it occurs, results in a supranuclear palsy on the opposite side.

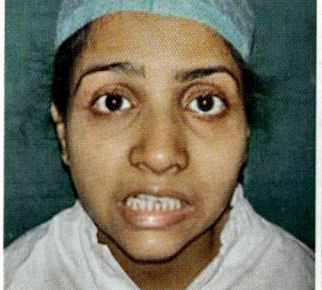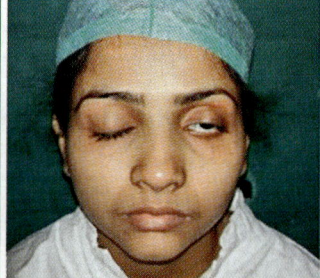

Fig. 12.10: Facial palsy

Treatment:
- *Supranuclear palsy:* Treatment is same as for temporal lobe abscess since this is the aetiology of the palsy.
- *Infranuclear palsy:* Mastoidectomy with facial nerve decompression at the earliest.

Ear

CHAPTER 13

Facial Nerve Paralysis

DEFINITION

Facial nerve paralysis is the paralysis of the VIIth cranial nerve (facial nerve).

CLASSIFICATION

- Supranuclear palsy.
- Infranuclear palsy due to lesions affecting the nerve after it emerges from the brain at the cerebello-pontine (CP) angle.

  It is a flaccid paralysis of the face on the side of the lesion including the upper portion of the face which is usually spared in a supranuclear palsy.

APPLIED ANATOMY

The facial nerve is the only cranial nerve in the body with the longest course through a bony canal (Fig. 13.1). Because of this, it is more prone to damage and compression due to disease or trauma.

It emerges from the CP angle and traverses a short course to enter the internal acoustic meatus. Here, it runs along with the VIIIth cranial nerve. It emerges from the internal auditory canal in its labyrinthine part when the geniculate ganglion gives out a branch (greater superficial petrosal nerve) and then the nerve turns at the first genu to enter the middle ear. It runs horizontally above the promontary on the medial wall of the middle ear in its tympanic course. Then, it turns downward behind the oval window at the second genu to run in its mastoid course. The nerve then, emerges into the neck after passing through the stylomastoid foramen to supply the following:

- Motor fibres to the muscles of facial expression, stylohyoid muscle, digastric muscle, buccinator and stapedius muscles.
- Secretomotor (parasympathetic) fibres to the lacrimal and nasal glands and the submandibular and sublingual salivary glands.
- Taste fibres to the anterior two-thirds of the tongue.

Labyrinthine segment	:	After leaving the internal acaustic meatus to the first genu.
Tympanic/ Horizontal segment	:	From first genu to second genu.
Mastoid/Vertical segment	:	From second genu to stylomastoid foramen.

It can be divided anatomically into three parts:

Intracranial course	:	From CP angle to geniculate ganglion.
Intratemporal course	:	From geniculate ganglion to stylomastoid foramen.
Extratemporal course	:	From stylomastoid foramen onwards in the neck and face.

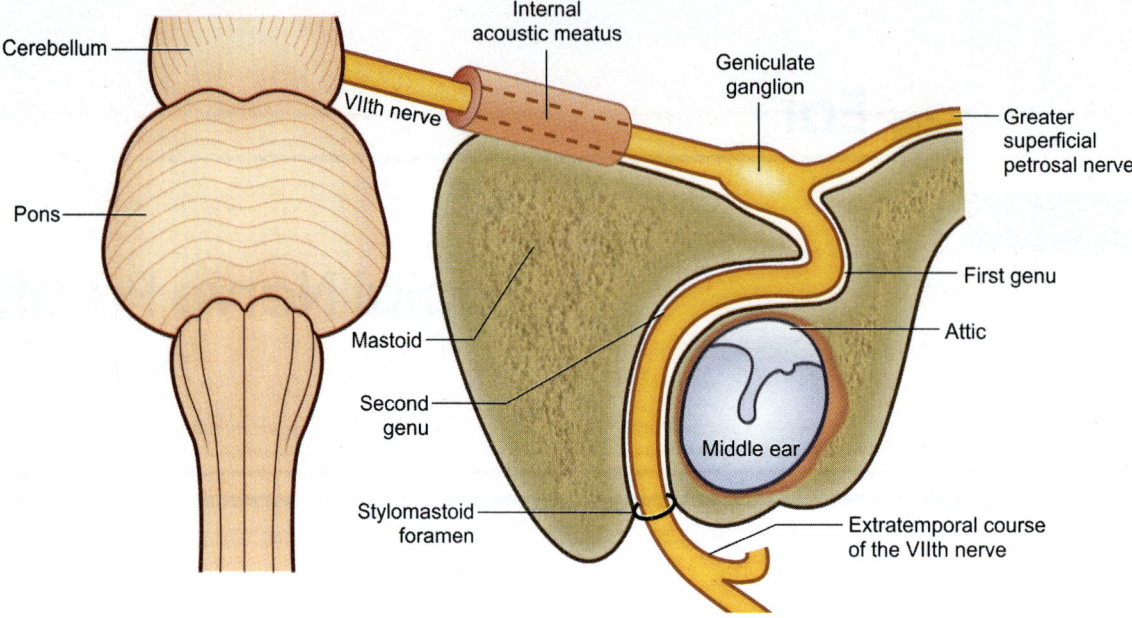

Fig. 13.1: Diagrammatic representation of the course of the facial nerve

FACIAL PALSY

- Classification: A broad classification of facial palsy is shown in the form of a Flowchart 13.1.
- Branches of facial nerve
    - Greater superficial petrosal nerve
    - Chorda tympani nerve
    - Nerve to stapedius
    - Sensory branch to EAC
    - Nerve to stylohoid muscle ⎤
    - Nerve to posterior belly of ⎬ After its exit from the stylomastoid foramen
      digastric muscle ⎪
    - Nerve to postauricular ⎦
      muscles

- Temporal branch ⎤
- Zygomatic branch ⎪
- Buccal branch ⎬ Terminal branches
- Marginal mandibular branch ⎪
- Cervical branch to platysma ⎦

- Aetiology:
    - Congenital or palsy at birth
    - Traumatic
    - Neoplastic
    - Inflammatory / Infective.
    - Idiopathic.

Flowchart 13.1: Classification of facial palsy

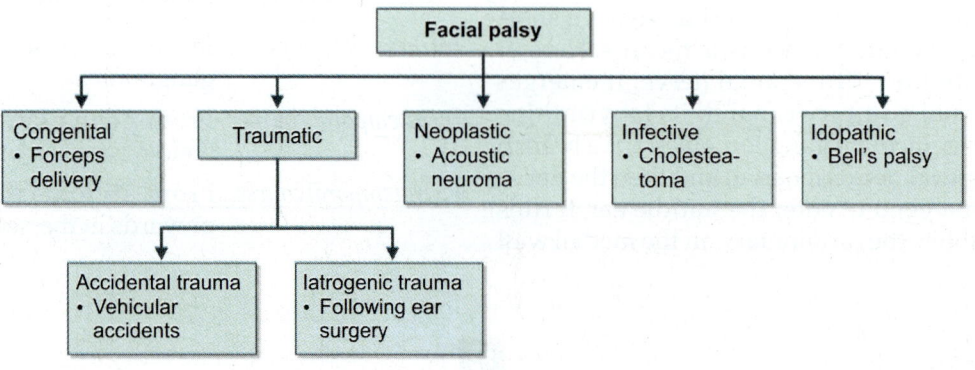

- Congenital causes or causes at birth
  - Moebius' syndrome
  - Forceps delivery
  - Trauma during delivery
- Traumatic causes
  - *Accidental trauma*
    - Vehicular accident
    - Head injury with fracture of temporal bone
    - Fall on head
    - Penetrating injury to middle ear
    - Barotrauma
      - high altitudes
      - scuba diving
  - *Iatrogenic trauma*
    - Following surgery on the ear and mastoid bone e.g. mastoidectomy, tympanoplasty, etc.
    - Following surgery of the neck and face like parotidectomy, dental or mandibular surgery.
- Neoplastic causes
  - Acoustic neuroma (VIIIth cranial nerve tumour usually occurring in the IAM).
  - Facial nerve neuroma.
  - Carcinoma of middle ear.
  - Malignant otitis externa (seen in elderly diabetics) not a true neoplasm, but an inflammatory condition.
  - Von Recklinghausen's disease.
- Inflammatory/Infective
  - Unsafe CSOM
  - Cholesteatoma
    - granulations
  - Mastoiditis
  - ASOM
  - Herpes zoster oticus (Ramsay Hunt syndrome).
  - Mumps
  - Tuberculosis
  - Mucormycosis
  - Syphilis
  - Leprosy
  - Malaria
- Idiopathic: Also known as Bell's palsy, the exact aetiology of this is not known.

Five common causes of infranuclear facial palsy in clinical practice

- Bell's palsy (Idiopathic)
- Head injury
- Unsafe CSOM
- Postoperative (Iatrogenic)
- Acoustic neuroma.

BELL'S PALSY

Synonym

- Idiopathic facial palsy
- This is the commonest type of facial nerve palsy seen in clinical practice.

Aetiology   The exact cause is not known.

- Age: It is common in the third and fourth decades of life.
- Sex: It is seen equally in both sexes.
- Ischaemic theory: It could be due to vasospasm of the blood vessels supplying the facial nerve near the stylomastoid foramen. This results in ischaemia of the nerve and subsequent palsy. This can occur due to exposure to extreme cold or chill winds. Vasospasm → ischaemia → oedema of the nerve → compression of the nerve in the rigid bony canal → more ischaemia.
- Viral theory: It has been thought to be of viral origin.
- Allergic theory: Allergy is thought to be a probable cause.
- Autoimmune disease is also thought to be a cause.

Pathophysiology   The commonly accepted theory of causation is that of autonomic imbalance, vasospasm primary ischaemia oedema of the facial nerve compression of the nerve in the rigid canal compression of the perineural vascular plexus secondary ischaemia worsening of the oedema and palsy.

Clinical features   The patient usually gives a history of exposure to cold like a cold blast of air on the face while travelling in a vehicle or washing the face with cold water followed by onset of facial palsy (Fig. 13.2):

- The onset is sudden.
- Dull pain in retroauricular region may be present.
- Involvement of one half of the face with inability to close the eye and upward movement of the eyeball on attempting closure of the eye (Bell's phenomenon).
- Inability to wrinkle the forehead on affected side.
- Epiphora due to:
  - Reflex increase in the secretions of the secretory glands due to exposure of sclera as a result of inability to close the eye, and
  - Eversion of lower eyelid due to palsy resulting in improper drainage of lacrimal fluid into the lower lacrimal punctum.
- Angle of the mouth deviates to the normal side of the face.
- Drooping of the angle of the mouth.
- Dribbling of saliva and liquids on attempts to drink.

- Collection of food in cheek as a result of paralysis of buccinator muscle and inability to blow or whistle.
- Loss of taste may be present due to involvement of the chorda tympani nerve.
- Hyperacusis may be present due to stapedius muscle palsy.
- Hearing is normal as seen on testing with tuning fork.
- Tympanic membrane is normal or occasionally there may be congestion of the chorda tympani nerve.

Site of lesion　　The exact site of lesion in Bell's palsy is not known. Previously, it was thought to be at the stylomastoid foramen or in the labyrinthine segment of the nerve. However, the recent thought is that there are multiple sites of involvement with 'skip areas' of normal nerve tissue in between. On this theory, the principle for decompression of the nerve from the labyrinthine segment to the stylomastoid foramen is based.

Prognosis　　Most cases of Bell's palsy recover with medical line of treatment within 3–6 weeks. Almost all cases of partial paresis recover completely.

Investigations in a case of facial palsy

- **Pure tone audiometry:** It reveals normal hearing in Bell's palsy, conductive deafness in CSOM or middle ear tumours and nerve deafness in mumps or acoustic neuroma.
- **Impedence audiometry and stapedial (acoustic) reflex:** These are to be performed only in Bell's palsy. Impedence audiometry is within normal limits and acoustic reflex is absent due to involvement of nerve to stapedius muscle.
- **The presence of stapedial (acoustic) reflex:** It is usually the first sign of recovery in Bell's palsy.
- **CT scan of the brain and temporal bone:** This helps to locate the site of lesion in tumours or trauma.
- **X-ray of the mastoid:** It is done in case of cholesteatoma or tumours of the middle ear and mastoid.
- **Facial nerve function tests**
  - *Electrodiagnostic tests:* These are the most important and reliable. These tests helps to test nerve conduction and status of the muscles supplied. These are of prognostic value.
    - Electromyography (EMG)
    - Strength–duration curve (SD curve)
    - Nerve excitability test (NET)
    - Electroneuronography (ENoG): This is the most recent test and most accurate.
  - *Topognostic tests:* These are of diagnostic value to detect the site of lesion. These include:
    - Schirmer's or Lacrimation test

- Test for taste or electrogustometry
- Salivatory flow tests
- Stapedial/Acoustic reflex, earliest indication of recovery of function

Treatment of facial palsy　　(1) Medical/conservative; (2) surgical, and (3) treatment of the cause of palsy.

- **Medical/Conservative treatment:**
  - *Steroids:* Oral prednisolone 40–60 mg daily in four divided doses and tapered off gradually over 2 weeks. They help by reducing the oedema.
  - *Vasodilators:* These help to reduce the vasospasm, e.g. intravenous or oral nicotinic acid derivatives.
  - *Vitamins:* Vit. B1, B6, B12 injections or orally.
  - *Care of the eye* with a pad bandage at night, dark glasses during the day and antibiotic eye drops to prevent exposure keratitis and corneal ulcers.

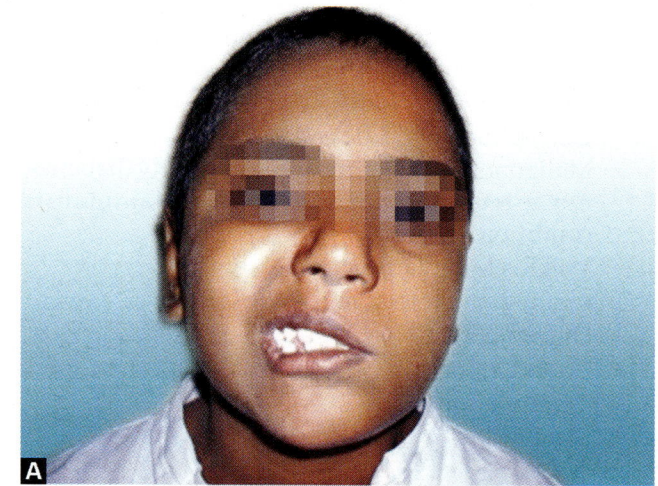

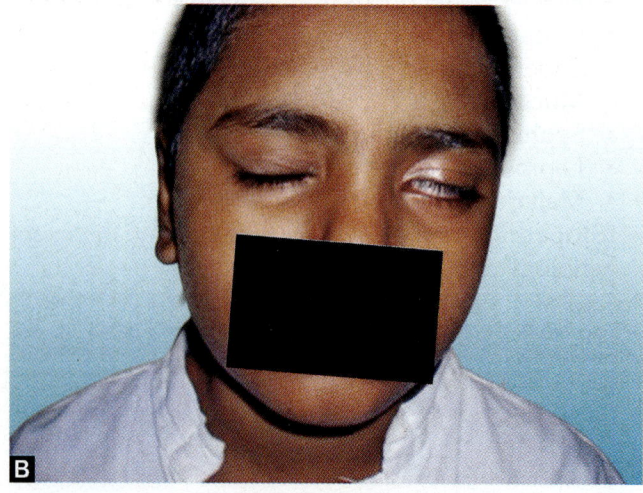

Fig. 13.2A and B: Facial palsy (Left)

- *Physiotherapy*
  - Active exercises
  - Passive physiotherapy in the form of massage and electrical stimulation of muscles
  - Short wave diathermy.
- Surgical treatment: In a case of Bell's palsy, if there is no recovery within 6–8 weeks with medical line of treatment, surgical decompression of the nerve is performed.

  A cortical mastoidectomy is performed with a posterior tympanotomy and the nerve is decompressed completely by removing the roof and the lateral walls of the fallopian (facial) canal from the labyrinthine segment (i.e. internal auditory meatus) to the stylomastoid foramen.

  Decompression is done also in case of post-traumatic palsy and palsy due to other causes or if facial palsy fails to recover in 6–8 weeks with medical line of treatment.

  Plastic surgery may be required, if the palsy is of several years duration for cosmetic improvement and protection to the eye.
- Treatment of the cause is of primary importance in case the cause is known.

CHAPTER **14**

Meniere's Disease

DEFINITION

Meniere's disease is a disease characterised by a triad of symptoms, which consist of vertigo, tinnitus, and fluctuating deafness.

- It is one of the commonest causes of otogenic vertigo.
- American academy of ophthalmology and otolaryngology [AAOO (1972)], defined Meniere's as committee on equilibrium.
- It is a disease of membranous inner ear characterized by deafness. Vertigo and tinnitus have their pathologic correlate in hydropic distention of endolymphatic system.

  Synonym: Endolymphatic hydrops.

AETIOLOGY

The exact aetiology is not known, but various factors are considered.

- Age: Common after third decade of life.
- Sex: Male:Female = 1:1.
- Endolymphatic hydrops → decrease in blood supply to the labyrinth → reduced absorption of endolymph. Due to ischaemia of endolymphatic sac → increased tension of endolymph in the labyrinth → distension of the endolymphatic system.
- Vasospasm reduced blood supply to the labyrinth.
- Vasomotor → imbalance due to sympathetic over-activity → spasm of internal auditory artery and/or its branches (thus interfering with functions of cochlear or vestibular nerve epithelium) →

anoxia of capillaries of stria vascularis → increased permeability transudation of fluid → increased production of endolymph.

- Histamine sensitivity → allergen food stuff or inhalant → excessive production of endolymph.
- Water and electrolyte imbalance in endolymph.
- Autoimmune disorders
- Viral cause
- Metabolic disorders, carbohydrate metabolism disorder.
- Hypothyroidism about 3% of cases of Meniere's disease are due to hypothyroidism.
- Hypoadrenalism and hypopituitarism, inadequate function of pituitary and adrenals are responsible for about 6% of the cases.
- Syphilis and cochlear otosclerosis can also produce endolymphatic hydrops.

PATHOPHYSIOLOGY

Ischaemia → reduced absorption of endolymph → increased volume of endolymph distension of the membranous labyrinth. The membranous labyrinth may rupture resulting in a chemical imbalance which may damage the organ of Corti and vestibular epithelium.

CLINICAL FEATURES

- Age of onset is 35–50 years.
- The disease is usually unilateral, but becomes bilateral later.

- It is characterised by a feeling of fullness in the ear, tinnitus, rotatory vertigo, nausea, occasionally vomiting and fluctuating deafness.
- The attacks initially occur at long intervals and subsequently increase in intensity and frequency.
- The duration of these attacks is for a few hours or even for a few days.
- During the interval between attacks the patient is normal and his/her hearing is normal.
- Nystagmus is seen during the attacks.
- The deafness is of the sensorineural type.
- Initially tinnitus disappears after the attack, but later, it becomes continuous.
- Perspiration, gastric upset and diarrhoea occur due to vagal stimulation. The patient looks anxious and may have hypotension during the attack.

INVESTIGATIONS

- Tuning fork tests will reveal sensorineural deafness.
- Pure tone audiometry, reveals sensorineural deafness in the low frequencies initially. It is normal in between attacks. Later, sensorineural deafness is seen in both low and high frequencies and may not disappear in between attacks.
- Recruitment tests are positive for the affected ear.
- Vestibular function tests reveal canal paresis on the affected side.
- Short increment sensitivity index (SISI): SISI score is better than 70% in two-thirds of patients.
- Electrocochleography is diagnostic. Normally, ratio of summating potential (SP) to action potential (AP) is 20%. In Meniere's disease SP/AP ratio is greater than 30%.
- Glycerol test during pure tone audiometry reveals transient improvement of hearing on taking glycerol orally. This is characteristic of Meniere's disease. Glycerol is a dehydrating agent. When given orally, it reduces endolymphatic pressure. Dose is 1.5 mL/mg.
- Bekesy audiometry shows a type II tracing.

DIFFERENTIAL DIAGNOSIS

- Labyrinthitis
- Acoustic neuroma
- Ototoxicity
- Trauma to labyrinth due to head injury
- Perilymph fistula

VARIANTS OF MENIERE'S DISEASE

- Cochlear hydrops: Here, only the cochlear symptoms, and signs of Meniere's disease are present. Vertigo is absent. It is only after several years that vertigo will make its appearance.
- Vestibular hydrops: Patients get typical attacks of episodic vertigo, while cochlear functions remain normal. It is only with time that a typical picture of Meniere's disease will develop.
- Lermoyez syndrome: Here, symptoms of Meniere's disease are in reverse order. First, there is progressive deterioration of hearing followed by an attack of vertigo, at which time the hearing recovers.

Secondary Meniere's disease   Endolymphatic hydrops with clinical picture resembling Meniere's disease has been observed in congenital or acquired syphilis, otosclerosis, Paget's diseases, and post-stapedectomy patients.

TREATMENT

Conservative   Aims to preserve hearing and control.

Destructive   Aims at eradication of vertigo and tinnitus vertigo and tinnitus at the cost of hearing.

Conservative Treatment
- Medical treatment.
- Labyrinthine exercises.
- General treatment.
- Conservative surgery.
- Medical treatment
  - *During the attack*
    - Complete bed rest.
    - Labyrinthine sedatives given systemically, injections stemetil or largactil or avomine or dramamine.
    - Vasodilators systemically, inhalation of carbagen (95% O_2 + 5 CO_2)
    - Nicotinic acid derivatives are used.
    - This is of empirical value.
    - Intravenous fluids
    - Histamine drip: Intravenous drip of 1 mL histamine (1:1000) in 1 pint of 5% dextrose is administered.
    - Diuretics are administered.
    - Tranquillizers, such as diazepam help to relieve anxiety and functional overlay.
    - Recently, betahistine dihydrochloride is considered to be most effective, as it acts by local vasodilation of the inner ear vessels (stria vascularis) and hence helps in rapid absorption of endolymph.

- ◆ *In between attacks*
  - Reassurance of patient and relatives
  - Salt and fluid restricted diet
  - Oral betahistine dihydrochloride (8 mg), 3 times a day
  - Oral vasodilators
  - Vitamin B1, B6, B12 orally
  - Oral diuretics
  - Caution the patient not to drive or swim
  - Histamine desensitization
  - Avoid carbohydrate rich diet
  - Diuretics furesamide 40 mg every alternate day with potassium supplements
  - Elimination of allergen
  - If hypothyroidism, hypopituitarism or hypo-adrenalism is found to be cause appropriate replacement therapy.
- Labyrinthine exercises: Cooksey–Cawthorne's head and neck exercises are taught to patients to help the normal labyrinth to adapt.
- General treatment
  - ◆ Stop smoking
  - ◆ Stop alcohol
  - ◆ Removal of septic foci if present.
- Conservative surgery
  - ◆ Stellate ganglion block
  - ◆ Cervical sympathectomy
  - ◆ Endolymphatic sac decompression
  - ◆ *Shunt operations like:*
    - Endolymphatic, mastoid shunt
    - Endolymphatic, subarachnoid shunt.

Destructive Surgery

- Partial destruction of the labyrinth by ultrasono-graphy or cryosurgery.
- Destruction of the labyrinth by laser
- Labyrinthectomy
- Vestibular nerve section.

MENIETT DEVICE

This is a device that is used for the treatment of Meniere's disease.

It employs intermittent micropressure therapy for the treatment of the same.

Initially a ventilation tube (grommed) is inserted in the posteroinferior quadrant (overlying the round window membrane).

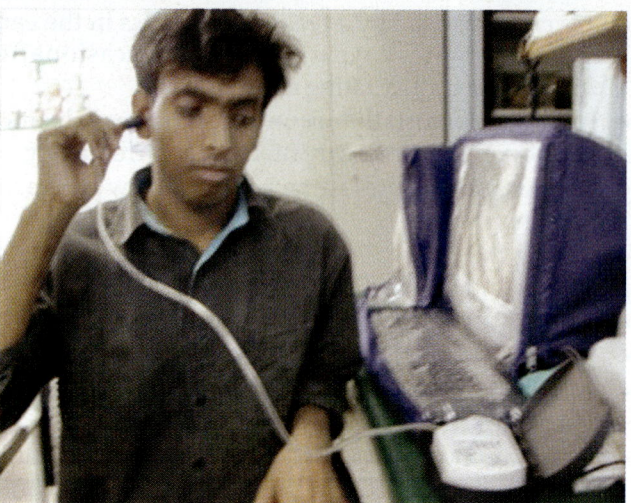

Fig. 14.1: Using a Meniett device

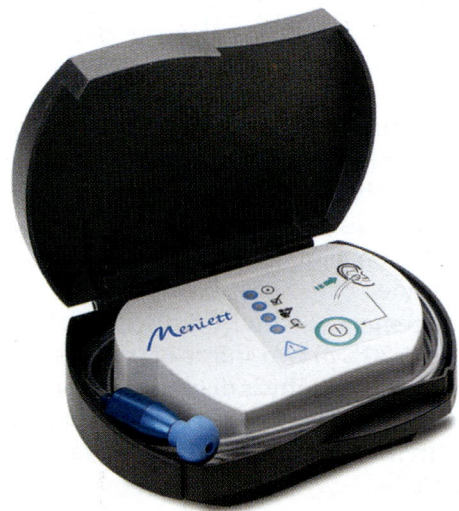

Fig. 14.2: Meniett device

Following that the Meniett device is used for a few minutes daily (at least 3–4 times).

The pressure impulses are transmitted via the ventilation tube, to the middle ear, from the middle ear to the round window membrane and forward to the perilymphatic and endolymphatic spaces.

It causes a redistribution of the endolymph in an attempt to dissipate the raised endolymphatic pressure.

It is given on an outpatient basis as the device is portable, and can be recommended for patients who stop responding to medical therapy, before considering any surgical procedure, which are usually of a permanent nature.

CHAPTER 15

Otosclerosis

INTRODUCTION

Otosclerosis is a disease that exclusively affects the human temporal bone.

DEFINITION

Otosclerosis is characterised by fixation of stapes footplate in the oval window, due to deposition of new-bone in the annular ligament of the stapes. The deposition of new-bone may also extend to the bony walls of the cochlea. It is a pathology, which characteristically affects the bone of the otic capsule.

AETIOLOGY

- **Age:** Most common in the second or third decade of life.
- **Sex:** It is very common in females and increases during pregnancy.
- **Heredity:** Fifty percent of cases have hereditary etiology.
- **Genetic/Racial factors:** It is common in white races and less common in Negros and Mongoloids. In India, it is most common in South Indians.
- **Blood group:** In a family usually affected members have same blood group.
- **Hormonal factors:** As it is more common in females specially during pregnancy, it is thought that hormonal factors play an important role in its aetiology.

- **Metabolic theory:** Disturbances of calcium metabolism are thought to be responsible for this disease.
- **Generalised osseous disease**
  - *Van-der-Hoeve Syndrome*: In this, otosclerosis is associated with:
    - Blue sclera, and
    - Osteogenesis imperfecta.
  - *Osteitis deformans:* Conductive deafness may be a feature of this disease.
- **Viral etiology:** It is suggested that a possible persistent measles virus infection similar to what occurs in the central nervous system in subacute sclerosing encephalitis could result in otosclerosis later in life.
- **Autoimmune:** Humoral autoimmunity to type II collagen has been implicated in the aetiology.
- **Biochemical factors or cytokines** are thought to arrest the secondary remodelling process in the otic capsule. Reactivation could result in otosclerosis.

PATHOLOGY

In otosclerosis, mature lameller bone is removed by osteoclasts and replaced by immature spongy bone of increased thickness, vascularity and cellularity. It affects the middle layer of the otic capsule.

Site/Types   Most common site is annular ligament of oval window, which leads to conductive deafness (stapedial otosclerosis). The process may spread to bony capsule of the labyrinth, which results in sensori-neural deafness (cochlear otosclerosis).

TYPES OF OTOSCLEROSIS

- **Stapedial otosclerosis:** Stapedial otosclerosis causing stapes fixation and conductive deafness is the most common variety. Here, the lesion starts first in front of the oval window in an area called 'fissula ante fenestram'. This is the site of predilection (anterior focus). The lesion may start behind the oval window (posterior focus), around margins of the stapes footplate (circumferential) in the footplate, but annular ligament being free (biscuit type). Sometimes, it may completely obliterate the oval window niche (obliterative type).
- **Cochlear otosclerosis:** It involves region of round window or other areas in the otic capsule and may cause sensorineural. Hearing loss probably due to liberation of toxic materials into the inner ear fluid.
- **Histologic otosclerosis:** This type of otosclerosis remains asymptomatic and causes neither conductive nor sensorineural hearing loss.

CLINICAL FEATURES

Symptoms

- **Deafness:** It is presenting symptom, especially it increases in pregnancy. It is bilateral and paradoxically the patient hears better in noisy surroundings (Paracusis Willisi).
- **Tinnitus:** It is frequently the presenting symptom.
- **Giddiness:** It is rarely seen.

Signs

- Eardrums are normal, but in active otosclerosis which is fast growing, a pink to red colouration of the eardrum (flamingo blush) near the umbo is seen due to presence of neo-vascularisation of the promontory (Schwartze sign).
- Eustachian tubes, nose, and throat are normal.

INVESTIGATIONS

- **Tuning fork tests:** Reveal bilaterally symmetrical conductive hearing loss and in cases with cochlear involvement, there is mixed hearing loss. In advanced cases, rarely there is severe sensorineural hearing loss.
- **Pure tone audiometry:** It confirms the results of tuning fork tests, i.e. bilaterally symmetrical conductive hearing loss/mixed hearing loss. It may show a Carhart's notch (Fig. 15.1), which is characterised by slight reduction (5–10 dB) in bone conduction at 2000 Hz. This is because of increase in the mass of the stapes footplate.
- **Impedance audiometry:** It shows normal middle ear pressure with reduced compliance. Stapedial reflex is absent. This is bilateral in majority of cases.

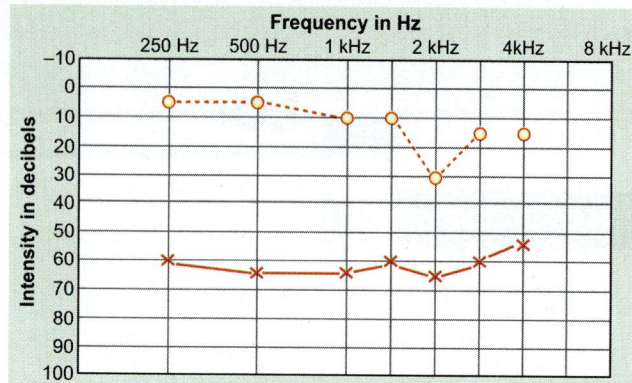

Fig. 15.1: Pure tone audiogram showing the characteristic Carhart's notch in bone conduction in a case of otosclerosis

DIFFERENTIAL DIAGNOSIS

Ossicular immobility

- **Congenital fixation of stapedial footplate:** Deafness is present since birth.
- **Tympanosclerosis:** It is characterised by the presence of white plaques in the eardrum and on the ossicles due to hyalin deposits, which may follow the healing of chronic suppurative otitis media. It may cause ossicular fixation.
- **Chronic adhesive otitis media,** i.e. stage IV atelectasis.

Ossicular discontinuity

- Head injury may cause incudostapedial joint dislocation.
- Chronic otitis media.

Generalised bone diseases

- Van der Hoeve's syndrome
- **Paget's disease:** When temporal bone is involved.

Middle ear infections

- Chronic otitis media with healed perforation
- Eustachian tube catarrah
- **Chronic secretory otitis media:** It is common in children, the eardrum is normal and a fluid level may be seen. Impedance audiometry and ear microscopy confirm the diagnosis.

TREATMENT

Medical

- **Sodium fluoride** 20 mg orally thrice a day is recommended for patients in whom surgery is contra-indicated. It has side-effects, like gastritis and fluorosis.
- **Hearing aid:** It is advised for patients who do not benefit from surgery or who are not willing for surgery or when surgery is contraindicated.

Surgical   Stapedotomy is the treatment of choice.

CHAPTER 16

Anatomy of the Nose and Paranasal Sinuses

THE NOSE

EXTERNAL NOSE

The shape of the external nose is pyramidal. It has a bony and cartilagenous supporting framework, which is derived from the nasal capsule.

The bony framework is formed by the following bones:
- The nasal bones
- The nasal processes of the frontal bones
- The frontal processes of the maxillae.

The cartilagenous framework is formed by:
- Paired upper lateral cartilages
- Paired lower lateral cartilages (alar cartilages)
- Quadrangular septal cartilage (in midline).

The upper bony part of the dorsum of the nose is called the bridge. The lower cartilagenous part forms alar folds which contain alar cartilages called alae nasi. The lower free border of nasal septum forms the columella which separates the anterior nares.

- Blood supply
  - Facial artery
  - External nasal branch of the ophthalmic artery
  - Infraorbital artery.
- Venous drainage
  - Facial vein
  - Ophthalmic vein.
- Lymphatic drainage
  - Preauricular lymphnodes
  - Submandibular lymphnodes.

NASAL CAVITIES

The nasal septum divides the nasal cavity into two halves (Fig. 16.1). Each nasal cavity communicates with:
- The exterior, through the anterior nares
- The nasopharynx, through the posterior-nares (choana)
- The paranasal sinuses, through their ostia.

Each nasal cavity is bounded by the floor, roof, medial wall, and lateral wall.

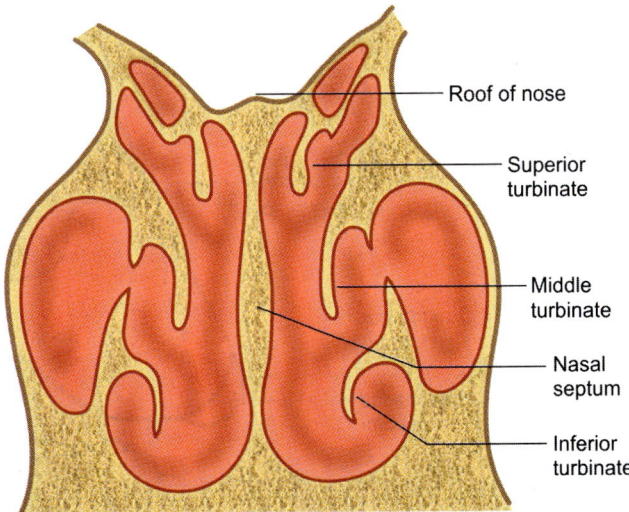

Fig. 16.1: Diagrammatic representation of coronal section through the nasal cavities

Development   Nose develops from the frontonasal process. Olfactory placodes on the frontonasal process become depressed to form the olfactory pit, which forms the nasal cavity. Primitive nasal septum divides the nasal cavity.

Paranasal sinus   The paranasal sinuses develop as the out-pouching of the nasal mucosa. The maxillary sinus is present at birth. It is fully developed after the eruption of the second molar tooth.

FLOOR

The nasal cavity is wide across the floor. The floor separates the nasal cavity from oral cavity. It is formed by:
- Anterior three-fourths by the palatine processes of the maxillae.
- Posterior one-fourth by the horizontal plates of the palatine bones.

ROOF

The roof is narrow, about 5 mm in width. It is concave in the anteroposterior direction. The roof separates the nasal cavity from the cranial cavity.

     It is formed by:
- Nasal bones and the supporting nasal septum forming the anterior sloping portion.
- Cribriform plate of the ethmoid in the centre.
- Floor of the sphenoid sinus forming the posterior sloping portion.

MEDIAL WALL

Nasal septum   It forms the medial wall of the nasal cavities (Fig. 16.2). It is formed by:
- Quadrilateral cartilage anteriorly
- Perpendicular plate of the ethmoid posterosuperiorly
- Vomer posteroinferiorly.

The **nasal septum articulates:**
- Anteriorly with
  - Nasal bones
  - Nasal spine of the frontal bone.
- Superiorly with
  - Rostrum of the sphenoid.
- Inferiorly with
  - Anterior nasal spine of the maxilla
  - Nasal crest of the maxilla
  - Nasal crest of the palatine bones.

The **nasal septum is divided into** three parts:
- Bony part
- Cartilagenous part
- Membraneous part which is the anteriormost portion lined by the skin.

LATERAL WALL

It is formed by the following bones (Fig. 16.3).
- Anteriorly
  - Medial (inner) aspect of the nasal bones
  - Frontal process of the maxilla
  - Anterior part of the body of the maxilla.

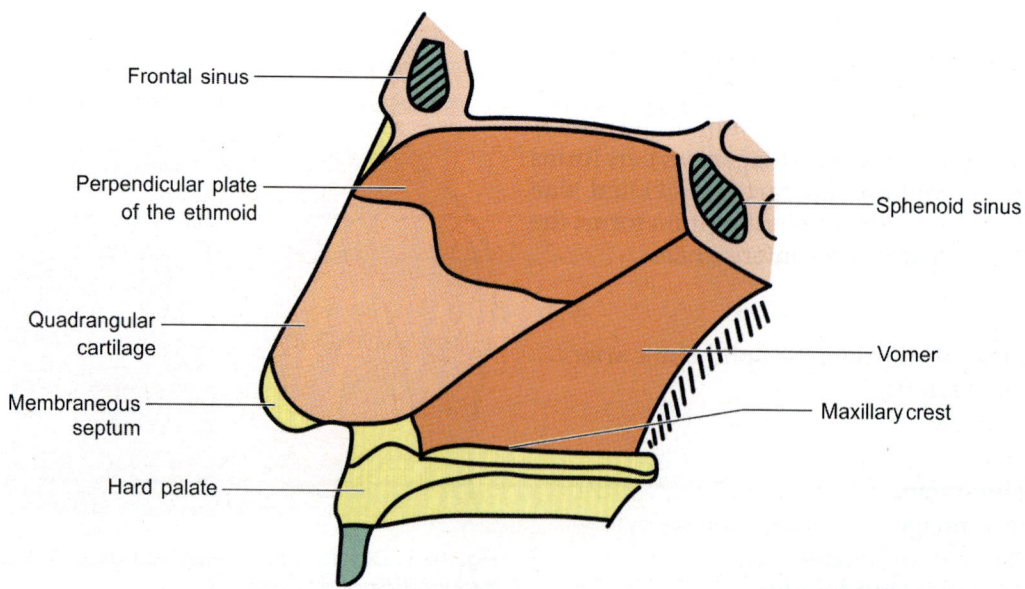

Fig. 16.2: Diagrammatic representation of the nasal septum and medial wall of the nose

- In the centre
  - Medial wall of the ethmoid in upper part.
  - Medial wall of the maxilla in the middle part.
  - Inferior turbinate in the lower part.
- Posteriorly
  - Perpendicular plate of the palatine bone.
  - Medial pterygoid plate.

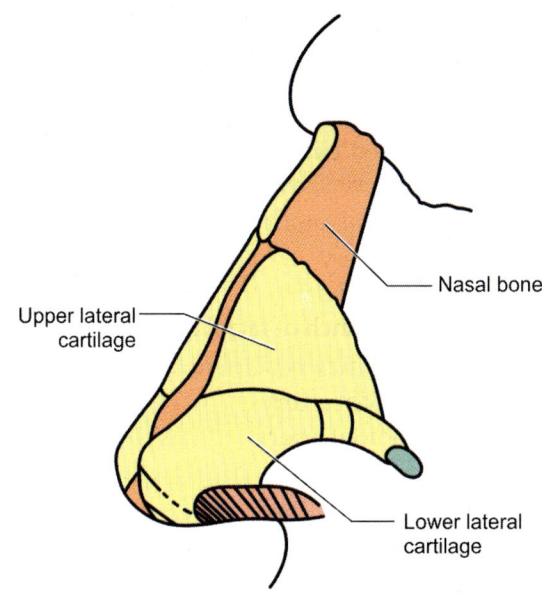

Fig. 16.3: Diagrammatic representation of the lateral nasal wall (nasal framework)

FEATURES OF THE LATERAL NASAL WALL

Nasal turbinates (conchae)   Lateral wall has a complex anatomical structure because of the presence of three shell-like projections directed downwards and medially (Fig. 16.4).

- **Superior turbinate:** It is a part of the ethmoid bone and is the smallest turbinate, situated about 1.25 cm below the cribriform plate.
- **Middle turbinate:** It is a part of the ethmoid bone. It extends anteriorly to articulate with frontal process of the maxilla. It extends posteriorly along the length of the lateral wall to the perpendicular plate of the ethmoid bone.
- **Inferior turbinate:** It is a separate bone. It extends from the body of the maxilla anteriorly and to the perpendicular plate of the palatine bone posteriorly.

Meatus   It is that space of the lateral nasal wall, which is overhung by the turbinates (Fig. 16.5).

- **Superior meatus:** It is the smallest meatus and has openings from the posterior ethmoid sinus.
- **Middle meatus:** It has following important landmarks and openings:
- **Uncinate process:** Sharp, curving ridge of bone projecting upwards from ethmoid.
  - *Bulla ethmoidalis:* It is a rounded projection produced by middle ethmoidal cells.

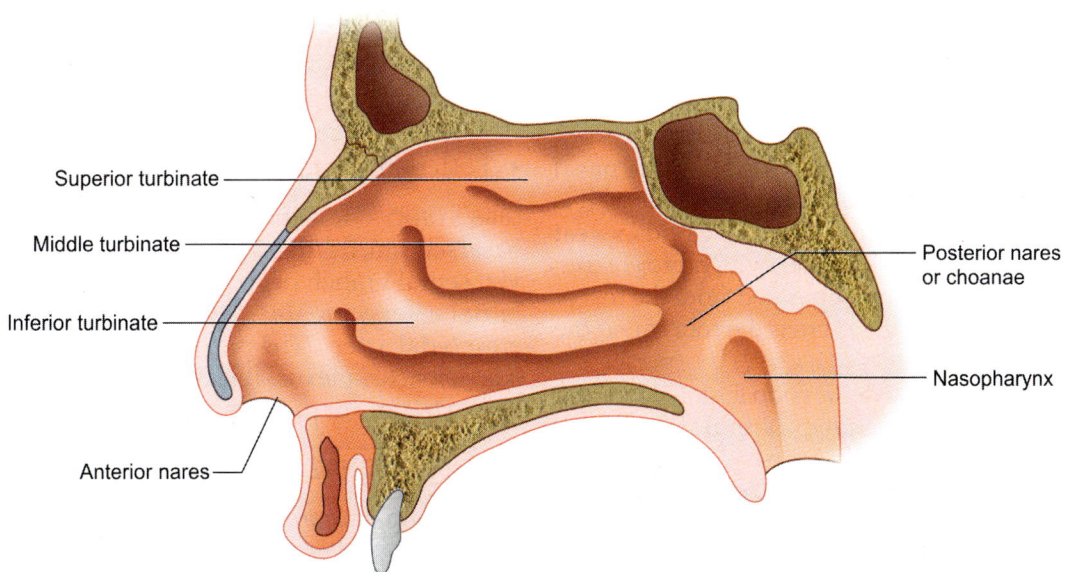

Fig. 16.4: Internal representation of the lateral wall of the nose

- *Hiatus semilunaris*: It is a semicircular fissure bounded by the edge of the uncinate process inferiorly and bulla ethmoidalis superiorly leading to the infundibulum.
- *Infundibulum*: It is a vertical groove between the lateral nasal wall and the uncinate process.
- *Opening of the*
  - Frontal sinus.
  - Maxillary sinus.
  - Anterior ethmoid sinus.
  - Middle ethmoid sinus.
- Inferior meatus: It is the largest meatus and the nasolacrimal duct opens into it.

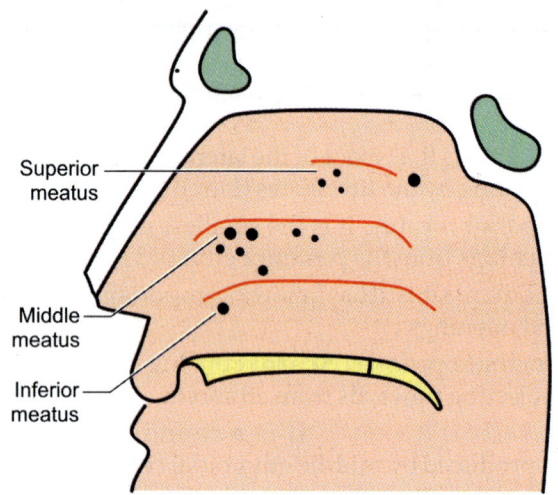

Superior meatus

Middle meatus

Inferior meatus

Fig. 16.5: Lateral wall of the nose showing the meatii (turbinates are removed)

Sphenoethmoidal recess   It is a small triangular depression present above and behind the superior turbinate. The sphenoid sinus opens in this recess.

Each nasal cavity can be divided into four parts:
- Vestibule: It is the anteriormost part of the nasal cavity, bounded laterally by the ala of the nose. It is lined by skin. Skin contains sebaceous glands, sweat glands, and stiff hair (vibrissae), which project into the vestibule. Vestibule is separated from the rest of the nasal cavity by a ridge across the roof called the limen nasi.
- Atrium: It is a shallow depression situated beyond the limen nasi. It lies anterior to the middle turbinate and below the ridge called agar nasi.
- Olfactory region: It is the upper part of nasal cavity in the region bounded by the roof, superior turbinate and upper one-third of the septum. It is lined by yellow olfactory neuroepithelium having bipolar sensory cells.

- Respiratory region: It includes the rest of the nasal cavity. It is lined by respiratory mucosa, which is formed by ciliated columnar epithelium. It is continuous with the mucosa of the sinuses, nasopharynx and Eustachian tube. The ciliary movements propel the nasal secretions backwards towards the choanae (posterior nares). Numerous goblet cells and secretory glands are present in the epithelium. The subepithelial tissue is very vascular and erectile, and it has functional importance in controlling nasal patency.

BLOOD SUPPLY

The nose is supplied by branches of the external and internal carotid arteries, which anastamose freely.

Branches of the external carotid artery
- Spehopalatine artery
- Greater palatine artery
- Superior labial branch of facial artery

Branches of the internal carotid artery
- Anterior ethmoidal artery
- Posterior ethmoidal artery

Blood supply of lateral wall
- Anterosuperior quadrant
  - Anterior ethmoidal artery
  - Posterior ethmoidal artery
- Anteroinferior quadrant
  - Superior labial branch of facial artery
  - Greater palatine artery
- Posterosuperior quadrant: Sphenopalatine artery
- Posteroinferior quadrant: Greater palatine artery

Blood supply of septum
- Anterosuperior part
  - Anterior ethmoidal artery.
  - Superior labial branch of facial artery.
- Posteroinferior part: Sphenopalatine artery.

Little's area   It is the anterior-inferior portion of the nasal septum. It is the site of anastomosis of four arteries viz. septal branch of sphenopalatine artery, superior labial artery, greater palatine artery, and anterior ethmoidal artery. The plexus, so formed is called the Kiesselbach's plexus. It is a common site for epistaxis due to trauma or picking of the nose (Fig. 16.6).

VENOUS DRAINAGE

- Sphenopalatine vein
- Anterior and posterior ethmoidal veins
- Anterior facial vein
- Cerebral veins

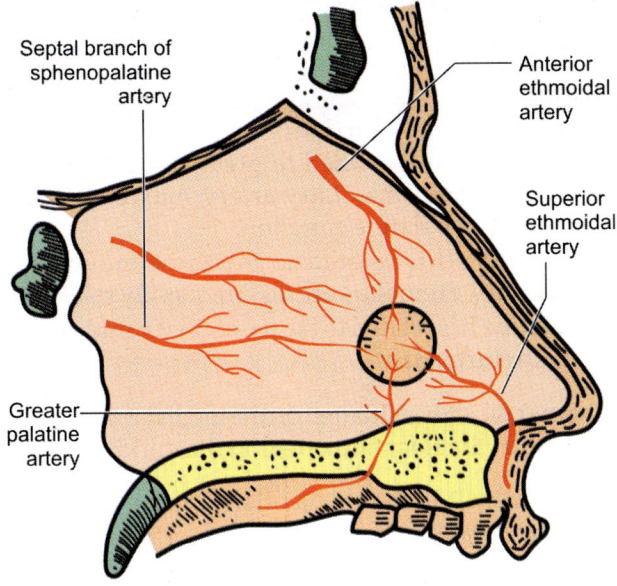

Fig. 16.6: Diagrammatic representation of the Little's area of the nasal septum

Flowchart 16.1: Components of autonomic nerve supply

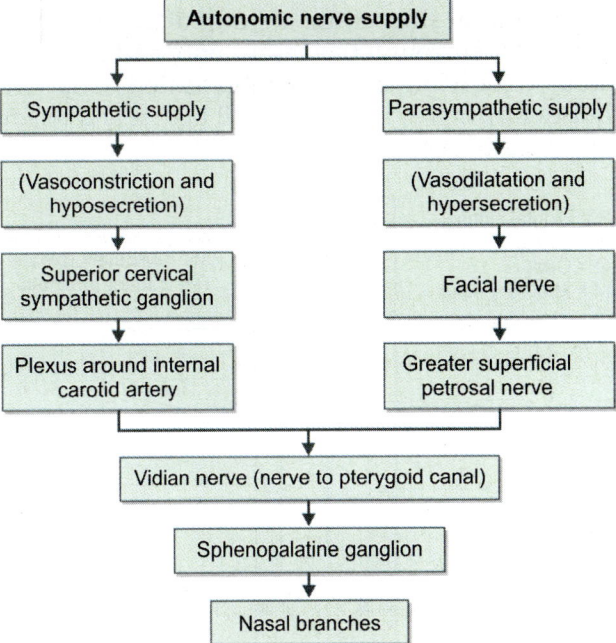

NERVE SUPPLY

Sensory

- **General sensory fibres** to the respiratory mucous membrane are supplied by the *trigeminal nerve* through the following branches:
  - *Ophthalmic division:* Anterior ethmoidal nerve supplies:
    - Anterosuperior part of septum
    - Anterosuperior quadrant of lateral nasal wall
  - *Maxillary division*
    - Anterior superior alveolar nerve supplies antero-inferior quadrant of lateral nasal wall
    - Branches of the sphenopalatine ganglion:
      - Greater palatine nerve
      - Short sphenopalatine nerve
      - Long sphenopalatine nerve
- **Olfactory nerves:** Carry the sense of smell.

Autonomic nerve supply Various components of autonomic nerve supply are shown in Flowchart 16.1.

LYMPHATIC DRAINAGE

External nose and anterior part of nose drain into the submandibular lymph nodes. Rest of the nasal cavity drains into the upper deep cervical lymph nodes.

APPLIED ANATOMY

- **Dangerous area of the face:** The lower part of external nose and the upper lip constitute the dangerous area of the face as infection may spread in a retrograde manner to the cavernous sinus through the inferior ophthalmic veins which do not have valves (Fig. 16.7).
- Nose is the most prominent feature of the face and as such is easily subject to **traumatic injury.**
- *Dangerous area of the nose:* The olfactory area of the nose may infect the meninges along the pia and anachnoid sheaths of the olfactory nerves passing through the cribriform plate of the ethmoid.

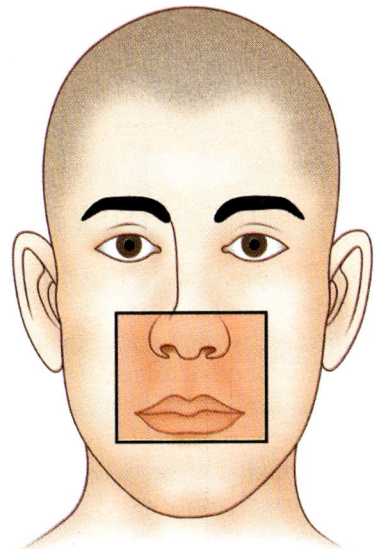

Fig. 16.7: Dangerous area of the face

PARANASAL SINUSES

The paranasal sinuses are a group of aircontaining spaces that surround the nasal cavity and are continuous with it through openings called ostia. The sinuses function to make the skull lighter and to add resonance to voice (Fig. 16.8).

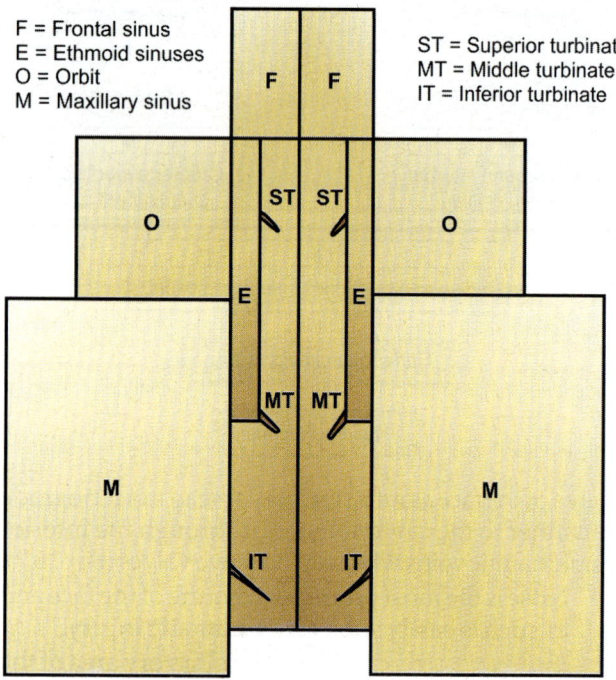

F = Frontal sinus
E = Ethmoid sinuses
O = Orbit
M = Maxillary sinus

ST = Superior turbinate
MT = Middle turbinate
IT = Inferior turbinate

Fig. 16.8: Diagrammatic representation of the paranasal sinuses

MAXILLARY SINUS (ANTRUM OF HIGHMORE)

It is the largest paranasal sinus and present within the body of the maxilla. It is pyramidal in shape. Capacity of adult maxillary sinus is approximately 15 cc.

Boundaries
- Apex: It lies in zygomatic process and directed laterally.
- Medial wall: It forms the base of the pyramid and formed by lateral wall of nose.
- Roof: It is formed by the floor of the orbit. It slopes downwards from medial to lateral. It is very thin and grooved by the infraorbital nerve.
- Floor: It is formed by the alveolar process and palatine process of the maxilla. It lies at or above the level of the floor of the nasal cavity in a child, while in adults it is at a lower level.
- Anterior wall: It is formed by the anterior surface of the maxilla. It has the infraorbital foramen.

- Posterior wall: It is formed by the posterior surface of the maxilla.

Relations
- Superiorly: It is related to orbit.
- Posteriorly: It is related to pterygopalatine fossa, which contains maxillary artery, maxillary nerve, and pterygopalatine ganglion.
- Inferiorly: It is related to the three molar teeth constantly. Premolars are less frequently related.
- Medially: It is related to the nasal cavity, middle, and inferior turbinate.

Maxillary ostium It is situated on the medial wall at a level higher than the floor and opens in the middle meatus.

Blood supply It is by the maxillary, infraorbital, facial and greater palatine arteries.

Venous drainage
- Anterior facial vein
- Pterygoid plexus of veins

Nerve supply   Branches of the maxillary division of the trigeminal nerve:
- Superior alveolar nerves (anterior, middle, and posterior).
- Anterior palatine nerve
- Infraorbital nerve

Lymphatic drainage
- Retropharyngeal lymph nodes
- Submandibular lymph nodes

Applied anatomy
- Caldwell Luc operation should not be performed in patients under the age of 12 years till the second molar erupts. Otherwise, dentition may be affected due to damage to the root of the tooth.
- The pterygopalatine fossa can be approached through the maxillary sinus for:
  - Ligation of the maxillary artery
  - Vidian neurectomy
  - Ethmoid sinus surgery
  - Sphenoid sinus surgery
  - Pituitary gland excision

FRONTAL SINUS

The frontal sinuses are situated in the frontal bone and are considered to be the upward outgrowths of the anterior ethmoidal sinuses.

The shape of the sinus is like a pyramid with the apex pointing upwards and the base is formed by the floor. Normally, there are two frontal sinuses, which are of unequal size and separated by an intersinus bony septum.

Capacity of the sinus is approximately 7 cc in adults.

Boundaries
- **Anterior wall:** It is formed by outer table of frontal bone.
- **Posterior wall:** It is thin and separates the sinus from the cranial cavity, formed by the inner table of the frontal bone.
- **Floor:** It separates the sinus from the orbit.
- **Medial wall:** It forms a septum between the two frontal sinuses.

It **drains** through the frontonasal duct which passes through the anterior ethmoidal sinus and opens in the middle meatus.

Blood supply
- Supraorbital artery.
- Anterior ethmoidal artery.

Nerve supply   Supraorbital nerve.

Lymphatic drainage   Submandibular lymph nodes.

ETHMOID SINUSES

These are situated in the ethmoid bone between the nasal cavity and the orbit. Each sinus consists of 3–18 ethmoid air cells.

Ethmoid air cells can be divided into two groups (Fig. 16.9):
- Anterior ethmoid group, which include the anterior and middle ethmoid sinuses.
- Posterior ethmoid sinus.

The septum which divides the ethmoid sinus into two groups is called the basal lamella.

Anterior group also contains middle ethmoid cells which forms the bulge called bulla ethmoidalis.

Drainage
- Anterior and middle ethmoid cells drain into the middle meatus.
- Posterior ethmoid cells drain into the superior meatus.

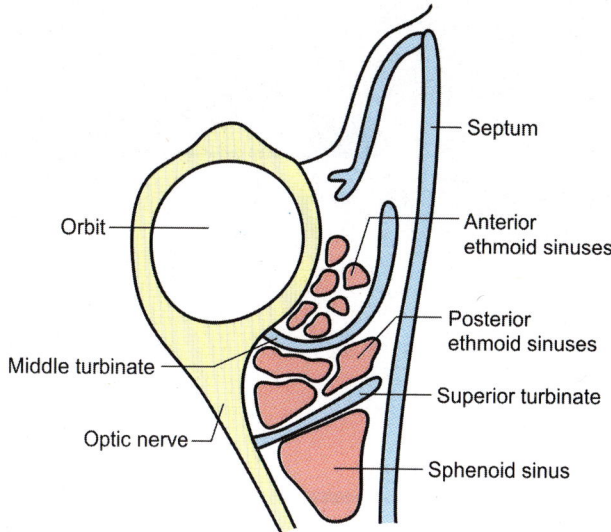

Fig. 16.9: Diagrammatic representation of ethmoid sinuses (axial section)

Relations
- **Superiorly:** Cranial cavity
- **Laterally:** Orbit and optic nerve
- **Medially:** Nasal cavity
- **Inferiorly:** Maxillary sinus
- **Posteriorly:** Sphenoid sinus

SPHENOID SINUS

There is one sphenoid sinus in the sphenoid bone, divided by a septum.

Drainage   It drains in the sphenoethmoidal recess.

Relations
- **Laterally**
  - Cavernous sinus containing IIIrd, IVth, Vth and VIth cranial nerves and the internal carotid artery.
  - Optic nerve
- **Superiorly**
  - Pituitary gland
  - Optic chiasma
  - Frontal lobe of cerebrum
  - Olfactory bulb
- **Inferiorly:** Nasopharynx
- **Anteriorly:** Nasal cavity

CHAPTER 17

Physiology of the Nose and Paranasal Sinuses

FUNCTIONS OF THE NOSE

The primary functions of the nose include the following:
- Respiration
- Airconditioning of the airstream
- Vocal resonance
- Filtration
- Olfaction
- Drainage
- Nasal reflex functions

Respiration The nasal passages serve as a natural airway, separate from the buccal cavity to enable respiration even during mastication. Neonates are essentially 'nose-breathers' and hence any nasal obstruction causes a difficulty in breathing or apnoea requiring insertion of an airway in between the gingiva to enable respiration through the mouth. If there is nasal obstruction in an individual, mouth-breathing is acquired, e.g. large adenoids, nasal polyps, etc.

Airconditioning The nasal cavities perform the function of warming and humidifying inhaled air prior to its passage into the lungs.

Vocal resonance The nasal cavities add resonance to the voice which is required for proper pronunciation of certain syllables.

Filtration The nasal cavities filter the inhaled air and protect the lower respiratory tract:
- The vibrissae filter coarse impurities

- The ciliae filter smaller impurities
- The mucous secretions help to remove impurities by trapping them. The mucous moves backwards to the pharynx and is swallowed.
- Lysosymes destroy bacteria
- Sneezing helps to eliminate irritants from the nasal cavities.

Olfaction Olfaction is a special sense performed by the olfactory mucosa lining the roof of the nasal cavities.

Drainage The paranasal sinuses and the nasolacrimal duct drain into the nasal cavities.

Nasal reflexes These include vasomotor reflex, olfactory reflexes and trigeminal reflexes. The olfactory reflexes are triggered off following the stimulation of olfactory receptors, which influence secretions of salivary, gastric and pancreatic glands.

Other nasal reflexes include reflex changes in pulmonary ventilation and changes in heart rate.

FUNCTIONS OF THE PARANASAL SINUSES

The exact functions are not known but, they are considered to perform the following functions:
- Reduce the weight of the skull
- Play a role in vocal resonance
- Protect the orbit
- Play a role in development of the face
- Humidification of air

Nose

CHAPTER 18

Examination of the Nose and Paranasal Sinuses

HISTORY TAKING

The chief symptoms include:
- Rhinorrhoea or nasal discharge
- Nasal obstruction
- Headache
- Sneezing
- Epistaxis or bleeding from the nose
- Change of smell/foul smell/loss of sense of smell

RHINORRHOEA

It is the term used to denote the discharge from the nose.

Features
- Continuous or intermittent
- Unilateral or bilateral
- Watery or purulent or blood stained
- Foul smelling or not
- Associated features
  - Headache
  - Sneezing, etc

Differential diagnosis of watery rhinorrhoea:
- Allergic rhinitis
- Vasomotor rhinitis
- Common cold
- Rhinitis medicamentosa
- CSF rhinorrhoea

Differential diagnosis of purulent rhinorrhoea:
- Rhinitis with bacterial infection
- Acute and chronic sinusitis
- Long standing foreign body in the nose
- Tuberculous or syphilitic infection of the nose
- Nasal granulomas
- Choanal atresia
- Atrophic rhinitis

Differential diagnosis of bloodstained rhinorrhoea:
- Rhinosporidiosis
- Acute or Chronic rhinosinusitis, rarely
- Atrophic rhinitis when crusts are dislodged
- Malignant tumour of the nose and paranasal sinuses
- Granulomas of the nose
- Inverted papilloma
- Nasal diphtheria

Differential diagnosis of unilateral discharge from nose:
- Foreign body in the nose
- Rhinolith
- Antrochoanal polyp
- Unilateral (secondary) atrophic rhinitis
- Granulomas or tumours involving only one nasal cavity.
- Unilateral choanal atresia.

NASAL OBSTRUCTION

Features
- Intermittent or Continuous
- Unilateral or Bilateral

- Associated features
  - Headache
  - Rhinorrhoea
  - Foul smell
- Physiological or Pathological.

Physiological nasal obstruction: It can be cyclic, reflex, or postural.
- **Cyclic:** One-nostril functions more than the other in a cyclic phase in a normal individual.
- **Reflex:** When the nose is exposed to cold, there is a reflex partial nasal obstruction to provide better humidification of air.
- **Postural:** Due to nasopulmonary reflexes, when an individual is lying down, the dependant nostril gets blocked gradually.

Differential diagnosis of nasal obstruction:
- Congenital
- Trauma
- Tumours
- Infections
- Foreign body
- Miscellaneous
- Congenital
  - Choanal atresia
  - Congenital tumours
- Trauma
  - Fractures of nasal bones
  - Dislocation of septum
  - Septal haematoma
  - Septal abscess
- Foreign bodies in the nose, e.g. bead, eraser, etc.
- Tumours of the nose and paranasal sinuses:
  - Nasopharyngeal angiofibroma
  - Rhinosporidiosis
  - Haemangioma
  - Malignancy
- Inflammation and infection
  - Allergic rhinitis
  - Vasomotor rhinitis
  - Atrophic rhinitis
- Miscellaneous
  - Nasal polyps
  - Deviated nasal septum
  - Adenoids
  - Turbinate hypertrophy
  - Rhinitis Medicamentosa
  - Use of snuff

- Smoking and alcoholism
- Hypothyroidism
- Use of hypotensive drugs

Differential diagnosis of unilateral nasal obstruction:
- Unilateral choanal atresia
- Deviated nasal septum
- Hypertrophied nasal turbinate
- Antrochoanal polyp
- Foreign body
- Rhinolith
- Rhinosporidiosis
- Synechiae and adhesions
- Tumours and granulomas in one nasal cavity

Differential diagnosis   Common causes of nasal obstruction in
- Children
  - Foreign body
  - Adenoid hypertrophy
  - Rhinitis
- Adults
  - Deviated nasal septum
  - Hypertrophied nasal turbinates
  - Allergic rhinitis
  - Vasomotor rhinitis
  - Nasal polypii
  - Rhinitis and sinusitis
  - Nasopharyngeal angiofibroma
- Elderly
  - Malignancy of the nose and / or paranasal sinuses
  - Carcinoma of the nasopharynx
  - Use of snuff
  - Use of hypotensive drugs
  - Rhinitis and sinusitis

Differential diagnosis of a nasal mass (*Refer to* Chapter 22; page 126)
- Antrochoanal polyp
- Ethmoidal polypii
- Rhinolith
- Rhinoscleroma (in the nodular stage)
- Rhinosporidiosis
- Deviated nasal septum
- Hypertrophied inferior turbinate
- Inverted papilloma
- Nasopharyngeal angiofibroma
- Malignant tumour
- Congenital tumours like meningocoele or encephalocoele

- Foreign body granuloma
- Granulomas of the nose
- Septal haemangioma

HEADACHE IN ENT

It can be continuous or intermittent and shooting or dull throbbing. Diseases of the nose and paranasal sinuses often result in headaches whereas diseases of the ear and throat cause a localised pain.

Aetiology
- Nose
  - DNS
  - Rhinitis
  - Migraine
  - Atrophic rhinitis
  - Nasal mass like granuloma, rhinolith, malignancy, etc.
  - Nasal polyps
- Paranasal sinuses
  - Sinusitis
  - Vacuum headache, due to obstruction to the ostia of the sinuses
  - Complications of sinusitis like mucocoele, pyocoele, etc.
- Ears
  - Only intracranial complications of unsafe CSOM can result in headache

SNEEZING

It is a normal reflex phenomenon due to nasal irritation.

Aetiology
- Allergic rhinitis
- Common cold
- Vasomotor rhinitis
- Ethmoidal polypii

EPISTAXIS

Refer to Chapter 20 for details on epistaxis.

HISTORY–TAKING IN BRIEF

CHIEF COMPLAINTS

Rhinorrhoea
- Duration (since when)
- Continuous/Intermittent
- Unilateral/Bilateral
- Consistency—watery/purulent/bloodstained
- Smell—whether foul smelling
- Associated with headache/sneezing

Nasal obstruction
- Duration
- Continuous/Intermittent
- Unilateral/Bilateral
- Diurnal variation
- Associated with headache/sneezing/foul smell

Headache
- Duration
- Continuous/Intermittent
- Dull throbbing/sharp shooting/heaviness of head
- Radiating
- Mild/Severe
- Localised/Generalised
- Diurnal variation
- Associated with sneezing/nasal obstruction/rhinorrhoea
- Aggravating/Relieving factors

Sneezing
- Duration
- Frequency of episodes
- Aggravating/Relieving factors
- Associated with headache/nasal discharge

Epistaxis
- Duration
- Frequency of episodes (how often)
- Quantity of blood lost in each episode
- Unilateral/Bilateral
- Number of episodes
- Spontaneous/Traumatic
- Aggravating/Relieving factors
- Similar family history
- Bleeding from other sites
- Any treatment taken

On direct questioning, ask for history of:
- Change of smell or loss of smell
- Loss of nasal twang to voice
- Fever
- Crusting in nose
- Lacrimation
- Diplopia or other visual disturbances
- Otalgia or otorrhoea
- Swelling over face
- Trauma

- Nose picking
- Allergy
- Bleeding tendencies in self/family
- Drug intake
- Cough
- Treatment for present complaints

PERSONAL HISTORY

- Alcoholism
- Smoking
- Snuff addiction
- Occupation in chrome/metal industry
- Residence in coastal India

FAMILY HISTORY

- Bleeding disorders
- Allergy
- Asthma

PAST HISTORY

- Drug intake.
- Treatment for similar complaints in the past.

EXAMINATION OF THE NOSE AND PARANASAL SINUSES

Examination of the nose includes the following:
- Examination of the external nose.
- Anterior rhinoscopy, for nasal cavity examination.
- Posterior rhinoscopy, for examination of the choana and nasopharynx.
- Palpation of the sinuses for tenderness.

Performed using a Bull's eye lamp and head mirror.

EXAMINATION OF EXTERNAL NOSE

Inspection of the nose for:
- Nasal bridge deformities like saddle-nose deformity or hump deformity of the nasal bridge.
- Swellings
- Ulcers
- Sinuses
- Growths on the skin
- Scars
- Broad nose due to long-standing nasal mass, like ethmoidal polyps or angiofibroma.
- Inflammation or cellulitis

Palpation of the nose for
- Detection of fracture of nasal bones, crepitations will be felt over the nasal bridge
- 'Woody' feel of the external nose in rhinoscleroma

ANTERIOR RHINOSCOPY

Performed using a Thudicum's nasal speculum in the left hand. The nasal speculum is held between the thumb and index finger with the spring action being controlled by the ring and middle fingers. It is introduced with the blades approximated and then gently opened in the nasal vestibule. Both nasal cavities are examined one after the other (Fig. 18.1).

In a child, the nasal cavities can be examined by lifting the tip of the nose as vibrissae (nasal hair) are absent in children, making examination easier.

Structures seen on anterior rhinoscopy
- Nasal mucosa, normally pink and moist.
- Inferior turbinate—anterior aspect
- Middle turbinate—anterior end
- Nasal septum
- Inferior meatus and middle meatus
- Nasal floor
- The nasal vestibule is visualised without the speculum by lifting the tip of the nose.

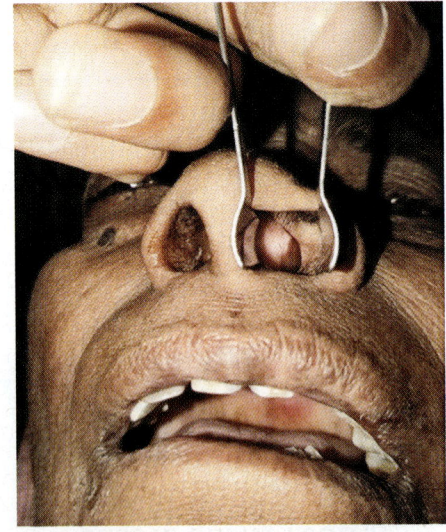

Fig. 18.1: Anterior rhinoscopy

The superior turbinate, meatus and nasal roof are not usually visualized except in a case of atrophic rhinitis, where the turbinates undergo atrophy.

Spatula test   This is used to test the presence of nasal obstruction. A metal spatula or a Lac's tongue depressor blade is placed after wiping it, clean near the anterior nares and the patient is asked to exhale through the nose on the spatula. The fogging created on the spatula by the blasts of air from both nostrils is compared. In a partially obstructed nostril, fogging is less and in a completely obstructed nostril, fogging is absent.

Cotton-wool test   It is done to detect patency of the nasal cavity. A wisp of cotton-wool is placed in front of the nostril. If the nostril is patent, the wisp will move on respiration, if not, it will not move.

Abnormal findings on anterior rhinoscopy include the following:

- Hypertrophied turbinates
- Inflammed nasal mucosa (rhinitis)
- Atrophic rhinitis
- Maggots (nasal myiasis)
- Polyps (antrochoanal or ethmoidal)
- Adhesions
- Foreign body
- Septal perforation
- Nasal mass, e.g. malignancy, granulomas, etc.

In case of hypertrophy of turbinates, a decongestant can be applied locally to cause blanching and shrinking and then examination is performed. This test is also performed to differentiate a hypertrophied turbinate from a polyp, since a polyp will not shrink.

Abnormal masses, polyps, secretions, adhesions, foreign bodies, etc., are to be noted.

Gentle probing is performed in case of a nasal mass to detect site of origin. However, a vascular mass (e.g. angiofibroma) is never probed.

POSTERIOR RHINOSCOPY

It is performed using a posterior rhinoscopy mirror, which is a bayonet shaped instrument with a plane mirror at its end (Fig. 18.2). Fogging on the mirror surface is prevented by the following measures:

- Dipping the *entire mirror* in warm water.
- Using a specially available demisting solution on the *mirror surface*.
- Dipping the mirror in cetavlon or savlon and wiping the *metal surface* dry, as this is an irritant and if a drop falls on the mucosa, it can result in a chemical mucositis (pharyngitis or laryngitis).
- Holding the *mirror surface* in front of the flame of a spirit lamp,
- Gently rubbing the mirror surface on the buccal mucosa of the patient so as to coat the mirror surface with a thin film of saliva.

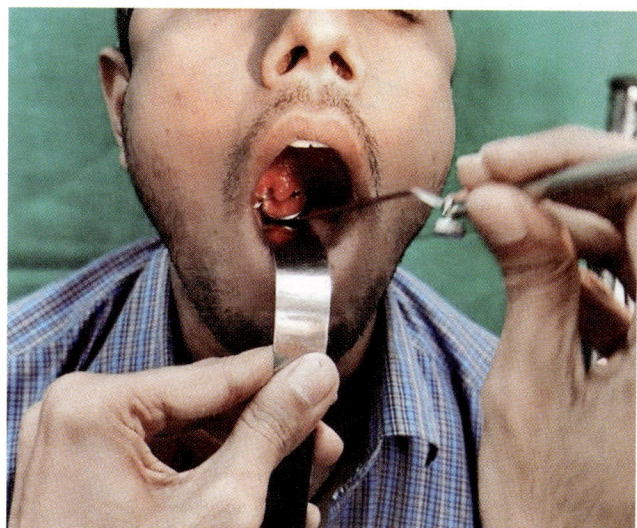

Fig. 18.2: Posterior rhinoscopy

Prior to introduction of the mirror into the mouth, the metal surface is tested on the back of the examiner's hand for temperature. The metal surface and NOT the mirror surface is tested because the metal surface gets heated faster and can result in scalding of the soft-palate mucosa.

The procedure (Fig. 18.3) is explained to the patient, as the patient's cooperation is most important for proper examination.

The anterior two-thirds of the tongue is depressed using a tongue depressor and the posterior rhinoscopy mirror is gently introduced with the mirror facing upwards till it lies in the oropharynx between the uvula and the posterior pharyngeal wall taking care not to touch the posterior pharyngeal wall as this elicits a gag reflex. The patient is asked to gently breathe through his nose as this helps to maintain the nasopharyngeal sphincter open and aids in visualization of the nasopharynx. Using the mirror, in this manner, the posterior nares and nasopharynx are examined.

The following structures are visualised (Fig. 18.4):

- Anteriorly
  - Posterior margin of the bony nasal septum.
  - Posterior ends of the inferior, middle, and superior turbinates.
  - Posterior nares or choanae.
- Laterally
  - Opening of the Eustachian tubes on either side with the tubal elevations are seen behind the posterior end of the inferior turbinate.
  - Fossa of Rosenmuller situated posterosuperior to the tubal elevations on either side.

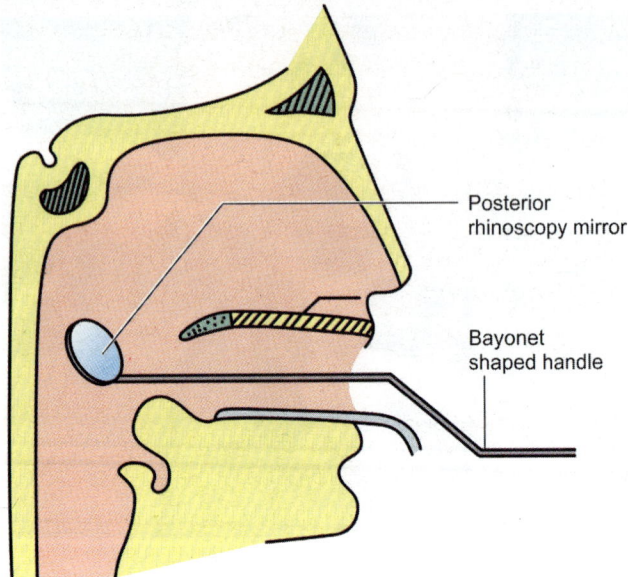

Fig. 18.3: Procedure of posterior rhinoscopy

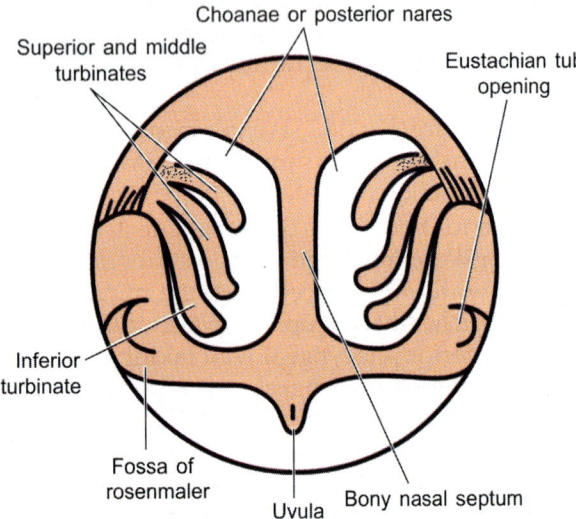

Fig. 18.4: Structures seen on posterior rhinoscopy

- Superiorly
  - Roof of nasopharynx
  - Superior part of posterior pharyngeal wall
- Anteriorly with tilt of the mirror
  - Nasal surface of the soft palate and uvula

Pathology like tumours, polyps, cysts, foreign body, and secretions are visualized if present.

Adenoids can be seen in children, but this procedure requires cooperation of the patient and, hence is not usually possible in children as a child does not usually cooperate for this procedure.

Problems encountered in posterior rhinoscopy

- Children do not usually cooperate
- It cannot be done in mentally retarded patients
- Excessive gagging may occur in a sensitive patient, this is prevented by surface anaesthesia with 4% lignocaine spray in the throat.

Uses of posterior rhinoscopy (Indications)

- Inspecting normal structures
- Detecting pathology in the nasopharynx
- Removing foreign body from the nasopharynx
- Taking a biopsy from a mass in the nasopharynx

For the last two indications, the forceps is manoeuvred through the nasal cavities.

Methods of examination of the nasopharynx

- Posterior rhinoscopy
- Digital palpation of the nasopharynx: Examiner stands behind the patient who is seated with neck flexed. He asks the patient to open his/her mouth and presses the left cheek of the patient between the patient's teeth with his/her left index finger. The nasopharynx is palpated with the index finger of the right hand, which is passed behind the uvula and soft palate through the oral cavity.

   Prior to digital palpation, the throat is sprayed with 4% lignocaine for surface anaesthesia and the procedure is explained to the patient.
- Use of a fibre-optic flexible nasopharyngoscope, which is passed along the floor of the nasal cavity.
- Use of a rigid Yaunkauer's nasopharyngeal speculum under general anaesthesia through the oral cavity.
- Recent advance: Use of a 120° nasal endoscope, which is passed through the nasal cavities.
- Under general anaesthesia, the soft palate is lifted forwards with a retractor or two rubber catheters passed through the nose and brought out through the mouth.
- X-ray of soft tissues of the nasopharynx.
- Xeroradiography of soft tissues of the nasopharynx.
- CT scan of base skull and nose with nasopharynx.

INSPECTION AND PALPATION OF THE PARANASAL SINUSES FOR TENDERNESS AND PATHOLOGY

The maxillary sinuses, ethmoidal sinuses and frontal sinus are inspected for superficial swelling, redness or fistula on the overlying skin.

   The site for palpation is the most superficial portion of the sinuses.

- **Maxillary sinuses:** Palpation over the canine fossa on the cheek with the index and middle fingers of the right hand or the thumb. The left hand steadies the patient's head. Examiner sits in front of the patient.
- **Frontal sinuses:** Palpation on the floor of the sinus just above the inner canthus of the eye with index and middle finger of right hand. Left hand steadies the patients head. Examiner stands to the right of the patient.

  Anterior wall of frontal sinus is not palpated, as it has two layers of bone.
- **Anterior ethmoid sinuses:** Palpation on the sides of the nose, midway between the inner canthus of the eye and nasion with the thumb and index fingers of the right hand. Left hand steadies the patient's head. Examiner sits in front of the patient.
- **Middle and posterior ethmoids and sphenoid sinuses** are situated deep and hence cannot be palpated. All sinuses should be palpated on both sides so as to compare tenderness.
- **Posture test:** It is not used nowadays, as it is not very reliable. It was used previously to differentiate between frontal and maxillary sinusitis. It is performed only in sinusitis with active nasal discharge. The nasal discharge is wiped clean and patient is asked to sit for 5 minutes. If discharge reappears, it indicates frontal sinusitis. If it does not reappear, patient is asked to lie down facing one side with the affected side up. Now, if the discharge appears, it indicates maxillary sinusitis.
- **Transillumination test:** This test is not performed nowadays and has been replaced by radiological investigations. It is performed in a darkroom. A battery operated lighted pencil-torch is placed in the oral cavity abutting against the hard palate and a glow is seen over the cheek. An 'infra-orbital crescent' of light is formed in a normal maxillary sinus. In the presence of sinusitis, this is absent. Polyps/Cysts will give a brilliant transillumination. For frontal sinusitis, two small pencil-torches are placed abutting against the floor of both frontal sinuses simultaneously and the glow on the forehead is compared. If a patient is wearing dentures, he/she is asked to remove them prior to the test.
- **Investigations**
  - X-ray paranasal sinuses—water's view for maxillary sinuses, Caldwell's view for ethmoidal and frontal sinuses. Water's view with mouth open for sphenoid sinus.
  - Proof puncture (antral puncture done for diagnostic purposes)
  - Nasal and sinus endoscopy
  - Examination under general anaesthesia
  - CT scan of nose and paranasal sinuses

Nose

CHAPTER 19

Conditions of the External Nose

Following may be the conditions of the external nose:
- Fracture of the nasal bones
- Fracture of the middle third of the face
- Vestibulitis
- Rhinophyma (potato nose)

FRACTURE OF THE NASAL BONES

Aetiology
- Trauma
- Direct trauma to nose due to fall or blow
- As a part of injury to the faciomaxillary region or head

Clinical features
- External nasal deformity: This is due to:
  - The fractured fragments which are dislocated.
  - Oedema of tissues due to trauma or haematoma.
- Skin over nasal bridge may be discoloured due to haematoma or lacerated.
- Palpation over the nasal bridge will elicit tenderness and bony crepitation.
- The bony injury is obscured by the oedema which sets in after 4–6 hours. Hence, the exact bony deformity can be assessed only within 2–4 hours of trauma or after 6–7 days, when oedema subsides.
- Epistaxis is often present and may be either profuse or scanty.
- Nasal obstruction: It is usually present due to blood clots, septal haematoma or septal deformity.

- Associated injury and haematoma of eyes, facio-maxillary region or head may be present.
- Watery nasal discharge is indicative of cerebrospinal fluid (CSF) leak due to a fracture of the cribriform plate in the roof of the nose.

Investigations
- X-ray of the nasal bones reveals the presence of a fracture with or without displacement of the bony fragments.

  X-ray in this case is also of medicolegal importance and for the purpose of documentation (Flowchart 19.1).

Flowchart 19.1: Investigations

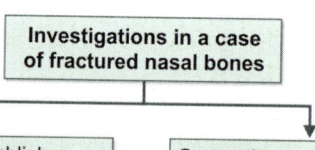

Investigations in a case of fractured nasal bones	
Specific to establish diagnosis	**Supportive**
• Radiographs which show fracture especially, lateral view (water's and Caldwell's view to rule out fracture of sinuses). • Anterior and posterior rhinoscopy to rule out blood clots, septal haematoma and DNS.	• Hb–to assess the blood loss. • Blood group and cross matching if haemoglobin is less than 10 g %. • X-ray skull and CT scan to detect associated head injury; if suspected. • Examination of eyes to rule out subconjunctival haemorrhage or other damage.

Treatment

- In case of vehicular accidents or head injuries, it is of primary importance to maintain the vital parameters of the patient.
- Epistaxis, if active and profuse, is treated by pinching the nose for 5–7 minutes or if required, an anterior nasal packing is done.
- Lacerations are cleaned and sutured.
- Antibiotics and anti-inflammatory analgesics are administered.
- If the fractured fragments are not dislocated, only conservative treatment is given. If they are dislocated reduction of fracture is required.
- In early cases i.e. the patient is seen immediately, before soft tissue oedema has occurred, the fracture is reduced under local anaesthesia.
- If the patient is seen within 4 weeks of trauma, the oedema is allowed to subside with anti-inflammatory analgesics and antibiotics. Then, the reduction of the fracture is performed under general anaesthesia using Ashe's forceps for the septum and Walsham's forceps for the lateral nasal wall.
- If the patient is seen after 4 weeks of trauma (i.e. after the tissue oedema subsides, and malunion of the fracture bone fragments has occurred) a rhinoplasty is required.
- This may be associated with a septal deformity or a septal haematoma, which is treated at the same time when the fracture is reduced.

FRACTURE OF THE MIDDLE THIRD OF THE FACE

Definition   It is the fracture of the facial bones between the supraorbital ridge and upper teeth.

Aetiology   It includes the following (Fig. 19.1):
- Severe blow to the face with hard object, e.g. stone, etc.
- Vehicular accidents
- Industrial accidents
- Fall on face from great heights

Classification   Depending on site of involvement:
- Central (nasomaxillary bones)
- Lateral (malar-maxillary bones)

Clinical features

- Central type: Le Fort's classification for central fractures is based on extent of bone involvement (Fig. 19.2).
    - *Le Fort I (transverse):* Transverse fracture of maxilla involving palate only.

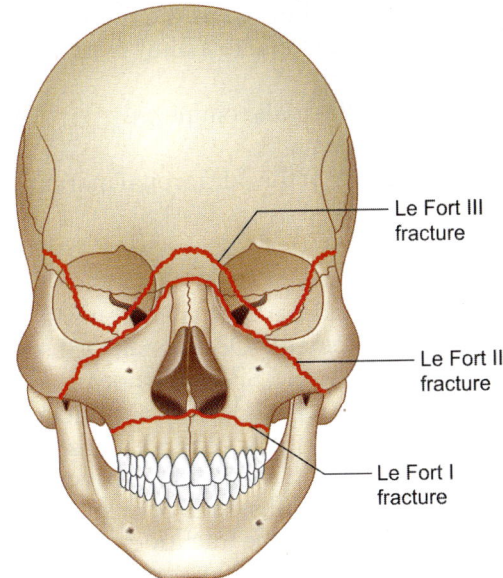

Fig. 19.1: Le Fort's fractures involving the middle one-third of the face

- *Le Fort II (pyramidal):* Fracture en bloc of the palate and middle third of face.
- *Le Fort III (craniofacial dysjunction):* This is the most severe of all the fractures and involves complete disruption of attachment of the facial skeleton from the cranium.

The following are the clinical features:
- *Nose*
    - Collapse of nasal bridge
    - Oedema of soft tissues
    - Epistaxis
    - Septal haematoma
    - Nasal obstruction
    - CSF rhinorrhoea
    - Anosmia
- *Maxillary sinuses*
    - Step-deformity of infraorbital margin due to fracture
    - Oedema of soft tissues
    - Anaesthesia or numbness over cheek, if infra-orbital nerve is involved in its foramen
- *Face*
    - Flattening of the face (dish-face deformity)
    - Malocclusion of the jaws
- *Eyes*
    - Epiphora
    - Subconjunctival haemorrhage
    - Diplopia
    - Enophthalmos

- **Lateral type:** Also known as the malar-maxillary complex and occurs due to a blow from the side of the face.
  - Flattening of the malar eminence
  - Soft tissue oedema
  - Step-deformity of the infraorbital margin
  - Enophthalmos
  - Diplopia
  - Trismus
- **Investigations:** Radiographs are diagnostic of fractures and displacements. Occasionally, CT scan may be required in cases of CSF rhinorrhoea.
- **Treatment for central and lateral face fractures:** The fracture is reduced under general anaesthesia and the reduced fragments are maintained in position by use of steel wires, splints, rods or even continuous traction depending on the fracture site.

VESTIBULITIS

Definition   It is the infection and inflammation of the nasal vestibule.

Aetiology   It includes the following (Fig. 19.2):
- Commonest cause is picking of the nose, which is habitual in some people.
- Diabetics are more prone to develop this condition.
- Causative organism, *Staphylococcus aureus*.

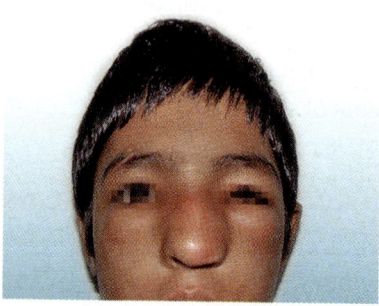

Fig. 19.2: Vestibulitis

Significance   Infection of the vestibule of the nose is potentially dangerous and can lead to life-threatening complications. The veins of the nose drain into the facial veins and inferior orbital veins which have no valves drain into the cavernous sinus. Thus, resulting in cavernous sinus thrombophlebitis and thrombosis with blindness. Cavernous sinus thrombosis may also be fatal.

Clinical features
- Furuncle in the nasal vestibule.
- Cellulitis of the nose in the region of the vestibule.
- Pain on the tip of the nose with tenderness on touch.

- Cellulitis of the face (mid-portion).
- Headache.
- Fever, malaise, and anorexia.

Complications
- Cellulitis of the face
- Blindness or blurring of vision
- Cavernous sinus thrombophlebitis and thrombosis, which may be fatal

Investigations
- Blood sugar to rule out diabetes mellitus
- Fundoscopy to rule out papilloedema

Treatment
- Antibiotics, parenterally initially and orally after 5 days.
- Anti-inflammatory analgesics
- Cold fomentation with magnesium sulphate locally over the external nose and face.
- Antibiotic ointment locally in the nasal vestibule.
- Patients are instructed not to pick the nose and maintain hygiene.

RHINOPHYMA

Synonym   Potato nose.

Aetiology   The exact aetiology is not known, but it is thought to be due to acne rosacea. There is hyperplasia of the sebaceous glands, connective tissue, and vessels of the skin with fibrosis.

Clinical features   The external nose shows thickening of the skin with pitting. The tip of the nose is hypertrophied and protuberant. It appears shiny and coarse (Fig. 19.3).

Treatment
- Treatment aims at being cosmetic.
- The excess tissue over the external nose is shaved off with a scalpel. The healing occurs without skin grafting by regeneration of the skin. Laser is the recent advancement in the treatment of this condition.

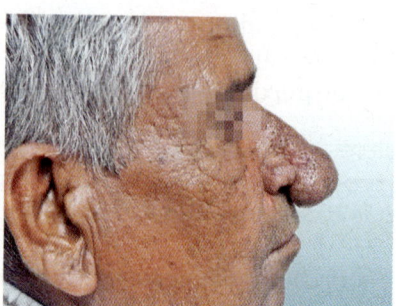

Fig. 19.3: Rhinophyma

Nose

CHAPTER 20

Epistaxis

DEFINITION

Epistaxis is defined as bleeding from the nose. It is not a disease, but it is a symptom as well as a sign.

AETIOLOGY/CAUSES

Aetiology or causes of epistasis are shown in Flowchart 20.1.

- Local
- Systemic
- Idiopathic

Local causes

- Congenital disorders
  - Osler-Weber Rendu syndrome (Hereditary telangiectasis).
- Infective/Inflammatory
  - *Acute*
    - *Specific:* Diphtheria
    - *Non-specific*
      - Acute vestibulitis
      - Acute rhinitis
      - Acute sinusitis
  - *Chronic*
    - *Specific*
      - Tuberculosis
      - Syphilis
      - Leprosy
      - Fungal, e.g. rhinosporidiosis

- *Non-specific*
  - Chronic rhinitis
  - Chronic sinusitis
  - Atrophic rhinitis
  - Rhinitis sicca
- Neoplastic
  - *Benign*
    - Nasopharyngeal angiofibroma
    - Angiomatous polyp arising from nasal septum 'Bleeding polypus of the nasal septum'.
    - Hemangiomas
  - *Malignant*
    - Carcinoma of the nose
    - Carcinoma of the nasopharynx
    - Carcinoma of the paranasal sinuses
- Traumatic
  - *Accidental trauma*
    - Vehicular accidents
    - Blows to face
    - Fracture of nasal bones
    - Nose picking especially in the region of Little's area
  - *Iatrogenic trauma*
    - Following any nasal surgery; primary, reactionary or secondary haemorrhage may occur.
- Miscellaneous
  - Environmental, very dry or very hot climate
  - Rhinolith

Flowchart 20.1: Investigations

```
                          ┌─────────────────────┐
                          │ Aetiology of epistaxis │
                          └─────────────────────┘
              ┌───────────────────┼───────────────────┐
     ┌──────────────┐     ┌──────────────┐     ┌──────────────┐
     │ Local causes │     │Systemic causes│     │  Idiopathic  │
     └──────────────┘     └──────────────┘     └──────────────┘
```

Congenital
- Osler-Weber Rendu syndrome

Infective

Neoplastic

Traumatic

Miscellaneous
- FB nose
- Rhinolith
- Maggots

Benign
- Angiofibroma
- Hemangioma
- Bleeding polyps of the septum

Malignant
- Ca nose
- Ca naso-pharynx
- Ca PNS

Accidental
- Vehicular accident
- Blows to face
- Fracture of nasal bones
- Nose-picking

Iatrogenic
- Following SMR, nasal polypectomy etc.

Acute

Chronic

Specific
- Diphtheria

Non-specific
- Acute vestibulitis
- Acute rhinitis
- Acute sinusitis

Specific
- Tuberculosis
- Syphilis
- Leprosy
- Fungal

Non-specific
- Chronic rhinitis
- Chronic sinusitis
- Atrophic rhinitis
- Rhinitis sicca

- Nasal myiasis (maggots)
- Foreign body in nose
- Vicarious menstruation

Systemic/General causes
- Hypertension
- Bleeding disorders
  - Haemophilia
  - Leukaemia
  - Agranulocytosis
  - Hodgkin's disease
- Exanthematous fevers
  - Measles
  - Chicken-pox
  - Influenza
  - Typhoid
  - Rheumatic fever
- Chronic diseases like kalazar, renal failure, uraemia, etc.
- Raised venous pressure as in mitral stenosis, superior mediastinal tumours, whooping cough, and pneumonia with excessive cough.

- Barotrauma, i.e. sudden change in atmospheric pressure, e.g. high altitudes, Caisson's disease.
- Drugs:
  - Aspirin used for long periods
  - Salicylates
  - Anticoagulants
  - Quinine

Idiopathic, where the cause is not known.

COMMON CAUSES IN CLINICAL PRACTICE

Common causes in children and adults are as follows:

In children	In adults
• Nose picking	• Hypertension
• Trauma	• Angiofibroma
• Exanthematous fevers	• Malignancy
• Diphtheria	• Trauma
• Foreign body	• Idiopathic

COMMON SITES OF EPISTAXIS

- Little's area: It is the commonest site (80%) of epistaxis especially in children.

- Anterior ethmoid artery: Above the middle turbinate.
- Woodruff's plexus: Behind the posterior end of the inferior turbinate.

CLINICAL FEATURES

- Usually of sudden onset: In some cases, there may be a history of the cause, e.g. hypertension, trauma, etc.
- The bleeding may be scanty, moderate or severe.
- It may arise anteriorly and drip through the anterior nares. In others, it may be more posterior and blood is seen in the oropharynx and oral cavity.
- The patient is anxious, if the bleeding is persistent or profuse.
- Haemoptysis is usually present.
- Haematemesis may occur, if blood is swallowed since it may act as irritant for gastric mucosa.
- Patient may be in a state of shock, if epistaxis is severe and persistent.

INVESTIGATIONS

- A detailed history should be taken which includes the amount, frequency, and duration of bleeding. Any similar episodes in the past, whether the epistaxis is unilateral or bilateral, anterior or posterior, whether it is from a particular nasal cavity. History of trauma, exanthematous fever, bleeding disorder in the family, hypertension, use of drugs, etc., should also be provided.
- Examination of the nose and nasopharynx: This helps to detect the cause of epistaxis and even the site occasionally.
- General examination including blood pressure (this helps to detect hypertension. A fall in blood pressure indicates that the blood loss is excessive and has resulted in hypovolaemic shock) and haemogram (anaemia indicates that the blood loss is chronic).
- Tests to rule out bleeding disorders, bleeding time, clotting time, prothrombin time, etc.
- CT scan if required, i.e. if a mass is suspected.
- X-ray of the nasal bones in case of trauma to rule out fracture of nasal bones.
- Biopsy of a nasal mass, if seen, such as rhinosporidiosis, angiofibroma, malignancy, etc.
- Electrocardiogram as a baseline, if the patient is above the age of 35 years or if the patient is in circulatory failure.
- Endoscopy of the nose and nasopharynx may also be helpful to detect the cause and site of epistaxis. However, it may not be possible, if epistaxis is severe as it will impede vision.

TREATMENT

- Local management of active epistaxis.
- Primary first-aid treatment.
- Systemic management of epistaxis.

The primary aim in the management of epistaxis is to stop the bleeding and monitor the vital parameters of the patient.

The blood pressure of the patient is checked to detect hypertension as a cause of the epistaxis. A fall in blood pressure or a rapid thready pulse with cold clammy extremities detects circulatory collapse and hypovolaemic shock. If the patient is in shock the treatment is aimed at management of the shock.

If the bleeding is active, the epistaxis is controlled by means of nasal packs.

Only after treating the epistaxis (if it is active) and management of the circulatory collapse, if present, should the cause be looked for and treated.

Primary first-aid treatment If medical facilities are not available, the following first-aid procedures may be performed:

- Application of an icepack on the nasal bridge—this helps by vasoconstriction.
- Pinching the nose—helps by compressing the vessels on Little's area and stops bleeding.
- Trotter's procedure is useful in hypertensive epistaxis. The patient is asked to sit up, slightly inclined forwards with the mouth open and breathe quietly. He is asked to spit out the blood and not swallow it. Also, forceful clearing of the nose is avoided to prevent clots from dislodging.

Local management of active epistaxis

- If the epistaxis is scanty, the blood clots may be cleared by suction under direct vision and the bleeding site is detected (usually it is the Little's area). This is cauterised using either a chemical cautery (silver nitrate or trichloroacetic acid) or an electrocautery after spraying the nose with 4% lignocaine solution.
- If the epistaxis is moderate and anterior, i.e. through the anterior nares, anterior nasal packing (Fig. 20.1) is performed using a Tilley's nasal packing forceps and a 0.5 inches ribbon gauze (approx. 1 metre long) lubricated with liquid paraffin, vaseline or antibiotic cream. The lubricant prevents the pack from sticking to the nasal mucosa, as it keeps the mucosa moist. This helps during removal of the pack. The nasal cavities are packed separately from the floor to the roof in layers, so that there is an equal distribution of pressure in all areas. The packs are removed after

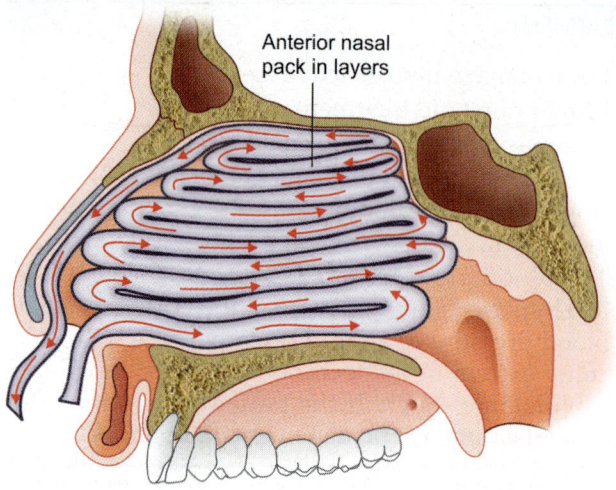

Anterior nasal pack in layers

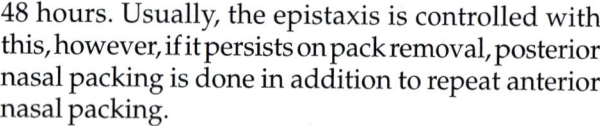

Fig. 20.1: Anterior nasal packing

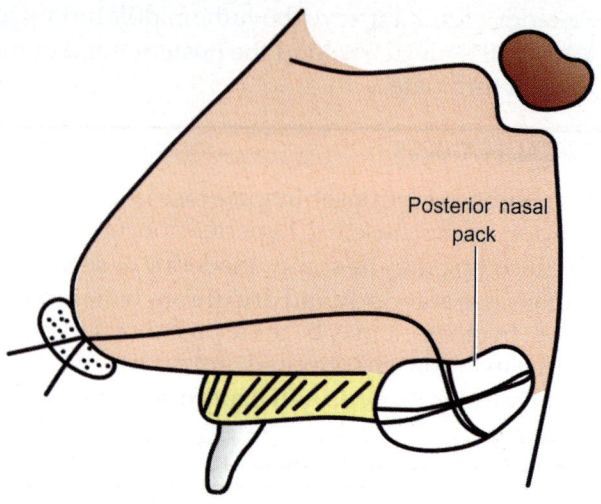

Posterior nasal pack

Fig. 20.2: Posterior nasal packing

48 hours. Usually, the epistaxis is controlled with this, however, if it persists on pack removal, posterior nasal packing is done in addition to repeat anterior nasal packing.

• **Posterior nasal packing** (Fig. 20.2) is preferably performed under general anaesthesia in the operation theatre. Two thin red rubber catheters (usually oxygen catheters), are passed from the nasal cavities, one on either side, along the floor of the nose and brought out through the mouth. The postnasal pack is actually, a roll of gauze soaked in an antibiotic ointment to which two linen tapes and one thread are tied. The two tapes are tied to the two rubber catheters at the oropharyngeal end. Now, the catheters are pulled through the nose along with the tapes and the pack is guided with a finger in position to fit snugly into the nasopharynx. The tapes are now tied across the columella after placing a small gauze between the knot and the columella. This has to be followed by anterior nasal packing. The pack is removed after 48 hours.

Adrenaline soaked packs are not advised, as this can further increase the blood pressure in hypertensive patients. Also, after sometime, there is a rebound congestion and this will result in further recurrence of epistaxis.

A Foley's catheter may also be used instead of a postnasal pack. It is introduced along the floor of one nasal cavity into the nasopharynx. It is inflated with air, when it is seen in the oropharynx and then pulled up so as to maintain pressure on the walls of the nasopharynx. However, it is secured with tapes on the cheek and this does not provide adequate

pressure at times. Also, unlike the gauze pack which confirms to the contour of the nasopharynx, it is smooth and spherical, hence all areas may not receive adequate pressure. The advantage is that this can be done under local anaesthesia or even without any anaesthesia.

Recently, synthetic sponge is used in the form of nasal tampons for anterior nasal packing. This has a central lumen to enable breathing.

• If in spite of this, bleeding is not controlled, the anterior ethmoidal or internal maxillary artery is ligated. The anterior ethmoidal artery is ligated through an incision taken below the medial portion of the eyebrow which is periosteum deep. Here, the artery is seen entering from the orbit into the nose and is ligated. The internal maxillary artery is ligated in the pterygopalatine fossa by a Caldwell Luc approach.

• However, external carotid artery ligation is preferred, as it is easily approached in the neck.

Systemic management in epistaxis

• Monitoring of pulse and blood pressure.
• Intravenous fluids and blood transfusion if required.
• Treatment of circulatory failure.
• Coagulants like vit. K and C.
• Sedatives to treat the anxiety.

Also, submucous resection of the nasal septum may be required in some cases to gain access to the site of bleeding, or as a treatment in case of epistaxis seen in hereditary telangiectasis.

Diseases of the Nasal Septum

DEVIATED NASAL SEPTUM

The nasal septum is deviated to one side in majority of individuals. However, correction is not required in all cases. Correction is considered only, if the deviated septum produces symptoms or a cosmetic nasal deformity.

Aetiology

- Age: The symptoms of deviated nasal septum (DNS), can occur at any age, however, they are common after the second decade of life, when the nasal septum is fully developed.
- Sex: There is no sex preponderance. Both the sexes are equally affected.
- Heredity: Heredity is considered to be one of the aetiologic factors in DNS.
- Trauma: DNS due to this cause is frequently seen in boxers. However, DNS may occur in any individual due to trauma to the external nose.
- Congenital: Abnormal intrauterine posture may result in compression of the nose and face resulting in DNS.
- Developmental: During the development of the face, the nasal septum, in some individuals, grows at a rate much faster than the rest of the face resulting in buckling of the septum to accommodate itself in the nose.
- High arched palate can result in buckling of the cartilagenous portion of the septum.

- Secondary: DNS can occur due to a mass (tumour/polyp) in one nasal cavity pushing the septum to the opposite side.

Pathology   Various types of septal deformities include (Fig. 21.1):
- Deviation: This is a smooth deflection of the septum away from the midline. It may be bony (posterior) or cartilagenous (anterior). It may be 'C' shaped or 'S' shaped and may involve the upper or lower half of the septum.
- Thickening: Following fracture of the cartilage or bony portion with subsequent healing in an irregular manner. The septum appears irregular and thick.
- Dislocation: This involves either the anterior edge which may be dislocated or the inferior edge (which rests on the maxillary crest), which may be displaced to one side. This involves only the cartilagenous septum and results in a DNS.
- Septal spur: This occurs at the junction of cartilage with bone, i.e. at the junction of quadrangular cartilage with septal bones or at the junction of cartilage with maxillary crest. It is an isolated thickening or deviation of bone.
- The DNS may be associated with a deformity of the external nose, e.g. hump, tip deformity, etc.
- Impacted septum: If the deviation is gross and results in the nasal septum touching the lateral wall of the nose it is termed as 'impacted' nasal septum.

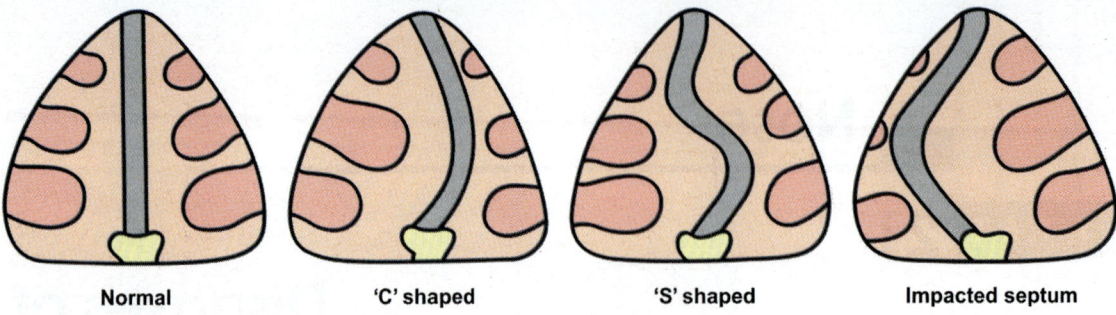

| Normal | 'C' shaped | 'S' shaped | Impacted septum |

Fig. 21.1: Types of deviated nasal septum

In case of DNS, the roomy nasal cavity, which faces the concave side of the septum shows hypertrophy of the turbinates especially the inferior turbinate. This is termed as 'compensatory' hypertrophy.

Also, the DNS may obstruct air entry on the affected side which increases during rhinitis as the mucosa is also oedematous and inflamed, thus resulting in complete obstruction of the nasal cavity on the convex side. Hence, patients may complain of nasal obstruction.

The DNS may further obstruct the drainage of the paranasal sinuses on the side of deviation resulting in sinusitis and headaches. The drainage on the other side may be obstructed by hypertrophied turbinates, resulting in bilateral sinusitis due to a DNS.

The Eustachian tube on the affected side too, may be obstructed due to recurrent infection following a DNS, resulting in serous otitis media and otalgia.

Clinical features
- Symptoms
  - *Asymptomatic:* Many patients with a DNS may not have any symptoms.
  - *Nasal obstruction:* It is the commonest symptom. It may be unilateral or bilateral (if the turbinates are hypertrophied on the opposite side).
  - *Headache:* It may be unilateral or bilateral. It may be due to the following causes :
    - *Vacuum headache:* It is the headache caused due to the vacuum created in the paranasal sinuses following absorption of air by the mucosa of the sinus due to obstruction to the drainage.
    - *Sinusitis:* It may be secondary to obstruction to drainage of sinuses as a result of DNS.
    - *Neuralgia:* Headache due to compression of the nerves in the lateral nasal wall, may occur in case of an impacted nasal septum.
  - *Epistaxis:* This is scanty and occasional. It occurs as a result of picking of crusts on the mucosa overlying the Little's area.
  - *Recurrent cold:* Due to stagnation of nasal secretions, as a result of obstruction to drainage or due to rhinitis and sinusitis.
  - *Anosmia* is rare but may occur occasionally, if the deviation is obstructing air flow to the nasal roof.
  - *External nasal deformity* may occasionally be present with a DNS. This is commonly seen following trauma.
- Signs
  - External nose may be deviated or deformed.
  - If the cause is trauma, a scar may be seen.
  - Anterior rhinoscopy will reveal the type of deviation of the septum or the presence of a mass in the nose, if it is the cause of DNS and the presence of compensatory hypertrophy of the turbinates.
  - Posterior rhinoscopy will reveal the presence of nasal mass or polyps, if they are the cause of deviation.
  - Sinus tenderness may be elicited over the maxillary, ethmoidal and frontal sinuses if there is acute sinusitis. It may be unilateral or bilateral.

Complications of Deviated Nasal septum
- **Sinusitis:** It is usually unilateral and as compensatory hypertrophy of the turbinates occurs, the sinusitis becomes bilateral.
- **Pharyngitis, laryngitis, and tracheobronchitis:** This occurs as a result of mouth breathing due to nasal obstruction.
- **Snoring** due to mouth breathing as a result of nasal obstruction.
- **Middle ear infection:** It occurs as a result of recurrent upper respiratory tract infection (URTI) affecting the Eustachian tube.
- **Atrophic rhinitis** may occasionally occur in DNS on the concave side, i.e. in the roomy nasal cavity.
- **Maggots** may occasionally occur in the roomy nasal cavity and may be associated with atrophic rhinitis.

- **Asthma:** DNS may occasionally trigger off bronchospasm.

Differential diagnosis
- Septal haematoma
- Hypertrophied inferior turbinates
- Nasal polypii

Treatment   The treatment of DNS is mainly surgical and indicated only if:
- The DNS is symptomatic.
- There are complications like sinusitis, epistaxis, and atrophic rhinitis.
- There are two types of surgery for DNS:
  - *Submucosal resection (SMR):* Here, the cartilagenous and bony septum is dissected from the mucous membrane and the cartilagenous septum with the deviated portion is removed.
  - *Septoplasty:* It is a more recent technique and is conservative in removal of the deviated portion of the nasal septum.

    Septorhinoplasty: This aims at simultaneously correcting the septal deformity and the external nasal deformity cosmetically. It includes septoplasty and rhinoplasty.

SUBMUCOSAL RESECTION AND SEPTOPLASTY

Submucosal reaction   Submucous resection of the nasal septum.

- Indications
  - Symptomatic DNS causing nasal obstruction.
  - Complications of DNS like recurrent sinusitis, URTI, epistaxis, headache, middle ear infection and serous otitis media (SOM).
  - As an approach to the sphenoid sinus, pituitary gland and vidian nerve.
  - Asthma may improve in a few patients after SMR.
  - To obtain a cartilage graft, which may be used for rhinoplasty, reconstructive ear surgery, etc.
  - As a treatment for epistaxis due to heriditary telangiectasis. Here, the cartilage is not removed but only mucoperichondrial flaps are elevated and replaced. This cause fibrosis submucosally and helps in preventing recurrent epistaxis.

All septal deviations anterior to an imaginary line passing from the nasal process of the frontal bone to the nasal spine of the maxilla are treated by septoplasty and all deviations posterior to this imaginary line are treated by SMR (Fig. 21.2).

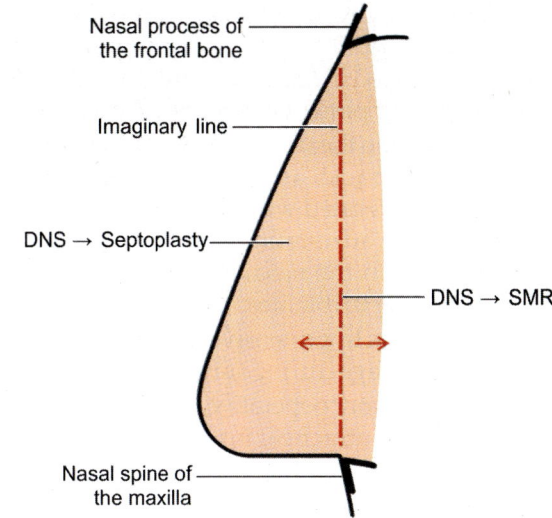

Fig. 21.2: The imaginary line for SMR and septoplasty

- Contraindications
  - *Acute rhinitis, pharyngitis or sinusitis:* These should be treated medically prior to surgical correction of the DNS, as acute URTI can result in haemorrhage during surgery.
  - *Age:* SMR is not performed in patients below 17 years of age, i.e. it is performed only after complete growth of the nasal septum has ceased. If done in younger individuals, it may hamper growth of the nasal septum or DNS may recur due to continued growth of the septum.
  - *Bleeding disorders:* These may result in excessive haemorrhage and difficulty in achieving haemostasis.
  - *Diabetes:* If present, should be controlled preoperatively.
  - *Hypertension:* It should be controlled, prior to surgery.
  - *Syphilis and tuberculosis,* if present should be treated preoperatively.
- Anaesthesia: SMR is always performed in an adult and hence preferred under local anaesthesia.

  Haemostasis is achieved better with local anaesthesia and intraoperative bleeding is minimal. Also, at the end of surgery, the patient can be asked to judge the relief obtained from nasal obstruction.

  The patient is sedated using 1 mL of fortwin (pentazocine lactate 30 mg) with 1 mL of phenargan (promethazine hydrochloride 25 mg) diluted to 10 mL in 5% dextrose. This is injected slowly intravenously with one hand on the patient's pulse. Alternatively, 10 mg (2 mL) calmpose (diazepam) can be used intravenously slowly.

The nose is sprayed with a solution of 4% lignocaine with 1:1,00,000 adrenaline and packed with gauze pack dipped in the same solution. This is done before taking the patient in the operation theatre.

In the operation theatre, the patient is first sedated, then the nasal packs are removed and the nasal cavities are infiltrated with 2% lignocaine solution with 1:1,00,000 adrenaline. Infiltration is done submucosally on the nasal septum on both sides and both inferior turbinates.

If the patient is hypertensive, adrenaline is not to be used at any stage during surgery.

If the patient is uncooperative, general anaesthesia is used with endotracheal intubation and a throat pack to prevent entry of blood into the air passage.

- **Preoperative preparation**
  - Written informed consent.
  - Injection atropine 0.6 mg intramuscular—½ hour preoperatively.
  - Injection tetanus toxoid 0.5 cc intramuscular.
  - Spray and pack nasal cavities with anaesthetic solution (4% lignocaine) as described previously.
- **Position of patient:** Patient lies supine on the operating table with head slightly extended. If under

local anaesthesia, the patient may be operated in a semi-sitting position to enable him to swallow or spit out secretions from the throat, thus preventing aspiration.

- **Procedure:** The procedure of SMR is shown in Fig. 21.3.
  - After infilteration anaesthesia, an incision is made using a no. 15 blade through the mucosa and perichondrium 2–3 mm behind the anterior free edge of the septal cartilage (Killian's incision). Incision is made on any one side, but preferably, it should be made on the concave side of the nasal septum to enable better visualisation of the field of surgery.
  - Mucoperichondrial flap is elevated with the help of a Freer's mucoperichondrial elevator on the side of the incision.
  - An incision is now made on the cartilage through its entire thickness (but not involving the perichondrium of the opposite side), a few millimeters posterior to the mucosal incision, and a mucoperichondrial flap is elevated on the opposite side.
  - The mucoperiosteal flaps over the bony septum and the maxillary crest on both sides, are also

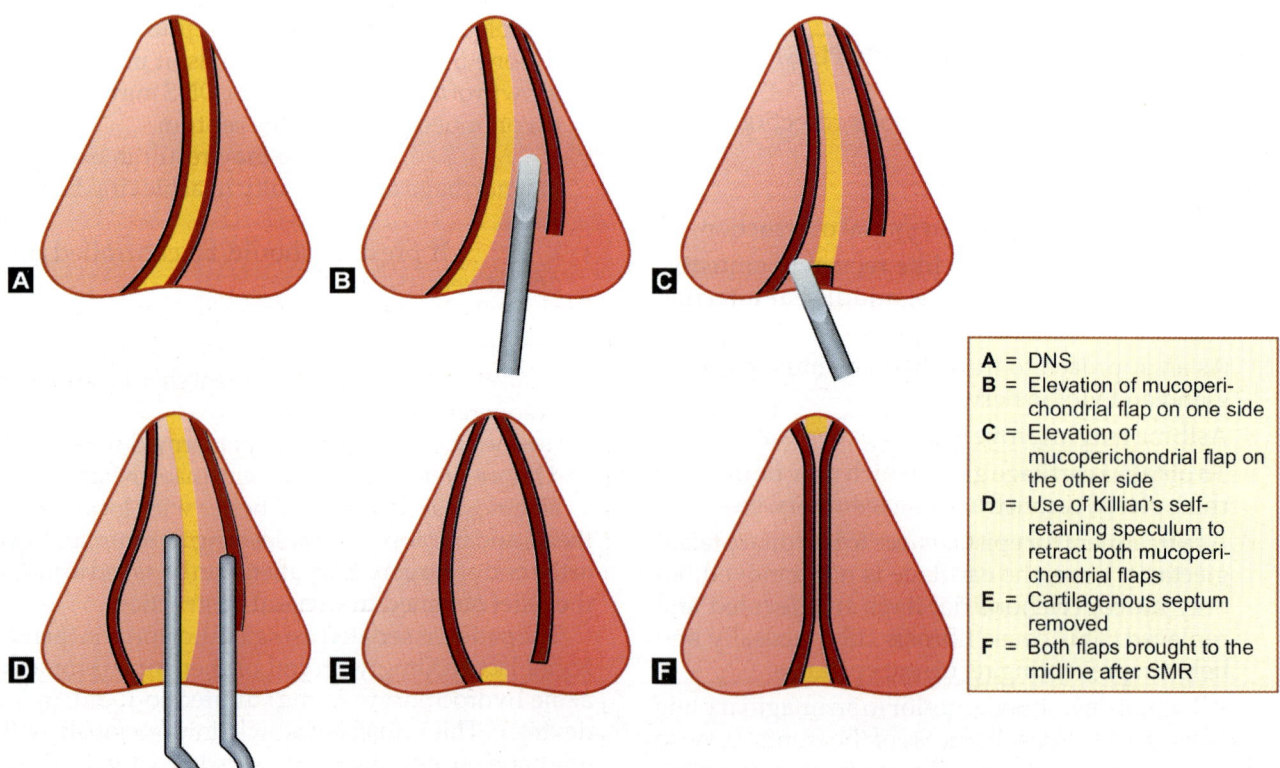

A = DNS
B = Elevation of mucoperi-chondrial flap on one side
C = Elevation of mucoperichondrial flap on the other side
D = Use of Killian's self-retaining speculum to retract both mucoperi-chondrial flaps
E = Cartilagenous septum removed
F = Both flaps brought to the midline after SMR

Fig. 21.3: Submucous resection of the nasal septum

elevated using a Killian's mucoperiosteal elevator which is different for the right and left sides of the septum.

♦ The mucoperichondrial and periosteal flaps are kept away from the cartilagenous and bony septum by insertion of a Killian's self-retaining nasal speculum.

♦ A small incision is made on the edge of the septal cartilage, 2–3 mm below the roof of the nose using a turbinectomy scissors.

♦ The blade of the Ballenger's swivel knife is now inserted into this nick and the knife is moved backwards, downwards, and forwards. The septal cartilage is removed as a whole piece using the Luc's forceps, leaving behind a 2–3 mm strip along the caudal end and the roof to maintain the shape of the external nose.

♦ All deviated portions of the bony septum and the maxillary crest are removed using the Luc's forceps or the gouge and hammer for the maxillary crest.

♦ The Killian's nasal speculum is removed and the flaps are brought to the midline. The incision in the mucoperichondrial flap is sutured using 3–0 chromic catgut in interrupted sutures.

♦ If under local anaesthesia, the patient is asked to judge the improvement in the nasal obstruction prior to packing of the nose.

♦ Anterior nasal packing is performed from the floor of the nose to the roof using roller gauze dipped in liquid paraffin or antibiotic ointment to help in lubrication during removal. If the pack is dry, removal is traumatic and painful and may result in dislodgement of dry crusts with bleeding.

• Postoperative care
  ♦ *Antibiotics orally*
    • Capsule ampicillin (500 mg) 4 times a day for 7 days.
  ♦ Anti-inflammatory analgesics orally for 7 days.
  ♦ Steam inhalation or tincture benzoin inhalations 4 times a day. This is required as the patient breathes by his/her mouth due to the nasal packs. It helps to humidify the air entering the respiratory tract and also helps to prevent halitosis.
  ♦ The nasal packs are removed gently after 48 hours.
  ♦ Liquid paraffin or vaseline nasal drops are put into the nasal cavities 4–5 times a day to loosen crusts, for 7 days.
  ♦ Rest is advised for a week following surgery.
  ♦ Trauma to the nose or forceful blowing of the nose is to be avoided for 3–4 weeks after surgery.

• **Complications:** Complications occurred are listed in Table 21.1:

TABLE 21.1: Immediate and delayed complications of SMR and septoplasty	
Immediate	*Delayed*
• Haemorrhage (primary). • Complications of anaesthesia. • Trauma to surrounding tissues, e.g. turbinates, mucoperichondrial flaps, etc. • Cerebrospinal fluid rhinorrhoea. • Flapping nasal septum.	• Reactionary or secondary haemorrhage. • Septal haematoma. • Septal abscess. • Septal perforation. • Infection. • Synechiae and adhesions. • Pain. • Persistence of nasal obstruction. • External nasal deformity.

• **Immediate complications**
  ♦ Complications of anaesthesia
    • Cardiac arythmias
    • Hypotension
    • Hypertension
  ♦ *Primary haemorrhage:* This usually occurs from the maxillary crest area and is controlled by use of dilute adrenaline packs or electrocautery. If not controlled, bone wax can be used to seal the bleeding site.
  ♦ *Trauma to surrounding tissues:* Surrounding tissues like the mucoperiosteal flaps or mucosa over the turbinates may be damaged and this can cause troublesome bleeding during surgery. If the mucoperiosteal flaps of both sides are torn at the same site, it results in a septal perforation.
  ♦ *CSF rhinorrhoea:* This is a rare complication and occurs due to damage to the cribriform plate of the ethmoid bone.

• **Delayed complications**
  ♦ Reactionary haemorrhage occurs within 48 hours of surgery and is usually due to the effect of adrenaline, wearing off in case of local anaesthesia or due to a rise in the blood pressure after surgery in case of general anaesthesia. It is controlled by firm anterior nasal packing.

  Secondary haemorrhage occurs after 48 hours of surgery and is due to infection. It is managed by repacking the nose, changing antibiotics, coagulants and if required replacement of blood loss.
  ♦ Septal haematoma occurs due to accumulation of blood between the two mucoperichondrial flaps

after healing of the incision. The septum is soft and swollen on either side. This results in nasal obstruction. Since the cartilage depends on its perichondrium for nutrition, if the haematoma persists for 2–3 days, the cartilage undergoes necrosis and absorption. It is treated by incision of one mucoperichondrial flap and drainage of the haematoma. A ribbon gauze is inserted in between the flaps and the nose is packed tightly for 48 hours (anterior nasal packing).

- Septal abscess develops due to infection of a septal haematoma (Fig. 21.4). It is associated with nasal obstruction, severe throbbing pain in the nose and if left untreated, it may even result in cavernous sinus thrombophlebitis or meningitis, as the nose lies in the dangerous area of the face. It is treated with urgent incision and drainage followed by placement of ribbon gauze and packing similar to a septal haematoma with hospitalization and intravenous antibiotics and analgesics.

In septal haematoma and abscess, the septal cartilage undergoes necrosis and hence, as a later complication, there is external nasal deformity.

- Septal perforation may occur, if both the muco-perichondrial flaps are torn at the same site. If asymptomatic, it need not be treated, small perforations may result in a whistling sound while breathing and are treated with surgery using local flaps of mucosa. Large perforations may predispose to atrophic rhinitis or maggots and are treated by obturators (prosthesis) made of silastic/teflon.
- Infection may occur if the pack is not removed within 48 hours postoperatively. It can also result in meningitis if the infection spreads through the cribriform plate.

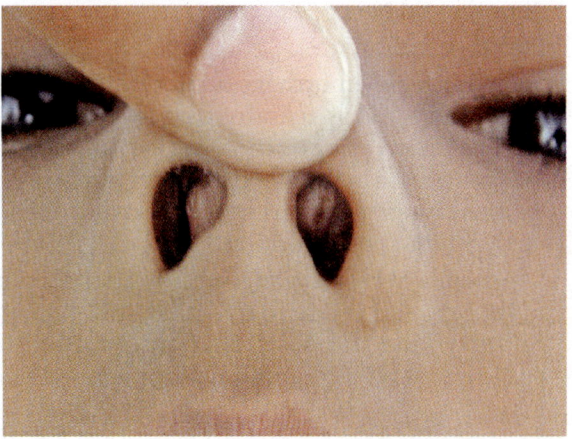

Fig. 21.4: Septal abscess

- Flapping nasal septum occurs, if there is excessive redundant mucosa left behind after removal of deviated septum. The septum postoperatively sags on one side, or the other making a flapping sound during respiration. However, the condition corrects itself after sometime due to fibrosis and scarring.
- Synechiae and adhesions develop between the septum and lateral nasal wall resulting in nasal obstruction postoperatively. These adhesions should be cut and a silastic sheet or an X-ray plate is inserted between the two raw areas for 2–3 weeks to enable healing without recurrence of adhesions.
- Pain may occur on touching the nose and may persist for several weeks postoperatively in a few cases.
- Nasal obstruction may persist postoperatively due to:
  - Synechiae,
  - Hypertrophied turbinates,
  - Allergy, or
  - Incomplete removal of the deviated portion of the septum.

    If SMR is performed in patients below the age of 17 years, recurrence of deviation may occur as the nasal bones grow.
- External nasal deformity may occur as a late complication of SMR, such as a supratip deformity, columellar retraction, saddle nose deformity, etc.

Septoplasty   It is a conservative procedure, where a deviation of the nasal septum is corrected by minimal removal of cartilagenous or bony septum.
- Indications
  - Symptomatic DNS causing nasal obstruction.
  - Patients below 17 years of age, who require correction of septal deviation.
  - Complications of DNS like recurrent sinusitis, URTI, epistaxis, headache, middle ear infection and SOM.
  - Wherever a rhinoplasty is required along with correction of a deviated nasal septum.

All septal deviations anterior to an imaginary line passing from the nasal process of the frontal bone to the nasal spine of the maxilla are treated by septoplasty and all deviations posterior to this imaginary line are treated with SMR operation.
- Contraindication: All those listed for SMR except age. This operation can be performed safely at any age.

- **Anaesthesia:** Same as for SMR except that if septoplasty is performed in a child or an uncooperative patient, general anaesthesia is required.
- **Preoperative preparation:** Same as for SMR.
- **Position of patient:** Same as for SMR.
- **Procedure:** The procedure of septoplasty is shown in Fig. 21.5.
  - After infiltration of anaesthesia, an incision is made at the caudal free border of the septum (Freer's or hemitransfixation incision) using a no. 15 blade.
  - Mucoperichondrial flap is elevated with the help of Freer's mucoperichondrial elevator only on the concave side of the deviated septum.
  - Using a Killian's mucoperiosteal elevator, mucoperiosteal flaps are elevated on either side of the maxillary crest. The flap on the concave side is joined with the already elevated mucoperichondrial flap.
  - Also, mucoperiosteal flaps are elevated on both sides of the bony septum using the Killian's elevator after separating the cartilage from the bony septum. The cartilage is also separated from the maxillary crest.
  - Now, the cartilagenous septum lies freely attached only to the lateral nasal cartilages and the mucoperichondrium of the convex surface.
  - The maxillary crest is removed and the deviated cartilage is straightened by criss-cross incisions not going through the whole thickness of the cartilage so as to break its inherent elasticity. Thus, the spring action of cartilage is lost and it remains in the midline.
  - Deviations in the bony septum are removed using a Luc's forceps.
  - The hemitransfixation incision is now sutured using 3–0 chromic catgut in interrupted sutures.
  - If under local anaesthesia, the patient is asked to judge improvement in the nasal obstruction.
  - Anterior nasal packing is performed.
  - Endoscopic septoplasty is performed today using the rigid nasal/sinus endoscope. It however required expertise as the surgeon has to operate visualizing the monitor.
- **Postoperative care:** Same as for SMR.
- **Endoscopic septoplasty:** It is performed nowadays using the Hopkin's regid nasal/sinus endoscope. However, it requires expertise as the region has to operate visualizing the monitor.
- **Complications:** Since this is a conservative procedure as compared to SMR, the complications are relatively less frequent.

Immediate	Delayed
• Primary haemorrhage.	• Reactionary or secondary haemorrhage.
• Complications of anaesthesia.	• Infection.
• Trauma to surrounding tissues.	• Synechiae and adhesions.
	• Pain.
	• Persistence of nasal obstruction.

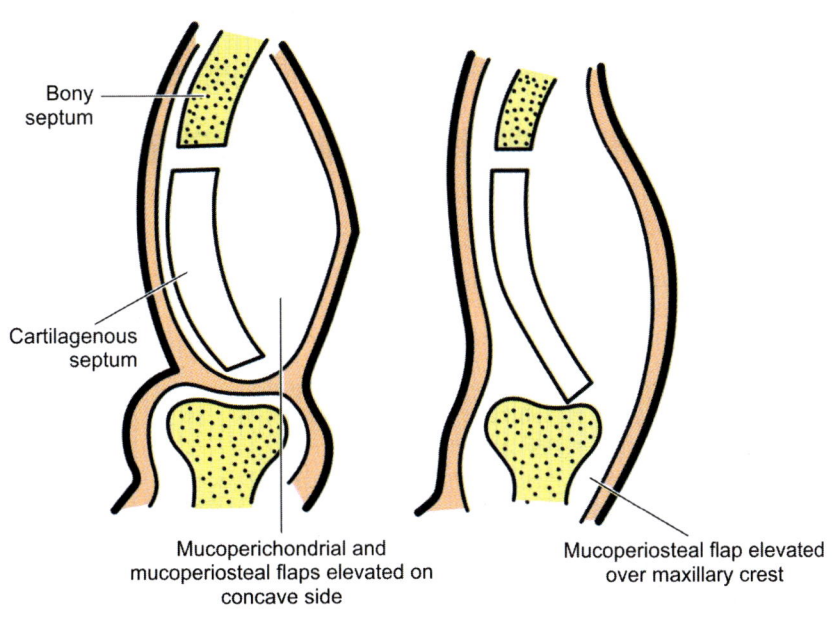
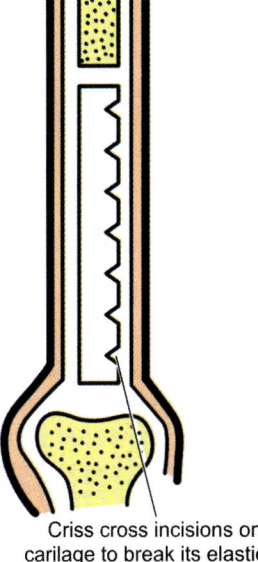

Bony septum

Cartilagenous septum

Mucoperichondrial and mucoperiosteal flaps elevated on concave side

Mucoperiosteal flap elevated over maxillary crest

Criss cross incisions on carilage to break its elasticity

Fig. 21.5: Steps in septoplasty operation

DIFFERENCE BETWEEN SMR AND SEPTOPLASTY

See Table 21.2.

SEPTAL HAEMATOMA

Definition   It is the accumulation of blood in between the two mucoperichondrial flaps of the nasal septum (Fig. 21.6).

Aetiology
* Trauma to nose, e.g. boxers or vehicular accident or blow to nose.
* Postoperatively after SMR operation.

Clinical features
* History of nasal trauma or surgery.
* Nasal obstruction.
* Pain and tenderness over nose.

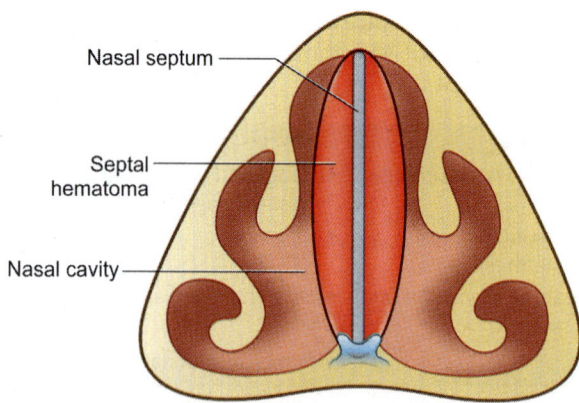

Fig. 21.6: Septal hematoma

* Anterior rhinoscopy reveals a biconvex swollen soft nasal septum obstructing the air entry.

Treatment
* Admission to hospital
* Intravenous antibiotics
* Anti-inflammatory analgesics
* Incision and drainage of haematoma by nicking the mucoperichondrium of only one side and introducing a suction canula. All necrosed pieces of cartilage are removed using a sinus forceps. A ribbon gauze wick is inserted between the two flaps to prevent recurrence and allow drainage. Anterior nasal packing is done on both sides. Packs and wick are removed after 48 hours.

Sequelae
* External nasal deformity, like saddle nose or supratip deformity.

Complications
* Septal abscess
* Facial cellulitis
* Meningitis
* Cavernous sinus thrombophlebitis

SEPTAL ABSCESS

Definition   It is the accumulation of pus in between the two mucoperichondrial layers of the nasal septum.

Aetiology
* Infected septal haematoma
* Furuncle of the nasal vestibule
* Diabetes mellitus predisposes to this condition

TABLE 21.2: Difference between SMR and septoplasty	
SMR	*Septoplasty*
• Radical surgery	• Conservative surgery.
• Not done below 17 years of age	• Can be done at any age.
• Entire cartilage except for a 2–3 mm strip at the caudal end and the roof is removed	• Only minimal removal of cartilage.
• Flaps elevated on both sides of cartilage	• Flap elevated only on concave side of cartilage.
• Caudal dislocation cannot be corrected	• Caudal dislocation is corrected.
• Trauma to cribriform plate resulting in CSF leak may occur	• Trauma to cribriform plate is rare.
• Chance of septal perforation is higher	• Perforation is rare.
• Septal haematoma and abscess may occur	• Haematoma and abscess is rarely seen.
• Supratip deformity, saddle nose deformity and columellar retraction may occur	• External nasal deformity postoperatively is rare.
• Revision surgery is difficult	• Revision surgery is relatively easier.
• Cannot be combined with rhinoplasty	• Can be combined with rhinoplasty (septorhinoplasty).
• Can be used to harvest cartilage as graft material	• Cannot be used, if cartilage graft is to be harvested.

Clinical features

- History of nasal trauma or surgery 3–4 days ago
- Nasal obstruction
- Worsening of pain
- Severe tenderness over nose
- Fever with chills
- Anterior rhinoscopy reveals a biconvex swollen nasal septum

Treatment   Same as for septal haematoma

Sequelae   Same as for septal haematoma

Complications   Same as for septal haematoma

SEPTAL PERFORATION

Definition   It can be defined as a breach in the continuity of the nasal septum, resulting in an abnormal communication between the two nasal cavities.

Classification

- Small or large (size)
- Anterior or posterior (site)

Aetiology

- **Trauma**
  - Accidental, nose-picking
  - Iatrogenic, following septal surgery (SMR)
- **Inflammatory or infective**
  - Septal abscess
  - Leprosy
  - Tuberculosis
  - Syphilis
- **Tumours:** Malignant neoplasms of nose
- **Granulomas**
  - Rhinosporidiosis
  - Rhinoscleroma in the nodular stage
  - Malignant granulomas of the nose

- **Irritants**
  - Snuff addicts
  - Asbestos fumes
  - Chrome fumes
  - Painters
  - Carpenters
  - Cocaine addicts
- Perforation of the nasal septum for wearing ornaments is performed in certain communities.

Clinical features

- It may be asymptomatic
- History of aetiological factor may be present.
- Crusting at the site of perforation.
- Epistaxis if crusts are removed
- Whistling sound with every breath if perforation is anteriorly placed and small.
- Atrophic rhinitis secondary to large perforation.
- Maggots secondary to atrophic rhinitis.

Treatment   Investigations to rule out:

- Diabetes
- Syphilis
- Tuberculosis
- Leprosy

Biopsy of nasal mass or granuloma if present.
- If asymptomatic, no treatment is required
- **Conservative management:**
  - Nasal lubricants like liquid paraffin or vaseline
  - Alkaline nasal douches to remove crusts
- **Surgical treatment**
  - Small perforations are closed by mobilization of local mucosal flaps.
  - Large perforations are closed using silastic or teflon obturators (prosthesis).

Nose

CHAPTER 22

Nasal Polyps

DEFINITION

A nasal polyp is a prolapsed pedunculated portion of the oedematous mucosa, lining the nose and paranasal sinuses.

It is not a true neoplasm, as it is inflammatory in origin and not neoplastic.

CLASSIFICATION

There are two types of nasal polyps:
- Antrochoanal
- Ethmoidal

AETIOLOGY

- Age: Antrochoanal polyp is common in children. Ethmoidal polyps are common in adults.
- Sex: Both the sexes are equally affected.
- Allergy: Ethmoidal polyps are usually of allergic origin.
- Infection: Antrochoanal polyps are of infective origin.
- Vasomotor imbalance: Polyps are thought to occur due to an imbalance in the sympathetic and parasympathetic system.
- Bernoulli phenomenon: When air passes through a narrow constriction, there is a fall in air pressure in the vicinity of this constriction. If this principle is applied to the paranasal sinuses and the ostium is considered as the constriction, a fall in pressure results in a suction like effect with subsequent oedema and prolapse of the mucosa in the vicinity and polyp formation.
- Polysaccharide changes in the ground substance of the mucosa may predispose to polyp formation.
- Recent theory is that polyps occur as a result of mast cell reactions in the mucosa of the nose and paranasal sinuses (PNS).
- It is thought to occur as a result of immunoglobulin changes.
- Around 20–40% of patients with polyps have a co-existing asthma.
- Aspirin hypersensitivity and polyps are seen to coexist in 8% of patients.
- Recurrence is common after excision.

PATHOLOGY

Gross (Macroscopic) Macroscopic or gross pathology is shown in Figs 22.1A and B).
- Antrochoanal (AC) polyp: It is characteristically solitary and 'trifoliate' in appearance with a pale pink smooth surface. It has three parts and one constriction; the smallest 'antral part', which is separated from the other parts by a constriction or the 'neck' which is the portion at the ostium. The largest portion is the 'choanal part' followed by the 'nasal part' which is relatively smaller. It can extend beyond the choana into the nasopharynx and oropharynx as it enlarges. The choanal portion is the largest, since the choanae are more roomy and allow expansion of the polyp without offering resistance.

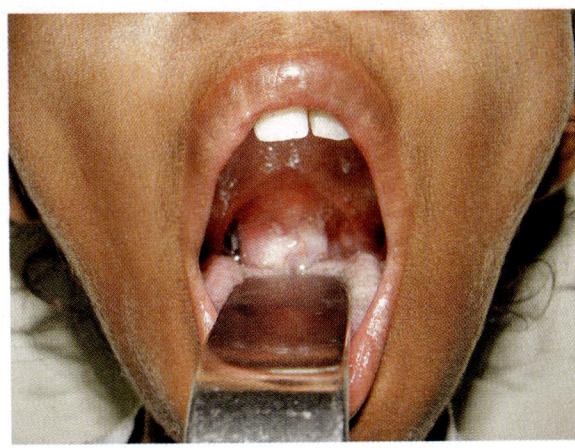

Fig. 22.1A: Polyp in oropharynx

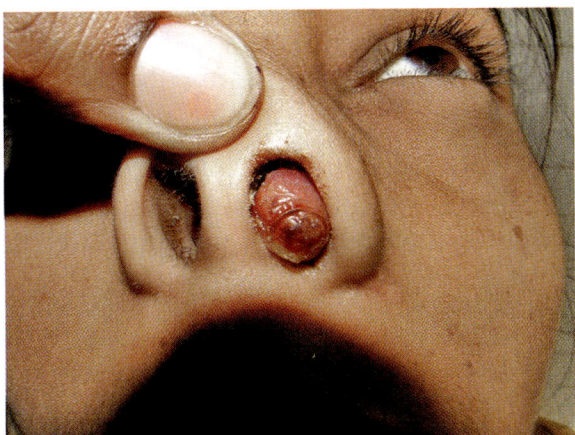

Fig. 22.1B: Infected AC polyp

- **Ethmoidal polypii:** These are characteristically multiple and bilateral and more anteriorly placed. They usually involve the choanae later. They appear pale and oedematous and resemble a 'bunch of grapes'.

Microscopic The lining mucosa is ciliated columnar epithelium with oedematous submucosa comprised of intercellular serous fluid and loose fibrillar stroma. With exposure to atmospheric air, the nasal portion may undergo metaplastic change. Submucosa contains few blood vessels and nerve fibres. Cellular infiltrate contains plasma cells, lymphocytes, macrophages, and a high concentration of eosinophils.

CLINICAL FEATURES

Symptoms
- Nasal obstruction which can be unilateral or bilateral and which is not relieved by nasal decongestants.

- Nasal discharge which is mucopurulent and unilateral in case of antrochoanal polyp or watery and bilateral in case of ethmoidal polyps.
- Sneezing is common in case of ethmoidal polyps as they are allergic in origin.
- Anosmia may be present due to bilateral nasal blockage.
- Expansion of the nasal bridge may occur due to long standing ethmoidal polyps.
- Mouth-breathing and snoring due to nasal obstruction.
- Headache may occur due to nasal obstruction (vacuum headache) or secondary sinusitis.
- Rhinolalia clausa, i.e. loss of nasal tone of voice due to bilateral nasal obstruction.
- Post nasal drip is usually present and mucopurulent in nature.
- Epiphora may be present due to blockage of the nasolacrimal duct by the polyp.
- Rarely blood tinged nasal discharge, if nose is forcefully cleaned in presence of acute infection.

Signs
- Broadening of the nasal bridge resulting in a 'frog-face' appearance.
- Rhinolalia clausa (hyponasal voice).
- Anterior rhinoscopy:
  - Shows the presence of the polyps, which may be unilateral or bilateral and appear smooth, pale, and pearly white. They are non-tender and do not bleed on touch. In a unilateral polyp, the nasal septum may be pushed to the opposite side.
  - The antrochoanal polyp on coming out of the maxillary ostium tends to grow backwards to the choana due to the fact that the ostium of the maxillary sinus faces backwards. Hence, in early cases, it may not be seen in an anterior rhinoscopy.
  - The ethmoidal polyps are multiple, bilateral, and appear like a bunch of grapes. These grow towards the anterior nares.
  - The part of the polyp in the nasal cavities may get inflamed or ulcerated due to exposure to air currents and bleed or undergo metaplastic change.
  - On probing, it is soft but firm in consistency, mobile and attached to the lateral nasal wall.
- Posterior rhinoscopy:
  - Usually, it is an antrochoanal polyp, which is seen in the nasopharynx on posterior rhinoscopy. It is pale-white in colour, smooth, and covered with mucopurulent discharge. If it has grown to huge proportions, it may push the soft palate forwards

and even be seen hanging in the oropharynx behind the soft palate on examination of the throat. Ethmoidal polyps rarely tend to grow towards the choanae, but are sometimes seen as multiple smooth masses. However, a posterior rhinoscopy examination may not be possible in a case of ethmoidal polyps if both nostrils are blocked, as the patient cannot breathe through his nose and this is mandatory for posterior rhinoscopy (PRS).

INVESTIGATIONS

- X-ray paranasal sinuses (Water's view and Caldwell's view): There will be an opacity involving either one or both nasal cavities with opacity of the affected sinuses. However, it is not uncommon to see haziness in all sinuses of the same side of the polyp even though, it may not involve them. This is due to a secondary sinusitis caused by blocking of their ostia due to the polyp in the nasal cavity. Even a unilateral antrochoanal polyp can cause sinusitis on the opposite side. This is due to obstruction to normal drainage of the sinuses through their ostium by a secondary DNS. Also, there may be a coexisting allergic sinusitis.
- X-ray soft tissue nasopharynx: The lateral view will show a soft-tissue opacity in the nasopharynx. This has to be differentiated from a nasopharyngeal angiofibroma by the fact that a 'crescent' shaped airspace is present between the roof of the nasopharynx and the polyp as it is not attached to the roof. This crescentic air-shadow is absent in an angiofibroma.
- Cytology of the nasal secretions may reveal an eosionophilia if allergy is the aetiologic factor.
- Biopsy is rarely performed, especially to rule out metastatic changes.
- CT scan of the nose, nasopharynx and paranasal sinuses with skull base is required in case of suspected complications or prior to functional endoscopic sinus surgery (FESS).

COMPLICATIONS

- Secondary sinusitis
- Epistaxis due to inflammation and infection
- Metaplastic changes due to trauma by the air currents in the nasal cavity
- Mucocoele and pyocoele formation secondary to sinusitis
- Deviation of septum to opposite side due to long-standing pressure
- Broadening of nasal bridge
- Hypertelorism

DIFFERENTIAL DIAGNOSIS OF A NASAL MASS

- Antrochoanal polyp
- Ethmoidal polyps
- Hypertrophic turbinates: These are tender to touch, pinkish red or pale blue (if allergic), and hard bone is felt on slight pressure. On application of a decongestant, they become pale and shrink.
- Rhinosporidiosis: It is a dark red and mulberry–like mass, with white or grey spots on the surface (sporangia). Bleeds on touch. Similar history is present in neighbours or family and usually patient is a farmer or from a coastal area.
- Inverted papilloma: Greyish in colour, firm in consistency, unilateral, and non-tender. It is known to be a premalignant condition and also known as a 'transitional cell tumour'.
- Nasal angioma: Red in colour, single, smooth, and bleeds on touch. Usually arises from the nasal septum (Fig. 22.2).
- Malignancy: Irregular surface with areas of slough and necrosis. Firm to hard in consistency, bleeds on touch, non-tender, and foul smelling. Patient is elderly. Bone destruction and rapid growth is characteristic.
- Angiofibroma: Common in young males. Torrential epistaxis which is spontaneous in onset. Patient is pale. Mass is bluish-red in colour and smooth. Always seen in posterior rhinoscopy, as it arises first in nasopharynx and then involves the nasal cavities. Biopsy is never performed.
- Rhinoscleroma in the nodular stage. Irregular red mass in nose with mucosa showing atrophic changes.

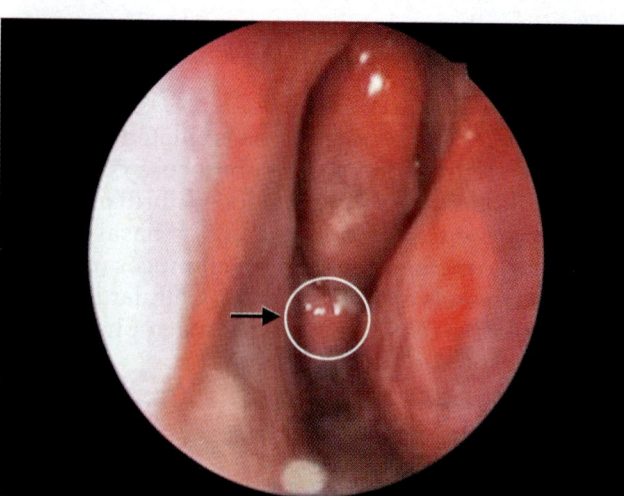

Fig. 22.2: Nasal angioma

- **Rhinolith:** It is common in children. An irregular red granulomatous mass with foul smelling discharge is found.
- **Nasal granulomas:** These are Wegener's and Ringertz tumours. These are characterised by rapidly destructive growth and in Wegener's tumour, there is a multi-system involvement.

Differences between antrochoanal and ethmoidal polyps

Distinction between antrochoanal and ethmoidal polys are shown in Table 22.1.

TABLE 22.1:	Differences between antrochoanal and ethmoidal polyps	
Criteria	*Antrochoanal polyp*	*Ethmoidal polyps*
• Number	Solitary	Multiple
• Side	Unilateral	Bilateral
• Aetiology	Infection	Allergy
• Arises from	Maxillary sinus	Ethmoidal sinuses
• Age	Common in children	Common in adults
• Extension	Backwards to the choanae (posterior nares)	Forwards to the anterior nares
• Shape	Trifoliate (initially *'dumbbell like'* due to antral and choanal parts only)	Grape like
• Size	Can grow to huge proportions and reach nasopharynx or oropharynx	Small and multiple
• Recurrence	Uncommon	Common
• Treatment	Caldwell Luc operation or functional endoscopic sinus surgery (FESS)	Ethmoidectomy or FESS

TREATMENT

Medical/Conservative   This is not of much use in an antrochoanal polyp, as it does not regress with medication. Ethmoidal polyps may regress with medication, but tend to recur.

However, preoperatively, antibiotics, and anti-inflammatory analgesics are given to control infection and hence, reduce intraoperative haemorrhage.

- Antibiotics orally
- Anti-inflammatory analgesics orally
- **Antihistaminics and nasal decongestants:** These are useful, especially in ethmoidal polyps since they have an allergic origin.
- **Steroids** orally are given in tapering doses as well as locally, as nose drops in combination with antibiotics. These help greatly in the regression of ethmoidal polyps.

Surgical   This is the mainstay of treatment and helps to prevent a recurrence if done adequately.

Polypectomy   The nasal polyps are avulsed using a Luc's forceps or a nasal snare. However, the cause which lies in the sinuses is not treated and hence, recurrences are common.

Caldwell Luc operation   It is performed to completely eradicate the antrochoanal polyp.

Ethmoidectomy   It is intranasal, external or transantral ethmoidectomy. If all the ethmoid aircells are exenterated, chances of recurrence is less as compared to nasal polypectomy. However, the cause of recurrence in ethmoidal polyps, is allergy and complex anatomy of the ethmoidal air cells system.

Functional endoscopic sinus surgery   It is the recent advancement in this field and an ethmoidectomy using FESS has considerably reduced incidence of recurrence.

Laser used with FESS is also a recent advancement.

PREVENTION OF RECURRENCE

Antrochoanal polyp   Caldwell Luc is better than nasal polypectomy. FESS is recently being preferred over Caldwell Luc, since it further reduces recurrence and is performed under vision. However, it requires expertise and experience.

Ethmoidal polyps   Recurrence of ethmoidal polyps is more common than with antrochoanal polyps and can be reduced by ethmoidectomy done meticulously using FESS, antihistaminics for 4–6 weeks after surgery, topical, and oral steroids for 3–4 weeks postoperatively.

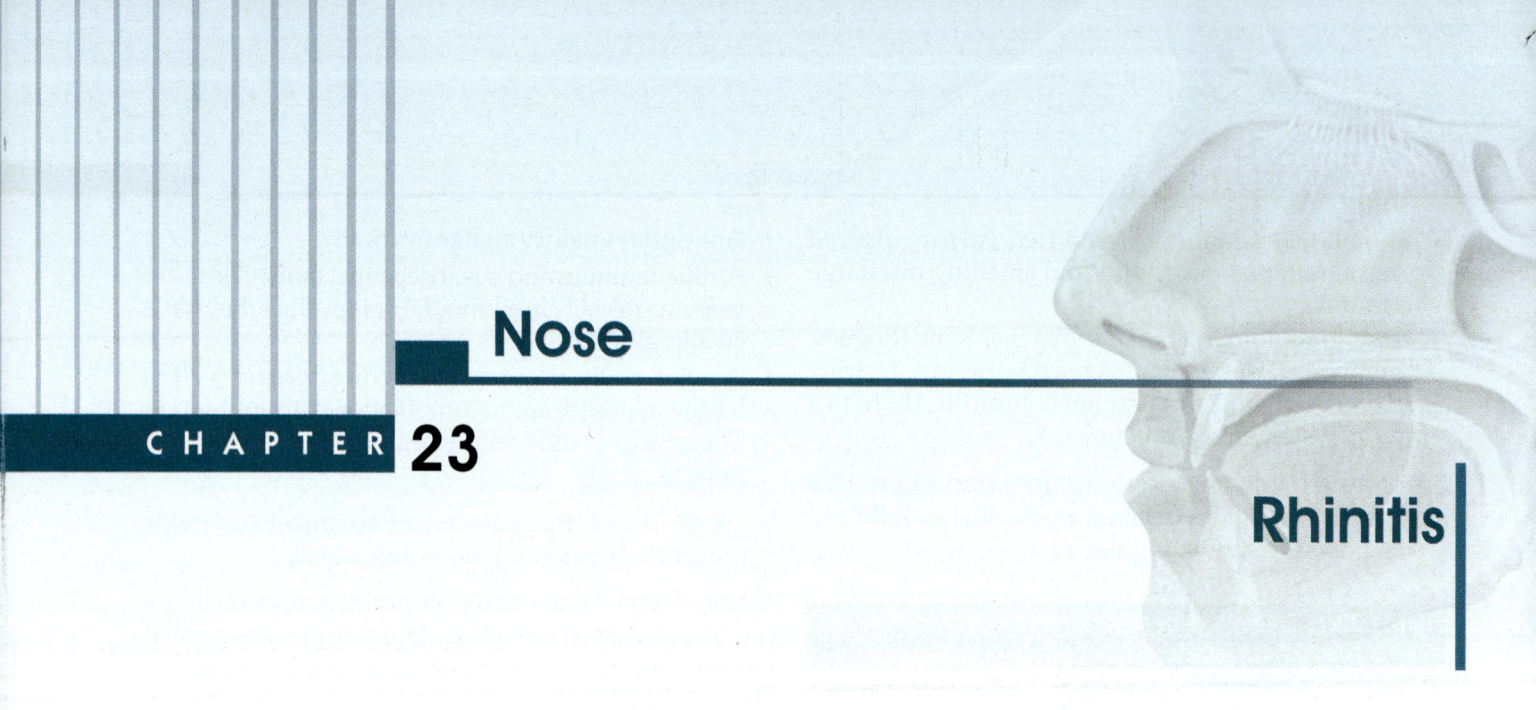

Definition Rhinitis is the inflammation of the nasal mucous membranes.

Classification *See* Flowchart 23.1.

DIPHTHERETIC RHINITIS/NASAL DIPHTHERIA

It is a specific form of acute infective rhinitis.

Aetiology
- Causative organism: *Corynebacterium diphtheriae* (Kleb-Loeffler's bacillus).
- Age: It is common in children
- Primary: It may affect the nose first without involvement of other tissues.

Flowchart 23.1: Classification of rhinitis

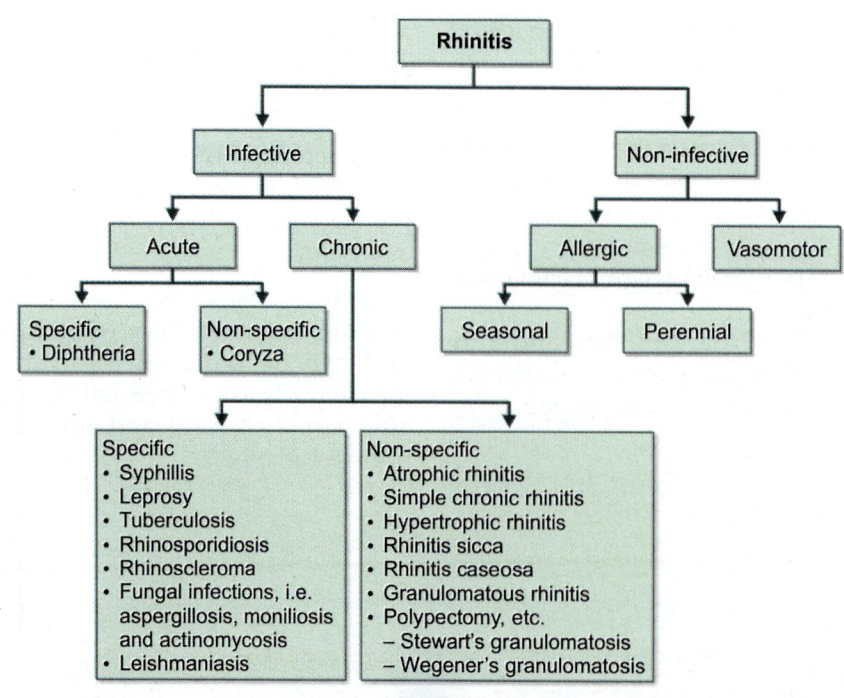

- **Secondary:** It may affect the nose secondary to faucial diphtheria.

Clinical features
- Blood stained watery rhinorrhoea
- Skin near the nasal vestibule may show excoriation due to continuous nasal discharge.
- Nasal obstruction
- Epistaxis
- Greyish-white membrane is seen on the turbinates or nasal septum. It is difficult to remove and bleeds on removal
- Constitutional symptoms such as fever, malaise, etc. are rare, hence the diagnosis is usually missed.
- Throat should be examined to rule out involvement of tonsils or pharynx

Investigations
- Swab culture will show diphtheria bacilli

Treatment
- Patient is hospitalised and isolated
- 10,000 units of antitoxin serum are given for nasal diphtheria, after a skin sensitivity test.
- Injection crystalline penicillin 5 lac units intramuscular (IM) 6 hourly or Injection ampicillin 250 mg (IM) 6 hourly to control bacterial infection. This is given for 5 days.
- Prophylactic dose of antitoxin is given to all contacts.

CORYZA

Coryza is an acute non-specific infective rhinitis. Also known as 'common cold'.

Aetiology
- Causative organism is a virus and may be either the influenza virus, rhinovirus or adenovirus.
- Spread is by airborne droplet infection or by direct contact.
- Secondary infection by bacteria may occur, e.g. streptococcus, staphylococcus, pneumococcus, *Haemophilus influenzae*, etc.

Pathology   Viral infection of the nasal mucosa → acute generalised hyperemia of the nasal mucosa → engorgement of secretory glands and goblet cells → profuse secretion. Involvement of sinuses → sinusitis. Involvement of Eustachian tube opening → acute suppurative otitis media (ASOM) and serous otitis media (SOM).

Clinical features   Four stages following an incubation period of 1–3 days.

- Ischaemic stage
  - Raw sensation and irritation in the pharynx
  - Irritation and dryness in the nose
  - Sneezing attacks
  - Malaise with chills
- Hyperaemic stage
  - Profuse watery rhinorrhoea
  - Blocking of nose
  - Congested nasal mucosa
  - Anosmia
  - Fever and malaise with chills
  - Headache and otalgia
- Stage of secondary infection
  - Nasal discharge becomes thicker and yellowish or greenish
  - Fever and malaise with chills
  - Headache
  - Otalgia
  - Congested nasal mucosa
- Stage of resolution
  - Resolution of uncomplicated cases occurs within 6–10 days
- Complications
  - Sinusitis
  - Acute otitis media
  - Pharyngitis
  - Laryngitis and tracheobronchitis
  - Pneumonia
- Treatment
  - Antibiotics orally for preventing or treating the secondary infection
  - Analgesics and antipyretics orally
  - Antihistaminics orally
  - Vitamin C orally (empirical value)
  - Rest and warmth
  - High protein diet
  - Nasal decongestants locally
  - Steam inhalations with tincture benzoin or menthol
  - Prophylaxis/Prevention
    - Avoid contact with infected individuals
    - Vaccines are not very effective. Surgical removal of focus of infection such as infected tonsils or adenoids help to reduce frequency of attacks.

ATROPHIC RHINITIS

Synonym   Ozaena

Definition   Atrophic rhinitis is a chronic inflammatory disease of the nasal mucosa which is characterised by progressive atrophy of the mucosa and turbinates, formation of crusts, and foul smell from the nose.

Classification
- Unilateral or Bilateral
- Primary or Secondary

Aetiology
- **Primary:** The exact aetiology is not known, but the probable predisposing factors include:
  - *Age:* It is common between 15–40 years. It usually occurs at puberty.
  - *Sex:* It is more common in females.
  - *Heredity:* There is a racial preponderance.
  - *Familial:* It is known to occur in members of the same family.
  - *Environmental:* It is common in the tropical countries.
  - *Nutritional:* It is common in undernourished persons. It is usually associated with vitamin A deficiency.
  - *Hormonal:* Hormonal factors are implicated, as it is seen to affect females more commonly and worsen during menarche, menopause, pregnancy, etc.
  - Autonomic imbalance has been implicated as a cause.
  - Infection of the nasal mucosa by organisms is also thought of as a cause. However, it is thought by some scientists that it is caused by *Klebsiella ozaenae*, Perez bacilli, Abel bacilli, and diphtheroid organisms.
  - Exanthematous disease in childhood predisposes to atrophic rhinitis due to altered immunity.
  - It is seen to occur more commonly in blood groups O and B.
  - Immunodeficiency is also thought to predispose to atrophic rhinitis.
  - Reflex sympathetic dystrophy syndrome (RSDS) has been implicated as a cause.
- **Secondary**
  - Deviated nasal septum results in atrophic rhinitis in the roomy nasal cavity on the concave side of the deviated nasal septum (DNS).
  - Chronic specific infections like syphilis, leprosy, lupus vulgaris, tuberculosis, and initial stages of rhinoscleroma may result in atrophic changes in the nasal mucosa.
  - Chronic sinusitis can lead to atrophic rhinitis. However atrophic rhinitis can also cause chronic sinusitis due to obstruction of the sinus ostia.

- Postoperatively, atrophic rhinitis may occur if a roomy nasal cavity is the result, e.g. over-correction of DNS will result in atrophic rhinitis on the roomy side; septal perforations which are large; removal of nasal polypii with a roomy nasal cavity as a result; turbinectomy; surgery for rhinoporidiosis removal; removal of nasopharyn-geal angiofibroma, etc.
- **Pathology:** It is a condition characterised by atrophic changes in all the nasal tissues:
  - Mucosa undergoes atrophy and metaplasia to cuboidal or stratified epithelium. Cilia and secretory glands also undergo atrophy with a resultant pale, dry, thin mucosa with thick scanty secretions. Secretions dry to form crusts which may bleed on removal.
  - Secondary infection usually supervenes resulting in a foul foetid smell.
  - Turbinates undergo atrophy resulting in loss of anatomical landmarks of the nose and a roomy nasal cavity.
  - Blood vessels undergo periarteritis and endarteritis resulting in ischaemia which causes atrophy of the mucosa and underlying bones.
  - Sensory nerves undergo atrophy and hence the patient may complain of nasal obstruction, as he does not feel the air passing through the nose.
  - Atrophy of the olfactory nerve endings results in anosmia.

Clinical features
- Symptoms
  - *Nasal obstruction:* It can be due to:
    - Crusts in nasal cavity.
    - Atrophy of sensory nerves which gives a false sense of nasal obstruction as patient cannot feel air passing through his/her nose, even in the absence of crusts.
  - *Crusting in nose (ozaena):* It occurs due to atrophy of secretory glands and goblet cells resulting in thick scanty secretions which dry to form crusts.
  - *Foul smell from the nose:* This is due to secondary infection of crusts in the nose. However, due to anosmia the patient usually cannot get this foul smell and it is detected by friends or relatives. (Hence, this anosmia is described by some researchers as a 'merciful anosmia').
  - *Anosmia or loss of sense of smell:* It occurs due to :
    - Atrophy of olfactory nerve endings.
    - Obstruction to the olfactory nerve endings by accumulation of crusts.

- ◆ *Epistaxis:* Scanty epistaxis occurs, if crusts are forcefully pulled out.
- ◆ *Headache and dryness* of nose and throat.
- Signs
  - ◆ *External nasal examination:* The bridge of the nose may be depressed (saddle shaped nose), due to atrophy of septal and nasal bones.
  - ◆ *Anterior rhinoscopy*
    - Nasal cavity is roomy.
    - Causative factor like DNS or septal perforation is seen.
    - Mucosa is pale, shiny, dry, and atrophic.
    - Crusts are seen.
    - Turbinates are atrophied and normal anatomical landmarks are not seen.
    - Nasopharynx and roof of the nose are easily seen due to atrophy of the turbinates.
  - ◆ *Posterior rhinoscopy:* In a patient of atrophic rhinitis, posterior rhinoscopy (PRS) is easy to perform, as there is diminished sensation of the mucosa due to atrophy of sensory nerve endings. PRS reveals crusts and dry mucosa.

Complications
- Sinusitis
- Middle ear infection
- Atrophic pharyngitis
- Maggots
- External nasal deformity
- Psychological complications due to foul smell from nose resulting in depression.

Differential diagnosis
- **Rhinitis sicca:** It is characterised by crusting only in the anterior aspect of the nose. No foul smell or atrophy is seen.
- Rhinoscleroma in the early stage may show atrophic change but mucosa is pink and turbinates are not affected. A biopsy is confirmatory.
- **Rhinitis medicamentosa:** Characteristic history of overuse of nasal decongestants is present.
- Syphilis, tuberculosis, and leprosy affecting the nasal cavity may cause atrophic changes or coexist with atrophic rhinitis.

Investigations
- X-rays of paranasal sinuses to rule out sinusitis which may be primary or secondary. The walls of the sinuses may be thickened.
- X-ray chest to rule out tuberculosis.
- Venereal disease research laboratory (VDRL) to rule out syphilis.

- Dermatological examination to rule out leprosy.
- Nasal smear to rule out leprosy or tuberculosis.
- Biopsy, if any other diagnosis is suspected, e.g. rhinoscleroma.
- Usually, the diagnosis is based only on clinical examination.

Treatment
- Treat the cause, i.e. DNS, septal perforation, etc.
- Conservative/Medical treatment.
- Surgical treatment.
- **Conservative/Medical treatment.**

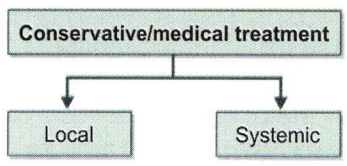

- ◆ *Aims:*
  - To reduce crusting
  - To prevent foetor (foul smell)
  - To keep the nasal cavity clean and moist
- *Local treatment*
  - ▪ *Nasal drops*
    - ◆ Twenty-five percent glucose in glycerine is used as nose drops. Glucose inhibits the growth of proteolytic organisms by getting fermented to lactic acid. Glycerine is hygroscopic and hence helps in retaining moisture of the nasal mucosa.
    - ◆ Ethylene oestradiol in arachis oil (1 : 10,000).
    - ◆ Chloramphenicol or Streptomycin nasal drops.
    - ◆ Kemicetine antiozaena nasal drops.
    - ◆ Liquid paraffin nose drops to soften crusts.
  - ▪ *Placental extract* has been used for local infiltration submucosally as well as for intramuscular injections. It helps by its hormonal effects.
  - ▪ *Alkaline nasal douches:* The nasal cavities are washed with a solution containing the following:
    - ◆ *Sodium bicarbonate:* It helps to loosen the crusts.
    - ◆ *Sodium biborate:* It is an antiseptic.
    - ◆ *Sodium chloride:* It makes the solution isotonic.
      A simple rubber catheter with a 20 cc plastic syringe or a glass asepto syringe or a Higginson's syringe is placed on the floor of the nose and the cavity is washed, so as to remove all crusts and clean the nasal cavities.

This is done twice a day till all crusts disappear and the nasal cavity mucosa is healthy.

- *Systemic treatment*
  - Antibiotics orally
  - High protein diet
  - Vitamin A orally
  - Vasodialators to increase the blood supply to the nose and hence increase secretions
  - Potassium iodide tablets orally to increase secretions

Surgical treatment

Aims

- To reduce the size of the nasal cavity, i.e. to make the nasal cavity narrow
- To decrease the air entry in the nasal cavity
- To increase secretion of nasal mucosa
- Surgery aimed to reduce the size of the nasal cavity
  - Submucosal implants of teflon, silastic, gold, ivory, cartilage, bone chips, liquid paraffin, dermofat or acrylic.
  - Submucosal injection of placental extract is given. It helps by mechanical narrowing of the nasal cavity in addition to the hormonal effects.
  - *Lautenslager's operation*: Medialisation of the lateral nasal wall.
- Surgery to decrease air entry into the nasal cavity (Fig. 23.1)
  - *Young's operation*: Closure of anterior nares using locally elevated mucosal flaps which are sutured together. This helps by giving rest to the nasal mucosa from the turbulent air currents and hence helps in regeneration of epithelium. Also, there

is a local hypoxia, which helps in regeneration of mucosa and proliferation of secretory glands and goblet cells. However, the patient has to breathe through the mouth, as both the nasal cavities has been blocked. This is uncomfortable for the patient and results in halitosis and snoring. The nares are re-opened after 9 months to one year after confirming recovery by posterior rhinoscopy, where healthy mucosa and absence of crusts are seen.

- *Modified Young's operation*: This involves partial closure of the anterior nares leaving behind a 3 mm opening. This enables breathing through the nares and hence the patient is more comfortable. Also, it helps the nasal mucosa to regenerate.
- Surgery to increase local nasal mucosal secretions
  - *Stellate ganglion block*: This results in local vasodialation, resulting in proliferation of secretory glands and goblet cells.
  - *Cervical sympathectomy*: This causes local vasodilation with subsequent proliferation of secretory glands and goblet cells.
  - *Transfer of Stenson's (parotid) duct to the maxillary sinus (Whitmack's operation)*: This improves lubrication of the nasal cavity. However, there is profuse rhinorrhoea during eating, which is troublesome and, hence the operation is not done nowadays.
  - *Transfer of maxillary antral mucosa to the nasal cavity (Raghav Sharan's operation)*: This helps to lubricate the nasal cavity. However, it is rarely performed.

CHRONIC SIMPLE RHINITIS

Aetiology

- Predisposing factors
  - Vasomotor rhinitis
  - DNS
  - Nasal polypii
  - Tonsillitis
  - Sinusitis
  - Smoking and alcoholism
  - Pollution, dust and smoke
  - Overuse of nose drops, occasionally
- Chronic rhinitis may result following recurrent attacks of acute rhinitis.

Clinical features

- Symptoms
  - Rhinorrhoea (mucopurulent)
  - Nasal obstruction

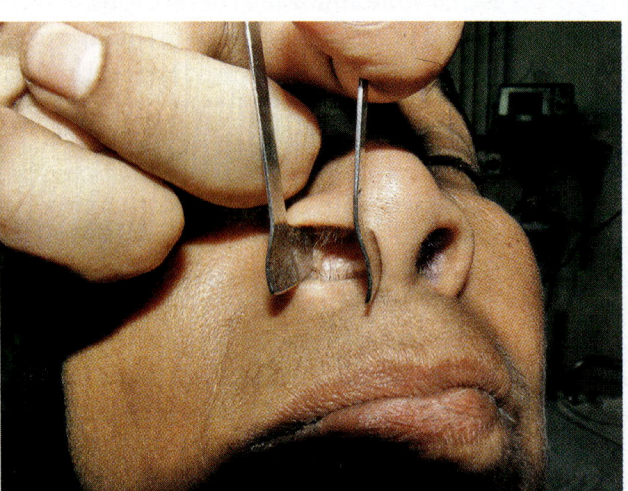

Fig. 23.1: Post Young's closure

- ◆ Headache
- ◆ Anosmia—rarely
- Signs
  - ◆ Hyperemic mucosa with oedema
  - ◆ Postnasal drip
  - ◆ Thick viscid mucopurulent nasal secretions
  - ◆ Pharyngitis
- Treatment
  - ◆ Alkaline nasal douching to clear the nose of thick viscid secretions
  - ◆ Treat the predisposing factors, if present
  - ◆ Stop smoking and alcohol

CHRONIC HYPERTROPHIC RHINITIS

Aetiology
- Usually, it results from recurrent attacks of acute rhinitis.
- Predisposing factors:
  - ◆ Vasomotor rhinitis
  - ◆ Sinusitis
  - ◆ Tonsillitis
  - ◆ DNS
  - ◆ Nasal polypii
  - ◆ Pollution, dust and smoke
  - ◆ Overuse of nasal drops
  - ◆ Alcoholism and smoking
  - ◆ Vitamin deficiency

Clinical features
- Symptoms
  - ◆ *Nasal obstruction*: This is due to hypertrophy of the turbinates
  - ◆ *Rhinorrhoea*: The nasal discharge is thick and viscid
  - ◆ *Anosmia*: It may be present
  - ◆ Dull headache
  - ◆ *Otalgia*: This is referred otalgia. Patients has no ear pathology
  - ◆ Sore-throat due to pharyngitis
- Signs
  - ◆ *Anterior rhinoscopy* reveals hypertrophied inferior nasal turbinates. The nasal mucosa is congested or in the presence of allergy, it will be pale and oedematous.
  - ◆ *Posterior rhinoscopy* reveals characteristic mulberry–like appearance of the posterior ends of the inferior turbinates.

Diagnostic features
The inferior turbinates are hypertrophic with congestion of nasal mucosa. They have to be differentiated from nasal polypii by the following:

- ◆ On probing, attachment to lateral nasal wall is detected.
- ◆ They are soft in consistency, but on pressure the underlying bone is felt.
- ◆ On application of decongestant nasal drops or dilute adrenaline solution to the surface of the turbinates, they will become pale and shrink temporarily. This is not seen in case of nasal polypii.

Treatment
- Removal or treatment of the predisposing factors.
- Local nasal decongestant drops: These help in relief of nasal obstruction. However, prolonged use is avoided, as this can cause a rebound congestion.
- Oral antihistaminics may be helpful.
- Surgical management for turbinate hypertrophy:
  - ◆ Submucosal cauterization of the turbinates performed by inserting a needle submucosally into the inferior turbinate and applying an electrocautery to it. It helps by producing deep tissue fibrosis.
  - ◆ Surface cauterization of the turbinate mucosa using an electrocautery also helps in shrinking the turbinates. However, the raw mucosa may develop adhesions with the nasal septum.
  - ◆ Cryosurgery may be used to shrink the turbinates.
  - ◆ Partial turbiznectomy may be performed surgically.
  - ◆ Laser may be used to either shrink the turbinate by coagulation or excise the turbinate.

RHINITIS SICCA

Definition
Rhinitis sicca is a disease of the nose characterised by drying and crusting, affecting only the anterior portion of the nasal cavity.

Aetiology
It is seen in persons working in dry, hot, and dusty environment like rubber factory workers, furnace workers, bottle factory workers, etc.

Clinical features
- Symptoms
  - ◆ Nasal obstruction due to crusting and drying of the secretions in the anterior portion of the nose.
  - ◆ Nasal irritation, due to crusting.
  - ◆ Epistaxis, due to picking of crusts.
- Signs
  - ◆ Anterior rhinoscopy shows dry, dark-red mucosa with crusts and ulcerations. Characteristically, only the anterior nasal cavity is affected.
  - ◆ Septal perforation may be seen.

- There is no foetid odour, as seen in atrophic rhinitis.
- Posterior rhinoscopy shows normal nasal mucosa without any crusts or drying.
- Treatment
  - Alkaline nasal douches for removal of the crusts.
  - Emollient nose drops like vaseline or liquid paraffin to moisten the nasal cavities and prevent crusting.
  - Change of environment or job helps to reverse the mucosal changes.

RHINITIS CASEOSA

Synonym   Cholesteatoma of the nose.

Definition   Rhinitis caseosa is a condition characterised by accumulation of a caseous (cheezy) material in the nasal cavity and maxillary sinus.

It is a rare condition affecting the nasal cavity.

Aetiology   The exact aetiology is not known but it is thought to occur as a result of failure of resolution of sinusitis, when the contents become inspissated; associated with inflammation and granulation of the lining mucosa. There may be erosion of the lateral nasal wall.

Clinical features
- Symptoms
  - Nasal obstruction
  - Foul smell from the nose
  - Headache
  - Thick viscid rhinorrhoea
- Signs
  - Presence of thick cheezy or caseous material obstructing the nasal cavity
  - Foetid odour
  - Involvement of maxillary sinus

Treatment   Caldwell-Luc operation to completely clear the maxillary antrum and nasal cavity of the caseous necrotic material and granulations. An inferior meatal antrostomy enables adequate drainage of the maxillary antrum.

GRANULOMATOUS RHINITIS

Granulomatous rhinitis is shown in Fig. 23.2.

Synonym   Malignant granulomas of the nose.

Classification/Types   Malignant granulomas of the nose are of two types.

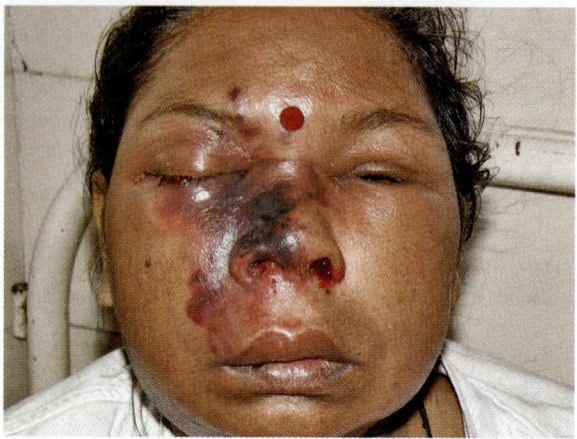

Fig. 23.2: Granuloma

- **Stewart's granuloma:** It is characterized by localised, rapidly progressive ulceration with granulation of the mucosa of the nose and paranasal sinuses. It may also extend to involve the pharynx. The disease rapidly and progressively destroys bones, cartilage, and soft-tissues, thus simulating a malignancy. Eventually, the entire nose is destroyed by the granuloma.
  Treatment: Curative (radiotherapy).
- **Wegener's granulomatosis:** It is a necrotising granulomatosis affecting the nose, lungs and kidneys. It is a multisystem disorder unlike Stewart's granuloma which is localised to the nose. It is characterised by focal necrotizing vasculitis involving the vessels of the lungs and kidneys with destructive granulomatosis of the nose.
  Treatment: It is a rapidly fatal disease and the following help in palliation :
  - Steroids
  - Cytotoxic drugs
  - Antimetabolites

RHINITIS MEDICAMENTOSA

Definition   Rhinitis medicamentosa is an iatrogenic condition affecting the nasal cavity characterised by hypertrophy of the nasal mucosa with rhinitis.

Aetiology   It occurs due to prolonged use of nasal decongestant drops, which results in a rebound phenomenon of congestion.

Clinical features
- Symptoms
  - Nasal obstruction
  - Irritation in nose
  - Scanty epistaxis
  - Headache occasionally

- **Signs**
  - Hypertrophied inflammed nasal mucosa with crusts is seen on anterior rhinoscopy and posterior rhinoscopy.
  - Hypertrophied inferior turbinates
- **Treatment**
  - Stop nasal decongestant drops
  - Steroid drops locally
  - Orally antihistaminics
  - Submucosal diathermy of turbinates, if required

RHINOSPORIDIOSIS

Definition Rhinosporidiosis is the infection of the nose by a spore-bearing fungus (Fig. 23.3).

It may affect sites other than the nose, such as conjunctiva, ear, skin, genitalia, etc.

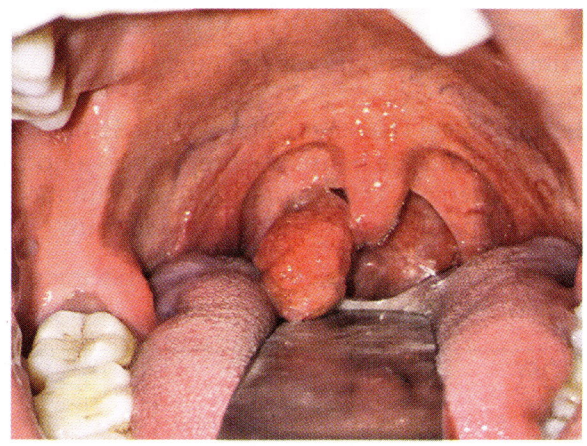

Fig. 23.3: Rhinosporidiosis

Aetiology
- **Age:** It is commonly seen in young adults. It can occur at any age.
- **Sex:** Males are affected more commonly
- **Occupation:** Common in farmers, country-dwellers, etc.
- **Trauma** is a probable predisposing factor
- **Geographical distribution:** It is commonly occur along the coastal areas of tropical countries like India, Bangladesh, Sri Lanka, Africa and South America. It was first seen in India and Sri Lanka.

  Causative organisms:
  - *Rhinosporidium seeberi*
  - *Rhinosporidium kinealyi*

  Mode of transmission: Waterborne and airborne

  The infective spores are transmitted by cattle and horses through faeces polluting water in ponds or air.

The spores are transmitted to humans while bathing in infected ponds, or inhaling polluted air.

Pathology Trauma to the nasal mucosa is a predisposing factor. The infective spores enter the traumatised mucosa and multiply in the submucosal layer to form sporangia which are oval or round chitinous cysts full of spores. The spores burst through the germinal pore and spill over into the tissues. This causes a reactive hyperplasia resulting in the formation of a polypoid vascular mass. Transmission to extranasal sites is usually through water or a contaminated finger-nail. It usually starts at the mucocutaneous junction of the anterior nares.

Clinical features
- **Symptoms**
  - Nasal obstruction
  - Epistaxis
  - Rhinorrhoea
  - Headache due to sinusitis
  - Nasal mass may be visible through the anterior nares
- **Signs**
  - The nasal cavity shows a vascular strawberry-like or mulberry-like polypoidal mass which is dark-red in colour with grey spots on its surface which are the sporangia.
  - The mass bleeds on touch.
  - It may extend to the other nasal cavity and pharynx.
  - The mass arises from the mucocutaneous junction near the nasal vestibule.
- **Treatment**
  - Surgery is the only form of curative treatment. A wide surgical excision with cauterization of the pedicle is performed. Recurrences are common.
  - Recently diaminodiphenyl sulfone orally, has been used following surgery to prevent recurrence.

RHINOSCLEROMA

Definition Rhinoscleroma is a chronic granulomatous disease affecting the nose characterised by sclerosis and stenosis of the nasal cavities.

It affects the nose and the respiratory tract and is known as 'scleroma' of the nasopharynx, oropharynx, larynx and rarely the tracheobronchial tree.

Aetiology
- **Age:** Usually seen beyond the second decade of life.
- Environmental factors include rural areas all over the world.
- Low socioeconomic status and poor housing conditions predispose to this disease.

- **Geographical distribution:** It is common in central Europe, South America, and tropical countries like India, Sri Lanka, etc. (North and Central parts).

Causative organism: Klebsiella rhinoscleromatis which is also known as the Frisch Bacillus.

Pathology   The disease is characterised by granulations which infilterate the mucosa and submucosa. There is a presence of Mikulicz cells, Russel bodies, and lymphocytes in dense fibrous tissue. Mikulicz cells are large vacuolated foamy cells with a central nucleus and containing acid-fast Frisch bacilli.

Stages   The disease process follows three stages:

- **Atrophic stage:** This stage is characterised by crusting, foul odour and nasal obstruction, but the nasal mucosa is pink in colour.
- **Nodular or Granular stage:** This stage is characterised by bluish-red nodular masses which are of rubbery consistency and are non-ulcerative. It may involve the upper lip secondarily.
- **Stage of cicatrization or fibrosis and stenosis:** This stage is characterised by nasal obstruction or adhesions and scarring with total stenosis of the nasal cavities. The process of obliteration of the nasal cavities starts from the anterior nares and progresses posteriorly.

Clinical features

- Symptoms
  - Nasal obstruction
  - Nasal discharge, which is thick and mucopurulent
  - Epistaxis occasionally
  - Mass seen in nose
  - Headache
- Signs
  - The external nose is hard in consistency (Woody nose)
  - Anterior rhinoscopy findings vary with the stage of the disease
  - The throat, oropharynx, larynx and trachea may be involved

Differential diagnosis

- Atrophic rhinitis
- Rhinosporidiosis
- Tertiary syphilis

Treatment

- In the first and second stages, antibiotics like streptomycin and tetracycline are given for a period of 9–12 months.

- Recently, rifampicin has been used with good results for regression of the disease
- Steroids given over a prolonged period of time help to prevent cicatrisation
- Surgical treatment is required in the third stage i.e. after fibrosis and stenosis and have occurred. Dilatation, recanalisation or plastic reconstruction may be required.
- Laser is a recent advance in treatment

SYPHILIS

Congenital

- **Early:** 'Snuffles' is characterised by nasal discharge and bleeding with crusting and fissure formation.
- **Late:** Deformities are similar to those seen in tertiary syphilis

Acquired

- **Primary and secondary stages** rarely manifest with nasal pathology.
- **Tertiary stage:** This stage is characterised by gumma formation on the bony nasal septum as a nodule which ulcerates. This results in septal perforation in the bony portion with saddle-nose deformity.

Treatment   Antisyphilitic therapy with systemic penicillin and nasal douching.

LEPROSY

Leprosy is a common disease in India. Leprosy affects the cartilagenous portion of the nasal septum in the form of a nodule, which later ulcerates to form a septal perforation with saddle-nose deformity.

TUBERCULOSIS

Tuberculosis rarely affects the nose primarily. It results in a granuloma (tuberculoma) affecting the cartilagenous septum with ulceration and subsequent septal perforation.

LUPUS VULGARIS

Lupus vulgaris is a tuberculous infection of low virulence. It is often associated with a cutaneous lesion. It commonly occurs in young females. The lesion occurs at the mucocutaneous junction of the nasal vestibule with ulceration and 'apple-jelly' nodule formation. There may rarely be a septal perforation of the cartilagenous septum.

CHAPTER 24

Allergic Rhinitis and Vasomotor Rhinitis

ALLERGIC RHINITIS

Definition   Allergic rhinitis is an inflammation of the nasal mucous membrane due to an allergic aetiology.

Classification
- Seasonal: That occurs in certain months.
- Perennial: That occurs throughout the year.

Aetiology
- Predisposing factors
  - *Environmental*: Variation in temperature and seasonal changes in humidity or pollution can make the nasal mucosa more susceptible to allergy.
  - *Emotional or psychological factors* predispose to allergy.
  - *Hormonal changes*, such as those seen during puberty, pregnancy, and menopause may also predispose to allergy.
  - *Heredity*: A family history is often present.
- Precipitating factors
  - *Exogenous allergens*
    - *Inhalants:* Dust, pollens, powders, tobacco-smoke, animal-odour, feathers, etc.
    - *Ingestants:* Eggs, fish, prawns, nuts, pineapple, etc.
    - *Contactants:* Powders, cosmetics, synthetic-clothes, etc.
    - *Drugs:* Aspirin, iodides, nasal-drops, etc.
    - *Infection:* Bacterial allergy.

  - *Endogenous allergens*
    - Intestinal helminths.
    - Tissue proteins in body fluids.

Pathogenesis   Allergens → Formation of reaginic antibodies → Release of histamine and histamine–like substances → Allergic reaction.

Pathology
- Oedema of submucosal tissue by allergic fluid (transudate).
- Infilteration by eosinophils and plasma cells.
- Vasodilation and engorgement of inferior turbinate.
- Increased activity of secretory glands of the nasal mucosa.
- Infection may occur secondarily.
- Prolapse of oedematous mucosa polyp formation.

Clinical features
- Symptoms
  - Nasal irritation
  - Sneezing episodes
  - Rhinorrhoea (watery and copious)
  - Nasal obstruction due to turbinate mucosal hypertrophy
  - Anosmia occasionally
- Signs
  - On anterior rhinoscopy, the nasal mucosa appears pale and oedematous with watery seromucinous

nasal secretions. The mucosa may appear bluish or purplish due to venous stasis. Mucosal changes are seen more on the inferior turbinates.

- *Polyps may be present:* Allergic rhinitis usually gives rise to ethmoidal polypii
- Superimposed infection may be present

Other features of allergy

- Eyes may be congested and watering
- Eustachian tube obstruction may result in secretory otitis media.
- Pharyngitis may occur due to continuous postnasal discharge.
- Patient may give history of asthma. Nasal allergy may precipitate attacks of asthma.

Investigations

- Detailed history including family history, previous episodes and probable cause of the attack.
- Complete blood count: Eosinophilia is present.
- Nasal smear may show eosinophils or mast cells.
- Stools are examined to rule out helminths.
- Tests to detect the allergen :
  - Detailed history.
  - Skin test: Intradermal test with allergens.
  - Provocative food test.
  - Nasal challenge test.
  - Radio allergo sorbent test (RAST): To measure concentration of immunoglobulin E (IgE) anti-bodies,
  - Cell degranulation test.

Treatment

- Avoid the allergen
- Local treatment
- Desensitization
- Systemic treatment
- Surgical treatment
- Avoiding the allergen is the best mode of preventing allergic rhinitis, however, in most cases, there is more than one allergen and they are not always detected. Hence, this is not practically possible.
- Local treatment
  - *Steroids*
    - Nasal drops or aerosol
    - Local injection of 0.5 cc hydrocortisone sub-mucosally into the inferior turbinates once a week for 5–6 times.
  - *Cryosurgery:* Cauterization of the inferior turbinates using a cryoprobe helps in improving the airway.

- *Surface electrocautery* of the inferior turbinates helps in improving the air way
- *Submucous diathermy* of the inferior turbinates improves the airway without the risk of developing adhesions.
- *Autohaem injections* submucosally in the inferior turbinates
- *Application of 15% silver nitrate* as surface chemical cauterization to inferior turbinates
- *Zinc ionisation:* It is not much in use nowadays. It decreases the sensitivity of the nasal mucosa to the inhaled allergen.
- *Disodium chromoglycate:* It is only of prophylactic value. It is used as drops or a spray locally, it can prevent an attack.
- Desensitization
  - Specific by use of specific vaccines, if the allergen is known
  - Non-specific by use of stock vaccines, if the allergen is not known
- Systemic treatment
  - Oral antihistaminics
  - Oral steroids
  - Vitamin C and calcium are used orally empirically.
  - Vitamin B complex.
- Surgical treatment: This aims at treating the nasal obstruction and improving the airway.
  - Treatment of nasal obstruction by:
    - Nasal polypectomy
    - Septoplasty for DNS
    - Turbinectomy of inferior turbinates, if hyper-trophy is present.
  - Removal of septic foci, like tonsils, adenoids, treatment of sinusitis, etc.

VASOMOTOR RHINITIS

Definition   Vasomotor rhinitis is an inflammatory condition of the nasal mucosa due to a reaction to certain stimuli in the absence of any specific allergen.

Aetiology   Autonomic imbalance is considered as the etiological factor, as allergens are not responsible for this condition.

Clinical features

- Symptoms:
  - Nasal obstruction.
  - *Rhinorrhoea (watery discharge):* It is one of the main clinical features.

- ◆ *Sneezing*: It is one of the main clinical features.
- Signs
  - ◆ Nasal mucosa is pale oedematous and occasionally pinkish due to vasodilation.
  - ◆ Eosinophilia is not a feature of vasomotor rhinitis.
- Treatment: Similar to that of allergic rhinitis except desensitization. Surgical treatment also includes :

- ◆ Vidian neurectomy.
- ◆ Sphenopalatine ganglion block.

DIFFERENCE BETWEEN ALLERGIC AND VASOMOTOR RHINITIS

Table 24.1 shows the differences between allergic and vasomotor rhinitis.

TABLE 24.1: Differences between allergic and vasomotor rhinitis	
Allergic rhinitis	*Vasomotor rhinitis*
• Usually starts from adolescence.	• Starts in third or fourth decade of life.
• Caused by allergens.	• Caused by vasomotor imbalance.
• History of exposure to allergens present.	• No such history present.
• Itchiness in nose and sneezing more frequent.	• Not so frequent.
• Conjunctival irritation and watering of eyes present.	• Not present.
• Raised eosinophil count in blood.	• Eosinophilia not present.
• Eosinophils seen in nasal smear.	• Absent.
• Skin tests positive.	• Negative.
• Mucosa bluish.	• Mucosa pale or pinkish.
• Blood IgE level raised.	• Not raised.
• Vidian neurectomy not effective.	• Vidian neurectomy effective.

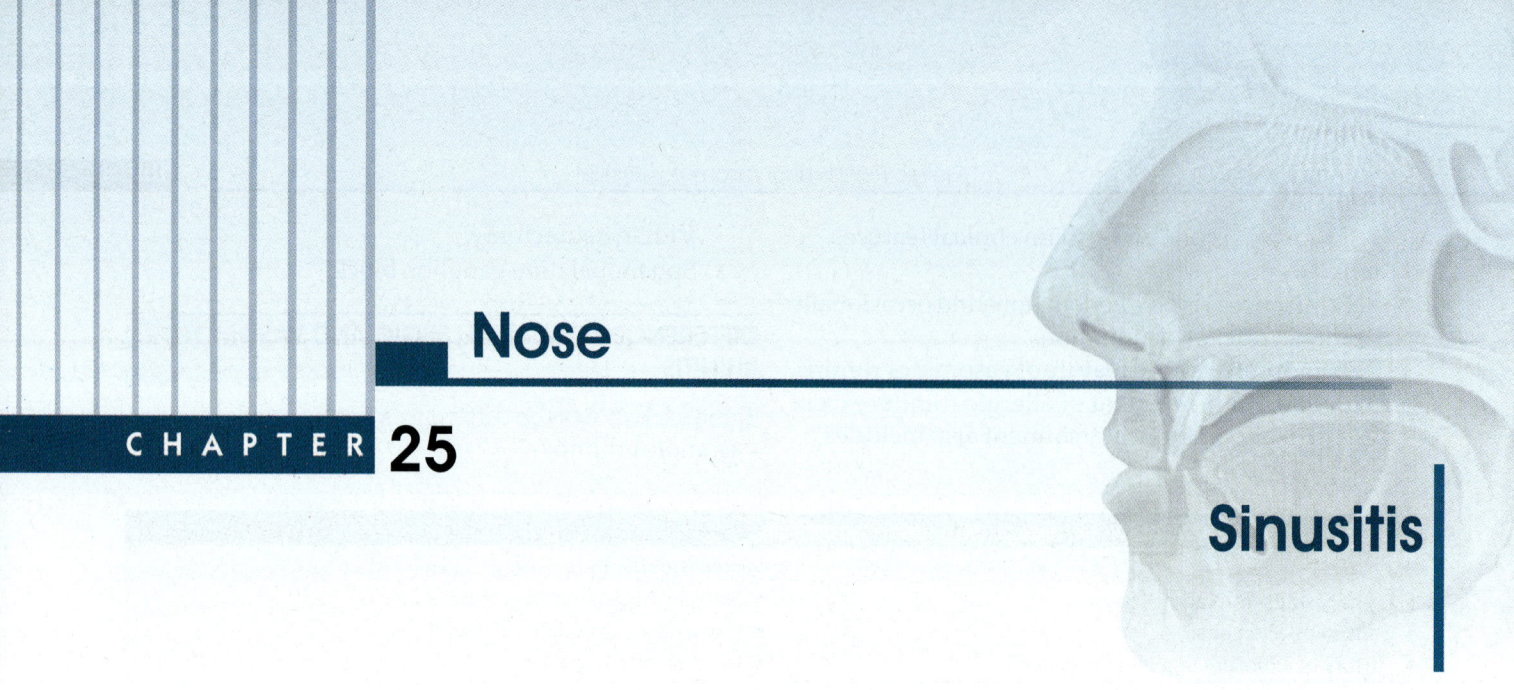

Nose

CHAPTER **25**

Sinusitis

DEFINITION

Sinusitis is an inflammation of the mucosa of the paranasal sinuses (maxillary, frontal, ethmoidal and sphenoidal).
- The infection may be acute or chronic.
- The maxillary sinus is most frequently affected.
- The inflammation may be suppurative or non-suppurative.

RELEVANT ANATOMY

The paranasal sinuses include two maxillary sinuses, two groups of ethmoidal sinuses, two frontal sinuses and a single sphenoidal sinus. These are lined by ciliated columnar epithelium, which contains secretory glands and goblet cells. The sinuses drain via their ostia into the nasal cavities.

AETIOLOGY

- **Age:** It can occur at any age, however, it is commonly seen above the age of 12–15 years. Maxillary sinusitis is common in children, whereas ethmoidal sinusitis is common in adults.
- **Sex:** Both the sexes are equally affected.
- **Secondary to rhinitis** due to a retrograde spread of infection through the ostia of the sinuses.
- **Allergy.**
- **Nasal obstruction** due to DNS, polyps or a nasal mass can result in inadequate drainage of secretions from the sinuses with subsequent stagnation and infection.

- **Swimming** predisposes to sinusitis as water enters the nose forcefully, especially during diving with entry of infection into sinuses through their ostia.
- **Barotrauma:** Either due to flying in an unpressurised aircraft or due to deep-sea diving.
- **Dental infection:** Infection of the roots of the upper premolar or molar teeth may result in spread of infection to the maxillary sinuses.
- **Trauma:** Vehicular accidents, etc. can result in fracture of the skull and facial bones with haematoma formation in the sinus cavity and subsequent infection.
- **Immunodeficiency, atmospheric pollution, and infection of adjacent tissues,** such as tonsillitis or adenoiditis may predispose to sinusitis.
- **Rarely infection of the sinuses may be bloodborne.**

Causative organisms
- Streptococcus
- *Haemophilus influenzae*
- Pneumococcus
- Staphylococcus

PATHOLOGY

Pathological changes are enhanced due to the following factors:
- The mucosa lines an aircontaining cavity.
- The ostium, which is responsible for adequate drainage, is small and gets blocked easily by oedema of the lining mucosa.

- In the maxillary sinus, the ostium is in a non-dependant position which is disadvantageous for adequate drainage of the sinus, in the presence of excessive secretions.

Stages   Sinusitis goes through the following stages:
- **Catarrhal stage:** It is characterised by congestion and oedema of the mucosa and hypertrophy of the secretory glands.
- **Stage of exudation:** The secretions of the goblet cells and secretory glands increase and collect in the sinus cavity. It is initially mucoid and later becomes mucopurulent.
- **Stage of infection:** Due to infection of the accumulated secretions and due to inadequate drainage through the blocked ostium, the stagnant exudate becomes mucopurulent. The cilia too may get destroyed or paralysed due to infection, this further prevents adequate drainage. The secretions collect under pressure in the sinus cavity resulting in 'acute empyma' of the sinus.
- **Stage of resolution:** If treated adequately, the infection resolves and further course of the disease is arrested.
- **Stage of complication:** If treatment is not adequate or the virulence of the organisms is high, complications may occur.

ACUTE SINUSITIS

Acute maxillary sinusitis
- **Definition:** It is an acute infection of the mucosa lining the maxillary sinus.
- **Aetiology:** As described previously in this chapter.
- **Pathology:** As discussed previously in this chapter.
- **Clinical features**
  - *Symptoms*
    - Nasal discharge which is mucopurulent and thick
    - Nasal obstruction
    - Pain in the maxillary region, which may radiate to the teeth, eyes, ear, and frontal sinus. It is aggravated on bending down, coughing or sneezing.
    - Change in taste sensation
    - Heaviness of the head
    - Fever and malaise
    - Dry cough
    - Epistaxis occasionally

  - *Signs*
    - Tenderness over the maxillary sinuses on palpation. Maximal over the canine fossa, as this is the most superficial part of the sinus.
    - Congested and oedematous nasal mucosa
    - Thick, mucopurulent nasal secretions
    - Postnasal discharge may be seen on the posterior pharyngeal wall on examination of the throat. This may result in pharyngitis.
    - Transillumination test helps in diagnosis of maxillary and frontal sinusitis. However, it is rarely done nowadays.
- **Investigations**
  - *X-ray of the paranasal sinuses:* Water's view is specific for the maxillary sinus and will show a 'ground-glass' haziness of homogenous density in the sinus cavity. In the presence of empyma, an air-fluid level is seen (i.e. a homogenous opacity with a concave upper border), in the maxillary antrum.
  - Nasal secretions may be sent for culture and antibiotic sensitivity.
  - *Transillumination test:* Not performed nowadays, as it is unreliable
  - CT scan of the paranasal sinus is performed, and is diagnostic
- **Differential diagnosis**
  - Tooth abscess
  - Cellulitis of the cheek
  - Angioneurotic oedema
  - Infraorbital neuralgia
  - Trigeminal neuralgia
  - Ca maxilla
  - Temporal arteritis
- **Treatment**
  - *Aims*
    - To treat infection and the cause, e.g. dental caries
    - To ensure adequate drainage through the natural ostium and regeneration of mucosal lining
    - Symptomatic relief
  - *Antibiotics:* Antibiotics are parenterally preferred, e.g. injection ampicillin (250 mg) with injection cloxacillin (250 mg) intravenously 6 hourly for 5 days. If antibiotic sensitivity of the nasal discharge is known, the appropriate antibiotic is started.
  - *Anti-inflammatory analgesics* orally or parenterally
  - *Antihistaminics* orally
  - *Nasal decongestant drops:* One percent ephedrine nose drops
  - *Steam inhalations* with tincture benzoin, menthol or eucalyptus oil to liquefy the secretions and aid in drainage.

- *Local heat to the sinus* by hot fomentation or short wave diathermy (dry heat).
- *Diet*: Plenty of fluids and high protein diet.
- *Vitamins*: A, E, B complex, and C.
- *Care of oral cavity*: Condy's gargles.
- *Proof puncture*: If all the above treatments fail to produce rapid relief from symptoms, the maxillary sinus is punctured through the inferior meatus under local anaesthesia and the stagnant secretions are drained out. However, this is rarely required nowadays due to availability of higher antibiotics.
- Endoscopic clearance of the mucosa is performed using a regid sinus endoscope. The mucos is collected in a sterile 'mucus aspirater' to be sent for culture and antibiotic sensitivity.

Acute frontal sinusitis

- **Definition:** It is the acute inflammation of the mucosa lining the frontal sinus.
- **Aetiology**
  - As described previously in the chapter except for 'dental infection'.
  - Acute frontal sinusitis usually occurs secondary to maxillary sinusitis.
- **Pathology:** As described previously in this chapter.
- **Clinical features**
  - *Symptoms*
    - Nasal obstruction.
    - Nasal discharge is thick and mucopurulent.
    - Pain in the frontal region, which radiates to the temporal and parietal regions. It is more in the morning and gradually decreases as the day progresses since the stagnant secretions drain slowly in the vertical position. In the initial stages, there is absorption of air from the sinus due to blocking of the frontonasal duct resulting in headache. This is characteristically called 'vacuum headache'.
  - *Signs*
    - Tenderness over the frontal sinus.
    - Congestion and oedema of the nasal mucosa.
    - Viscid, mucopurulent secretions in the nasal cavity.
    - Oedema of the upper eyelid is rare.
    - Transillumination test is not done nowadays.
- **Investigations**
  - *X-ray of the paranasal sinuses*: Caldwell's view is specific for frontal sinus and shows a characteristic 'ground-glass' haziness of the frontal sinuses.
  - Culture and antibiotic sensitivity of the nasal discharge.

- *Transillumination test*: It is not of much value.
- CT scan of the paranasal sinus is diagnostic.
- **Differential diagnosis**
  - Ophthalmic headache
  - Migraine
- **Treatment**
  - Same as for acute maxillary sinusitis except 'proof puncture'
  - In severe persistent cases, the frontal sinus is drained through a trephine hole, in the floor of the sinus at its medial end. A polythene tube is inserted into this hole to enable intermittent irrigation of the sinus with antibiotic solution.
  - Endoscopic clearance of the mucosa is performed using a regid sinus endoscope. The mucus is collected in a sterile 'mucus aspirator', to be sent for culture and antibiotic sensitivity.

Acute ethmoiditis and sphenoiditis

- These occur as a part of generalised sinus infection (pansinusitis).
- Acute ethmoiditis causes pain in between the eyes on the nasal bridge. This is also the site for testing ethmoid tenderness.
- Acute sphenoiditis causes a characteristic deep seated continuous central headache with radiation to retroorbital region.
- **Treatment:** Same as for 'acute maxillary sinusitis' except for 'proof puncture', which cannot be performed for these conditions.

CHRONIC SINUSITIS

Chronic maxillary sinusitis

- **Definition:** It is a chronic inflammation of the mucosa of the maxillary sinus.
- **Aetiology**
  - Following recurrent attacks of acute maxillary sinusitis.
  - As described previously in the chapter.
- **Pathology:** The mucosa shows hypertrophy, atrophy or papillary changes. It may be pale and oedematous in case of allergy.
- **Clinical features**
  - *Symptoms*
    - Nasal obstruction
    - *Rhinorrhoea:* Viscid and mucopurulent, if infective aetiology and watery if allergic aetiology.
    - Dull continuous headache
    - Heaviness of the head

- Sorethroat due to postnasal drip
- Hawking, due to postnasal drip
- Change of taste
- Foul smell from nose
- Malaise and occasionally low grade fever
- Hyposmia or Cacosmia
- *Signs*
  - Anterior rhinoscopy reveals congested, hypertrophied nasal mucosa.
  - Turbinates may be hypertrophied
  - Mucopurulent discharge is seen in the nasal cavity
  - Mucopurulent discharge may be seen on the posterior pharyngeal wall
  - Posterior rhinoscopy shows pus in the middle meatus region
  - Transillumination test is rarely done nowadays
- Investigations
  - *X-ray paranasal sinuses*: Water's view is specific for maxillary sinuses. It will show 'ground-glass' homogenous haziness of the maxillary antrum, mucosal thickening or polypoidal hypertrophy of the lining mucosa and occasionally osteitis or sclerosis and thickening of the bony walls.
  - CT scan of the paranasal sinus is diagnostic.
  - Nasal and sinus endoscopy is diagnostic.
  - *Postural test*: Patient is in siting position and the pus from middle meatus is cleaned and if it reappears, it is from the frontal sinus. If it is does not reappear, the patient's head is placed sidewards with the affected sinus up. As the maxillary ostium becomes dependent, pus will reappear in the middle meatus, in case of maxillary sinusitis.
- Treatment
  - *Aims*: Same as those for acute maxillary sinusitis.
  - Conservative treatment.
  - Surgical treatment.
  - *Conservative treatment*: Same as for acute maxillary sinusitis except 'proof puncture' which is not done in chronic maxillary sinusitis.
  - *Surgical treatment*
  - Treatment of the cause, e.g. septoplasty for DNS, polypectomy for nasal polypii, etc.
  - Inferior turbinate cauterization for hypertrophied inferior turbinates.
  - Antral puncture
  - Intranasal antrostomy, if all conservative treatment fails and if three repeated antral punctures are persistently purulent.

- Caldwell Luc operation, if antrostomy or three consecutive antral punctures fail to cure this condition.
- However, today functional endoscopic sinus surgery (FESS) is performed to clear the maxillary sinus of all diseased mucosa and widen its ostium, so as to facilitate drainage.

Chronic frontal sinusitis

- Definition: It is a chronic inflammation of the frontal sinus mucosa
- Aetiology
  - Due to recurrent attacks of acute frontal sinusitis
  - As a part of pansinusitis
  - All other aetiology, as in acute frontal sinusitis
- Pathology: The mucosa, lining the frontal sinus is hypertrophied and polypoidal
- Clinical features
  - *Symptoms*
    - Nasal obstruction
    - Nasal discharge is thick and mucopurulent
    - Dull ache in the region of the frontal sinus, which is continuous in nature
  - *Signs*
    - Congestion and hypertrophy of the nasal mucosa
    - Hypertrophied nasal turbinates
    - Mucopurulent discharge in the nasal cavity
    - Transillumination is rarely done nowadays
- Investigations
  - *X-ray of the paranasal sinuses*: Caldwell's view is diagnostic
  - Postural test helps in diagnosis
  - Pus is seen in the anterior part of the middle meatus which is cleaned. The pus will reappear in a few minutes, if it is from the frontonasal duct, when patient is in the sitting position.
  - Transillumination is rarely performed
  - CT scan of the paranasal sinus is diagnostic
- Treatment
  - Surgical treatment
    - Howarth's operation (clearance of frontal sinus disease via external approach)
    - Frontal sinus trephining and catheterization for washes with antibiotic solution
    - Functional endoscopic sinus surgery (FESS) to clear disease and enable drainage

Chronic ethmoidal sinusitis

Usually occurs as a part of pansinusitis or following obstruction to drainage due to ethmoidal polypii, DNS, nasal mass, etc.

- Treatment
  - *Aims and conservative treatment:* Same as for chronic maxillary sinusitis.
  - *Surgical treatment*
    - Intranasal ethmoidectomy.
    - External ethmoidectomy.
    - Transantral ethmoidectomy.
    - Functional endoscopic sinus surgery (FESS) to clear disease and enable drainage.

COMPLICATIONS OF SINUSITIS

The paranasal sinuses are in close proximity to the nose, eyes and brain. Hence, spread of infection beyond their bony walls can result in grave complications.

Orbital complications
- Orbital cellulitis
- Orbital abscess
- Retrobulbar neuritis
- Superior orbital fissure syndrome
- Orbital apex syndrome

Intracranial complications
- Meningitis
- Encephalitis
- Extradural abscess
- Subdural abscess
- Brain abscess: Frontal lobe abscess
- Cavernous sinus thrombophlebitis and thrombosis

Osteomyelitis of the bony walls with formation of fistulae (oroantral fistula) and external sinuses on the facial skin overlying the sinuses.

Dental complications
- Dental pain
- Oroantral fistula
- Dental abscess
- Dental cyst

Nasal complications
- Chronic simple rhinitis
- Chronic hypertrophic rhinitis
- Nasal polyposis
- Secondary atrophic rhinitis

Pharyngeal and laryngeal complications
- Simple pharyngitis
- Granular pharyngitis
- Tonsillitis
- Laryngitis and tracheobronchitis—rarely occurred

Ear complications
- Eustachian tube catarrh
- Middle ear effusion (SOM)
- Atelectasis
- Chronic suppurative otitis media (CSOM)

Miscellaneous
- Mucocoele
- Pyocoele
- CT scan of the paranasal sinus (plain and contrast) is performed for diagnostic

Oroantral Fistula

Definition: It is an abnormal communication between the oral cavity and the maxillary antrum

Aetiology
- Dental extraction of upper molars or premolars
- Trauma to palate
- Gunshot wounds
- Osteomyelitis of the floor of the maxillary antrum
- Iatrogenic–After Caldwell-Luc surgery or after the palatal fenestration operation
- Ca maxilla

Sites
- Sublabial
- Palatal
- Alveolar–through the tooth socket

Clinical features
- Change of taste or foul taste in the mouth due to drainage of pus into the oral cavity
- Nasal regurgitation of fluids if the fistula opens into the floor of the nose (oronasal fistula)
- History of tooth extraction or surgery prior to symptoms
- On examination, the oral opening of the fistula is seen

Investigations
- Fistulogram—instillation of a radio-opaque dye into the fistula followed by X-ray to detect the inner opening of the fistula.
- Diagnostic nasal and sinus endoscopy can be performed and saline washes given to confirm presence of the fistula.

Treatment
- Keep the site clean by regular Condy's gargles.
- Antibiotics to counter the infection.
- Inferior meatal antrostomy to enable adequate drainage and giving antibiotic washes to the antrum.

Usually, the above results in closure of a small fistula by granulation and healing by secondary intention.

- Use of local flaps from the palate or buccal mucosa for surgical closure if the above mentioned methods fail.
- If detected immediately during dental extraction it can be closed primarily with sutures.
- Endoscopic clarance of all debris from the maxillary sinus is done and the fistula is then closed using local flaps.

Mucocoele and Pyocoele

Definition: **Mucocoele** is a cystic swelling lined by epithelium and containing sterile fluid. It is seen to occur in the paranasal sinuses (maxillary, ethmoidal, frontal or sphenoidal).

Infection of the mucocoele results in accumulation of pus in this cyst and it is characterised by inflammatory changes. This is now known as a **pyocoele**.

It commonly occurs in the frontal sinuses and occasionally in the ethmoidal sinuses.

The mucocoele contains straw-coloured or white mucous fluid with cholesterol crystals.

Aetiology: It occurs due to obstruction to the ostium of the sinus with resultant accumulation of secretions and formation of a cyst—mucocoele. When infected, it is known as a pyocoele.

Pathology: This swelling is expansile in nature and gradually erodes the bony walls of the sinus due to osteomyelitis resulting in compression of the neighbouring orbital contents.

Clinical features
- Symptoms
  - Initially asymptomatic.
  - Later, there is a dull continuous pain.
  - Headache.
  - Progressively increasing painless swelling in the region of the affected sinus.
  - Diplopia.
- Signs: On examination, a tense, smooth, non-tender, swelling is seen in the region of the orbital roof (floor of frontal sinus) pushing the eyeball. Expansion and thinning of the bone with erosion gives rise to an 'eggshell crackling' feel on palpation.

Investigations
- X-ray paranasal sinuses Caldwell's view shows haziness in the frontal sinus.

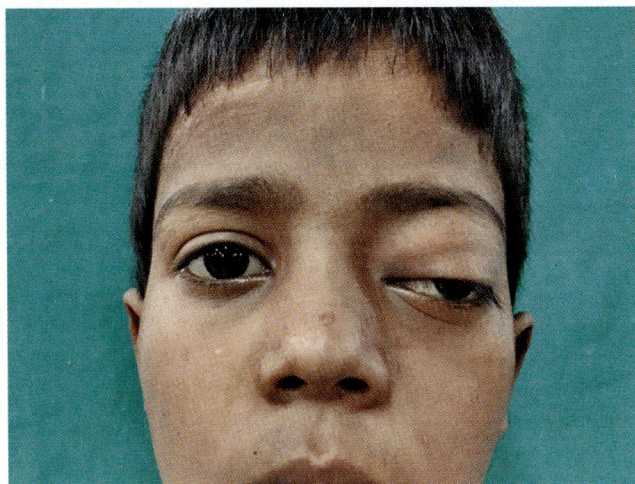

Fig. 25.1: Left frontoethmoidal mucocele

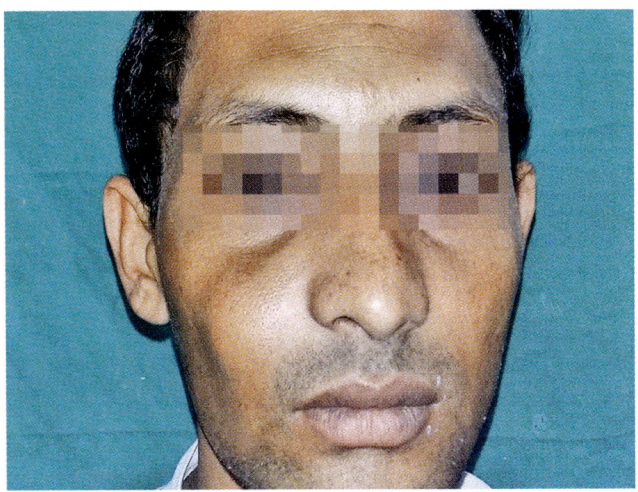

Fig. 25.2: Right maxillary mucocele

- CT scan of the paranasal sinus is diagnostic.
- Loss of scalloping of the superior border of the frontal sinus,
- Bony erosion may be present.

Treatment
- Complete removal of the cystic mass with adequate drainage into the nasal cavity.
- *Frontoethmoidal mucocoele:* Lynch Howarth operation (Fig. 25.1).
- *Maxillary mucocoele:* Caldwell Luc operation (Fig. 25.2).
- Endoscopic drainage of the mucocele/pyo-coele with marsupialisation is performed nowadays.

CHAPTER 26

Tumours and Cysts of the Nose and Paranasal Sinuses

Flowchart 26.1: Tumours and their classification

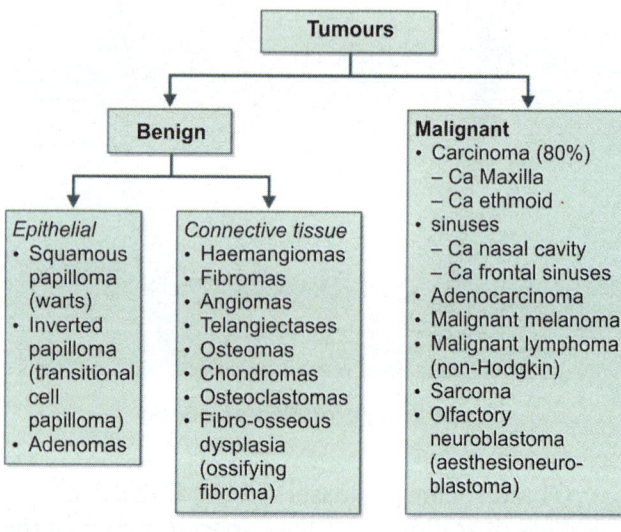

CYSTS

These can be:
- Congenital cysts
- Mucocoeles and pyocoeles
- Cystic odontomas
- Dermoids
- Bone cysts

INVERTED PAPILLOMA

- **Definition:** Inverted papilloma is a transitional-cell tumour seen in the nasal cavity or the paranasal sinuses.

- **Synonym:** Transitional-cell tumour, Ringertz tumour.
- **Site of occurance:** Nasal cavity or paranasal sinuses.
- **Aetio pathogenesis:** Thickening of the epithelial layer with infolding and formation of a solid papillomatous mass. The characteristic feature is that the basement membrane is intact. It is common in males and seen in the third or fourth decade of life. It is a premalignant condition.
- **Clinical features:** It presents with unilateral nasal obstruction, rhinorrhoea, and epistaxis (scanty). On examination, a greyish-white papillomatous mass is seen in the nasal cavity.
- **Treatment:** Complete excision, usually via a lateral rhinotomy approach. This has to be followed by a histopathological examination of the specimen to rule out malignant change.

  Nowadays, with the advent of angled endoscopes and specific instruments, complete excision is possible endoscopically in most cases. However, the comfort and expertise of the surgeon plays a major role in the approach used surgically.

SQUAMOUS PAPILLOMAS

- **Synonym—Warts:** These occur in the vestibule of the nasal cavities. They may be single or multiple. They are thought to be premalignant lesions.
- **Treatment:** Treatment is excision with cauterization of the base. Histopathology to rule out a malignant change is important.

ANGIOMA OF THE SEPTUM

- Synonym—*bleeding polypus of the septum:* It is a smooth red vascular polyp arising from the nasal septum. It is really a capillary haemangioma arising from the Kisselbach's plexus in the Little's area. It is characterised by episodes of epistaxis.
- Treatment: Excision with cauterisation of the pedicle.

OSTEOMA

It can be of two types:

- Localised ivory (compact) osteoma: It commonly occurs in the frontal sinus and is ivory hard in consistency. It is seen as a dense opacity in an X-ray PNS Caldwell's view. Usually, asymptomatic, when no treatment is required. Rarely, it causes headache and requires excision through the floor of the frontal sinus or an osteoplastic flap approach.
- Cancellous osteoma: It occurs commonly in the maxillary and ethmoidal sinuses. If symptomatic, it is excised.

FIBRO-OSSEOUS DYSPLASIA

- Synonym—ossifying fibroma: It is caused by increased activity of the bone mesenchyme. It can be localised or diffuse. It may involve one bone (monostotic) or multiple bones (polyostotic).
- Treatment: It involves shaving off excess bone for cosmetic purpose. If there is no cosmetic deformity, no treatment is required.

CARCINOMA OF THE MAXILLA

Definition   It is a malignant tumour occurring in the maxillary sinus.

Aetiology

- Age: It is ommonly seen after the fourth decade of life.
- Sex: Males are affected more than females.
- Smoking
- Wood-dust: Common in carpenters especially due to sawdust.
- Snuff: The Bantu tribe of South Africa is more prone to this pathology, probably due to use of home-made snuff.
- Nickel or chrome dust.
- Fumes, e.g. in the rubber industry.
- Chronic sinusitis—probable rare causes.
- Dental sepsis
- Exposure to ionising radiation.

Classification

- Primary or Secondary
  - *Primary*: Arising from the maxilla (90% are squamous cell carcinomas).
  - *Secondary:* Involving the maxilla from surrounding structures, like the nose, alveolus, palate, ethmoids, parotid, etc.
- Ohngren's classification: Based on anatomical site of tumour:
  - *Inferomedial:* Least dangerous and causes early symptoms—good prognosis
  - Inferolateral—poor prognosis
  - Superolateral—poor prognosis
  - *Superomedial:* It spreads rapidly to important structures, worst prognosis

  Division is by an imaginary line from the inner canthus of the eye to the angle of the mandible and a vertical imaginary line dropped down from the pupil of the eye in the neutral position.
- Lederman's classification: Based on anatomical site:
  - Superior group
  - Middle group
  - Inferior group

  Division is by two imaginary horizontal lines, passing through the floor of the orbit and floor of the maxillary antrum. Prognosis is best for the inferior group and worst for the superior group of tumours.
- Broder's classification: Based on histology of the tumour:
  - Grade I < 25% cells are malignant.
  - Grade II < 50% cells are malignant.
  - Grade III < 75% cells are malignant.
  - Grade IV 75% or more than 75% cells are malignant.
- Tumour, node and metastases (TNM) classification: TNM classification is not much is use for Ca maxilla.
- The American Joint Committee on Cancer (AJCC) system of classification for Ca of the maxillary antrum is the only accepted classification at present.

Spread

- Spread by continuity: Tumour may spread by erosion to the orbit, cribriform plate, anterior cranial fossa, alveolus, palate, cheek, nose, nasopharynx, infratemporal region, and pterygoid muscles.
- Lymphatic spread: The first group of lymph nodes to be involved are the retropharyngeal lymph nodes of Rouviere. These are difficult to detect clinically and require CT scan for detection of involvement. These drain into the lower deep jugular group of lymph nodes in the neck which then get involved.

- Haematogenous spread: This is late to occur and may involve distant organs like liver, spleen, lungs, kidneys or brain.

Pathology   Eighty percent of the primary malignancies of the maxilla are squamous cell carcinomas.

Others are adenocarcinoma, malignant melanoma, non-Hodgkin's lymphoma and sarcoma.

Clinical features
- Symptoms
  - *Early*
    - Dull pain over the maxillary sinus, which increases on bending forwards or straining
    - Bloodstained nasal discharge
    - Ipsilateral watering of the eye (epiphora)
    - Anaesthesia over the malar region
    - Nasal obstruction
    - Toothache
  - *Late*
    - *Medial spread to nose*
      - Nasal obstruction
      - Anosmia or parosmia
      - Mass in nose
      - Foul smelling unilateral rhinorrhoea
    - *Superior spread to orbit*
      - Diplopia
      - Loss of vision
      - Proptosis
    - *Anterior spread to cheek*
      - Swelling in malar region
      - Fungating (proliferative) growth involving the cheek
      - Infraorbital neuralgia
    - *Posterior spread to pterygoid region*
      - Trismus
    - *Inferior spread to alveolus and palate*
      - Painless loosening and falling off of teeth
      - Dentures become ill-fitting
      - Fungating growth involving palate
    - *Cachexia and loss of appetite*
- Signs
  - *Early*
    - Infraorbital anaesthesia over the malar region.
    - Loose teeth
    - Empty sockets of fallen teeth
  - *Late*
    - *Medial spread to nose*
      - Granulomatous mass obliterating the nasal cavity

- Bleeds on touch
- *Superior spread to orbit*
  - Proptosis
  - Obliteration of the infraorbital margin
- *Anterior spread to cheek*
  - Fungating or ulceroproliferative growth on the cheek
- *Posterior spread to pterygoid region*
  - Trismus
- *Inferior spread to alveolus and palate*
  - Oroantral fistula
  - Fungating or ulceroproliferative growth involving the hard palate
- *Lymph node metastases in the neck presenting as hard fixed swellings*

Investigation
- X-ray paranasal sinuses: Water's and Caldwell's view:
  - Haziness of the maxillary sinus and/or ethmoid sinus
  - Erosion of bony walls
  - *CT scan*: It shows extent of tumour invasion.
  - *Biopsy* of the tumour from the nasal cavity or from the maxillary sinus in the absence of a nasal mass using a sinus endoscope or via Caldwell-Luc approach.
  - *Cytology* of an antral lavage may be done in the absence of a nasal mass for detection of malignant cells. However, sinus endoscopy is the preferred method for biopsy nowadays.
  - *Contrast radiography and polytomography* have been replaced by CT scan.
- Differential diagnosis: Similar to maxillary sinusitis or a nasal mass/polyp.
- Treatment
  - *Surgery*
    - *Maxillectomy*
      - Partial
      - Total
      - Extended with exenteration of eyeball and removal of palate when involved
    - *Radical neck dissection* if lymph nodes are involved
      Maxillectomy is performed via an extended lateral rhinotomy or Weber Fergusson's incision. In maxillectomy, following structures are removed:
- Maxilla
- Ethmoidal sinuses
- Lateral nasal wall

- Ipsilateral palate, if involved
- Eyeball

Contraindications to surgery
- Distant metastases
- Involvement of pterygoid bones (base skull)
- Nasopharyngeal involvement
- Intracranial involvement
- Poor general condition of patient
- Medical contraindications to surgery like hypertension, diabetes, etc.

♦ *Radiotherapy*
- Curative dose of radiotherapy is given in early cases—5000 to 6000 rads over 5–6 weeks. 200 rads per day for 5 days in a week.

- Preoperative radiotherapy is given by some surgeons.
- Postoperative radiotherapy is preferred by most surgeons.

♦ *Chemotherapy*
- Methotrexate or 5–fluorouracil or antimetabolites are given systemically.
- Carcinoma of the ethmoidal and frontal sinuses are not common, and clinical features are similar to those of Ca maxilla. Orbital and intracranial involvement is early.

Various types of cysts of the nose and nasal mass are shown in Figs 26.1–26.5.

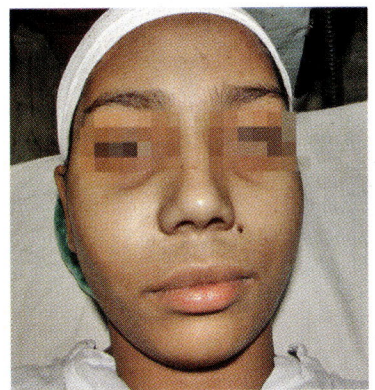

Fig. 26.1: Right dentigerous cyst

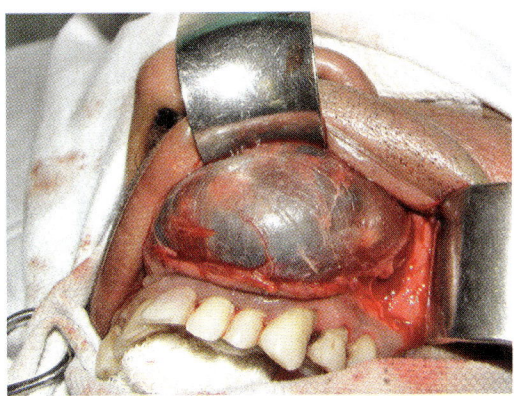

Fig. 26.2: Dentigerous cyst seen intraoperatively

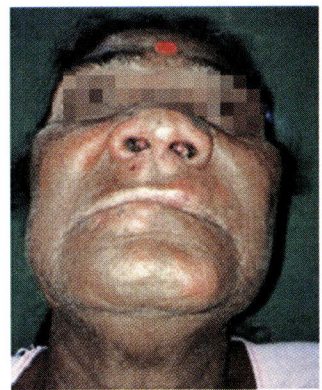

Fig. 26.3: Nasal mass

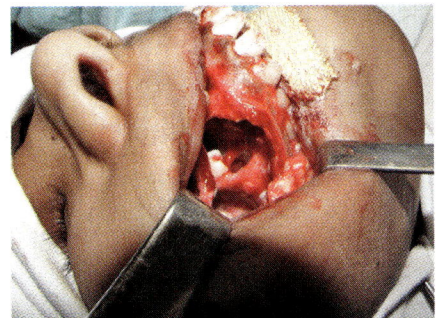

Fig. 26.4: Dentigerous cyst excised

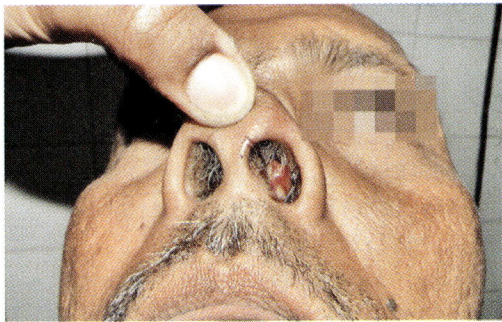

Fig. 26.5: Unilateral nasal mass (Left side)

Nose

CHAPTER 27

Miscellaneous Conditions of the Nose

Miscellaneous conditions of the nose involves:
- Foreign bodies in nose
- Maggots in the nose (nasal myiasis)
- Rhinolith
- Rhinolalia
- Choanal atresia
- Proptosis
- Cerebrospinal fluid (CSF) rhinorrhoea
- Disturbances of smell

FOREIGN BODIES IN THE NOSE

Aetiology
- **Age:** It is common in children, as they insert small foreign bodies through the anterior nares.
- Following bony sequestration in situ.
- Following trauma to nose, e.g. in vehicular accidents splinters of wood may get lodged in the nose.
- Foreign bodies like bullets may enter directly.
- **Iatrogenic:** Following nasal surgery, gauze or cotton swabs may be left behind in the nasal cavity.
- Maggots may enter the nasal cavity.
- Rhinolith may develop in the nasal cavity.
- Mentally retarded patients are more prone to insert foreign bodies into their nose.

Clinical features
- Nasal obstruction—unilateral
- Unilateral nasal discharge which is:
  - Purulent
  - Foul smelling
  - Yellowish-green in colour at times
- History of insertion of foreign body, may or may not be present.
- On anterior rhinoscopy, the foreign body may be seen or may be hidden behind granulations.

Types of foreign bodies
- **Living:** Maggots (myiasis)
- **Non-living**
  - *Organic*: Seeds, peas and grass.
  - *Inorganic*: Paper, buttons, cotton, gauze, beads, etc.

Complications
- Formation of rhinolith.
- It may slip into the nasopharynx and may enter into the tracheobronchial tree or into the oesophagus.

Investigations
X-ray of the nose will help to reveal only radio-opaque foreign bodies.

Treatment
The foreign body is removed in the OPD using a blunt hook or a vectis in case of round smooth objects, e.g. beads, peas, etc., and by using a forceps in case of irregular rough foreign bodies, e.g. paper, buttons, etc. The child's head is to be held properly by an assistant to prevent any movement.

The Eustachian tube catheter may also be used for a smooth round foreign body. The tip of the hook/vectis/Eustachian catheter is carefully inserted into the nasal cavity beyond the foreign body. Then, the tip is brought down to touch the floor of the nasal cavity and the foreign body is lodged in the angle of the vectis. The foreign body is brought out by gently withdrawing the vectis while keeping the tip on the nasal floor. In case of an uncooperative child or mentally retarded patients, general anaesthesia is required for removal. Rarely, if it cannot be removed, through the anterior nares, it may be pushed into the pharynx through the posterior nares and removed. However, care should be taken to see that the foreign body is not aspirated into the airway.

Sometimes, endoscopic removal of a posteriorly situated foreign body may be required.

NASAL MYIASIS

- **Synonym:** Maggots in the nasal cavity.
- **Definition:** Myiasis is an infestation of the nose by maggots, which are the larvae of a fly (Genus, Chrysoma).
- **Aetiology**
  - Atrophic rhinitis is the most important predisposing factor.
  - Leprosy and syphills predispose to this infestation.
  - Large roomy nasal cavity following operation, such as removal of nasal polypii, rhinosporidiosis, angiofibroma, etc.
  - After surgery for Ca maxilla.
  - Poor hygiene.
  - Poor nutritional status.
- **Pathogenesis:** Flies (Genus Chrysoma), lay eggs in the nasal cavity. These eggs hatch into larvae (maggots) with superadded secondary bacterial infection. The paranasal sinuses are also invaded by maggots.
- **Clinical features**
  - Nasal obstruction
  - Pain in nose
  - Nasal discharge with foul smelling
  - History of crawling sensation in nose and maggots coming out of the nasal cavity.
  - On anterior rhinoscopy, maggots are seen crawling in the nasal cavity and even crawling out of the nose.
  - Cellulitis may develop over the nose and face.
  - Fever, malaise, headache, and toxaemia may also be present.
- **Treatment**
  - Removal of the maggots with a nasal dressing forceps.
  - Irrigation of the nasal cavities with dilute chloroform or ether, this stupefies the maggots which are then washed out.

- Instillation of liquid paraffin in the nasal cavities.
- Nasal cavities are packed with a ribbon gauze soaked in turpentine for 24 hours.
- Antibiotics to control secondary infection.
- Maintenance of nasal hygiene with alkaline nasal douches.

RHINOLITH

Definition   Rhinolith is a concretion in the nasal cavity formed around a foreign body, blood clot or inspissated mucus or pus. It is a deposit of calcium and magnesium carbonate with phosphate salts (Fig. 27.1).

Aetiology
- Foreign body
- Blood clots
- Inspissated pus
- Inspissated mucus

Clinical features
- Nasal obstruction—unilateral.
- Rhinorrhoea—unilateral, foul smelling, and blood stained.
- Anterior rhinoscopy reveals a brownish or blackish mass obstructing one nasal cavity.
- Probing reveals a stony-hard consistency usually.

Pathology   A rhinolith is usually hard and sometimes friable. It occurs due to deposition of layers of carbonates and phosphates of calcium and magnesium around the foreign body.

Investigations   X-ray of the nose and paranasal sinuses (Water's view) shows the rhinolith which is radio-opaque.

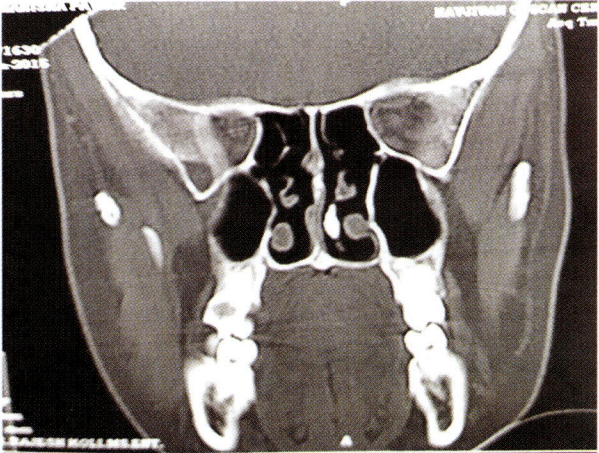

Fig. 27.1: Rhinolith in left nasal cavity

Treatment Removal of the entire mass under general anaesthesia either as a whole or piecemeal, by the transnasal route. Rarely, if the mass is very big, a lateral rhinotomy is required.

CHOANAL ATRESIA

Definition It is the failure of canalization of the posterior nares and is congenital in origin.

Classification
- Unilateral or bilateral
- Complete or incomplete
- Bony or membraneous

Aetiology It is developmental in origin and occurs due to a persistance of the bucconasal membrane.

Clinical features
- Bilateral choanal atresia is detected at birth more so if it is complete, as neonates are essentially nose-breathers:
  - Asphyxia and cyanosis
  - Difficulty in suckling and cyanosis during suckling.
  - The characteristic feature is that the neonate gets cyanosed during rest and starts crying. When he cries the cyanosis disappears, as the child inhales through the open mouth during crying.
- Unilateral choanal atresia is detected at any age, but usually presents by 5–10 years of age with unilateral nasal obstruction and foul smelling nasal discharge.

Investigations
- A soft simple rubber catheter when passed along the floor of the nose posteriorly, cannot be passed through the posterior nares (choanae) into the pharynx.
- Choanogram: Instillation of a radio-opaque dye into the nasal cavity followed by radiographs will reveal the site and type (complete or incomplete) of atresia.
- CT scan is required to detect the type (membraneous or bony) and thickness of the atretic plate.

Treatment
- Endotracheal intubation or tracheostomy is performed in case of severe asphyxia. Usually, a temporary oropharyngeal airway is used followed by emergency surgery.
- The atretic plate is perforated either by the transnasal or transpalatal approach.
- Use of endoscope to visualise and perforate the atretic plate.

- Laser is a recent advance used for perforation of the atretic plate.

PROPTOSIS

Definition It is defined as the forward displacement of the eyeball.

It may be axial (straight forward) or to one side.

Aetiology
- Trauma: This may occur following faciomaxillary trauma.
- Infections of the nose and paranasal sinuses, can also lead to proptosis due to formation of orbital cellulitis, subperiosteal abscess or cavernous sinus thrombosis.
- Neoplasms: Nasopharyngeal angiofibroma, Ca maxilla, Ca of ethmoid sinuses, nasopharyngeal Ca, etc.
- Mucocoele or pyocoele of the frontal or ethmoid sinuses.
- Fibro-osseous dysplasia.

Clinical features
- Diplopia
- Protrusion of eyeball
- Features of the causative pathology

Investigations
- X-rays of orbit
- X-rays of paranasal sinuses
- CT scan
- Biopsy, if a neoplasm is present.

Treatment Mainstay of treatment is to treat the cause.

CEREBROSPINAL FLUID RHINORRHOEA

Definition Cerebrospinal fluid rhinorrhoea is the flow of cerebrospinal fluid from the nose.

Site of CSF leak
- Cribriform plate of the ethmoid.
- Frontal sinus
- Ethmoid sinus
- Sphenoid sinus

Aetiology
- Congenital: Dehiscence in the roof of the nose, it is rare.
- Traumatic
  - Head injury resulting in fractures.
  - *Iatrogenic:* Following operations on the nose and paranasal sinuses, like endoscopic sinus surgery,

ethmoidectomy, SMR, transnasal sphenoidectomy or transphenoidal hypophysectomy, etc.

- **Spontaneous CSF leak:** It is due to prolonged raised intracranial tension (ICT) as in hydrocephalus or due to erosion of bone by destructive lesions like tumours.

Clinical features

- **Rhinorrhoea:** Watery, clear, scanty or profuse, increases on sneezing or coughing or straining.
- **Headache:** Either before the rhinorrhoea, when it is relieved by rhinorrhoea or after the rhinorrhoea. The former is due to raised ICT and the latter is due to reduced ICT.
- **Meningitis:** Rarely is the presenting feature. However, patient may have history of meningitis in the past.

Investigations

- Nasal discharge is collected in a sterile test tube and examined for glucose and chlorides. If present, it indicates CSF.
- A white cotton handkerchief is soaked in the nasal discharge. If it is CSF, it will not stiffen on drying as the discharge does not contain mucous. If it is nasal discharge, it contains mucous and hence, the cloth will stiffen on drying.
- X-ray of skull bones to detect fracture.
- CT scan of skull and paranasal sinuses, to see the site of fracture and its extent. CT scan with a contrast medium (metrizamide), which is specific for CSF to detect the exact site of the CSF leak.
- Dye tests using fluorescene, which is introduced by lumbar puncture into the intrathecal space (CSF) to detect site of leak in the nasal cavity.
- Nasal endoscopy is used recently to detect the site of leakage.

Treatment

- Complete bed rest with 30° head high.
- Avoid straining, sneezing, blowing of nose or coughing.
- No nasal drops (to prevent meningitis).
- No nasal packing (to prevent meningitis).
- Antibiotics, which cross the blood-n-dash brain barrier are given.
- Mannitol and acetazolamide to reduce the intra-cranial pressure.
- Treatment of the cause.
- Repair of the fistula using fascia or muscle graft via the intranasal, transethmoid or intracranial route.

This is required, if spontaneous healing does not occur with above measures or if there are recurrent episodes of meningitis.

DISTURBANCES OF SMELL

- **Anosmia:** It is the loss of sense of smell. It is noticed only if it is bilateral.
- **Hyposmia:** It is a diminished sense of smell.
- **Cacosmia:** It is the perception of bad odour.
- **Parosmia:** It is the sensation of unpleasant smell in the absence of any stimulus, i.e. perversion of sense of smell.
- **Hyperosmia:** It is an increase in the sense of smell.

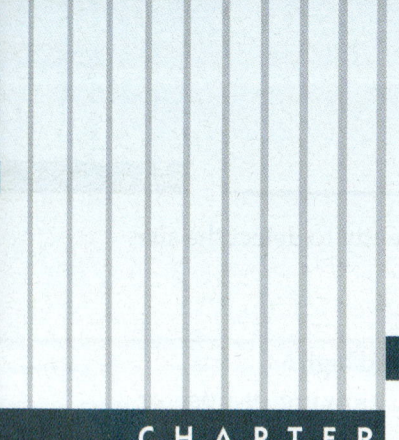

CHAPTER 28

Anatomy of the Oral Cavity and Pharynx

ANATOMY OF THE ORAL CAVITY AND PHARYNX

Embryology of the oral cavity The hard palate develops from the horizontal processes of the maxillary and palatine bones whereas, the oral cavity develops from the primitive stomatodaeum.

Boundaries The oral cavity is bounded by the following:

- *Anteriorly* : the lips.
- *Posteriorly* : the soft palate.
- *Laterally* : the cheeks and buccal mucosa.
- *Superiorly* : the hard palate, which also forms the floor of the nose.
- *Inferiorly* : the muscles of the floor of the mouth covered by mucosa.

Contents It forms the uppermost portion of the digestive tract, and comprises of the following structures:

- Lips: They form the anterior boundary of the oral cavity.
- Buccal mucosa: It lines the inner surface of the cheeks and lips.
- Gingivae (gums): They cover the upper and lower alveolar ridges and the roots of the teeth.
- Gingivo-labial and gingivo-buccal sulcii (upper and lower): These are the grooves formed between the gingivae and the labial mucosa and the gingivae and the buccal mucosa, respectively.

- Hard palate with its mucosa: It forms the roof of the oral cavity.
- Oral tongue: This includes only the anterior two-thirds of the tongue. This portion of the tongue lies in the oral cavity and it is the mobile portion of the tongue. It has the following parts—tip, dorsum, under-surface and lateral borders.
- Floor of the mouth: It is the area which lies in-between the undersurface of the tongue and the lower gingivae. It is examined by asking the patient to open his mouth and raise his tongue to touch the hard palate. It contains the sublingual papillae with the openings of the sublingual ducts and the frenulum with the lingual veins on either side.

Retromolar trigone It is a triangular region comprising of the mucosa which overlies the ascending ramus of the mandible. Its base is posterior to the lower last molar and its apex is adjacent to the maxillary tuberosity.

It is of surgical importance since malignancy in this region is very difficult to treat surgically since it is impossible to remove the primary tumour with adequate tumour free margins. Also a malignancy in this region involves the base of the skull rapidly making complete surgical excision impossible. Hence, most surgeons prefer to treat a malignancy in this region by radiotherapy.

THE PALATINE (FAUCIAL) TONSILS

These are a part of the lymphoid tissue which forms the Waldeyer's ring in the upper aerodigestive tract.

Embryology The palatine tonsils develop from the second pharyngeal pouch.

- **Site, size, shape and structure**
  - They are bilateral and situated submucosally in the oropharynx in the tonsillar fossa, between the anterior and posterior pillars. They lie between the soft palate above and the lateral border of the base of the tongue below.
  - The size varies from that of an apricot or walnut to that of an almond and they are almond shaped. The size usually increases in childhood and regresses after 15–16 years of age. They are usually small and fibrosed in adults beyond 20 years of age and hypertrophied in children.
  - They are covered by a true fibrous capsule which sends fibrous septae into the tissue of the tonsil. These crypts are lined by stratified squamous epithelium and surrounded by lymphoid tissue.
- **Poles**
  - *The upper pole*: At the insertion of the two pillars in the soft palate.
  - *The lower pole*: At the insertion of the two pillars in the base of the tongue.

  It also contains the insertion of the palatoglossus muscle.
- **Surfaces:** (Fig. 28.1)
  - *Medial surface*: It faces the oral cavity. It is irregular,

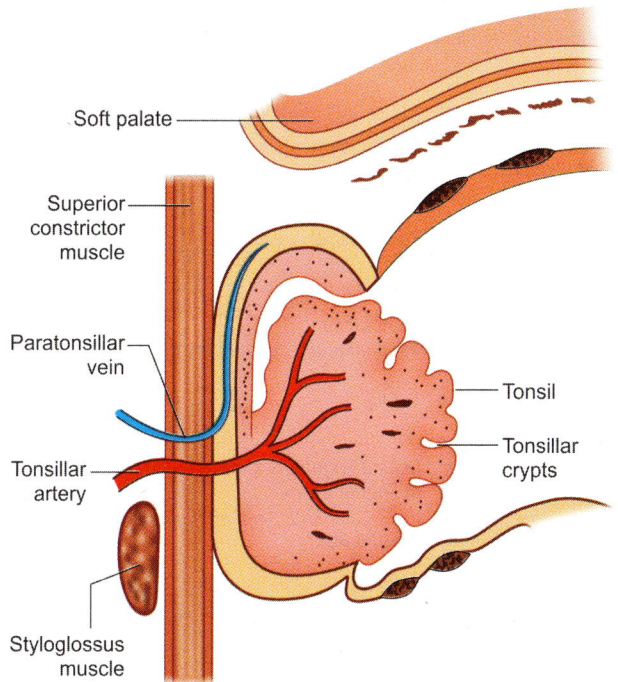

Fig. 28.1 : Coronal section of the faucial tonsil

submucosal and has 15–20 crypts, which end bluntly in the tonsillar tissue. The crypts run into the tonsil tissue and may even reach the capsule at the lateral surface. The largest crypt is called the crypta-magna or the intra-tonsillar cleft (the term 'supra-tonsillar cleft' used by some is incorrect as this crypt is in the tonsil and not above it).
  - *Lateral surface*: It is smooth and capsulated. It lies facing the tonsillar fossa and is covered by the bucco-pharyngeal fascia with the superior constrictor muscle.
- **Borders:** Each tonsil has two borders:
  - Anterior, and
  - Posterior.
- **Pillars:** These are arches of mucous membrane between which each tonsil lies:
  - *Anterior*: It receives the insertion of the of the palatoglossus muscle at its base,
  - *Posterior.*
- **Folds:** There are twofolds of mucous membrane at the upper and lower poles of each tonsil:
  - *Plica semilunaris*: It joins the two pillars at the upper pole.
  - *Plica triangularis*: It lies at the lower end of the anterior pillar.
- **Relations:** (Fig. 28.2)
  - *Anteriorly* : Anterior faucial pillar
  - *Posteriorly* : Posterior faucial pillar
  - *Superiorly* : Soft palate
  - *Inferiorly* : Lateral border of the posterior one-third of the tongue
  - *Laterally* : From medial to lateral the following structures form the lateral boundary of the faucial tonsil:
    - Loose areolar tissue and para-tonsillar vein,
    - Pharyngeal aponeurosis,
    - Superior constrictor muscle,
    - Bucco-pharyngeal fascia,
    - Glossopharyngeal nerve,
    - Pterygoid muscles,
    - Mandible.
- **Blood supply** (Fig. 28.3)
  - Tonsillar branch of the facial artery—near the lower pole—it is the main blood supply to the tonsil
  - Ascending pharyngeal artery.
  - Descending palatine artery.
  - Dorsalis linguae artery.
  - Ascending palatine artery.
- **Venous drainage:** The venous drainage of tonsils is as follows:

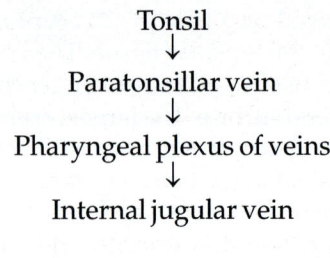

Tonsil

↓

Paratonsillar vein

↓

Pharyngeal plexus of veins

↓

Internal jugular vein

- **Lymphatc drainage:** The tonsils do not receive afferent lymphatics. The efferents drain into the jugulodigastric lymph nodes.
- **Nerve supply**
  - Glossopharyngeal nerve.
  - Lesser palatine nerves.

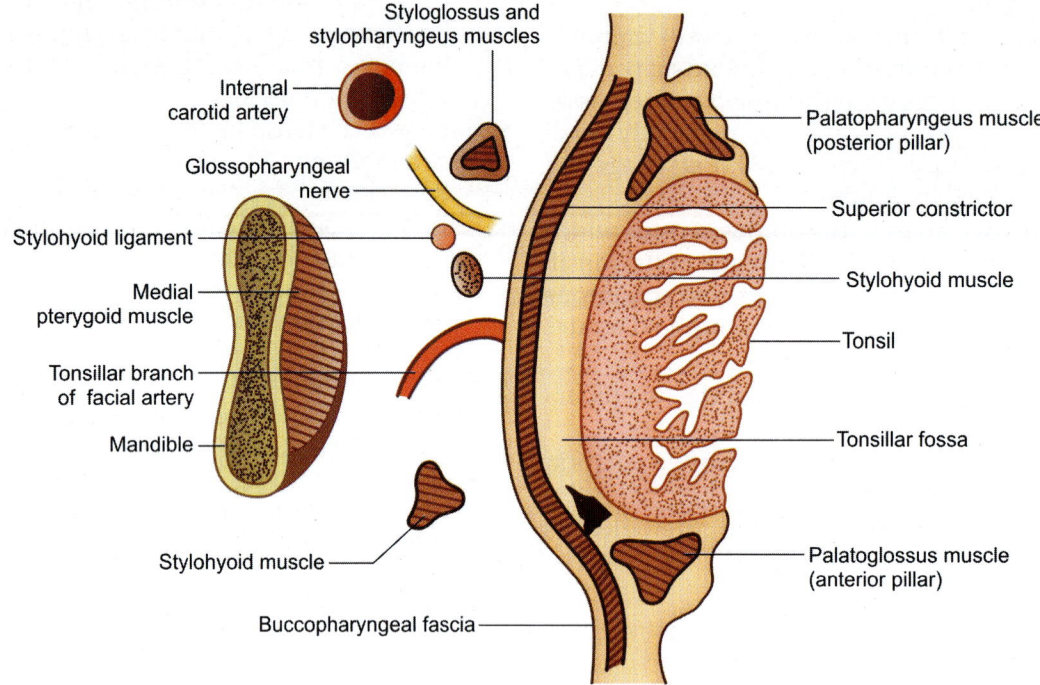

Fig. 28.2 : Relations of the faucial tonsil

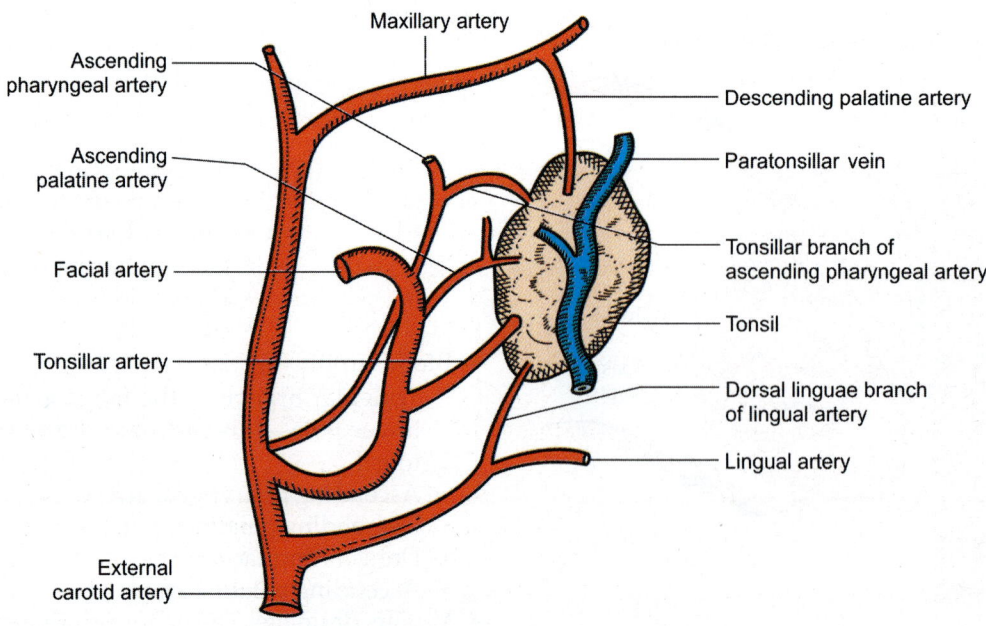

Fig. 28.3 : Blood supply of the tonsil

- **Pedicle:** The pedicle of the tonsil lies at the lower pole and it is the only attachment of the tonsil which is not dissected during tonsillectomy. After the tonsil is dissected free from its fossa it remains attached to the lower pole only by its pedicle which has to be clamped, crushed and cut with a tonsillar snare.

  The pedicle contains the following:
  - Loose fibroareolar tissue,
  - Tonsillar artery, vein, nerves and lymphatics,
  - Insertion of the palatoglossus muscle.

- **Functions of the tonsil**
  - Immunity.
  - Lymphocyte formation.
  - First line of defence against infection as a part of the Waldeyer's ring.
  - Formation of antibodies.
  - The crypts increase the surface area in contact with foreign bodies.

- **Applied anatomy**
  - Referred otalgia after tonsillectomy is via the glossopharyngeal nerve which innervates both the tonsil as well as the ear.
  - Severe haemorrhage during or after a tonsillectomy occurs from the paratonsillar vein.
  - The plane of dissection in tonsillectomy is between the capsule of the tonsil (pharyngeal aponeurosis) and the fossa containing loose fibroareolar tissue.
  - Obstruction to and infection of the intratonsillar cleft result in a peritonsillar abscess (quinsy). Following this there is scarring, fibrosis and adhesion formation making subsequent tonsillectomy difficult.
  - Haemostasis after tonsillectomy is by the contraction and retraction of blood vessels in the tonsillar fossa (like the uterus). Hence, presence of a clot in the fossa prevents haemostasis and needs to be urgently removed to prevent further blood loss.
  - Recurrence of tonsillitis or even quinsy after a tonsillectomy is due to hypertrophy and infection of tonsillar tags which may have been left behind or hypertrophy and infection of the lingual tonsils.
  - Tonsillectomy is preferably not to be performed below the age of five years since the tonsils are very important in the immune mechanism of the body and blood loss as well as general anaesthesia may not be well tolerated in a very small child.

THE NASOPHARYNGEAL TONSIL OR THE ADENOID

Site and structure It is the subepithelial group of lymphoid tissue forming a part of the Waldeyer's ring (Fig. 28.4).

It is situated on the postero-superior wall of the nasopharynx as three or more vertical ridges in the midline. The tubal tonsils lie on either side of the adenoids.

Lymphatic drainage It has no afferents. The efferents drain into the lateral retropharyngeal lymph node of Rouviere situated in the fossa of Rosenmuller and from there to the upper deep cervical group of lymph nodes in the posterior triangle of the neck.

Blood supply The adenoids are supplied mainly by the ascending pharyngeal artery.

Venous drainage They are drained by the pharyngeal plexus of veins.

THE PHARYNX

Embryology The pharynx develops from the anterior end of the primitive foregut.

Size, shape and extent The pharynx is approximately 10–12 cm long in a normal adult. It is a funnel shaped fibromuscular tube which is broad above and narrow below. It extends from the base of the skull to the sixth cervical vertebra (C6).

It is narrowest at the point of entry into the oesophagus and this portion is called the *cricopharyngeal sphincter* which is also the narrowest portion of the gastrointestinal tract.

Parts The pharynx is divided into three parts (Fig. 28.5):
- The nasopharynx, which is in communication with the choanae and the nasal cavities anteriorly.

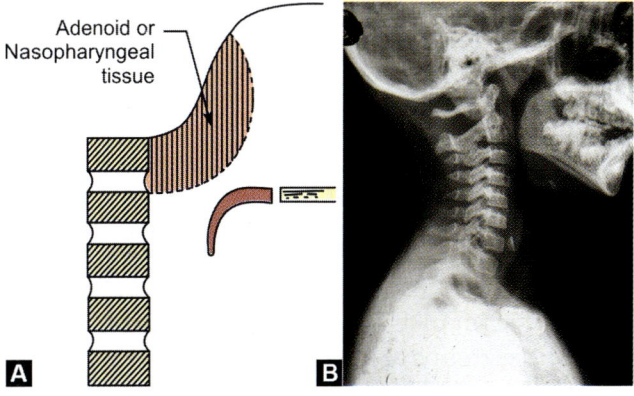

Adenoid or Nasopharyngeal tissue

Fig. 28.4: Anatomy of the adenoid

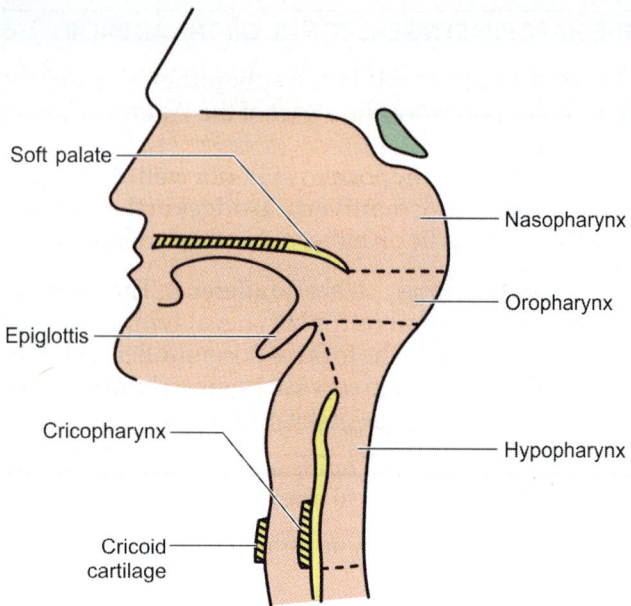

Fig. 28.5 : Anatomy of the pharynx

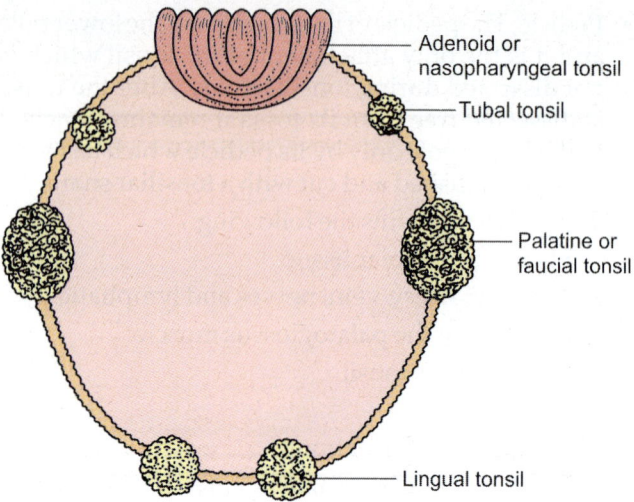

Fig. 28.6 : Waldeyer's ring

- The oropharynx, which communicates with the nasopharynx superiorly, the hypopharynx inferiorly and the oral cavity anteriorly.
- The hypopharynx or the laryngopharynx, which communicates with the oropharynx superiorly and the oesophagus inferiorly through the cricopharyngeal sphincter. It is the common pathway for deglutition and respiration.

Layers of the pharynx   The pharynx has the following five layers from the lumen outwards:

- **Mucous membrane:** The upper half of the naso-pharynx is lined by ciliated columnar epithelium. The lower half of the nasopharynx is lined by transitional epithelium. The oesophagus and hypopharynx are lined by stratified squamous epithelium.
- **Submucous lymphoid tissue (Waldeyer's ring)** (Fig. 28.6): The subepithelial collection of lymphoid tissue in the pharynx forms the first line of defence against infections. It comprises of the following—nasopharyngeal tonsil, tubal tonsils, faucial tonsils and lingual tonsils. These are known as the Waldeyer's ring. They have no afferents. Efferents drain into the cervical lymph nodes. All the tonsils are in pairs except the adenoid which is a midline structure.

  In addition to these, there are vertical groups of lymphoid tissue situated in the submucosal plane of the posterior pharyngeal wall.

  These groups of lymphoid tissue increase in size till puberty and then gradually regress till the age of 20 years, after which they remain constant in size.

- **Pharyngeal aponeurosis:** It is a layer of connective tissue between the submucosal and muscular layers of the pharynx and it is thickest in its superior portion which is also known as the pharyngo-basilar fascia.
- **Muscular layer:** It comprises of:
  - The inner group of muscles which include the stylopharyngeus, the palatopharyngeus and the salpingopharyngeus muscles.
  - The outer group of muscles which include the superior, middle and inferior constrictor muscles.
- **Buccopharyngeal fascia:** It covers the outer surface of the muscular layer.

Blood supply of the pharynx
- Branch of the facial artery.
- Ascending pharyngeal artery.
- Descending palatine artery.
- Greater palatine artery.
- Dorsalis linguae artery.

Venous drainage of the pharynx   The pharynx drains into the pharyngeal plexus of veins which drains into the common facial vein and then into the internal jugular vein.

Nerve supply of the pharynx   The pharynx is supplied by the pharyngeal plexus of nerves which is formed by the IX, X, and XI cranial nerves. The nasopharynx is supplied by the Vth cranial nerve.

Lymphatic drainage   The pharynx drains into the retropharyngeal group of lymph nodes and then into the jugulodigastric nodes and the deep cervical lymph nodes.

Applied anatomy

- A pharyngeal pouch (Fig. 28.7) can develop due to prolapse of the mucous membrane through the Killian's dehiscence. The Killian's dehiscence is a potential gap between the two parts of the inferior constrictor muscle; the thyropharyngeus and the cricopharyngeus.

  - *Thornwaldt's bursitis*: Is the infection and inflammation of the thornwaldt's cyst which may occur in the nasopharynx. The clinical features resemble adenoid infection but, it is usually seen in adults. It is also known as the nasopharyngeal bursa.

  - *Sinus of morgagni*: It is the space between the base of the skull and the upper border of the superior constrictor muscle. The Eustachian tube enters the nasopharynx through it.

  - *Passavant's ridge*: It is a muscular ridge formed by contraction of the horizontal fibres of the palatopharyngeus muscle (the vertical fibres form the posterior pillar of the faucial tonsil). It lies submucosally in the posterior pharyngeal wall at the level of the hard palate. It is of utmost importance in the closure of the nasopharyngeal (velopharyngeal) sphincter since the soft palate makes contact with this ridge for closure of the sphincter. Dynamic pharyngoplasty is based on the surgical principle of augmenting this ridge for the treatment of velopharyngeal insufficiency.

- Tubal tonsils when enlarged can cause Eustachian tube obstruction and otitis media.

- Rathke's pouch is represented as a dimple in the roof of the nasopharynx and a craniopharyngioma may arise from it.

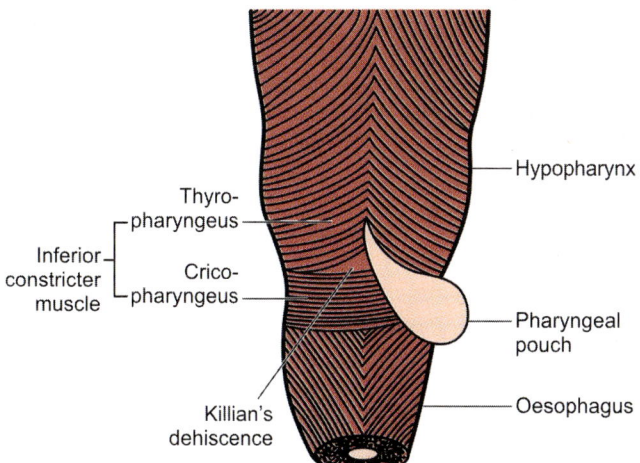

Fig. 28.7: Killian's dehiscence through which a pharyngeal pouch has been formed

THE NASOPHARYNX

It extends from the base of the skull to the soft palate, anterior to the body of the first cervical vertebra. It communicates anteriorly with the nasal cavities through the choanae. Inferiorly, it is in communication with the oropharynx. The adenoids are located in its roof and posterior wall. Its lateral wall contains the openings of the Eustachian tubes on either side approximately 1cm behind the posterior end of the inferior turbinates. The fossa of Rosenmuller is situated behind the tubal openings and it contains the lymphnode of Rouviere. The tubal tonsils are also situated in the lateral wall of the nasopharynx on either side.

The soft palate forms the anterior wall of the nasopharyngeal isthmus, which closes the nasopharyngeal sphincter during swallowing or speech. The nasopharyngeal isthmus is formed by; the soft palate anteriorly, the posterior pharyngeal wall posteriorly (which forms the Passavant's ridge) and the lateral pharyngeal walls on each side.

THE OROPHARYNX

It extends from the soft palate to the tip of the epiglottis, from the second to the third cervical vertebrae. It communicates with the oral cavity anteriorly. The tonsils are situated submucosally between the anterior and posterior faucial pillars. The anterior faucial pillar contains the palatoglossus muscle and the posterior faucial pillar contains the palatopharyngeus muscle. The posterior wall contains the pharyngeal lymphoid tissue submucosally.

The valleculae are situated between the base of the tongue and the lingual surface of the epiglottis. They are bounded by the lateral glosso-epiglottic folds on either side and separated by the median glosso-epiglottic fold.

THE LARYNGOPHARYNX OR HYPOPHARYNX

It extends from the tip of the epiglottis to the cricopharynx, from the third to the sixth cervical vertebrae. It has three parts:
- pyriform fossae on either side,
- posterior pharyngeal wall,
- cricopharynx.

The pyriform fossae are bilateral, pyramidal recesses situated on either side of the laryngeal inlet. The internal branch of the superior laryngeal nerve lies in the floor of the fossa. It is bound medially by the aryepiglottic fold and laterally by the thyroid cartilage and thyrohyoid membrane.

Parapharyngeal space   It is a potential space lying on either side of the pharynx. It is triangular in cross-section (Fig. 28.8).

- Boundaries
  - *Laterally*   : Upper part—parotid gland and ramus of the mandible.
  -            : Lower part—sternomastoid muscle.
  - *Medially*   : Buccopharyngeal fascia.
  -            : Prevertebral fascia and muscles.
  - *Superiorly* : Base of the skull.
  - *Inferiorly* : Mediastinum.
- Contents
  - IXth, Xth, XIth, and XIIth cranial nerves.
  - Ascending palatine and ascending pharyngeal arteries.
  - Great vessels of the neck.
  - Cervical sympathetic trunk.
  - Deep cervical lymph nodes.
- Applied anatomy: Infection from the oral cavity or the oropharynx can spread to this space and result in:
  - Parapharyngeal abscess,
  - Mediastinitis,
  - Intracranial spread of infection along the carotid sheath.

The bucco-pharyngeal fascia is tough and usually prevents medial spread of the abscess.

The Retropharyngeal Space

- Synonym
  - Gillette's space: It lies behind the pharynx and is divided into two compartments by a median partition.
- Boundaries
  - *Anteriorly* : Bucco-pharyngeal fascia Posterior pharyngeal wall.
  - *Posteriorly* : Prevertebral fascia and prevertebral muscles.
  - *Laterally*   : Buccopharyngeal fascia.
- Contents: It contains the retropharyngeal group of lymph nodes which atrophy by 4–5 years of age. They drain the nose, pharynx, palate and Eustachian tubes.
- Applied anatomy: Retropharyngeal abscess can occur due to two reasons:
  - Due to suppuration of the retropharyngeal lymph nodes. Such an abscess is usually uni-lateral due to the median partition which prevents spread of the abscess across the midline.
  - Due to caries of the cervical vertebral bodies. Such an abscess is usually situated in the prevertebral space and hence is seen as a midline swelling. It is not in the true retro-pharyngeal space of Gillette.

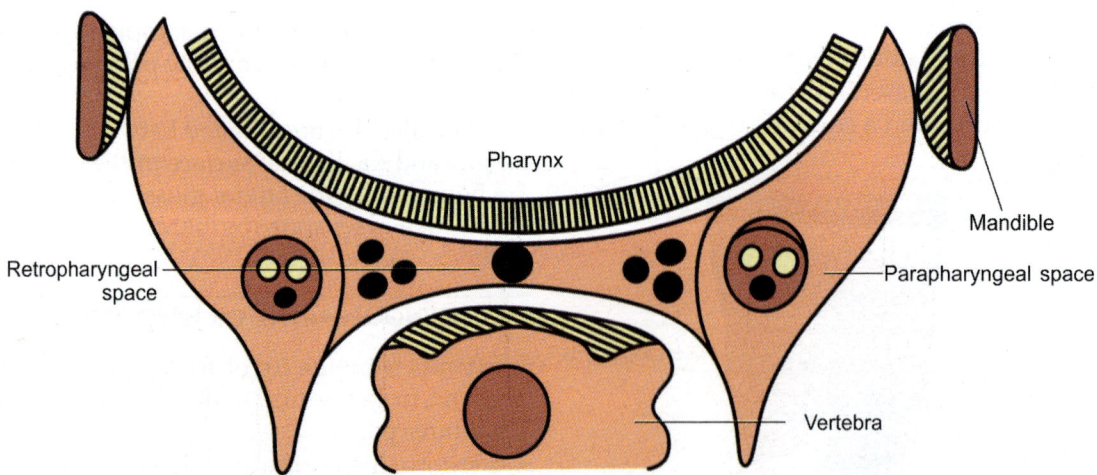

Fig. 28.8 : Retropharyngeal and parapharyngeal spaces

Oral Cavity and Pharynx

CHAPTER 29

Physiology of the Oral Cavity and Pharynx

FUNCTIONS OF THE ORAL CAVITY

- Mastication.
- Mixing saliva with food.
- Directing feed and liquids into the oropharynx and oesophagus.
- Saliva keeps the mucosa of the pharynx and mouth moist.
- Lubricating and moistening the mucosa of the mouth for speech.
- Saliva aids in digestion of starch.
- Antibacterial activity of saliva.
- Taste.
- Speech: It helps in articulation.

FUNCTIONS OF THE PHARYNX

- Deglutition: The pharynx plays a role in the second stage of deglutition.
- Mucous glands of the pharyngeal mucosa lubricate the pharynx.
- Speech: The pharynx plays a role in speech production.
- Respiration: The pharynx forms a part of the upper airway.
- Taste: The oropharynx has a few taste buds which help in taste.
- The nose and middle ear drain into the pharynx.
- Immune defence mechanism: The pharyngeal lymphoid tissue plays a role in immune defence of the body.

- The pharynx plays an important role in the opening and closing of the Eustachian tube.
- Thirst sensation is referred to the pharynx.

FUNCTIONS OF THE TONSILS

- Immunity: The function of the tonsils in the immune defence mechanism is most important before the age of 5 years.
- Antibody formation
- Lymphocyte formation
- Barrier against infection: They form a part of the Waldeyer's inner ring and perform a protective function.

PHYSIOLOGY OF MASTICATION

Mastication of solid food is an essential prerequisite to deglutition.

The solid food is crushed and disintegrated in the mouth by the action of the teeth and jaws. Saliva plays an important role in bolus formation. The muscles of mastication are assisted by the tongue, lips and cheeks. The tongue and cheeks place the food between the occlusal surfaces of the upper and lower jaws. The movements occur at the temporomandibular joint. There are three varieties of movements, which occur at this joint:

- Hinge-like movements for biting food
- Protrusion and retrusion
- Lateral movement for grinding food

The food, once crushed and made into a bolus is passed backwards into the pharynx for deglutition.

PHYSIOLOGY OF DEGLUTITION

Deglutition is a complex coordinated reflex action, which is initiated voluntarily and which is carried out by a series of involuntary reflexes. For description purposes, it is divided into three stages:

- Oral
- Pharyngeal
- Oesophageal

However, deglutition is a continuous and integrated act and initiation of the first phase inevitably leads to the automatic completion of the whole process.

Oral stage (voluntary)

It involves propulsion of the food bolus from the mouth through the oropharyngeal isthmus into the oropharynx.

Lips close and the cheeks are compressed against the teeth. The bolus lies on the dorsum of the tongue. A small inspiratory movement of the diaphragm occurs, known as the 'respiration of swallowing'. Floor of the mouth is elevated. Tongue moves backwards and the bolus is forced backwards into the pharynx. The palatoglossus muscles contract to close the oropharyngeal isthmus along with the tongue, thus, preventing the bolus from coming back into the oral cavity.

For liquids, the tongue is moulded to form a longitudinal groove, which abuts against the hard palate to form a tubular space containing the liquid. The dorsum of the tongue is forced upwards from the anterior end to the posterior, thus, squirting the liquid backwards into the oropharynx.

Pharyngeal stage (involuntary)

The food passes through the pharynx to the upper end of the oesophagus. Since, the pharynx is common to both the respiratory and alimentary passages, the passage of food is accompanied by closure of the nasal, oral and laryngeal inlets. The bolus travels along the epiglottis into the pyriform fossae and reaches the cricopharynx.

The cricopharynx relaxes to permit the entry of food into the oesophagus. This phase of swallowing is a reflex mechanism elicited by the stimulation of the receptors in the pharyngeal mucosa.

Oesophageal stage (involuntary)

- The food passes through the oesophagus into the stomach by peristalsis and gravity, if the patient is in the erect position.
- Respiration is transiently inhibited during deglutition.
- The centre for deglutition is situated in the medulla near the Xth cranial nerve nucleus.
- Afferent fibres for deglutition, are carried by the Vth, IXth and Xth cranial nerves.
- Efferent fibres are carried by the Xth and XIth cranial nerves.

CHAPTER 30

Examination of the Throat and Pharynx

EXAMINATION OF THE NASOPHARYNX

This has been described in details in Chapter 18, examination of the nose and paranasal sinuses.

EXAMINATION OF THE ORAL CAVITY AND OROPHARYNX

On examination of the oral cavity the structures seen are shown in Fig. 30.1.

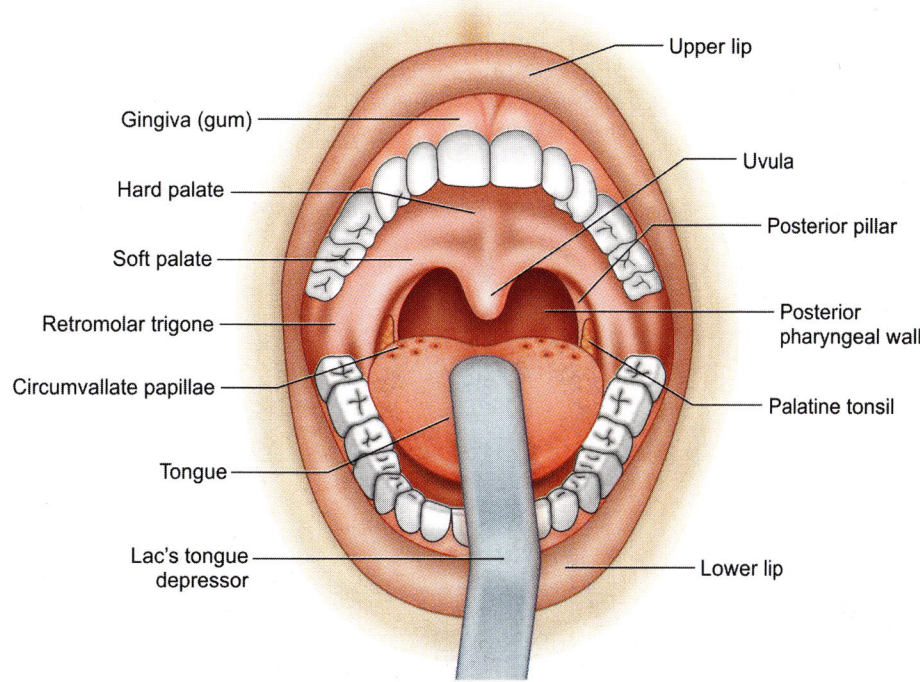

Fig. 30.1: Structures seen on examination of the oral cavity

Upper lip

Gingiva (gum)

Hard palate

Soft palate

Retromolar trigone

Circumvallate papillae

Tongue

Lac's tongue depressor

Uvula

Posterior pillar

Posterior pharyngeal wall

Palatine tonsil

Lower lip

Symptoms associated with diseases of the oral cavity and oropharynx include the following:

Odynophagia   Pain occurs during swallowing. It can be intermittent or continuous ; unilateral or bilateral, and may be referred to the ipsilateral ear.

Foreign-body sensation in the throat or irritation in the throat is seen commonly due to the following:
- Postnasal drip
- Allergic pharyngitis
- Granular pharyngitis
- Foreign-body, e.g. fish bone
- Stylalgia or Eagle's syndrome
- Malignancy involving the pharynx

Increased salivation   It usually occurs due to failure to swallow, as a result of the pain (odynophagia) or as a result of dysphagia. The saliva may be foul smelling in the presence of infection or bloodstained in the presence of malignancy.

Dysphagia   It is difficulty in swallowing, seen in hypopharyngeal or oesophageal pathology, e.g. inflammation, swelling, tumours, etc.

Nasal twang and nasal regurgitation Nasal twang is also known as rhinolalia aperta. It is usually associated with nasal regurgitation of liquids or solids during deglutition. It occurs due to the incomplete closure of the nasopharyngeal sphincter (velopharyngeal sphincter) or an abnormal communication between the oral and nasal cavities, e.g. cleft palate, short palate,

palatal paralysis, palatal perforation and malignancy involving the soft palate or after surgery on the palate, where the soft palate is damaged, e.g. surgery for sleep apnoea.

Postnasal discharge   It is seen in inflammatory conditions of the nose, paranasal sinuses or nasopharynx and results in hawking (clearing of the throat), which further increases the inflammation.

Feeling of a lump in the throat   It is seen in malignancy, cricopharyngeal spasm, cervical spondylosis, pharyngeal pouch, or it may be functional (globus hystericus).

Muffled voice   It is common in tumours involving the oropharynx (base of the tongue), hypopharynx (pyriform fossae) or supragottic larynx (epiglottis). It is characteristically known as *hot-potato speech*.

Decreased hearing   This may occur, if a nasopharyngeal mass obstructs the Eustachian tube resulting in serous otitis media.

Halitosis or foul smell   Foul smell from the oral cavity occurs in the presence of poor oral hygiene, e.g. in dental caries, aphthous ulcers, malignancy, etc.

Signs

Examination is carried out using illumination from a Bull's eye lamp, reflected to the site using a head mirror.

The patient is asked to open his/her mouth and the tongue is depressed using a Lac's tongue depressor. The tongue depressor is placed only on the anterior

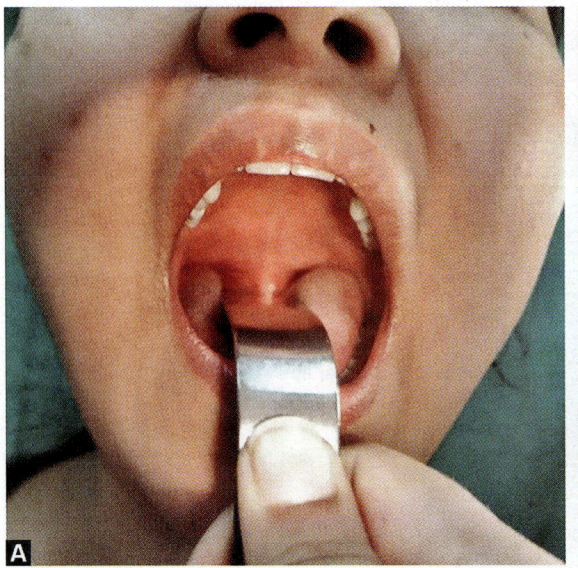
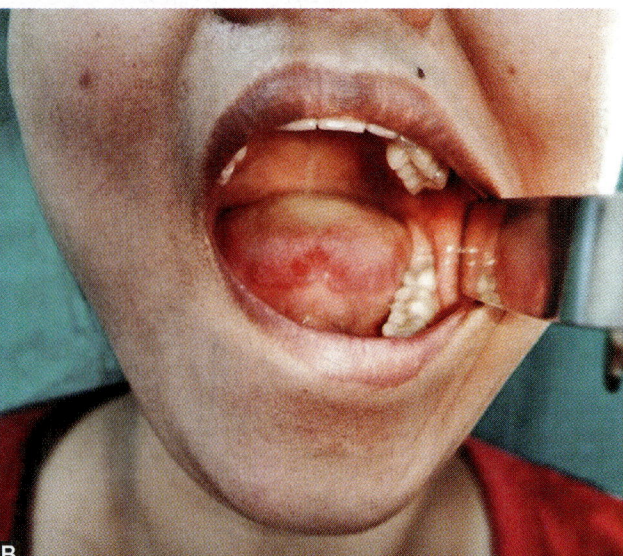

Fig. 30.2: Examination of the oral cavity

two-thirds of the tongue, since only this portion of the tongue is mobile and also depression of the posterior one-thirds results in a gag reflex being elicited.

The structures examined in the oral cavity are lips, buccal mucosa, gums, hard and soft palate, teeth, tongue, and floor of the mouth (Fig. 30.2).

The following structures are examined in oropharynx:

- Anterior pillars
- Palatine or Faucial tonsils
- Posterior pillars
- Soft palate and uvula
- Tonsillolingual sulcus
- Posterior pharngeal wall

The movements of the soft palate are noted during phonation. The gag reflex is tested using a Lack's tongue depressor to touch the posterior pharyngeal wall.

The tonsillolingual sulcus is one of the sites referred to as the surgeon's graveyard, since malignancies in this region can be easily missed, if not examined properly especially by palpation.

Palpation is required in all cases of malignancy to detect surrounding induration which is indicative of microscopic infiltration or in a case of suspected malignancy of the oral cavity, foreign body or elongated styloid process.

Surgeon's Graveyard

The following sites are referred to as the surgeon's graveyard since, if these sites are not kept in mind during examination of the oral cavity and pharynx, a lesion at these sites can be easily missed. These regions are not directly in the surgeon's line of vision during a routine examination. These should be specifically kept in mind during examination.

- Tonsillolingual sulcus
- Valleculae
- Pyriform fossae
- Floor of the mouth
- Nasopharynx

These areas are to be thoroughly examined in case of suspected malignancy.

EXAMINATION OF THE HYPOPHARYNX

Described in detail in Chapter 39, examination of the larynx.

INVESTIGATIONS

Radiological examination

- X-ray soft tissue nasopharynx or neck–(lateral view), is helpful to detect foreign bodies, tumours, abscesses, etc.
- Barium swallow detects pharyngeal pouches or webs.
- X-ray of the base of the skull helps in diagnosis of nasopharyngeal tumours.

Haematological investigations   Anaemia is often seen in pharyngeal pouch, inflammations, webs or Plummer-vinson syndrome due to either odynophagia or dysphagia.

Biopsy   It is the best means to confirm the diagnosis.

Computed tomography (CT scan)   It is the most recent and accurate diagnostic investigation and often used with a biopsy for confirmatory diagnosis.

CHAPTER **31**

Diseases of the Tonsils and Adenoids

The diseases associated with tonsils and adenoids include:

- Acute tonsillitis
- Chronic tonsillitis
- Adenoid hypertrophy
- Peritonsillar abscess (quinsy) and peritonsillitis

ACUTE TONSILLITIS

Definition   Acute tonsillitis is the acute inflammation and infection of the faucial tonsil (palatine tonsils) (Fig. 31.1).

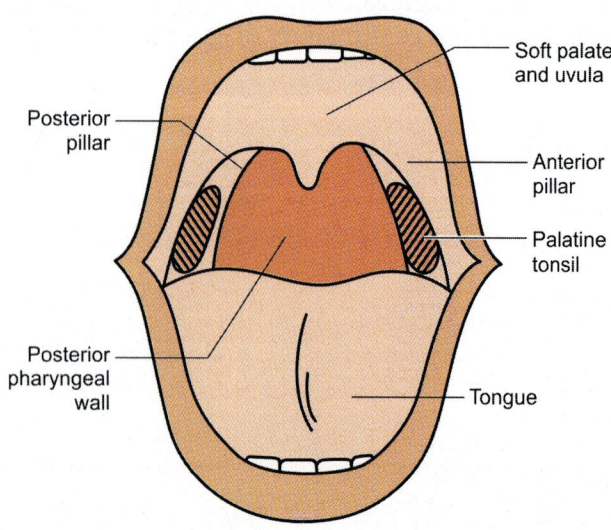

Fig. 31.1: Diagrammatic representation of the palatine tonsils

Aetiology
- Age: It is common up to the age of 13–14 years (adolescence). However, it can occur at any age.
- Sex: There is no sex preponderance.
- Predisposing factors
  - *Exogenous factors*
    - Contact with individuals having the infection can cause tonsillitis
    - Pollution
    - Overcrowding
    - Vasoconstriction in the throat by the local effect of cold eatables or cold drinks can lower resistance.
    - Foreign body, embedded in the tonsil may get infected
  - *Endogenous factors*
    - Preexisting chronic tonsillitis
    - Upper respiratory tract infection
    - Postnasal discharge in rhinitis or sinusitis
    - Immunodeficiency
    - Residual tags after tonsillectomy may get infected
    - Lowered resistance due to blood dyscrasias

Causative organisms
- Viral infection
- Streptococcus
- Staphylococcus
- Pneumococcus
- Diphtheroids

Pathological types

- Acute parenchymatous tonsillitis: Tonsils are congested, inflamed, and enlarged.
- Acute follicular tonsillitis: Tonsils are congested, inflamed, and have multiple follicles (crypts studded with pus).

Clinical features

- Symptoms
  - Sore throat or a raw sensation in the throat is the commonest symptom.
  - *Odynophagia:* Pain in the throat on swallowing.
  - *Refusal to eat food:* This is seen in younger children who usually do not complain of pain in the throat, but refuse to eat.
  - Fever, malaise, and headache are present.
  - Enlarged and painful jugulodigastric lymph nodes.
  - Bilateral earache (otalgia).
- Signs
  - Child is toxic and febrile.
  - Tonsils are enlarged and congested. In the follicular type, they show multiple yellow follicles on the medial surface.
  - Anterior pillars are congested.
  - Halitosis is present.
  - Tongue is coated.
  - Jugulodigastric lymph nodes are enlarged and tender.

Differential diagnosis

- Diphtheria
- Vincent's angina
- Peritonsillitis
- Peritonsillar abscess (quinsy)
- Glandular fever (infectious mononucleosis)
- Thrush
- Scarlet fever
- Herpes
- Agranulocytosis can result in gangrenous tonsillitis
- Tonsillar keratosis

Sequelae and complications

- Peritonsillitis
- Peritonsillar abscess (quinsy)
- Parapharyngeal abscess
- Retropharyngeal abscess
- Laryngeal oedema
- Acute otitis media
- Septicaemia

- Chronic tonsillitis following repeated attacks of acute tonsillitis
- Infected tonsils may act as a septic focus and aggravate subacute bacterial endocarditis, acute nephritis or rheumatism.

Treatment

- Bed rest
- Soft bland warm diet
- Avoid cold, oily, and spicy foods
- Antibiotics for 5–7 days, e.g. capsule ampicillin (250 mg) QDS.
- Anti-inflammatory analgesics to reduce pain, fever, and inflammation, e.g. oral paracetamol 500 mg TDS.
- Condy's gargles (1:4000 potassium permanganate) or warm saline gargles for local antiseptic and soothing properties.
- Vitamin C orally
- Multivitamins orally

CHRONIC TONSILLITIS

Definition   Chronic tonsillitis is the chronic inflammation and infection of the palatal (faucial) tonsils.

It is characterised by recurrent attacks of acute tonsillitis. A history of at least three to four attacks of acute tonsillitis in a year should be present to label it as "chronic".

Aetiology   Same as for acute tonsillitis.

Causative organisms   Same as for acute tonsillitis.

Pathological types

- Chronic parenchymatous tonsillitis: Tonsils are enlarged with recurrent attacks of acute tonsillitis. It is usually seen in children and adolescents.
- Chronic fibrotic tonsillitis: Tonsils are small, shrunken, and fibrotic with recurrent attacks of acute tonsillitis. It is usually seen in adults.

Clinical features

- Symptoms
  - Recurrent history of sore throat, odynophagia, and fever with symptom-free interval between two such attacks.
  - Halitosis.
  - Change of taste.
  - Hawking due to irritation in the throat.
  - Dry cough.
  - Failure to grow, seen in children.
- Signs
  - Tonsils may be enlarged (parenchymatous type) or fibrotic and small (follicular type).

- Yellowish cheesy material is seen in the tonsillar crypts, which oozes out when the tonsils are squeezed using a tongue depressor.
- Anterior pillars are congested.
- Enlarged jugulodigastric lymph nodes.
- Occasionally, yellowish cystic swelling (retention cysts) may be seen on the surface of the tonsils.

Treatment
- Nutrition of the patient is improved with good diet and multivitamins.
- Treatment of acute attack, if present.
- Tonsillectomy, if there are three to four attacks of acute tonsillitis per year.

ADENOID HYPERTROPHY

Relevant anatomy The adenoids are a group of lymphoid tissue situated at the junction of the roof and posterior wall of the nasopharynx, posterosuperiorly. They are a part of the Waldeyer's ring (Fig. 31.2) which forms the first line of defence against infection in the body. Adenoids usually undergo atrophy by the age of 13–14 years (puberty). However, in some children the hypertrophied adenoid tissue may produce symptoms, and then treatment is required.

Synonym Adenoid is also known as the nasopharyngeal tonsil.

Aetiology
- **Age:** It is common between 3–10 years of age.
- Infection, which may be non-specific or specific like tuberculosis.

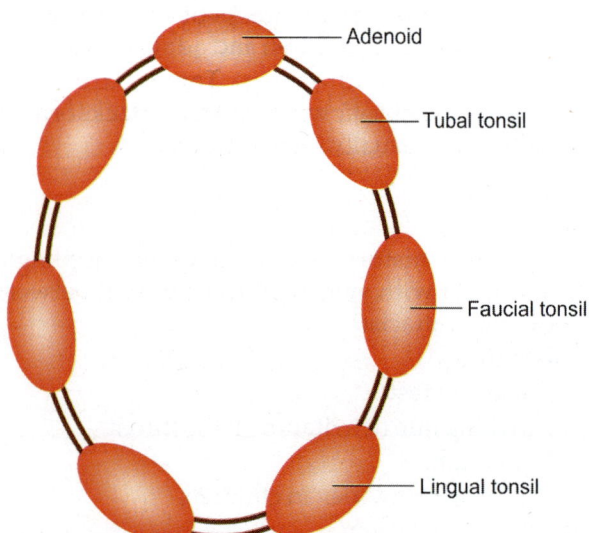

Fig. 31.2: Diagrammatic representation of Waldeyer's ring

- Associated with infection of the tonsils usually.
- Physiological hypertrophy is seen between 3–10 years of age, but this is asymptomatic. Only, if symptoms are present, treatment is required.
- Predisposing factors are similar to those of acute tonsillitis.

Clinical features
Symptoms and signs occur due to the following:
- Due to nasal obstruction
- Due to Eustachian tube obstruction
- Due to mouth breathing
- General manifestations

- **Clinical features due to nasal obstruction**
  - Mouth breathing
  - Snoring or noisy breathing in sleep
  - Drooling of saliva
  - Difficulty in breathing
  - Change of voice—rhinolalia clausa
  - Rhinitis and sinusitis
- **Clinical features due to Eustachian tube obstruction**
  - Otalgia
  - Acute otitis media
  - Secretory otitis media
  - Chronic otitis media
  - Atelectasis
- **Clinical features due to mouth breathing**
  - Difficulty in feeding
  - Failure to grow
  - Drooling of saliva
  - Halitosis
  - High arched palate
  - Crowded teeth and protrusion of upper incisors
  - Chronic pharyngitis and laryngitis
- **General manifestations**
  - 'Adenoid facies'
    - Pinched and narrow nose
    - Loss of nasolabial groove
    - Mouth remains open
    - Noisy breathing
    - Drooling of saliva from mouth
    - Dull facial expression
    - Protruding teeth
    - Overcrowded teeth
    - High arched palate
  - Poor nutrition–malnourished poorly built child
  - Pigeon chest

- Protuberant abdomen
- Flat toneless voice due to lack of nasal tone:
  - Rhinolalia clausa

Investigation   Detection of adenoid tissue by:
- Posterior rhinoscopy (difficult in a child)
- Digital palpation of adenoids in the nasopharynx. However, in a small child, this may not be possible.
- X-ray soft tissue nasopharynx is also useful to detect the adenoids.
- Examination under general anaesthesia

Differential diagnosis
- Nasal obstruction due to other causes, like DNS, Nasal polyps, etc.
- Thornwaldt's cyst or Thornwaldt's bursitis (inflammation of the cyst).
- Orthodontic abnormality: High-arched palate with protruberant teeth.

Treatment
- Medical or conservative treatment
  - Antibiotics
  - Anti-inflammatory analgesics
  - Antihistaminics
  - Local nasal decongestents
  - Improvement in nutrition
- Surgical treatment
  - Adenoidectomy under general anaesthesia
  - Myringotomy with grommet insertion for SOM, if present

PERITONSILLITIS AND PERITONSILLAR ABSCESS

Synonym   Quinsy

Definition   It is defined as the collection of pus in the peritonsillar space, i.e. between the tonsillar capsule and the superior constrictor muscle.

Initially, there is an inflammation of the peritonsillar tissues, known as peritonsillitis followed by suppuration and abscess formation resulting in quinsy. It is usually unilateral.

Aetiology:
- Recurrent attacks of tonsillitis can result in obliteration of the intratonsillar cleft (crypta magna) with infection reaching the peritonsillar space followed by abscess formation.
- Foreign body embedded in the tonsil can result in peritonsillitis and quinsy.
- Residual tonsillar tag after tonsillectomy can get infected, leading to peritonsillitis and quinsy.

- **Age:** It is common in adults in the second and third decades of life.
- **Sex:** It is common in males.

Pathogenesis   It is shown in Flowchart 31.1

Flowchart 31.1: Pathogenesis of peritonsillitis and peritonsillar abscess

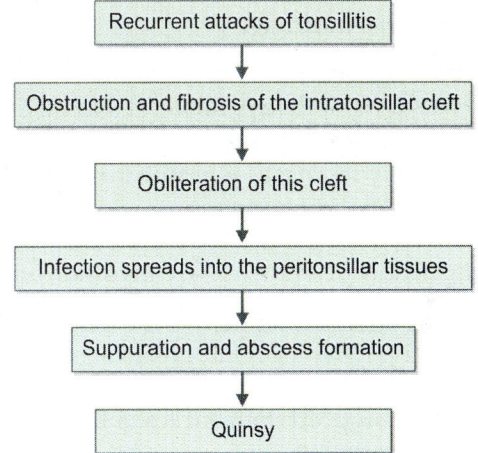

Clinical features
- Symptoms
  - Severe sore throat, unilateral pain in throat.
  - Odynophagia
  - Unilateral referred otalgia
  - Fever, malaise and bodyache
  - Trismus due to spasm of pterygoid muscles
  - Dribbling of saliva
  - Speech is thick and muffled
- Signs
  - Anterior pillar is congested and swollen
  - Tonsil is congested and pushed medially and downwards
  - Uvula is oedematous, congested, and pushed to the opposite side
  - Halitosis
  - Trismus
  - Coated tongue
  - Ipsilateral cervical lymphadenitis may be present
  - Patient looks ill and toxic, and may be febrile
  - Spontaneous rupture of the abscess may occur, if untreated

Complications
- Parapharyngeal abscess
- Retropharyngeal abscess
- Laryngeal oedema

- Cellulitis of the neck
- Thrombophlebitis of internal jugular vein
- Septicaemia
- Aspiration of the pus into the tracheobronchial tree, if abscess ruptures spontaneously
- Supraglottic oedema resulting in airway obstruction can occur occasionally
- Rarely, necrosis of the wall of the internal carotid artery with haemorrhage

Differential diagnosis

- *Acute tonsillitis*—Always bilateral. No evidence of oedema or congestion of soft palate and uvula.
- *Malignancy of the tonsil*—chronic in onset and less painful. No fever or toxaemia.
- *Parapharyngeal abscess*: It may push the tonsil medially, making it more prominent. No congestion of tonsils.

Treatment   Patient is admitted to the hospital.

- **Conservative/Medical:** Only given for peritonsillitis where abscess has not formed. Once abscess (quinsy) has formed, surgical treatment is required in addition to medial treatment:
  - Antibiotics—intravenously, e.g. injection ampicillin (500 mg) IV 6 hourly.
  - Anti-inflammatory analgesics and antipyretics to relieve the pain, inflammation, and fever.
  - Maintenance of oral hygiene with Condy's gargles.
  - Intravenous fluids as patient fails to take oral feeds adequately.
  - Soft bland warm diet.
- **Surgical:** Incision and drainage (I and D) of the abscess is the treatment of choice.

  The throat is sprayed with 4% lignocaine solution and the patient is explained the procedure. The patient is kept in the sitting position for the I and D. Sedation or general anaesthesia is not used, as patient may aspirate the purulent material.

  A quinsy forceps or a guarded 11 no. stab knife is used for the I and D. The patient is asked to open his mouth and the tongue is depressed using a Lack's tongue depressor, so as to visualise the site of the abscess.

  The site of incision is either:
  - At the site of maximum pointing of the abscess,
  - At the junction of a horizontal imaginary line running through the base of the uvula and a vertical imaginary line along the anterior pillar (Fig. 31.3), or
  - In the intratonsillar cleft.

  After incision, drainage is performed by use of sinus forceps or a nasal dressing forceps.

  After I and D, the patient is asked to gargle with dilute hydrogen peroxide or Condy's solution.
- Tonsillectomy is performed after 4–6 weeks to prevent a recurrence of quinsy.
- Rarely, tonsillectomy is performed at time of draining the quinsy. However, it is not recommended, as it can cause excessive bleeding or thromboembolism. It is known as 'Quinsy tonsillectomy'.

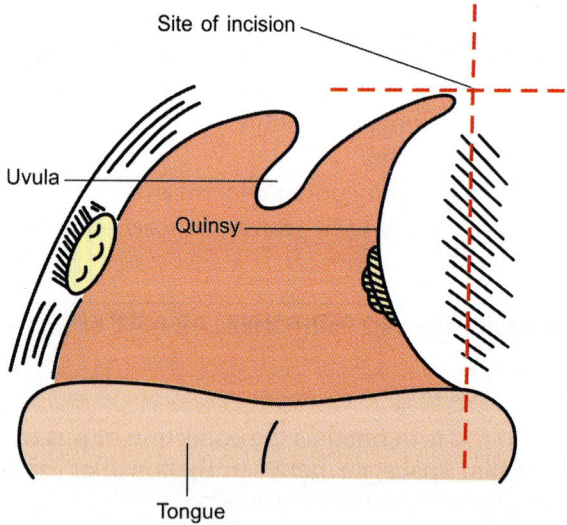

Fig. 31.3: Site of incision and drainage of quinsy

CHAPTER 32

Miscellaneous Diseases of Tonsils and Pharynx

Miscellaneous diseases associated with tonsils and pharynx include:
- Tonsillar keratosis or pharyngeal keratosis
- Tonsillolith
- Tonsillar cyst
- Foreign body in the pharynx
- Pharyngeal pouch
- Globus hystericus
- Stylohyoid syndrome (Eagle's syndrome)
- Patterson-Brown-Kelly syndrome
- Sleep-apnoea syndrome
- Neurological disorders

TONSILLAR KERATOSIS

Tonsillar keratosis is commonly associated with pharyngeal keratosis and both these terms are often used as synonyms.

Definition   It is a non-inflammatory condition characterised by multiple yellowish-white outgrowths which project from the mucosa of the tonsils, base-tongue, pharynx and larynx.

Aetiology   The exact aetiology is not known. However, smoking, alcoholism, tobacco chewing, vitamin 'A' deficiency, fungal infection and immunodeficiency are predisposing factors.

Clinical features
- Usually asymptomatic.
- White or yellowish-white keratinised epithelial outgrowths are seen over the mucosa of the tonsils, posterior pharyngeal wall, base tongue and larynx.

- Irritation or foreign body sensation in throat.
- Change of taste or foul taste in mouth.
- Halitosis

It is a benign condition characterised by absence of inflammation and it is self-limiting. Usually discovered accidentally by the patient.

Treatment
- If asymptomatic, no treatment is required, only reassurance, that the condition is self-limiting and benign.
- Condy's gargles 4–5 times daily.
- Mandl's throat paint is applied to the affected areas 4–5 times daily.
- Multivitamins are empirically given, as the condition is thought to be due to vitamin deficiency.

TONSILLOLITH

Definition   Tonsillolith is a condition, which occurs due to calcification of inspissated pus in the crypts of the tonsils.

Clinical features
- Hard white structures are seen to project out from the tonsils.
- Foreign-body sensation in the throat.
- May be asymptomatic at times.

These are felt as hard masses in the tonsils and may be mistaken for malignancy or elongated styloid process.

Treatment

- If asymptomatic, only reassurance is required.
- Tonsillectomy is performed for tonsilloliths producing symptoms.

TONSILLAR CYST

Tonsillar cyst occurs due to infection of the tonsils. Cysts develop from the crypts of the tonsils and are yellowish in colour. They may be single or multiple and are usually asymptomatic.

Treatment

- No treatment is required, if asymptomatic.
- Tonsillectomy is performed, if symptomatic.

FOREIGN BODY IN THE PHARYNX

Accidental ingestion of a foreign body, which lodges itself in the pharynx is seen commonly.

Common types of foreign bodies

- Fish bone—commonest
- Chicken bone
- Metal pin
- Dentures
- Needles, etc.

Common sites of lodgement

- Tonsils
- Base tongue
- Vallecula
- Posterior pharyngeal wall
- Pyriform fossa

Clinical features

- History of accidental ingestion of foreign body
- Foreign-body sensation or pricking sensation in throat
- Odynophagia
- Retching and sometimes vomiting
- On examination of throat or on indirect laryngoscopy, the foreign body may be visualised impacted in the tonsil or pharyngeal mucosa.

Investigations

- X-ray soft tissue of neck, lateral and anteroposterior view will reveal a radio-opaque metallic foreign body. However, fish bone is not seen well on X-ray.

Treatment

- Removal of the foreign body at the earliest with the help of a forceps.
- Removal is done in the OPD in cases of superficial foreign bodies, which are easily visible, e.g. on tonsil, base tongue, or posterior pharyngeal wall.

- Removal requires direct laryngoscopy in cases of foreign bodies embedded in the valleculae or pyriform fossa. Attempts to remove a foreign body with indirect laryngoscopy should be done with caution, since there are chances of its slipping into the air or food passages.
- Foreign-bodies like coins, etc., usually pass into the oesophagus, and removal under general anaesthesia using an oesophagoscope is required.

PHARYNGEAL POUCH

Synonyms

- Pharyngeal diverticulum (Fig. 32.1)
- Hypopharyngeal pouch.

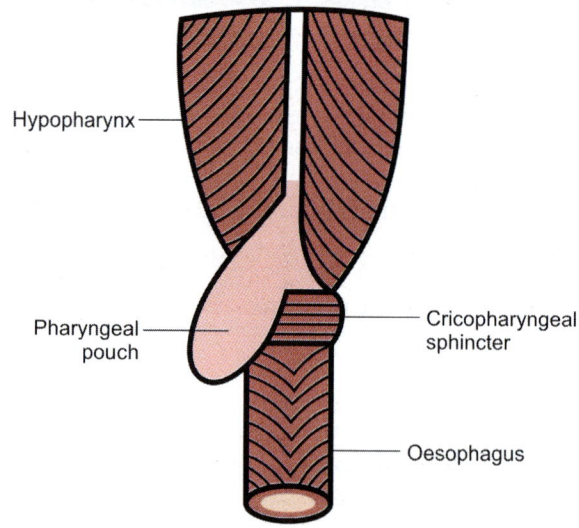

Fig. 32.1 : Pharyngeal pouch

Definition   It is the herniation of the pharyngeal mucosa through a dehiscence in the posterior pharyngeal wall (Killian's dehiscence).

Aetiology

- Congenital Killian's dehiscence may be present in the posterior pharyngeal wall.
- Neuromuscular incoordination of the posterior pharyngeal wall during swallowing, can result in the formation of a diverticulum.

Pathogenesis   It is shown in Flowchart 32.1.

Clinical features

- Common in elderly patients, as muscle tone is reduced in elderly.
- Chronic dysphagia.
- Loss of weight.
- Regurgitation of undigested food material.

Flowchart 32.1: Pathogenesis of formation of pharyngeal pouch

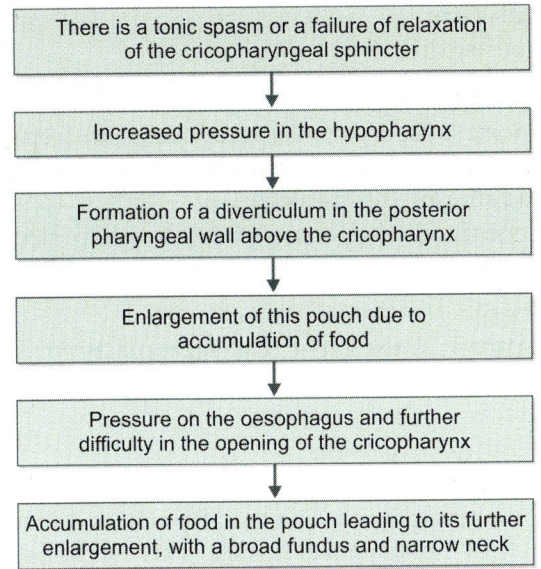

- Swelling may be seen on the left side of the neck, which is reducible on external pressure.
- Aspiration on coughing may occur due to regurgitation of fluids from the pouch.
- Rarely, a malignant change may occur.

Investigation   Barium swallow is diagnostic. A pouch is seen arising from the posterior pharyngeal wall, containing barium mixed with food particles.

Treatment
- Excision of the pouch with repair of the defect, is carried out through an external approach (via the neck).
- **Dohlman's operation:** Endoscopic division of the wall between the pouch and the oesophagus is the recent advance. Division is done either by using diathermy or using laser.

GLOBUS HYSTERICUS

Definition   Globus hystericus is a functional disorder characterised by the feeling of a lump in the throat.

Aetiology   It is a functional disorder due to psychological imbalance or cancerphobia.

Clinical features
- Commonly seen in adults
- Females are commonly affected
- Feeling of a lump in the throat
- Clinical examination is normal

Treatment
- Reassurance
- Psychiatric treatment

STYLOHYOID SYNDROME

Synonyms
- Eagle's syndrome.
- Stylalgia.

Aetiology
- Elongated styloid process.
- Calcified stylohyoid ligament.

Pathogenesis

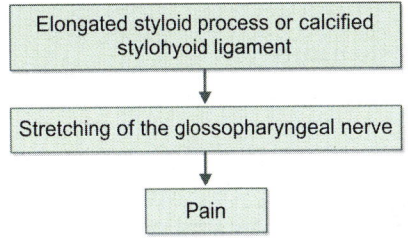

Clinical features
- Commonly unilateral, can be bilateral.
- Common in adults.

Characterised by a triad of:
- Pain in throat with referred otalgia.
- Foreign-body sensation in throat on the affected side.
- Palpable-elongated styloid process through the tonsillar fossa.

Investigations
- X-ray of styloid process shows presence of elongated styloid process.
- Injection of 0.5 cc of 2% lignocaine at the site (tonsillar fossa) will give relief within a few minutes, if the cause is in the glossopharyngeal nerve. This is diagnostic.

Treatment
- Analgesics and anti-inflammatory agents.
- Tranquillizers.
- **Styloidectomy:** It is the excision of the styloid process through the tonsillar fossa. Tonsillectomy is a pre-requisite to this surgery.
- Rarely, in case of persistent neuralgia, glosspharyngeal nerve sectioning (neurectomy) is required.

PATTERSON-BROWN-KELLY SYNDROME

Synonym
- Plummer–Vinson syndrome
- It is a precancerous lesion

Aetiology
- **Sex:** It is commonly seen in females

- Age: It is common in the fourth decade of life
- Iron deficiency anaemia
- Immunodeficiency
- Vitamin deficiency
- Autoimmune disease
- Chronic inflammatory disease of the bowel, e.g. chronic oesophagitis

Clinical features
- Dysphagia–more to solids than liquids
- Feeling of a lump in the throat
- Glossitis
- Angular stomatitis
- Koilonychia
- Pallor
- Sometimes, carcinomatous change may occur
- Indirect laryngoscopy is normal
- Cricopharyngoscopy and oesophagoscopy will reveal a web formation at the cricopharynx (post-cricoid region). This is the most helpful in confirming the diagnosis.

Diagnostic investigations
- Barium swallow: It shows the presence of a web in the postcricoid region
- Cricopharyngoscopy and oesophagoscopy are diagnostic
- Complete blood count will reveal an iron deficiency anaemia

Treatment
- Treatment of the iron deficiency anaemia helps to relieve symptoms in most cases. Ferrous sulphate and folic acid are given orally.
- Multivitamins
- Regular follow-up is required, as this is a pre-cancerous condition
- Dialatation of the web using a cricopharyngoscope is rarely required

SLEEP APNOEA SYNDROME

Definition   Sleep apnoea syndrome is characterised by apnoeic spells during sleep. There should be at least thirty apnoeic episodes lasting for 10 seconds or more during a 7-hour sleep period.

Aetiology
- It occurs due to obstructive pathology in the upper airway, e.g. deviated nasal septum, adenoids, enlarged tonsils, bulky and lax hypopharyngeal soft tissues (commonly seen in fat people).
- Age: It is common in four decade of life.

- Sex: It is common in males.
- Obesity
- Alcoholism
- Hypertension

Clinical features
- Apnoeic spells occur, when the patient is in deep sleep causing him/her to wake up breathless and sweating.
- Loud snoring during sleep.
- Apnoea is relieved, once patient is awake or sleeping lightly.

Treatment
- Treatment of the cause, e.g. septoplasty for DNS, tonsillectomy for enlarged tonsils.
- Reduction of body weight.
- Control hypertension.
- Stop alcohol.
- In an obese patient, this usually occurs due to lax and bulky pharyngeal tissues. This can be treated by surgery.
  - Uvulopalatopharyngoplasty (UPPP).

NEUROLOGICAL DISORDERS OF THE PHARYNX

Aetiology   Neurological disorders of the pharynx occurs due to lesions of the superior or recurrent laryngeal nerves causing symptoms.

Clinical features
- Due to sensory involvement
  - Anaesthesia
  - Paresthesia
  - Hyperaesthesia
  - Neuralgia, e.g. glossopharyngeal neuralgia due to elongated styloid process.
- Due to motor involvement
  - Pharyngeal palsy with absent gag reflex and dysphagia.
  - Aspiration due to pharyngeal palsy can cause cough during swallowing with cyanosis and occasionally aspiration pneumonia.
  - Palatal paralysis which is either unilateral or bilateral with nasal regurgitation and rhinolalia aperta (nasal twang to the voice).

Treatment
- Treatment of the cause, e.g. styloidectomy in case of an elongated styloid process.
- Ryle's tube feeding
- Tracheostomy
- Gastrostomy

CHAPTER 33

Infections of the Pharynx

Infections of the pharynx are listed in Flowchart 33.1.

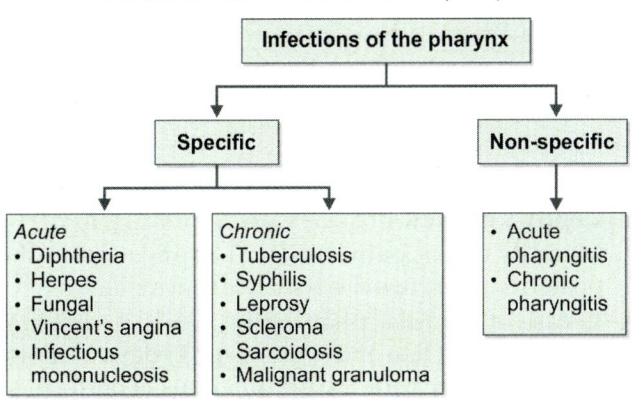

Flowchart 33.1: Infections of the pharynx

Infections of the pharynx

Specific

Acute
- Diphtheria
- Herpes
- Fungal
- Vincent's angina
- Infectious mononucleosis

Chronic
- Tuberculosis
- Syphilis
- Leprosy
- Scleroma
- Sarcoidosis
- Malignant granuloma

Non-specific
- Acute pharyngitis
- Chronic pharyngitis

ACUTE PHARYNGITIS

Definition   Acute pharyngitis is the acute non-specific infection of the pharynx.

Aetiology   The exact aetiology is unknown. It is commonly associated with cold. It is common in typhoid, influenza, measles, etc. It may occur after administration of certain drugs. Mouth-breathing, dental caries, etc., are predisposing factors.

Causative organisms   It is usually viral in origin. However, bacterial infection due to *Streptococcus haemolyticus*, pneumococcus, and *Haemophilus Influenzae* can also cause this condition.

Clinical features
- Symptoms
  - Sore throat or a raw sensation in the throat with halitosis.
  - Fever, malaise
  - Odynophagia
  - Dry, irritating cough
  - Slightly hoarse voice
- Signs
  - Catarrhal type is characterized by oedema, congestion, and inflammation of the posterior pharyngeal wall and soft palate.
  - Purulent type is characterised by the presence of a mucopurulent discharge on the posterior pharyngeal wall.
  - Ulcerative or gangrenous type is characterised by ulcerations and sloughing of the posterior pharyngeal wall. It is rare and may occur in an immunocompromised or diabetic individual. It may be associated with acute tonsillitis.

Differential diagnosis
- Diphtheria.
- Agranulocytosis: In this, the constitutional symptoms are much more severe.
- Exanthematous fevers may be associated with acute pharyngitis.

Treatment
- Bed rest and improvement of oral hygiene.
- Soft bland diet with plenty of fluids.

- Antibiotics
- Anti-inflammatory analgesics
- Condy's gargles (1 : 4000 potassium permanganate) as a local antiseptic.

CHRONIC PHARYNGITIS

Definition   Chronic pharyngitis is a chronic non-specific infection of the pharynx.

Aetiology
- Following infections of the nose and paranasal sinuses, such as:
  - DNS causing nasal obstruction and mouth-breathing
  - Rhinitis especially allergic rhinitis
  - Sinusitis
  - Postnasal discharge due to rhinitis or sinusitis
  - Atrophic rhinitis
- Following recurrent attacks of acute pharyngitis
- Following infections of the throat, such as:
  - Tonsillitis
  - Dental caries and sepsis
  - Stomatitis
- Following tonsillectomy operation, granular pharyngitis may be exaggerated due to hypertrophy of pharyngeal lymphoid tissue on exposure to allergens.
- Following bronchitis, bronchiectasis or asthma.
- Intestinal parasites can cause chronic pharyngitis.
- Tropical eosinophilia can cause chronic pharyngitis.
- Atmospheric pollution.
- Alcohol, acts as local irritants
- Smoking, acts as local irritants
- Tobacco chewing, acts as local irritants
- Emotional trauma can predispose to or aggravate this condition.

Classification
- Catarrhal pharyngitis
- Granular (hypertrophic) pharyngitis
- Atrophic pharyngitis

Clinical features
- Symptoms
  - Raw sensation in the throat
  - Hawking
  - Dry cough
  - Odynophagia
  - *Change in voice*: The voice breaks during speech and tires out.

- Rarely, blood-streaked sputum may be seen in case of granular pharyngitis.
- Signs
  - *Catarrhal type* will show oedema and congestion of the posterior pharyngeal wall.
  - *Granular type* will show presence of red granulations and hypertrophied lymphoid tissue on the posterior pharyngeal wall with congestion and dialated blood vessels.
  - Occasionally, yellowish cysts may be present due to cystic changes in the mucosal glands.
  - *Atrophic type* shows presence of thin, dry, glazed atrophic mucosa and is usually associated with atrophic rhinitis.

Investigations
- Haemogram with total and differential blood counts to rule out anaemia and eosinophilia.
- X-ray paranasal sinuses to detect sinusitis.
- X-ray chest to rule out tuberculosis, bronchitis or bronchiectasis.
- Throat swab for bacteriology, culture and antibiotic sensitivity.

Treatment
- Treatment of the cause.
- Antibiotics systemically.
- Anti-inflammatory analgesics.
- Condy's gargles.
- Mandl's throat paint for local application to the posterior pharyngeal wall, three times a day.
- In case of granular pharyngitis, which is resistant to the medical line of treatment for 15 days or more, chemical cautery of the granulations is performed using dilute (15%) silver nitrate or dilute (10%) trichloroacetic acid (TCA).
- Tincture benzoin or menthol in steam inhalation for a local soothing effect—3–4 times a day.

VINCENT'S ANGINA

Synonym
- Acute membraneous pharyngitis.
- Trench mouth.

Definition   Vincent's Angina is an acute ulcerative infection of the pharynx due to gram negative fusiform bacilli and a spirochaete.
- Site of involvement: It commonly affects the oropharynx especially both the tonsills, soft palate and gums.

Aetiology
- Causative organisms
  - Gram negative fusiform bacillus.
  - Spirochaete (spirochaeta denticola).
- Predisposing factors
  - Poor oral hygiene
  - Dental caries and abscess
  - Malnutrition
  - Immunosuppressed individuals
  - Diabetes mellitus

Clinical features
- Symptoms
  - High grade fever with chills
  - Pain in the throat
  - Odynophagia
  - Halitosis
- Signs
  - Poor oral hygiene
  - Foetor from the mouth
  - Ulcerative areas on tonsils, soft palate, and gums covered by a greyish membraneous slough. The base of this ulcer is granular and bleeds on touch.
  - Patient appears toxic
  - Cervical lymphadenitis is present

Differential diagnosis
- Faucial diphtheria
- Infectious mononucleosis
- Tertiary syphillis
- Agranulocytic angina

Diagnostic investigation
A hanging-drop preparation of the smear, which will demonstrate the organisms.

Treatment
- **Antibiotics systemically:** Penicillin is the drug of choice in this condition
- Antiseptic gargles using dilute hydrogen peroxide or Condy's gargles
- Anti-inflammatory analgesics and antipyretics
- Local application of chromic acid may help

ACUTE DIPHTHERETIC PHARYNGITIS

Synonym Pharyngeal diphtheria

Definition Acute diphtheretic pharyngitis is an acute specific infection of the pharynx by diphtheritic bacilli

Aetiology
- Causative organism—*Corynebacterium diphtheriae*
- It commonly occurs due to the lack of immunisation in children

- **Age:** It is common between 1–5 years of age.
- **Mode of spread:** Airborne or Droplet infection.

Clinical features
- Symptoms
  - Sore throat.
  - Fever, mild to moderate.
  - Tachycardia and weak pulse, which are out of proportion to the fever.
  - Mild pain or no pain.
- Signs
  - Child may look toxic.
  - *Presence of a greyish-white membrane,* which is seen to cover the tonsil and adjacent structures like the pillars, soft palate, pharyngeal wall, etc. This membrane is not easily separable and leaves behind a raw bleeding surface. It may even extend to the larynx causing respiratory obstruction and death.
  - *Cervical lymphadenopathy*: Massively enlarged bilateral tender cervical lymph nodes due to infection (Bull's neck).
  - *Neurological and cardiological complications* like neuritis, myocarditis, etc., can occur.

Differential diagnosis
- Acute ulcerative tonsillitis
- Vincent's angina
- Thrush

Investigation   Swab for bacteriological culture.

Treatment
- Hospitalization and isolation.
- Complete bed rest and good diet.
- **Antitoxin:** Antidiphtheretic serum (ADS) is administered at the earliest even without waiting for the bacteriology report. 20,000 to 100,000 units of ADS are administered depending on the extent and severity of the disease.
- **Systemic antibiotics:** Penicillin is the drug of choice. Erythromycin can also be used.
- All contacts are immunized.
- Tracheostomy may be required in case of involvement of larynx with respiratory distress.

FUNGAL PHARYNGITIS

The commonest fungal infection affecting the oral cavity is thrush.

Aetiology
- **Causative organism:** *Candida albicans*.
  - It is common in children and elderly.

- ◆ Diabetes mellitus, predisposing factors
- ◆ Malnutrition, predisposing factors
- ◆ Immunosuppression, predisposing factors

Clinical features

- • Symptoms
  - ◆ Burning sensation in the mouth
  - ◆ Odynophagia
  - ◆ Halitosis
- • Signs
  - ◆ Poor oral hygiene
  - ◆ Halitosis
  - ◆ White cotton-like patches on the oral mucosa, which can be peeled off easily and do not bleed.

Treatment

- • Local: Application of 1% gentian violet or nystatin solution.

  Recently—clotrimazole solution can be applied locally to hasten recovery.
- • Systemic: Secondary infection is controlled by administration of a broad spectrum antibiotic like penicillin.

HERPETIC PHARYNGITIS

Herpetic pharyngitis can occur due to herpes simplex or herpes zoster infection.

Clinical features

- • Herpes simplex
  - ◆ Small vesicles filled with clear fluid are seen on the oral mucosa and may even involve lips and face.
  - ◆ Pain
  - ◆ Fever
  - ◆ Odynophagia
  - ◆ Small, shallow and painful ulcers are formed due to rupture of the vesicles.
- • Herpes zoster
  - ◆ Small vesicles filled with clear fluid are seen on the oral mucosa. But they are unilateral and are in rows. It may involve the mucosa of the palate.
  - ◆ Pain is very severe
  - ◆ Otalgia (referred)
  - ◆ Odynophagia
  - ◆ Fever

Treatment

- • Condy's gargles for antiseptic purpose
- • 2% lignocaine solution or gargles with lignocaine viscous prior to meals will reduce pain
- • Bed rest
- • Nutritious diet

- • Analgesics
- • Rarely, antiviral agents, like acyclovir
- • Sometimes steroids under antibiotic cover can be used for severe cases

INFECTIOUS MONONUCLEOSIS

Synonym   Glandular fever

Definition   Infectious mononucleosis is a viral infection caused by the Epstein–Barr virus.

Clinical features

- • Sore throat
- • Fever
- • Odynophagia
- • Lymphadenopathy of the cervical, axillary, and other group of lymph nodes
- • Splenomegaly

Investigations   Paul Bunnel test is positive. It is the main diagnostic investigation.

Treatment   Symptomatic treatment.

TUBERCULOSIS OF THE PHARYNX

Classification

- • Chronic tuberculous ulcer: Usually single, shallow, and very painful
- • Tuberculoma: Exophytic lesion on the mucosa, which is very painful
- • Lupus: It is commonly associated with lupus of the nose and face, seen as nodules on the fauces, soft palate, and uvula; called 'apple-jelly' nodules. These nodules break down and ulcerate followed by healing and scar formation.
- • Acute miliary tuberculosis: Painful multiple small shallow ulcers are seen on the soft palate, fauces and posterior pharyngeal wall, which later coalesce.

  Usually, occurs secondary to pulmonary tuberculosis. Initially, the tonsils were thought to be the focus of infection, but tonsillar tuberculous infection usually results in cervical lymphadenopathy (tuberculous).

Diagnosis   Biopsy of the lesion for histopathology will confirm the diagnosis.

Treatment   Antituberculous drugs for a period of 9 months to 1 year.

SYPHILIS OF THE PHARYNX

It is rarely seen nowadays.

Classification

- **Primary:** It is seen as a chancre on the tonsil. There may be a unilateral painless enlargement of the tonsil, which is hard on palpation. The jugulodigastric lymph node is enlarged on the affected side. Primary syphilitic pharyngitis is rarely seen.
- **Secondary:** It is characterised by:
  - Greyish mucous patches.
  - Snail-track ulcerations.
  - Skin rash with lymphadenopathy.
- **Tertiary:** It is characterised by a gummatous ulcer on the soft palate, hard palate, or pharynx. There may be perforation of the soft palate or hard palate.

DIFFERENTIAL DIAGNOSIS OF MEMBRANEOUS LESIONS OF THE PHARYNX

- Acute follicular tonsillitis
- Vincent's angina
- Diphtheretic pharyngitis
- Fungal infection (thrush)
- Keratosis pharyngitis
- Infectious mononucleosis
- Agranulocytosis
- Streptococcal pharyngitis

CHAPTER 34

Pharyngeal Abscesses

Pharyngeal abscesses are of two types:
- Retropharyngeal abscess:
  - Acute
  - Chronic
- Parapharyngeal abscess

RETROPHARYNGEAL ABSCESS

Definition   Retropharyngeal abscess is an accumulation of pus in the retropharyngeal space of Gillette (Fig. 34.1).

Classification
- Acute retropharyngeal abscess
  - *Aetiology:* It occurs due to infection and suppuration of the retropharyngeal group of lymph nodes by pyogenic organisms.

    These lymph nodes drain the nasopharynx, oropharynx, and part of the upper respiratory tract. They atrophy by the age of 5–8 years.
    - *Age:* It occurs in children and is common below 1 year of age.
    - *Nasopharyngeal infections:* Adenoids, postnasal discharge, etc.
    - *Pharyngeal infections:* Tonsillitis, pharyngitis, etc.
    - Foreign body embedded in the posterior pharyngeal wall, which gets infected.
    - Upper respiratory tract infections.
  - *Causative organisms*
    - Streptococcus
    - *Staphylococcus aureus*

- *Clinical features*
  - *Symptoms*
    - Dysphagia
    - Fever, malaise
    - Sore throat
    - Refusal to eat
    - Dribbling of saliva
    - Croupy cough
    - Neck is held rigid. Occasionally, there is torticollis.
    - Nasal obstruction due to spread of oedema to the nasopharynx.
  - *Signs*
    - Examination of the oral cavity reveals:
      - Unilateral smooth bulge on the posterior pharyngeal wall.
      - Congestion and oedema of the pharyngeal wall mucosa.
      - Spread is upwards to the nasopharynx and downwards to the cricopharynx, but it does not cross the midline due to the presence of the median pharyngeal raphe.
    - Examination of the neck reveals:
      - Enlarged and tender jugulodigastric or upper deep cervical lymph nodes.
- *Complications*
  - Spontaneous rupture of the abscess may result in inhalation of the pus and pulmonary complications, asphyxia, or even sudden death.
  - Laryngeal oedema may require a tracheostomy.

- Severe malnutrition and dehydration due to dysphagia may occur.
- ◆ *Differential diagnosis*
  - Tuberculous cold abscess of the retropharyngeal lymph nodes.
  - Tuberculous cold abscess of the vertebral column.
- ◆ *Investigations*
  - Diagnostic investigation is a plain X-ray of the neck (lateral view) which will show a soft tissue density shadow with widening of the retropharyngeal space. Rarely an air-fluid level may be seen. Also, there is loss of normal anatomical curvature of the cervical spine. But vertebral bodies are intact.
  - After incision and drainage of the abscess, the pus is sent for bacteriological culture and sensitivity to antibiotics.
- ◆ *Treatment*
  - Patient is admitted to the hospital.
  - Systemic antibiotics to cover anaerobes and aerobes.
  - Anti-inflammatory analgesics.
  - Incision and drainage of the abscess at the earliest. It is done transorally and preferably without anaesthesia, as an endotracheal intubation may result in rupture of the abscess and aspiration of pus with asphyxia. The child is wrapped in a sheet or a towel and the mouth is opened gently with a mouth gag. The head is held steady by an assistant in the head-low position to prevent aspiration. The abscess is incised and purulent material is cleared by use of suction apparatus.

    Tracheostomy is required if:
    - The child is in severe respiratory distress due to laryngeal oedema.
    - The general anaesthesia is to be given for incision and drainage of the abscess.
- Chronic retropharyngeal abscess
  - ◆ *Aetiology*
    - Secondary to cold abscess of the retropharyngeal lymph nodes.
    - Secondary to cold abscess of the cervical vertebrae.
  - ◆ *Classification*
    - *Lateral:* It begins on one side and is due to abscess of the retropharyngeal lymph node.
    - *Medial:* It begins in the midline and spreads on both sides. It is due to cold abscess of the cervical vertebrae, which spreads to the prevertebral space.

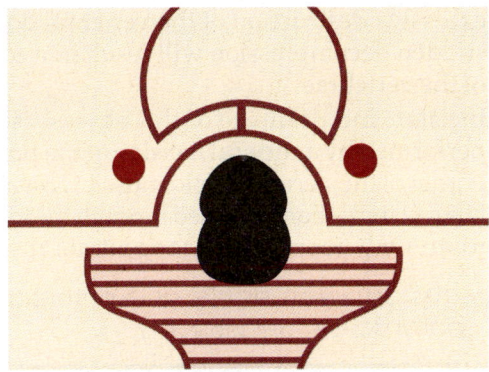

Fig. 34.1 : Retropharyngeal abscess

- ◆ *Clinical features*
  - *Age:* Chronic retropharyngeal abscess secondary to cold abscess of the retropharyngeal lymph nodes, is common in children, as these lymph nodes atrophy after 5–8 years of age. Retropharyngeal abscess due to cold abscess of the cervical vertebrae occurs at any age.
  - Patient complains of dysphagia.
  - Examination of the oral cavity will reveal a smooth bulge in the posterior pharyngeal wall which may be central or laterally situated without features of inflammation.
  - Cervical lymphadenitis may be present.
  - In case of tuberculous abscess of the cervical spine, there may be restriction of neck movement.
- ◆ *Differential diagnosis:* Refer to the DD of acute retropharyngeal abscess .
- ◆ *Investigations*
  - X-ray cervical spine lateral view will reveal straightening of the cervical spine with loss of normal curvature and destruction of the body of the cervical vertebrae and a soft tissue density shadow widening the retropharyngeal space.
  - X-ray chest–PA view may reveal pulmonary Kochs in some patients.
  - Complete haemogram and erythrocyte sedimentation rate (ESR).
  - Pus, after incision and drainage is sent for bacteriological culture and antibiotic sensitivity.
- ◆ *Treatment*
  - *Antituberculous therapy:* The regime is given for a period of 12–14 months.
  - Caries of the cervical spine will require orthopaedic treatment.
  - Aspiration of the abscess through the oral cavity with a thick needle, may be done to progressively decompress the cervical spine, as in cases of

excessive destruction of the vertebral bodies, a sudden decompression will result in a collapse of the vertebrae.

- Incision and drainage of this abscess is rarely performed by a cervical incision at the posterior border of the sternomastoid muscle. This abscess is never incised and drained through the intraoral route. Only aspiration is done intraorally.

Differences between acute and chronic retropharyngeal abscess   *See* Table 34.1

TABLE 34.1: Differences between acute and chronic retropharyngeal abscesses

Acute retropharyngeal abscess	Chronic retropharyngeal abscess
• Occurs in children below 3 years of age.	• Occurs in older children and adults.
• Involves the true retropharyngeal space of Gillette.	• Involves the prevertebral space.
• Pyogenic organisms are the causative agents.	• Tuberculous bacilli are the causative organisms.
• Acute in onset.	• Insidious in onset.
• Associated with constitutional symptoms like fever.	• No constitutional symptoms.
• Dyspnoea is common.	• Dyspnoea is rare.
• Dysphagia is acute.	• Chronic dysphagia.
• Abscess is unilateral.	• Abscess is in midline.
• Signs of acute inflammation are present.	• No signs of acute inflammation are seen.
• *Treatment:* Incision and drainage through transoral route with antibiotics for the causative organism.	• *Treatment:* Aspiration is preferred to incision and drainage. If incision and drainage is performed, it is always through the external approach. Anti-Kochs therapy is given.

PARAPHARYNGEAL ABSCESS

Definition
Parapharyngeal abscess is the accumulation of pus in the parapharyngeal space (Fig. 34.2).

Aetiology
- **Age:** It may occur at any age.
- Oral cavity infections may spread to involve the parapharyngeal space e.g. tooth abscess, infected last molar, quinsy, etc.
- Predisposing features
  - Poor general condition
  - Diabetes mellitus
  - Immunosuppressed patients

Clinical features
- Symptoms
  - Pain in the throat

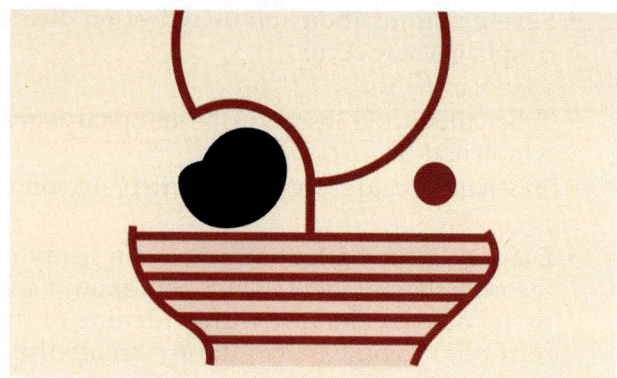

Fig. 34.2 : Parapharyngeal abscess

- Trismus
- Odynophagia
- Constitutional symptoms: Fever, malaise, etc.
- Swelling in the neck.
- Signs
  - Diffuse swelling and inflammation in the neck at the site of the parapharyngeal space.
  - On examination of the throat, the tonsil is pushed medially and lateral pharyngeal wall is inflamed and oedematous.

Differential diagnosis
- Quinsy
- Retropharyngeal abscess
- Benign tumour of the tonsil

Complications
- Spread may occur upwards along the carotid sheath to the cranial cavity resulting in meningitis.
- Downward spread may occur to the mediastinum resulting in mediastinitis.
- Laryngeal oedema may occur.
- Thrombophlebitis of the internal jugular vein may occur resulting in toxemia, pyaemia and septicaemia.
- Rarely, sloughing off of the wall of the carotid artery may occur resulting in fatal haemorrhage.

Treatment
- Admission to hospital
- Tracheostomy, if there is severe respiratory distress
- Systemic antibiotics
- Systemic anti-inflammatory analgesics
- Incision and drainage either via the transoral or external route (neck), at the site of maximum bulging. Internal oral drainage requires good suction and is to be performed preferably without anaesthesia to prevent aspiration of pus into the tracheobronchial tree.

CHAPTER **35**

Tumours of the Pharynx

Tumours that may appear in pharynx are listed in Flowchart 35.1

Flowchart 35.1: Tumours of the pharynx

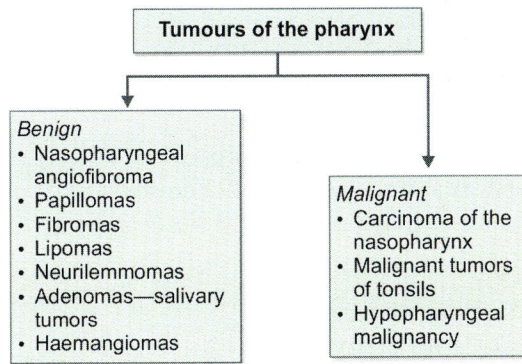

NASOPHARYNGEAL ANGIOFIBROMA

Definition Nasopharyngeal angiofibroma is a very vascular benign tumour with fibrous stroma and a rapid destructive growth occurring in the nasopharynx and commonly seen in adolescent males.

Hence, it is correctly known as the 'juvenile naso-pharyngeal angiofibroma'.

Aetiology The exact cause is not known, but various theories have been put forward.

- Age: It is common in the ages between 10 and 15 years.
- Sex: It is common in males.
- Site of origin: Sphenopalatine foramen in the naso-pharynx, is considered to be the site of origin.

- Hormonal theory: This theory suggests that the angiofibroma occurs due to oestrogen and androgen imbalance.
- Fibroblastic theory: According to this theory, the tumour occurs as an abnormal proliferation of various tissues in the nasopharynx. For example:
  - Facia basalis
  - Periosteum of the nasopharyngeal wall
  - Embryonic occipital cartilage
- Hamartomatous theory: It suggests that the tumour originates from the nasal erectile tissue.

Pathogenesis It is a rapidly expanding benign tumour, which consists of blood vessels and fibrous tissue. The blood vessel walls do not have the tunica media, which helps the vessel to contract and retract. Hence, there is torrential haemorrhage from the tumour. The tumour expands and destroys the surrounding tissues, like the nasal septum, maxillary sinus, sphenoid sinus, pterygopalatine fossa, and cranial fossae. The blood supply is usually from the ipsilateral internal maxillary artery.

Clinical features

- Symptoms
  - Nasal obstruction
  - *Epistaxis*: Spontaneous and profuse.
  - Usually, the patient is a male between 10–25 years of age.
  - Swelling over the cheek
  - Rhinolalia clausa, i.e. loss of vocal resonance

- ◆ Bulging of the soft palate
- ◆ Ipsilateral otalgia and blocking of the ear.
- ◆ Diplopia or headache may occur due to expansion.
- Signs
  - ◆ Pallor
  - ◆ Swelling over the malar region
  - ◆ Anterior rhinoscopy may reveal a bluish-red mass which is smooth and bleeds torrentially, if touched accidentally.
  - ◆ Soft palate is pushed forward by the mass.
  - ◆ Posterior rhinoscopy reveals a bluish-red smooth mass in the nasopharynx.
  - ◆ Examination of the ears may reveal secretory otitis media due to Eustachian tube obstruction.
  - ◆ Proptosis may be present due to retro-orbital spread.

Investigations

- Haemogram will reveal anaemia.
- X-ray of the skull: Lateral view shows a forward bowing of the posterior wall of the maxilla with a soft tissue, shadow in the nasopharynx.
- X-ray of the paranasal sinuses: Water's view shows widening of the distance between the maxilla and mandible on the side of the tumour.
- Computed tomography (CT) scan is the most important diagnostic tool today. It is performed with and without contrast medium to detect the site, extent, vascularity of the tumour and destruction caused by the tumour.
- Angiography is performed to detect the feeding vessels and for purpose of embolisation prior to surgery. This helps to reduce the intraoperative haemorrhage.
- Biopsy is never performed as this results in torrential haemorrhage.

Treatment

- Surgical excision of the tumour in toto is performed after ligating or embolising the feeding blood vessels. At least two or three pints of blood are cross-matched and kept ready preoperatively. Today with the advent of angled rigid Hopkin's nasal endoscopes, high definition camera system and accurate/precise embolisation techniques by interventional neuroradiologist, many surgeons perform complete excision of the angiofibroma endoscopically. This however, requires expertise and good equipment and instruments.
- Radiation therapy is palliative and used in cases with extensive intracranial spread, where surgery is not possible.

Prognosis   It is seen that natural regression of the tumour occurs after 25 years of age. However, it may not always be possible to wait for a natural remission, as there may be excessive blood loss associated with this tumour or there may be intracranial extension which may be fatal. Recurrence after excision is known to occur.

CARCINOMA OF THE NASOPHARYNX

Definition   Carcinoma of the nasopharynx is a malignant squamous cell tumour.

Aetiology

- Age: It has a bimodal peak and is common between 20–30 years and 40–70 years of age.
- Sex: It usually occurs more in male than female.
- Geographical distribution: It is commonly seen in Cantonese Chinese.
- Common in population which consume smoked fish in large quantity.
- Probably occurs due to use of joss sticks and inscence sticks in religious practices.
- Ebstein–Barr virus has been implicated as an aetiological factor.
- Household smoke may predispose.
- Chinese herbal medicines are thought to be predisposing factors.
- Tobacco smoke may predispose.
- Wood-dust and industrial chemicals like rubber fumes, etc., may predispose to its development.

Pathology

- Gross: It may be either:
  - ◆ Ulcerative or invasive
  - ◆ Proliferative.
  - ◆ Verrucous, which spreads on the surface.
- Microscopic: It is usually a moderately well-differentiated squamous cell carcinoma.

Site of origin   It commonly arises from the postero-superior wall or the lateral wall of the nasopharynx.

The lymph node of Rouviere in the fossa of Rosenmuller is the first site for drainage and gets enlarged. Obliteration of the fossa of Rosenmuller on CT scan of nasopharynx, is the first sign of nasopharyngeal carcinoma.

Clinical features

- Symptoms
  - ◆ Nasal obstruction is common, if growth is proliferative

- ◆ Epistaxis is common, if growth is ulcerative
- ◆ Rhinorrhoea
- ◆ Pain due to involvement of cranial nerves
- ◆ Diplopia due to spread to ophthalmic nerves
- ◆ Serous otitis media (SOM) and conductive deafness due to involvement of Eustachian tube usually unilateral initially and later bilateral. Unilateral SOM in an adult male should alert the surgeon to rule out nasopharyngeal tumour.
- ◆ Trismus due to pterygoid involvement
- ◆ Swelling in the neck on both sides may occasionally be a presenting feature

- • Signs
  - ◆ Bilateral enlarged metastatic lymphadenopathy in the posterior triangle of the neck.
  - ◆ Ophthalmic spread will result in opthalmoplegia and proptosis.
  - ◆ Intracranial spread will cause Horner's syndrome and paralysis of IXth, Xth and XIth cranial nerves.
  - ◆ Cranial nerve involvement results in paralysis of Vth, VIth, IXth and Xth nerves.
  - ◆ Trotter's triad:
    - • Pain on ipsilateral side of face.
    - • Ipsilateral palatal palsy.
    - • Ipsilateral conductive deafness.
    - • Posterior rhinoscopy reveals the tumour with an irregular surface and areas of slough and necrosis.

Diagnostic investigations

- • Posterior rhinoscopy will reveal the carcinoma with necrosis and slough.
- • Fibreoptic nasopharyngoscopy with biopsy.
- • Rigid nasopharyngoscopy using Yaunkaur's naso-pharyngoscope, not done nowadays due to the advent of the fibreoptic scope, as it requires general anaesthesia.
- • X-ray soft tissue nasopharynx may reveal a proli-ferative growth.
- • CT scan of nasopharynx and base skull with and without contrast medium, is most important in diagnosis and for detecting extent of tumour.
- • Obliteration of the fossa of Rosenmuller on CT scan is one of the first diagnostic features of Ca nasopharynx in the absence of other signs and symptoms.
- • Examination of the nasopharynx, under general anaesthesia with biopsy is diagnostic.

Treatment

- • Prognosis is very poor.
- • Radiotherapy is the treatment of choice. Surgery is not possible, since the tumour is at the base skull which is not easily accessible. Also, patients present late and with metastasis, making surgical treatment impossible.

  Radiotherapy: 5000–6000 rads over 5–6 weeks in the dose of 200 rads per day for 5 days a week. Neck metastases are also given in radiotherapy.
- • Chemotherapy is not preferred.

CHAPTER 36

Differential Diagnosis of Dysphagia

Dysphagia is defined as a difficulty in swallowing. It is a symptom and not a disease.

Odynophagia is defined as pain during swallowing.

Aetiology   It is shown in Flowchart 36.1

Flowchart 36.1: Aetiology of dysphagia

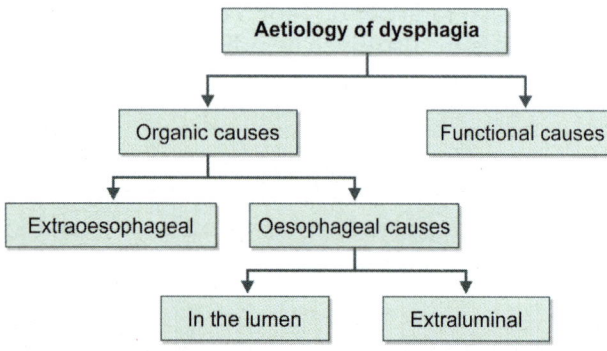

ORGANIC CAUSES

Extraoesophageal causes of dysphagia

- Pharyngeal tumours:
  - Carcinoma
  - Haemangioma
- Pharyngeal trauma: Scarring following scalding by corrosives or steam.
- Paralysis of the palate or pharynx
- Cleft palate
- Retropharyngeal or parapharyngeal abscess

- Quinsy
- Carcinoma of the supraglottic larynx
- Laryngeal oedema
- Trismus
- Ludwig's angina
- Nasal obstruction due to tumours, adenoids or nasal packing

Oesophageal Causes

Intraluminal causes (in the lumen and the wall):
- Congenital
  - Stricture
  - Web
  - Tracheo-oesophageal fistula
- Neoplastic
  - Carcinoma
  - Benign neoplasms such as a leiomyoma
- Infective
  - Oesophagitis
- Traumatic
  - Corrosive poisoning resulting in oesophagitis immediately and stricture formation later.
  - Iatrogenic trauma resulting in an oesophageal fistula or a tracheo-oesophageal fistula, e.g. following neck surgery like thyroidectomy, tracheostomy, etc.
- Neurological
  - Spasm of the cricopharyngeal sphincter
  - Paralysis of oesophagus

- ◆ Myasthenia gravis
- ◆ Tetanus
- Miscellaneous
  - ◆ Oesophageal diverticulum
  - ◆ Plummer—Vinson syndrome (Patterson–Brown Kelly syndrome)
  - ◆ Achalasia cardia
  - ◆ Hiatus hernia

Extraluminal pressure (outside the oesophagus causing dysphagia due to compression):
- Causes of pressure compression of the cervical oesophagus
  - ◆ Malignancy of the thyroid gland.
  - ◆ Pharyngeal pouch.
  - ◆ Cervical lymph node metastases.
  - ◆ Cervical spondylosis may cause dysphagia (cervical dysphagia) due to pressure on the oeso-phagus by osteophytes.
- Causes of pressure compression of the thoracic oesophagus
  - ◆ Retrosternal goitre.
  - ◆ Pressure due to an aberrant blood vessel running across the oesophagus (dysphagia lusoria).
  - ◆ Aortic aneurysm.
  - ◆ Mediastinal tumours (enlarged lymph nodes due to malignancy, Hodgkin's disease or tuberculosis).
  - ◆ Cardiomegaly or pericardial effusion.
- Causes of pressure compression of the abdominal oesophagus.
  - ◆ Hepatomegaly.

FUNCTIONAL CAUSES

- Globus hystericus

DIFFERENTIAL DIAGNOSIS OF ODYNOPHAGIA

- Stomatitis
- Glossitis
- Tonsillitis
- Pharyngitis
- Peritonsillitis
- Foreign body in the pharynx

History taking in a case of dysphagia
- Age: Certain diseases have a prediliction for a partic-ular age. For example:
  - ◆ Malignancy of the oesophagus is more common between the fourth to sixth decade of life.
  - ◆ Achalasia cardia affects patients between the age of 20–40 years.

- ◆ The Plummer–Vinson's syndrome is seen to occur in the fourth decade of life.
- Sex: The Plummer-Vinson's syndrome is seen commonly in females.
- Past history
  - ◆ History of ingestion of corrosive liquids should be asked.
  - ◆ History of ingestion of foreign body and type of foreign-body is asked.
  - ◆ History of anaemia is important in Plummer-Vinson's syndrome.
  - ◆ History of smoking or alcohol ingestion is important in malignancy.
  - ◆ History of poliomyelitis, diabetes, diphtheria, and tuberculosis is asked.
  - ◆ Patient with hysteria is prone to develop globus hystericus.

Examination of a patient of dysphagia   It includes the following:
- Symptoms
  - ◆ Acute dysphagia can occur due to foreign bodies or ingestion of corrosives.
  - ◆ Chronic, gradually progressive dysphagia is seen in malignancy of the oesophagus or a stricture.
  - ◆ Dysphagia to solids is common in malignancy.
  - ◆ Dysphagia to liquids is common in achalasia cardia.
  - ◆ Vertigo and hearing loss are common in cervical spondylosis.
  - ◆ Pain occurs in the presence of inflammation or on ingestion of corrosives. Epigastric burning occurs in reflux oesophagitis. Retrosteral pain or sharp pain radiating to the back between the shoulder blades occurs in oesophageal perforation.
  - ◆ Haematemesis occurs in trauma or infection or malignancy.
  - ◆ Cachexia is seen with malignancy and also with chronic dysphagia.
  - ◆ Regurgitation of food is seen in cardiospasm, pharyngeal diverticulum or malignancy.
- Signs
  - ◆ Associated glossitis or stomatitis.
  - ◆ Evidence of anaemia.
  - ◆ Evidence of psychiatric disturbances.
  - ◆ A detailed general, local and systemic examination should be performed to diagnose the cause of dysphagia.

Specific Investigations in a patient of dysphagia
- Haemoglobin: Hypochromic microcytic anaemia is seen in the Patterson-Brown-Kelly syndrome.

However, anaemia may be the result of chronic dysphagia.

- Complete blood count.
- Venereal disease research laboratory (VDRL) test: To rule out syphilis.
- Blood sugar: To rule out diabetes mellitus, which can affect the nerves and cause dysphagia.
- Radiological investigations
  - Barium swallow
  - X-ray chest to rule out opaque foreign bodies, mediastinal masses or cardiomegaly, etc.
- Neurological examination, if a neurogenic cause is suspected.
- Computed tomography (CT) scan of neck and thorax to detect a space occupying lesion.
- Pan endoscopy with biopsy: Direct laryngoscopy, oesophagoscopy, bronchoscopy, and nasopharyngoscopy.

Treatment
- Treat the cause, e.g. correction of anaemia in Plummer-Vinson syndrome, removal of foreign body, surgery for stricture, etc.
- Management of nutritional deficiency, which is seen in patients with chronic dysphagia.
- Ryle's tube feeds.
- Feeding gastrostomy, if passage of a ryle's tube is not possible to treat the chronic nutritional deficiency.

DIFFERENTIAL DIAGNOSIS OF DYSPHAGIA

Plummer Vinson syndrome
- Synonym: Patterson-Brown-Kelly syndrome
- Definition: It is a syndrome comprising of chronic and gradually progressive dysphagia to solids associated with a hypochromic microcytic anaemia.
- Aetiology
  - *Age*: It is common in the fourth decade of life.
  - *Sex*: It is common in females.
  - Nutritional deficiency, especially iron deficiency can result in this condition.
- Clinical features
  - Dysphagia
    - Gradually progressive.
    - More to solids than liquids initially.
  - Patient is usually a female aged 40 years or so.
  - Pallor due to an iron deficiency anaemia.
  - Angular stomatitis.
  - Glossitis.
  - Koilonychia (spoon-shaped nails).

- Splenomegaly.
- Presence of an oesophageal web in the region of the cricopharynx.
- Sequelae: Occasionally, this condition may progress to a postcricoid carcinoma. Hence, this condition is thought to be precancerous.
- Investigations
  - *Haemogram*: Hypochromic microcytic (iron deficiency), anaemia is present.
  - Barium swallow shows the characteristic feature of a cricopharyngeal web.
  - Oesophagoscopy confirms presence of a web and helps to take a biopsy and if malignant change is suspected.
  - On gastric analysis, achlorhydria is detected.
- Treatment
  - Iron and folic acid orally.
  - Vitamin supplements.
  - Dialatation of the web using oesophagoscopy, if dysphagia is severe.
  - Regular follow-up to rule out a malignant change.
- Dysphagia lusoria: An aberrant blood vessel in the mediastinum, may form a loop around the thoracic oesophagus resulting in compression and a resultant dysphagia. The vascular anomalies can be any of the following:
  - Right aortic arch.
  - Double aortic arch.
  - Aberrant right subclavian artery.
  - Anomalous innominate artery.
  - Patent ductus arteriosus.
- Diagnosis is by aortography and magnetic resonance imaging (MRI).
- Treatment is by cardiovascular thoracic surgery.

Achalasia cardia
- Synonym: Cardiospasm.
- Definition: It is a condition characterised by a failure of relaxation of the lower oesophageal sphincter during deglutition.
- Aetiology: The exact aetiology is not known. Factors implicated include:
  - Degeneration of Auerbach's plexus
  - Abnormal pinchcock mechanism of the right crus of the diaphragm.
  - Ischaemia during rotation of the gut in utero.
  - Chaga's disease (trypanosomiasis).
  The lower third of the oesophagus, shows a marked elongation, tortuosity and dialatation.
- Pathology: Pathology is shown in Flowchart 36.2.

Flowchart 36.2: Pathology of achalasia cardia

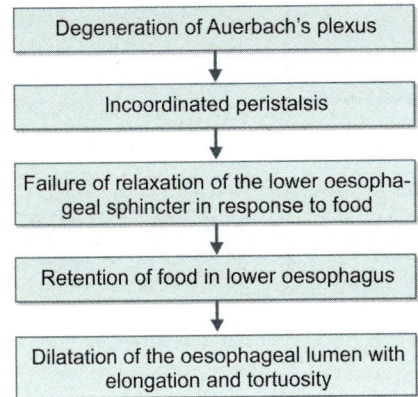

- Degeneration of Auerbach's plexus
- Incoordinated peristalsis
- Failure of relaxation of the lower oesophageal sphincter in response to food
- Retention of food in lower oesophagus
- Dilatation of the oesophageal lumen with elongation and tortuosity

- **Clinical features**
  - *Age:* It is common in young adults.
  - *Sex:* It affects both sexes equally.
  - Progressive dysphagia more to liquids than solids.
  - Epigastric discomfort or burning.
  - Regurgitation of undigested food.
  - Aspiration may cause pulmonary complications.
  - Sometimes, there may be some weight-loss.
- **Investigations**
  - *Barium swallow is diagnostic:* A characteristic fusiform smooth dilatation of the lower oesophagus is seen with a fluid level and particles of food stagnant. The gastric gas-shadow is absent.
  - *On oesophagoscopy:* A sudden smooth dialatation is seen in the lower oesophagus with the presence of undigested food.
- **Sequelae:** This is a premalignant condition and pre-disposes to malignancy of the oesophagus.
- **Treatment**
  - Anti-cholinergic drugs orally before meals help the sphincter to relax, e.g., amyl nitrate tablets.
  - Oesophagoscopic dialatation of the sphincter using bougies.
  - Patients can also perform the dialatation themselves using Hurst mercury bougies.
  - Surgical relaxation of the sphincter by a cardiomyotomy (Heller's operation).

Anatomy of the Larynx

DEVELOPMENT

Develops from the tracheobronchial groove, which is a ventral midline diverticulum of the foregut. The thyroid, cricoid, and arytenoid cartilages are derivatives of the 4th, 5th, and 6th arches respectively.

ANATOMY

Situation   Midline of neck. Anterior to the third to sixth cervical vertebrae (C3 to C6).

Constitution   Formed by a cartilagenous skeleton held together by ligaments. It is moved by muscles and lined by mucous membrane.

CARTILAGENOUS SKELETON

Cartilagenous skeleton (Fig. 37.1) of larynx comprises of:
- Paired cartilages
- Unpaired cartilages

Paired cartilages
- Arytenoid cartilages
- Corniculate cartilages
- Cuneiform cartilages

Unpaired cartilages
- Epiglottis
- Thyroid cartilage
- Cricoid cartilage
- Thyroid cartilage
  - Largest
  - Hyaline in nature

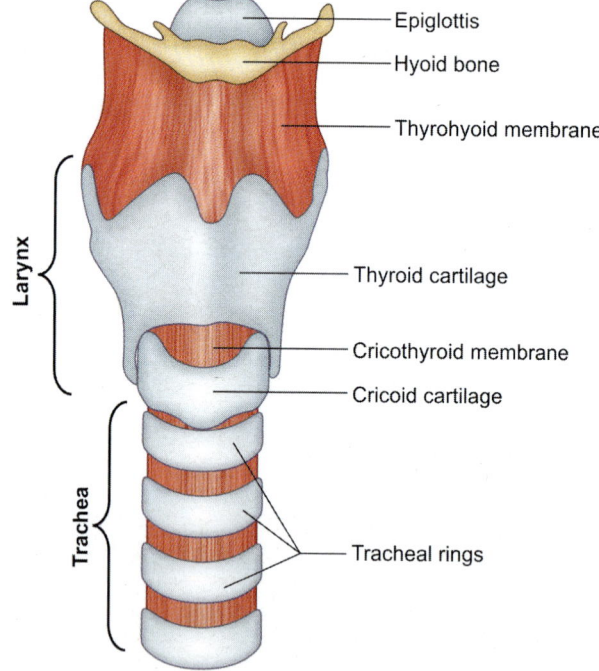

Fig. 37.1 : Diagrammatic representation of the larynx

- It consists of two flattened quadrangular alae, which are fused in the midline to form an angle of:
  - 90° in males,
  - 120° in females.

    In males, the fused anterior border projects in the midline, more prominently, seen subcutaneously as 'The laryngeal prominence' or 'The Adam's apple'.

- A 'V' shaped 'thyroid notch' is present above the laryngeal prominence.
- Two prominences, 'The superior and inferior cornua' project from the posterior border of each alae.

- Cricoid cartilage
  - It lies below the thyroid cartilage
  - 'Signet-ring' shaped
  - It is the only complete cartilagenous ring in the larynx
  - It consists of:
    - A narrow anterior arch
    - A posterior quadrate lamina
      The superolateral aspect of the posterior quadrate lamina articulates with the base of the arytenoid cartilage. Also, there is a prominent articular facet present at the junction of the arch with the lamina for articulation with the inferior cornua of thyroid cartilage.
  - Its internal surface is lined by mucous membrane
  - It is a hyaline cartilage with variable ossification

- Arytenoid cartilage
  - It is pyramidal in shape
  - It articulates with the upper and lateral border of the cricoid lamina
  - It has:
    - Three surfaces
      - Medial surface
      - Anterolateral surface
      - Posterior surface
    - Base
    - An apex
      The base has an anterior projection, called the vocal process, which gives attachment to vocal ligament. It also has a lateral projection called the muscular process, which gives attachment to the various muscles.

- Corniculate cartilage/Cartilage of Wrisberg
  - It is a fibroelastic cartilage
  - It is conical in shape
- Cuneiform cartilage/Cartilage of Santorini
  - Very small club-shaped cartilage
  - It is present in the free margins of the aryepiglottic folds
- Epiglottis/Epiglottic cartilage
  - It is a fibroelastic cartilage, it never ossifies
  - It is slightly curved, flattened, and leaf-like in shape

- It consists of:
  - Two ends
    - Free upper end
    - Long distal end/petiole
  - Two surfaces
    - Anterior surface
    - Posterior surface
  - *Two sides:* On which the aryepiglottic fold is present.
    A number of dehiscences are present in the cartilage, which provide an important pathway for the spread of cancer to the preepiglottic space.

LARYNGEAL ARTICULATIONS

- Cricothyroid joint (synovial joint)
- Cricoarytenoid joint (synovial joint)

MUSCLES OF THE LARYNX

- Extrinsic
- Intrinsic

Extrinsic muscles of larynx
- Elevation of larynx during deglutition and phonation
  - Anterior and posterior digastric
  - Mylohyoid
- Depress and fix the larynx
  - Thyrohyoid
  - Sternohyoid
  - Omohyoid
- Relaxation of cricopharyngeal sphincter
  - Cricopharyngeus
  - Middle and inferior constrictor

Intrinsic muscles of the larynx
All the intrinsic muscles of the larynx, are paired except the transverse arytenoid muscle.
- Adductors of vocal cords
  - Lateral cricoarytenoid—main adductor
  - Transverse arytenoids
  - Cricothyroids
  - Thyroarytenoids
- Abductors of vocal cords
  - Posterior cricoarytenoid muscle
- Tensors of the vocal cords
  - Cricothyroid muscle
- Relaxes the vocal cord
  - Thyroarytenoid
  - Vocalis
- Opens the laryngeal inlet
  - Thyroepiglottis

- Closes the laryngeal inlet
  - Oblique arytenoids
  - Aryepiglottis

LARYNGEAL MEMBRANES

- Conus elasticus
- Quadrangular membrane
- Thyrohyoid membrane
- Mucous membrane

Conus elasticus

- It extends from lower border of thyroid cartilage to cricoid cartilage
- Its free upper border is thickened and forms the vocal ligament.

Quadrangular membrane

It is attached from the sides of the epiglottis to the vocal process/corniculate cartilage.

Thyrohyoid membrane

- It is attached from hyoid bone above to thyroid cartilage
- It is pierced by superior laryngeal nerves and vessels

Mucous membrane   Two folds of mucous membrane are present:

- False vocal cords are formed by ventricular ligament/vestibular fold of mucous membrane
- True vocal cords are formed by vocal ligament/vocal fold of mucous membrane

LINING OF THE LARYNX

Stratified squamous epithelium   It is present on:

- Vocal cords
- Epiglottis, upper part
- Aryepiglottic folds

Pseudostratified ciliated columnar epithelium lines the rest of the larynx.

CAVITY OF THE LARYNX

Cavity of larynx consists of the following three parts:

Vestibule

- It is the upper portion
- It lies between laryngeal inlet and vestibular folds (false vocal cords)
- The laryngeal inlet is bounded:
  - Anteriorly by free border of epiglottis
  - Laterally by aryepiglottic folds
  - Posteriorly by corniculate cartilage and upper part of arytenoid muscles

Ventricle

- It is the middle part.
- It lies between true and false vocal cords.
- Rima glottidis is a slit between the margins of the vocal cords.

Subglottic part

- It is the lower portion.
- It lies between the true vocal cords and the lower border of the cricoid cartilage.

ANATOMIC DIVISIONS OF LARYNX

Digrammatic view of anatomic divisions of larynx is shown in Fig. 37.2. These divisions are:

- Supraglottis
- Glottis
- Subglottis

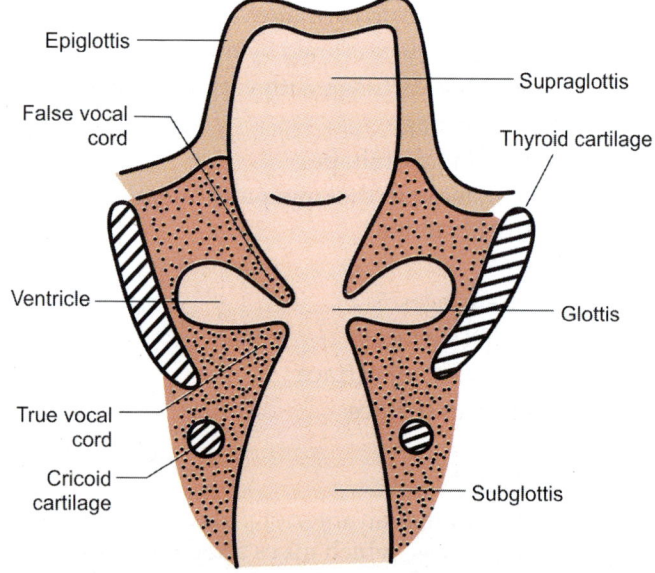

Fig. 37.2 : Coronal section of larynx (diagrammatic)

BLOOD SUPPLY

The larynx is divided at the level of the glottis into two segments by an imaginary line.

- Superior segment
- Inferior segment

Arterial supply

- Superior segment: Superior laryngeal artery (branch of superior thyroid artery).
- Inferior segment: Inferior laryngeal artery (branch of inferior thyroid artery).

Venous drainage

- **Superior segment:** It drains into superior laryngeal vein which drains into superior thyroid vein and then into internal jugular vein.
- **Inferior segment:** It drains into inferior thyroid vein, then into left brachiocephalic vein.

NERVE SUPPLY OF LARYNX

Supplied by branches of the vagus nerve (Xth cranial nerve).

Sensory supply

- Above the vocal cords/superior segment: Superior laryngeal nerve.
- Below the vocal cords/inferior segment: Recurrent laryngeal nerve.

Motor supply

All intrinsic muscles of the larynx are supplied by the recurrent laryngeal nerve except for the cricothyroid muscle. This muscle is supplied by external laryngeal nerve (branch of superior laryngeal nerve).

LYMPHATIC DRAINAGE

Supraglottic portion

- Pre-epiglottic lymph nodes.
- Upper deep cervical lymph nodes.

Glottis

Scanty lymphatic drainage, hence, spread of vocal cord cancer to regional lymph nodes is very late.

Subglottic portion

- Prelaryngeal lymph nodes.
- Pretracheal lymph nodes.
- Lower deep cervical lymph nodes.

DIFFERENCES OF LARYNX OF AN INFANT AND AN ADULT

The differences between the larynx of an infant and an adult are given in the Table 37.1.

TABLE 37.1: Differences in larynx of an infant and an adult	
Infant	*Adult*
• Situated high up.	• Situated opposite C3–C6
• Size: Equal in both sexes.	• Males: Larger in size than females.
• Laryngeal cartilages: Softer.	• Laryngeal cartilages: More rigid.
• Narrowest portion is the supra-glottis (larynx is funnel shaped).	• Glottis is the narrowest part.
• Epiglottis: Narrow and folded.	• Epiglottis: Leaf-like.
• Submucous space: More space, therefore, more chances of developing oedema secondary to infections.	• Less submucous space.

Physiology of the Larynx

Physiology of larynx include:
- Functions of the larynx
- Physiology of phonation

- Oropharynx and oral cavity with nose and paranasal sinuses (PNS) = Articulators → Quality of voice

FUNCTIONS OF THE LARYNX

Respiration and airflow regulation The larynx forms an important part of the upper respiratory tract and it regulates air flowing through the respiratory tract by movements of the vocal cords.

Protection The larynx prevents entry of foreign bodies into the lower respiratory tract by a reflex cough mechanism.

Sphincteric action During swallowing and vomitting, the glottis closes by its sphincteric mechanism.

Fixation of the thorax The larynx helps to fix the thorax for strenuous work, such as lifting heavy weights, climbing, childbirth, straining during defecation, etc.

Circulatory function The larynx helps in promoting venous return to heart.

Phonation and speech The glottis plays an important role in phonation and speech.

Production of Speech
- Lungs = Reservoir of air → Intensity of voice
- Vocal cords = Phonaters → Pitch of voice (number of vibrations per second)

PHYSIOLOGY OF PHONATION

Physiology of phonation is shown in Flowchart 38.1.

Flowchart 38.1: Physiology of phonation

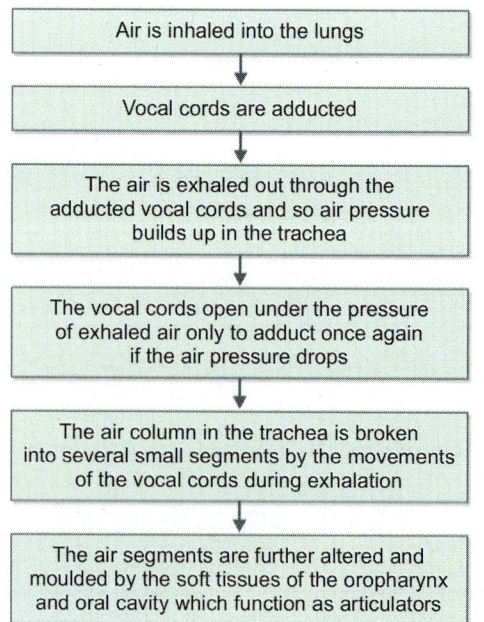

Air is inhaled into the lungs

Vocal cords are adducted

The air is exhaled out through the adducted vocal cords and so air pressure builds up in the trachea

The vocal cords open under the pressure of exhaled air only to adduct once again if the air pressure drops

The air column in the trachea is broken into several small segments by the movements of the vocal cords during exhalation

The air segments are further altered and moulded by the soft tissues of the oropharynx and oral cavity which function as articulators

Larynx

CHAPTER 39

Examination of the Larynx

The examination of larynx include:

(A) History taking

(B) Examination
- External examination
- Laryngoscopy:
  - Indirect
  - Direct
  - Microlaryngoscopy
  - Fibreoptic laryngoscopy
- Radiology

HISTORY TAKING

Following are the important symptoms of laryngeal disease:

Hoarseness of voice (roughness of voice)   This is the commonest disorder resulting from disease of the larynx. Profession of the person is important as chronic laryngitis and vocal cord nodules may be due to abuse of voice. Age of the patient is important, as hoarse voice or hoarse cry, since childhood suggests congenital pathology. Hoarseness below fourth decade is generally of inflammatory etiology and hoarseness over fifth decade suggests malignancy.

Altered voice production   These consist of alterations of strength, pitch, tone, and quality.

Dysphagia   Difficulty or obstruction in swallowing may be a feature of laryngopharyngeal and/or oesophageal disorder. Dysphagia occurs in laryngeal disorders when the extrinsic portion of the larynx is involved.

Pain   It may occur due to injury, infection or malignancy. Pain of laryngeal origin may be referred to the ear.

Stridor (noisy breathing)   Stridor occurs due to some obstructive pathology in the larynx. Stridor of laryngeal origin is of inspiratory type and must be carefully differentiated from the expiratory dyspnoea seen in lower respiratory tract pathology.

Inspiratory stridor	Expiratory dyspnoea
• Inspiration is prolonged.	• Expiration is prolonged.
• Pathology is in upper respiratory tract.	• Pathology is in lower respiratory tract.

Sudden onset of difficulty in breathing may indicate laryngeal edema, foreign body, etc. Progressive difficulty in breathing suggests neoplasm.

Cough   Irritating cough with expectoration is seen in laryngeal disorders. Foul smelling, purulent, blood-strained sputum is seen in malignancy.

Foreign body sensation in throat and constant clearing of the throat (hawking)   This may be seen in early malignancy and vocal cord polyps. Such conditions should be suspected, when this is associated with hoarse voice.

Swellings in neck   It may be caused by lymph node enlargement, perichondritis, and tumour.

Relevant Past and Personal History

Enquiry about:
- Smoking
- Tobacco chewing
- Voice abuse: Voice abuse is seen in teachers, hawkers, and singers. Enquiry should be made, if the environment of residence and work is noisy and also about the presence of deaf relative in the house, as this usually requires the patient to talk loudly.
- History of tuberculosis
- History of syphilis

GENERAL EXAMINATION

- Cachexic patient suggests presence of tuberculosis, malignancy, or chronic dysphagia.
- Presence of neck nodes suggests tuberculosis (matted nodes) or malignancy (hard nodes).

LOCAL EXAMINATION

External examination

- Inspection: It may reveal the presence of a mass or fullness in the neck. Laryngeal framework may be distorted in certain tumours and inflammatory conditions.

  When there is laryngeal obstruction, larynx tends to move downwards during inspiration due to inspiratory dyspnoea, but with tracheal obstruction such movements do not occur.

- Palpation: The examiner should stand behind the patient who should remain comfortably seated with the head slightly flexed, so as to relax the neck muscles. Examination of the neck should be done methodically and it is best to examine it in triangles.

  The examiner should look for palpable lymphnodes, position of trachea, laryngeal crepitus, and evidence of perichondritis.

Laryngoscopy

- Indirect laryngoscopy: This is an OPD procedure. It is a very important diagnostic procedure. The procedure is called as 'indirect' as the larynx and hypopharynx are visualised indirectly through a plane mirror, illuminated by a reflected ray of light.
  - *Instruments required*
    - Light source
    - Indirect laryngoscopy (IDL) mirror
  - *Position of patient and examiner*: Both, the patient and the examiner are in sitting position, facing each other.

- *Procedure*: This is shown in Fig. 39.1 (digrammatic) and Fig. 39.2 (clinical).
  - Patient is explained about the procedure.
  - Indirect laryngoscopy mirror is warmed with hot water or a flame to prevent fogging (due to condensation of water vapour during expiration of the patient).
  - The warmth of the mirror is tested by touching the back of the mirror to the examiner's hand. It is very reassuring to the patient, as he will know that the hot mirror will not burn his mouth.

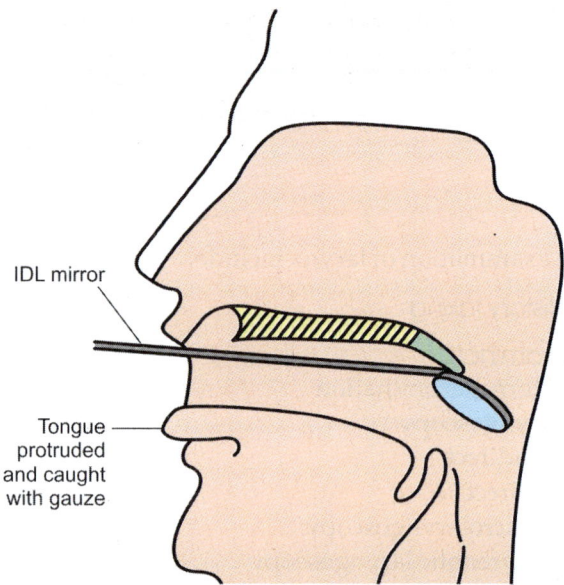

IDL mirror

Tongue protruded and caught with gauze

Fig. 39.1 : Indirect laryngoscopy (diaphragmmatic)

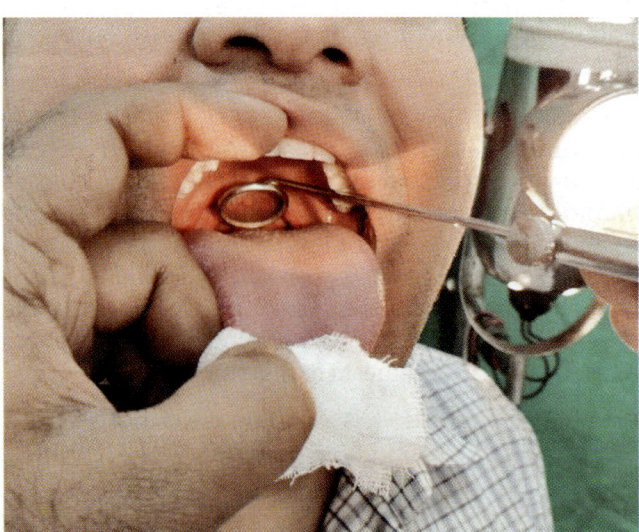

Fig. 39.2 : Indirect laryngoscopy (clinical)

- Patient is asked to swallow saliva and make his/her mouth dry.
- Patient is asked to open his/her mouth and protrude his/her tongue. The tongue is held lightly with a piece of gauze with the left hand of the examiner between the middle finger and thumb. The index finger retracts the upper jaw.
- Patient is asked to breathe quietly through his mouth. This helps as the soft palate moves up during mouth-breathing and hence more area is available for mirror placement.
- The warmed mirror is held in a pen-like fashion in the right hand and gently introduced into the mouth, taking care that it is not soiled by saliva.
- With the mirror facing downwards, it is gently placed against the soft palate and uvula, and these structures are gently elevated, bringing into view the larynx.
- Movement of the cords during phonation may be seen by asking the patient to say 'ee'.

- *Structures seen on indirect laryngoscopy:* The structures seen on IDL are shown in Fig. 39.3 and are listed as follows:
  - Base of tongue
  - Vallecula
  - Lingual (anterior) aspect of epiglottis
  - Arytenoids
  - Aryepiglottic folds
  - Vestibular folds or false cords
  - Anterior commissure (sometimes)
  - Posterior commissure
  - True vocal cords and rima glottidis

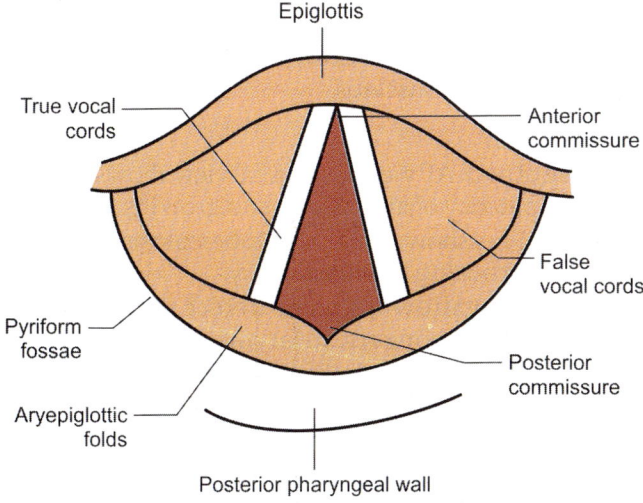

Labels: Epiglottis; True vocal cords; Anterior commissure; False vocal cords; Pyriform fossae; Posterior commissure; Aryepiglottic folds; Posterior pharyngeal wall

Fig. 39.3 : Structures seen on IDL

- Subglottis and few rings of trachea
- Pyriform fossa

- *Therapeutic indications of IDL*
  - Removal of embedded foreign body (fish bone) from posterior one-third of tongue, vallecula, and pyriform fossa.
  - To take biopsy from tumours or pathology in the hypopharynx and larynx.

- *Difficulties encountered in IDL*
  - *Uncooperative patients:* Some apprehensive patients and children may not cooperate for the examination. It is not possible in mentally retarded patients.
  - *Sensitive throat:* This may be overcome with application of 4% lignocaine spray in the throat.
  - *Anatomical problems:* Overhanging epiglottis may obstruct the view of larynx.
  - In *obese patients with short neck,* indirect laryngoscopy is very difficult.
  - *Hidden areas:* Anterior commissure, ventricle and subglottic area may not be properly visualised.

- Direct laryngoscopy: In the procedure of disect laryngoscopy (DLS), the larynx is visualised directly under general anaesthesia using a rigid direct laryngoscope. It differs from indirect laryngoscopy:
  - *Indications of direct laryngoscopy*
    - *Diagnostic*
      - When indirect laryngoscopy fails or is inadequate to make the diagnosis.
      - For taking biopsy
      - As a part of panendoscopy
    - *Therapeutic*
      - For removal of vocal cord nodule, polyps and foreign body from larynx.
      - Direct laryngoscopy is performed before doing a bronchoscopy and oesophago-scopy especially in children.
  - *Contraindications of direct laryngoscopy.*
    - *Laryngospasm and stridor:* In such conditions it is advisable to perform tracheostomy first and then follow it up with direct laryngoscopy.
    - Trismus or ankylosis of the temporomandibular joint.
    - Diseases of cervical vertebra may make this process hazardous as there are chances of dislocation leading to quadriplagia.
    - General contraindications like hypertension, cardiac abnormalities, diabetes etc. should be properly brought under control preoperatively.

◆ *Position of patient:*
- Patient is in supine position with extension of head. A pillow is placed under the shoulders.
- The examiner stands at the head end of the table.

◆ *Anaesthesia for dissect laryngoscopy:* General anaesthesia with endotracheal intubation is required for this procedure.

◆ *Steps of dissect laryngoscopy:*
- Patient is supine under general anaesthesia.
- Examiner stands at the head end.
- The upper teeth are protected with a gauze piece.
- Laryngoscope is held in right hand and is gently introduced taking care not to injure the lips and structures of oral cavity.
- The following structures are visualised, as the direct laryngoscope is gradually introduced:
  - Tonsillar pillars and tonsils
  - Soft palate
  - Base of the tongue
  - Posterior pharyngeal wall
  - Valleculae
  - Pyriform fossae
  - Epiglottis
- On reaching the epiglottis, *the epiglottis is elevated using the tip of the direct laryngoscope* and the following are visualised:
  - True vocal cords
  - False vocal cords
  - Anterior commissure
  - Posterior commissure
- After visualising all these structures, the direct laryngoscope is gently withdrawn and removed.
- Unlike the microlaryngoscope, which is introduced, so as to abut against the true vocal cords, *the direct laryngoscope is introduced only upto the epiglottis* to visualise the supraglottis and glottis.

◆ *Complications of direct laryngoscope*
- Trauma to lips, gum, teeth, and tongue.
- Damage to cervical spine.
- Laryngospasm and stridor may be precipitated.
- Improper or inadequate surgery due to non-availability of sufficient time.
- Anaesthetic complications like respiratory and cardiac arrest due to vagal stimulation.

- Differences between indirect and direct laryngoscopy: *See* Table 39.1

TABLE 39.1: Differences between indirect laryngoscopy and direct laryngoscopy

Indirect laryngoscopy	Direct laryngoscopy
Mirror is used for visualisation.	Direct visualisation
Inverted image seen.	True image seen.
2D image is seen on mirror.	3D visualisation is possible.
Vocal cord movements are seen better.	Not seen as patient is under general anaesthesia.
OPD procedure.	OT procedure.
Visualisation of anterior commissure, ventricle and subglottic area is not good.	Good visualisation of entire larynx is possible.
Overhanging epiglottis is a problem.	No such problem is faced.

- **Microlaryngoscopy:** This is a procedure, which is a refinement of direct laryngoscopy. It differs from direct laryngoscopy in several aspects.
  ◆ Examiner gets adequate time to perform the procedure.
  ◆ The microlaryngoscope is introduced, so as to *just abut against the true vocal cords.*
  ◆ Laryngoscope is self-retaining and can be fixed with a chest-piece. Hence, both the hands of the surgeon are free.
  ◆ Magnification is achieved by using an operating microscope with a 400 mm objective lens.
  ◆ Photography and video recording can be done.
  ◆ Teaching can be done by attaching a side-tube or a TV monitor to the operating microscope.
  ◆ Laser surgery can be performed.
- **Fibre-optic laryngoscopy:** This has been a recent development. A flexible fibreoptic laryngoscope is passed through the nose to the larynx via the nasopharynx. It is an OPD procedure and the movements of the vocal cords can be visualised as the patient is conscious.

Radiography
- X-ray of neck AP view and lateral view shows foreign body, patency of air passage and growths.
- Chest X-ray shows associated tuberculosis or masses in lungs causing laryngeal palsy.
- Barium swallow helps to detect carcinoma of oesophagus giving rise to laryngeal palsy.
- Tomograms demonstrate extent of tumours.
- Cine radiography.
- Contrast laryngography.
- Computed tamography (CT) scan.

Infections of the Larynx

Synonym   Laryngitis

Definition   It is defined as an inflammation of the larynx.

Classification   It is shown in Flowchart 40.1.

Flowchart 40.1: Classification of laryngitis

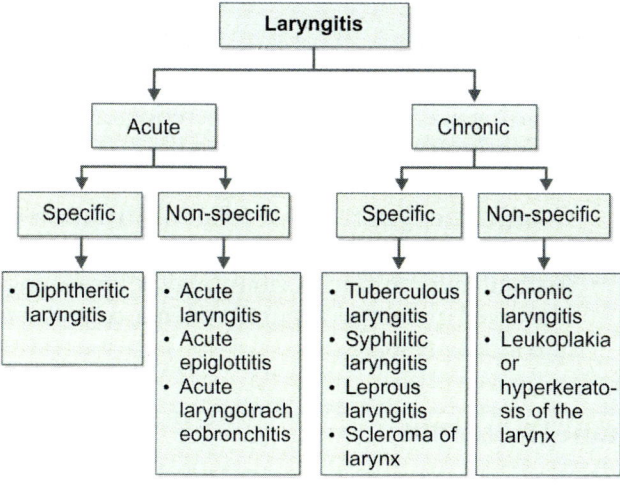

DIPHTHERITIC LARYNGITIS

Synonym   Laryngeal diphtheria.

Definition   Diphtheritic laryngitis is an infection of the larynx, usually secondary to faucial diphtheria.

Causative organism   *Corynebacterium diphtheriae.*

Pathogenesis   It is characterised by the presence of a greyish-white membrane formed over the tonsils, valleculae, and laryngeal inlet. If it gets detached, it can result in laryngospasm or even laryngeal obstruction with fatal consequences.

Clinical features
- Symptoms
    - Patient appears toxic
    - Low grade fever, tachycardia, and weak pulse
    - Hoarse croupy cough
    - Hoarseness of voice
    - Dyspnoea
- Signs:
    - Stridor—inspiratory
    - Greyish-white membrane is present on the tonsils and may be seen to extend on the vallecula and epiglottis. Indirect laryngoscopy will show a membrane on the vocal cords. Removal of this membrane will result in bleeding.

Differential diagnosis
- Acute laryngitis
- Acute laryngotracheobronchitis
- Foreign body in the larynx
- Tracheobronchial foreign body
- Laryngismus stridulus
- Multiple laryngeal papillomas (laryngeal papillomatosis)
- Allergic laryngitis

Investigations   Laryngeal swab showing presence of *C. diphtheriae* in smear and culture is diagnostic.

Treatment

- Tracheostomy is performed for relief of stridor and to prevent aspiration. Endotracheal intubation is preferably avoided, as it can push the membrane or its fragments into the lower respiratory tract.
- Oxygen is administered.
- Intravenous (IV) fluids for nutrition.
- Antitoxin is administered after a test dose, 40,000–1,00,000 units of injection anti-diphtheria serum (ADS) in a single dose.
- Injectable antibiotics: Penicillin in high doses. If patient is sensitive to penicillin; erythromycin is used.
- Steroids are used undercover of antibiotics to reduce laryngeal oedema.
- Other relatives in contact with the patient are immunised.

ACUTE NON-SPECIFIC LARYNGITIS

Synonym   Acute simple laryngitis

Definition   Acute non-specific laryngitis is acute superficial non-specific inflammation of the laryngeal mucosa.

Aetiology

- Age: It can occur at all ages, but it becomes life-threatening in children, since they have a small glottic inlet, which is easily blocked by oedema or membrane; their larynx is more excitable and goes into spasm easily and their cough reflex is weak, so aspiration occurs more easily than in adults.
- It may occur due to spread of tonsillitis, sinusitis, or bronchitis.
- It commonly occurs due to viral infections, like common cold. It may occur due to bacterial infection in some cases.
- Smoking and alcohol predispose to laryngitis.
- Overuse or misuse of voice can cause laryngitis.
- Changes in the climate or sudden exposure to cold can cause laryngitis.
- Inhalation of irritant fumes.
- Exanthemata or immunodeficiency predispose to laryngitis.
- Iatrogenic causes of laryngitis include prolonged intubation and endolaryngeal surgery.

Clinical features

- Symptoms
  - Hoarseness of voice
  - Aphonia

- Raw feeling or irritation in the throat
- Pain
- Irritating dry cough
- Dyspnoea and stridor
- Fever and malaise
- Signs: Indirect laryngoscopy will reveal features of acute laryngitis:
  - Oedema of the epiglottis and vocal cords
  - Congested and red vocal cords
  - Sluggish/Poor movements of the vocal cords
  - Presence of whitish plaques on the vocal cords:
    - 'Fibrinous laryngitis'
  - Presence of sticky and mucoid secretions on the larynx, which may become purulent.
    - 'Septic laryngitis'

Treatment   The patient should preferably be hospitalised and given bed rest.

- General treatment
  - Intravenous antibiotics
  - Intravenous fluids to maintain nutrition
  - Anti-inflammatory analgesics
  - Steroids under antibiotic cover
  - Syrup linctus codeine to reduce the irritant cough
  - Soft bland diet
  - Stop smoking and alcohol
- Local treatment:
  - Voice rest
  - Tincture benzoin steam inhalation as a local soothing agent and to loosen secretions. Menthol or Eucalyptus oil can also be used.
  - Hot fomentation of the neck
  - Cough lozenges for local relief of irritation in throat
  - In small children, tracheostomy may be life-saving. However, it is temporary until oedema, congestion and stridor resolve.

ACUTE EPIGLOTTITIS

Definition   Acute epiglottitis is a condition characterised by acute inflammation of the epiglottis.

Aetiology   Same as that of acute laryngitis.

Clinical features:

- Change of voice: 'Hot potato' speech or muffled speech.
- Dyspnoea and stridor
- Odynophagia
- Pain in the throat

- Indirect laryngoscopy reveals congestion and oedema of the epiglottis. However, it is done with caution, since it can cause reflex laryngeal spasm and apnoea.

Investigations   X-ray soft tissue of the neck, lateral view reveals a swollen and enlarged epiglottis, 'Thumb sign' is characteristic of acute epiglottitis.

Treatment   Admission and bed-rest is of primary importance.
- Intravenous antibiotics
- Anti-inflammatory analgesics
- Voice rest
- Steroids
- Steam inhalation using tincture benzoin, menthol or eucalyptus oil for soothing effect.
- Rarely, in severe cases, a tracheostomy is required temporarily for relief of respiratory distress.

ACUTE LARYNGOTRACHEOBRONCHITIS

Definition   Acute laryngotracheobronchitis is an acute inflammation of the mucosa of the respiratory tract.

Aetiology
- Age: It is common in infants and children.
- Immunocompromised patients are predisposed.
- Causative organism is usually *Streptococcus haemolyticus* or *Haemophilus influenzae* and occasionally, a virus.
- Debilitating illness predisposes

Pathogenesis   The entire respiratory tract mucosa is inflamed and congested. There are sticky secretions in the mucosa and these form crusts resulting in respiratory obstruction especially in the subglottis.

Clinical features
- Symptoms
  - High grade fever
  - Malaise
  - Severe toxaemia
  - Croupy cough
  - Hoarseness of voice
  - Dyspnoea and stridor
- Signs
  - Expiratory stridor
  - Rales and ronchi in the chest on auscultation
  - Indirect laryngoscopy shows congested and oedematous laryngeal mucosa with tenacious secretions and crusts in the glottis and subglottis.

Treatment   Admission to hospital and bed rest.
- General
  - Intravenous antibiotics.
  - Anti-inflammatory analgesics.
  - Oxygen.
  - Steroids.
  - Intravenous fluids.
- Local
  - Steam inhalation with menthol or tincture benzoin for loosening crusts and liquifying secretions.
  - Fibreoptic or Rigid bronchoscopy for tracheobronchial toilet.
  - Rarely, tracheostomy for relief from respiratory distress and for tracheobronchial toilet.

TUBERCULOUS LARYNGITIS

Definition   Tuberculous laryngitis is an infection of the larynx by pulmonary tuberculosis.

Aetiology
- Age: Common in the age group of 20–40 years.
- Secondary to pulmonary tuberculosis: This is the commonest cause of laryngeal tuberculosis and occurs due to stasis of sputum after bouts of coughing.
- Infection may also reach the larynx from other sites in the body via the lymphatics or bloodstream.
- As a part of generalised miliary tuberculosis, however, this is rare.

Pathogenesis

Flowchart 40.2: Steps of pathogenesis

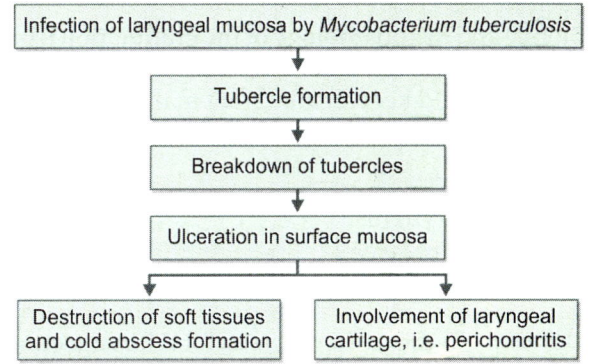

The commonest site of involvement is the posterior commissure, as maximum stagnation of infected sputum occurs at this site.

Clinical features
- Symptoms
  - Hoarseness of voice
  - Intermittent weakness of voice and aphonia
  - Cough with expectoration

- History of pulmonary tuberculosis.
- Fever, malaise and anorexia
- Odynophagia and dysphagia
- Referred otalgia
- Signs
  - Dyspnoea
  - Inspiratory stridor
  - Indirect laryngoscopy shows:
    - Sluggish movements of the vocal cords or even vocal cord palsy due to local involvement of muscle, recurrent laryngeal nerve palsy or fixation of cricoarytenoid joint due to infection.
    - Pale vocal cords with tubercles on them, especially in the posterior one-third part.
    - Presence of irregular heaped up granulation in the interarytenoid region—granuloma formation which may be misdiagnosed as malignancy.
    - Shallow irregular ulceration on the free margins of the posterior one-third of the vocal cords extending to the interarytenoid region giving it a characteristic 'mouse-nibbled' appearance.
    - Oedema of false cords
    - Perichondritis (pseudo-oedematous appearance), swelling of arytenoids and epiglottis.
    - Tissue necrosis with cold abscess formation is seen in late stages of the disease.

Investigations
- X-ray chest shows pulmonary tuberculosis.
- Sputum examination shows presence of acid-fast bacilli.
- Biopsy and histopathology of the granulation tissue confirms the diagnosis.
  One should keep in mind that malignancy of the larynx and tuberculosis are known to coexist.

Differential diagnosis
- Syphilitic laryngitis.
- Malignancy of larynx.
- Non-specific chronic laryngitis.

Treatment
In the earlier days, a total laryngectomy was performed for laryngeal tuberculosis as anti-Koch's therapy was not very well known and usually patients used to come in the advanced stage of the disease. Today, this condition is not very common and the treatment is conservative.
- Anti-tuberculous drug therapy for 12–14 months.
- Voice rest.
- Steam inhalation for soothing effect.
- Analgesics and anti-inflammatory agents.

- Rarely, a tracheostomy is required for relief of respiratory distress.
- In case of cartilage necrosis, arytenoidectomy or laryngectomy may be required.

SYPHILITIC LARYNGITIS

Definition   Syphilitic laryngitis is an infection of the larynx by *Treponema pallidum*.

Congenital syphilis   It is very rare and rarely affects the larynx.

Acquired syphilis
- Secondary syphilis is rare and may be seen as a serpinginous ulcer on the epiglottis and arytenoids.
- Tertiary syphilis is seen to affect the larynx in the form of a gumma. It commonly affects the anterior commissure, anterior one-third of vocal cords and epiglottis.

Tertiary syphilis
- Clinical features
  - *Symptoms*
    - Hoarseness of voice—presenting symptom.
    - Dyspnoea.
    - Inspiratory stridor.
  - *Signs:* Indirect laryngoscopy will reveal the following:
    - The entire larynx may show diffuse hypertrophy of mucosa.
    - A gummatous ulcer may be seen in the anterior aspect of the glottis or on the epiglottis, a deep ulcer with wash-leather slough.
    - Perichondritis, scarring, and stenosis are seen later.
- Investigations
  - Venereal disease research laboratory (VDRL) test.
  - Biopsy with histopathology.
- Treatment
  - Antisyphilitic treatment.
  - Tracheostomy is required, if respiratory distress is present.
  - If there is a stenosis, plastic surgical reconstruction is performed after the active infection is treated.

LEPROUS LARYNGITIS

Definition   Leprous laryngitis is an infection of the larynx by the organism *Mycobacterium leprae*. It is very rare.

Clinical features

- There may be a diffuse nodular involvement of the supraglottis (epiglottis, arytenoids and false vocal cords) with dyspnoea and stridor.
- Later on, stenosis may occur.

Treatment Antileprosy drug therapy.

SCLEROMA OF THE LARYNX

Definition Scleroma of the larynx is an infection of the larynx secondary to rhinoscleroma by the organism *Klebsiella rhinoscleromatis*. It commonly affects the subglottis.

Pathogenesis Submucosal infiltration of the subglottis results in dyspnoea and stridor due to subglottic stenosis.

Clinical features

- Patient will have features of rhinoscleroma, which is the associated feature.
- Dyspnoea.
- Inspiratory stridor.
- Change of voice.

Treatment

- Steroids to reduce fibrosis and scarring, as the subglottic lumen is narrow and stenosis will result in severe impedence to airflow.
- Streptomycin and doxycycline are given.
- In case of stenosis, laryngeal dialatation, or plastic surgical reconstruction may be required.

CHRONIC NON-SPECIFIC LARYNGITIS

Definition Chronic is a chronic non-specific inflammation of the laryngeal mucosa.

Aetiology

- **Age:** It is common in the second to fourth decade of life.
- **Sex:** Usually, more in males than females.
- **Predisposing factors**
  - Excessive faulty use or misuse of voice especially by teachers, hawkers, actors, etc.
  - Smoking.
  - Alcohol.
  - Recurrent acute laryngitis.
  - Allergy to pollution, dust, chemical fumes, etc.
  - Excessive chronic cough as seen in chronic bronchitis.
  - Septic focus, like chronic tonsillitis, nasal catarrh, sinusitis, dental sepsis, may cause laryngitis.

Clinical features

- **Symptoms**
  - Hoarseness of voice is usually the presenting symptom. Characteristically, it is worse in the mornings due to stagnant secretions and again worsens towards the evening due to vocal fatigue.
  - Irritation in throat.
  - Dry cough.
  - Hawking and raw sensation in throat due to stagnant secretions causing irritation.
- Signs: Both vocal cords show the following changes on indirect laryngoscopy:
  - Hyperemia—congested vocal cords which are pinkish or red,
  - Hypertrophy and hyperplasia of true and false vocal cords,
  - Oedema of both vocal cords—they appear pale and oedematous,
  - Granulations over vocal cords occur in late stages,
  - Vocal cords may occasionally undergo atrophy in the later stage,
  - Thick viscid secretions are seen in the supraglottis and glottis. These cause consistent irritation and patient clears the throat often which worsens the laryngitis.

Differential diagnosis

- Tuberculous laryngitis.
- Syphilitic laryngitis.
- Malignancy of larynx.
- Vocal cord nodules/Benign tumour.
- Vocal cord palsy.
- Leukoplakia of larynx.
- Acute laryngitis.

Treatment

- Eradicate the aetiological factors, e.g. smoking, alcohol, pollution, fumes, etc.
- Voice rest.
- Steam inhalation for soothing the inflamed larynx and liquifying secretions.
- Speech therapy is most important to prevent recurrence of this condition.
- Syrup linctus codeine for relief of dry cough.
- Antibiotics to treat infections, like sinusitis, rhinitis, etc.
- Surgery: Stripping of the hypertrophied vocal cords using microlaryngoscopy and instruments.
- Microlaryngoscopic stripping of vocal cords using laser (recent advance).

LEUCOPLAKIA OF LARYNX

Synonym
- Laryngeal hyperkeratosis.
- Laryngeal keratosis.

Definition
Leucoplakia of larynx is a localised patchy hyperkeratosis of the surface epithelium of the vocal cords resulting in 'white patches' on the vocal cords.
It is a premalignant condition.

Aetiology
The exact aetiology is not known. However, various factors are implicated:
- Age: It is common after 35 years of age.
- Sex: Usually, more in males than females.
- Smoking.
- Alcohol.
- Syphilis.

Clinical features
- Symptoms: Hoarseness of voice, which worsens gradually.
- Signs: Indirect laryngoscopy reveals both the vocal cords to be mobile and presence of raised whitish patches on the surface of the vocal cords, especially in the anterior two-thirds portion.

Investigations
Biopsy and histopathology are required to confirm the diagnosis and rule out a malignant change.

Treatment
- Eradication of the aetiological or aggravating factors, like alcohol, tobacco, etc.
- Voice rest.
- Steam inhalation for its soothing effect.
- Vitamin A has been used empirically.
- A regular follow-up is required, as this is a precancerous condition and may undergo carcinomatous change.
- Excision of the patches with microlaryngoscopy.
- In extensive cases, stripping of the vocal cords is carried out using microlaryngoscopy.
- Rarely, excision of the vocal cord is required.
- If malignant change has occurred (as detected by histopathology), it is treated with surgery or radiotherapy as for cancer of larynx.
- Recent advance in therapy is excision with the use of laser and microlaryngoscopy.

For differential diagnosis of laryngeal disorders *see* Table 40.1 and for differences between laryngeal diphtheria and acute laryngotracheo-bronchitis *see* Table 40.2.

TABLE 40.1: Differential diagnosis of laryngeal disorders

	Laryngeal tuberculosis	Syphilitic laryngitis	Non-specific Chronic laryngitis	Malignancy of larynx
Voice	Weak with episodes of aphonia	Hoarse	Hoarse	Hoarse.
Swallowing (deglutition)	Odynophagia	Normal	Normal	Dysphagia.
Pain in throat	Severe	Absent	Absent	May be present.
Cachexia	Present	Absent	Absent	Present.
Site of lesion	Posterior one-third of vocal cords and posterior commissure	Anterior one-third of vocal cords and anterior commissure	Entire vocal cords and supraglottis	Supraglottis, glottis or subglottis or transglottic.
X-ray chest	Evidence of pulmonary TB	Normal	Normal	Lung metastases in late stage (cannon-ball appearance).
VDRL	Negative	Positive	Negative	Negative.
Sputum examination	Acid-fast bacilli present	Negative	Negative	Negative.

TABLE 40.2: Differences between laryngeal diphtheria and acute laryngotracheo-bronchitis

	Laryngeal diphtheria	Acute laryngotracheo-bronchitis
History of exposure to diphtheria	Present	Absent.
Fever	Low grade	High.
Stridor	Inspiratory	Inspiratory and Expiratory.
Throat Examination	White membrane may be present on tonsils	Tonsillitis may be present.
Chest	Clear	Rales & ronchi on auscultation.
Indirect laryngoscopy	Whitish membrane present on larynx	Congestion and edema of laryngeal mucosa.

CHAPTER 41

Neurological Affections of the Larynx

The classification of neurological affections of the larynx is shown in Flowchart 41.1.

RELEVANT ANATOMY

Course of right recurrent laryngeal nerve:
- It has a shorter course.
- Arises from vagus in front of the subclavian artery (from fourth branchial arch).
- Hooks around subclavian artery.

- Runs up medially towards larynx in close relation to inferior thyroid artery and enters the tracheo-oesophageal groove.
- Enters the larynx behind the cricothyroid joint, by piercing the cricothyroid membrane.

Course of left recurrent laryngeal nerve
- It has a longer course.
- Arises from the vagus in front of the aorta.
- Hooks around the arch of aorta and ligamentum

Flowchart 41.1: Classification of the neurological affections of the larynx

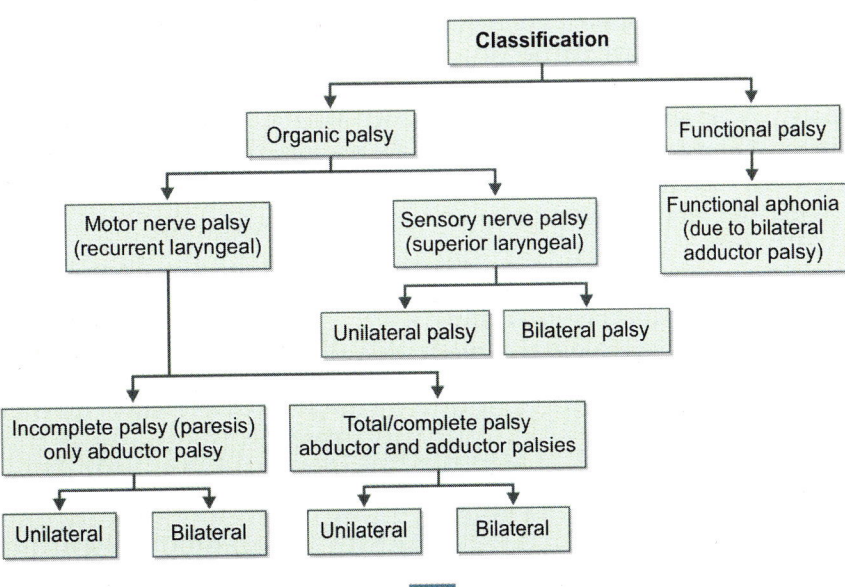

arteriosum (sixth arch derivative) to pass upwards into the neck.
- It lies in the tracheo-oesophageal groove and enters the larynx by piercing the cricothyroid membrane.

Surgical Importance   The right recurrent laryngeal nerve is more prone to injury in neck lesions and the left recurrent laryngeal nerve is more prone to injury in chest lesions (e.g. pulmonary TB with fibrosis, etc.).

Semon's law and Wagner and Grossmans theory are associated with paralysis of the vocal cords.

- Semon's law: This law postulates that in all progressive organic lesions of the recurrent laryngeal nerve, the abductor muscles are the first to be affected and the last to recover. It also states that purely adductor palsy of the vocal cords is functional in aetiology.

    However, it is not very acceptable nowadays.

    The possible explanation for abductors being affected first, is that the nerve fibres supplying the abductors develop later and hence, lie surrounding those supplying the adductors. This makes them more prone to damage. Also, the adductors are stronger muscles and hence resist palsy.

- Wagner and Grossman theory: This theory explains the position of the vocal cords in a case of laryngeal paralysis. If the vocal cord is in the paramedian position, it is due to paralysis of the recurrent laryngeal nerve. If the vocal cord is in the lateral (cadaveric) position, it is due to combined paralysis of the superior and recurrent laryngeal nerves.

Aetiology of vocal cord paralysis
- Central causes: These are less common and affect both, the superior and recurrent laryngeal nerves:
    - Supranuclear lesions have to be bilateral in order to cause nerve palsy, as the larynx has a bilateral representation in the motor area of the cortex.
    - Nuclear lesions result in bilateral involvement, e.g. Bulbar poliomyelitis, dyphtheria, motor neuron disease, syringobulbia, etc.
- Peripheral causes: See Flowchart 41.2.

    Paralysis of the superior laryngeal nerve usually occurs in association with recurrent laryngeal nerve palsy and is rarely seen alone. The vocal cord lies in the cadaveric position and appears lax (bowing of the vocal cord).

DIAGNOSIS

- Position of vocal cords (Fig. 41.1).
- Indirect laryngoscopic diagnosis of vocal cord palsy.

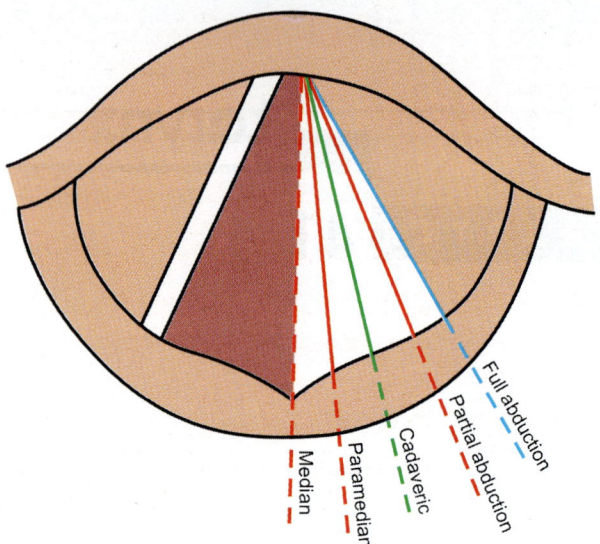

Fig. 41.1 : Position of the vocal cord in palsy

CLINICAL FEATURES

Clinical features are listed in Table 41.1.

TABLE 41.1: Clinical features of neurological affections				
	Unilateral recurrent nerve palsy		Bilateral recurrent nerve palsy	Superior and recurrent nerve palsy
	Complete	Incomplete		
Voice	Hoarseness or normal	Normal	Normal	Rough and easily fatigued
Dyspnoea	Absent	Absent	Presents with inspiratory stridor	Absent
Aspiration into larynx while swallowing	Absent	Absent	Absent	Present
IDL–vocal cord position	Paramedian	Median	Median or paramedian	Cadaveric and sagging

IDL, indirect laryngoscopy

- Unilateral vocal cord palsy
    - *Complete (Both adductor and abductor palsy)*
        - Dyspnoea on exertion.
        - Hoarse voice initially, which improves with time due to compensatory movement of normal vocal cord.
        - *Indirect laryngoscopy:* Vocal cord is in the cadaveric position and immobile with a phonatory gap.
    - *Incomplete:* (Only abductor palsy)
        - Asymptomatic patient. No dyspnoea and normal voice.

- *Indirect laryngoscopy:* Vocal cord is in median position.
- Bilateral abductor palsy
  - Severe dyspnoea and inspiratory stridor.
  - Voice is good.
  - *Indirect laryngoscopy:* Both vocal cords are in the median or paramedian position.
- Bilateral adductor palsy
  - Aphonia or A weak whispering voice.
  - *Indirect laryngoscopy:* Bowing of vocal cords on phonation.
- Complete bilateral palsy
  - Aphonia.
  - No respiratory difficulty.
  - *Indirect laryngoscopy:* Both the vocal cords are in the cadaveric position.
- Superior laryngeal nerve palsy
  - Rarely seen alone, usually seen with recurrent nerve palsy. However, when it occurs, it results in aspiration of food into the larynx as it is a sensory nerve. Patient complains of cough, while swallowing. Voice is rough and fatigues easily. No dyspnoea.
  - *Indirect laryngoscopy (IDL):* On phonation, the vocal cords appear at different levels, due to sagging of the affected cord as a result of tensor muscle weakness.

INVESTIGATIONS

- X-ray chest PA view to rule out a mediastinal lesion, tuberculosis, metastases, or enlarged left atrium of the heart.
- Barium swallow to rule out oesophageal malignancy.
- Blood sugar to rule out diabetes.
- Venereal disease researh laboratory (VDRL) test, to rule out syphillis.
- Erythrocyte sedimentation rate (ESR).
- Neurological investigations.
- Cardiovascular investigations.
- Panendoscopy to rule out malignancy.
- Computed tomography (CT) scan of head, neck, and chest for space occupying lesions.

Flowchart 41.2: Peripheral causes of vocal cord paralysis

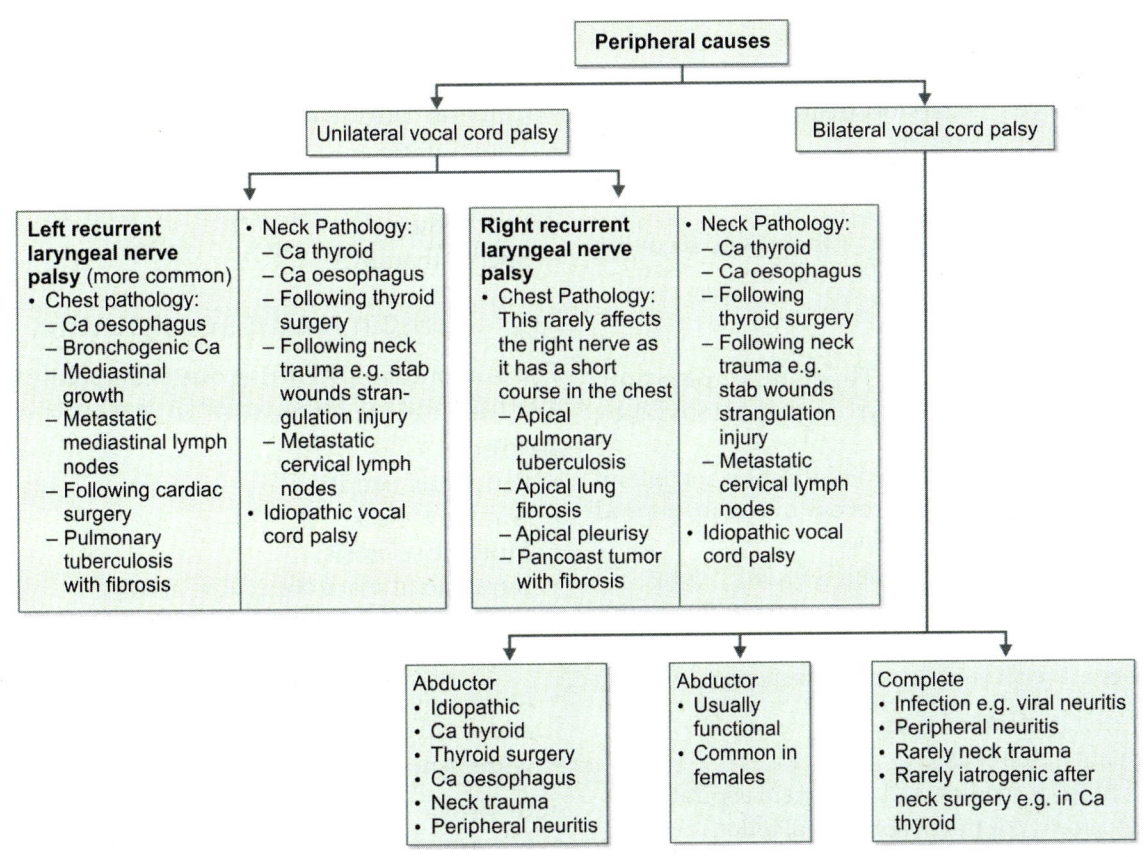

TREATMENT

Unilateral vocal cord paralysis
- Treatment of the cause.
- Asymptomatic patient—no treatment.
- Medical/Conservative treatment: For 6–9 months:
  - Speech therapy.
  - Vitamin B1, B6, and B12 orally.
  - Voice rest.
  - Tincture benzoin in steam inhalations.

    Usually, there is either a compensatory movement of the normal vocal cord towards the paralysed side or the paralysed cord recovers. However, if this does not occur or if the palsy is of a long duration, surgical treatment is required.
- Surgical treatment: Usually performed after 6–9 months of medical treatment.
  - Injection of teflon paste or liquid silicone into the paralysed vocal cord to push it medially. This eliminates the phonatory gap during speech and improves the quality of voice.
  - Implantation of cartilage into the displaced cord can be done to medialise the cord.
  - Arytenoidopexy is also useful.
  - Laser is the recent advance in surgery.

Bilateral vocal cord palsy
- Treatment of the cause.
- If there is a severe respiratory distress, an emergency tracheostomy is required.
- Medical treatment is given for 6–9 months, same as for unilateral cord palsy.
- Surgical treatment is given, if there is no recovery after 6–9 months of medical treatment:
  - Arytenoidopexy.
  - Cordectomy.
  - Arytenoidectomy by Thornell's operation, where the arytenoid cartilage is removed by microlaryngoscopy.
  - Woodmann's operation, mobilisation and lateral fixation of the vocal process of the arytenoid cartilage to the thyroid alae.
  - Nerve muscle transposition is recently done.
    Usually, the tracheostomy can be removed after this surgery.
  - Laser is the recent advance in surgery.

Superior laryngeal nerve palsy
- Treatment of the cause.
- Ryle's tube for feeding and to prevent aspiration.
- Tracheostomy for tracheobronchial toilet.

Bilateral adductor paralysis   Psychotherapy is required. Speech therapy.

FUNCTIONAL APHONIA

Synonym   Bilateral adductor palsy of the vocal cords.

Aetiology:
- Age: It is common in the teenage years or even later.
- Sex: Females are commonly affected.
- Psychological/Emotional shock usually results in functional aphonia.

Clinical features
- Symptoms
  - Sudden aphonia or a sudden change in voice to a whisper.
  - Throat pain.
  - No hoarseness of voice.
  - Cough reflex is normal.
  - History of emotional shock prior to aphonia.
- Signs
  - Patient appears depressed or in a state of emotional shock.
  - *Indirect laryngoscopy:* Vocal cords are normal, but there is phonatory gap and sluggish movement.

Differential diagnosis
- Aphasia.
- Cerebral concussion.
- Cerebral space occupying lesion.

Treatment
- Psychotherapy.
- Speech therapy.

SENSORY PARALYSIS OF THE LARYNX

This is a condition occurring due to the paralysis of the internal branch of the superior laryngeal nerve.

Aetiology
- Peripheral neuritis.
- Trauma to neck.
- Multiple sclerosis.
- Intracranial space occupying lesions.

Clinical features
- History of coughing or choking while swallowing.
- Indirect laryngoscopy: Larynx is insensitive to touch and vocal cords are sagging.
- Diminished cough reflex.

Treatment
- Described earlier in this chapter.

CHAPTER **42**

Carcinoma of the Larynx

Definition
- It is a malignant tumour affecting the larynx.
- Ca larynx is relatively common in India.

Relevant anatomy
- The larynx can be anatomically divided into three parts: Supraglottis, glottis and subglottis.
- The larynx is very closely related to the pyriform fossae on either side and hence, spread of laryngeal malignancy to the pyriform fossae occurs rapidly. The posterior commissure is also in close relation to the cricopharyngeal sphincter.

Aetiology
- Age: It is usually seen after the fourth decade of life.
- Sex: Usually, more in males than females.
- Precipitating factors
  - Smoking.
  - Alcohol (usually results in epiglottic Ca).
  - Environmental pollution.
  - Occupational exposure to asbestos dust, etc.
- Therapeutic radiation for neck malignancy can predispose to Ca larynx.
- Premalignant conditions
  - Leukoplakia.
  - Erythroplakia.
  - Keratosis of larynx.
  - Laryngeal papillomatosis.
  - Polyp.
  - Chronic laryngitis.

- Genetic factors are implicated, since Ca larynx has a racial prediliction.

Classification
- According to site

Internal	External
(Ca confined to the larynx only)	(Ca extending to structures adjacent to the larynx)
• Supraglottic (Fig. 42.1)	• Posterior one-third of tongue.
• Glottic (Fig. 42.2)	• Vallecula.
• Subglottic (Fig. 42.3)	• Pyriform fossa.
	• Postcricoid region.
	• Posterior pharyngeal wall.

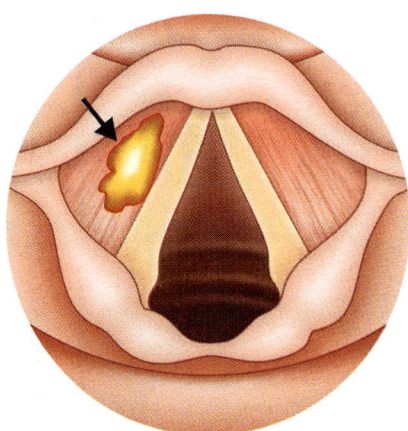

Fig. 42.1: Diagrammatic representation of supraglottic Ca larynx on IDL

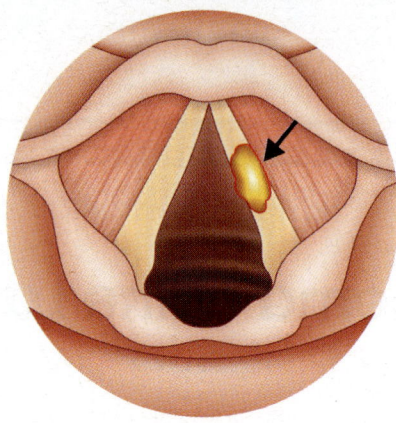

Fig. 42.2 : Diagrammatic representation of glottic Ca on IDL

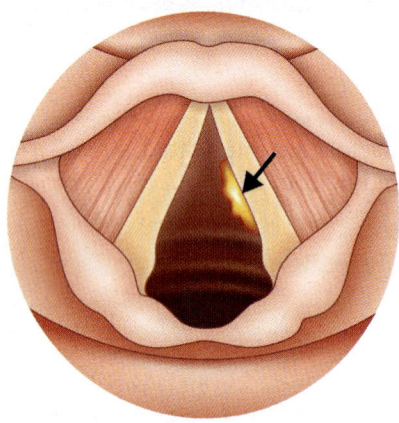

Fig. 42.3 : Diagrammatic representation of subglottic Ca on IDL

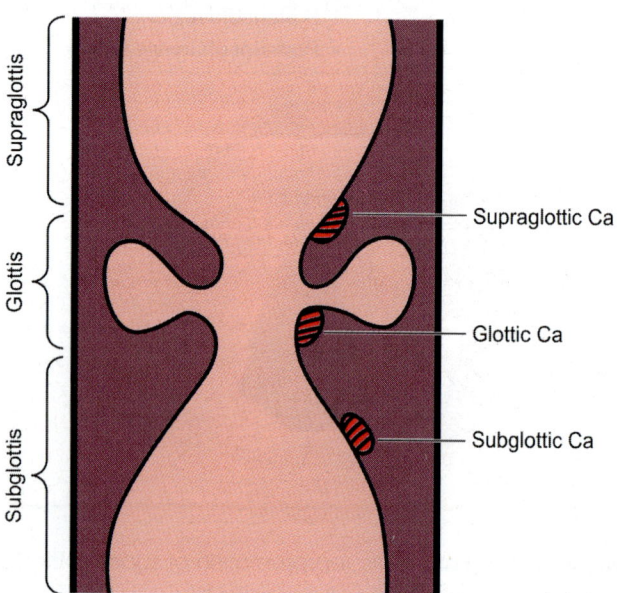

Fig. 42.4 : Diagrammatic representation of Ca larynx (coronal view)

Broder's classification It is based on the histopathology of the tumour and various grades are given:
- Grade I : 25% of cells are anaplastic.
- Grade II : 50% of cells are anaplastic.
- Grade III : 75% of cells are anaplastic.
- Grade IV : More than 75% cells are anaplastic.

Histological classification
- Squamous cell carcinoma (95%).
- Adenocarcinoma.
- Sarcoma.

Tumour-Node-Metastases (TNM) classification It is of prognostic value and most commonly used in clinical practice to decide the mode of treatment and the prognosis of the tumour.
- Primary tumour (T)
  - T_{is} : Carcinoma in situ.
  - T_1 : Tumour confined to one anatomic site.
    - T_{1a} : Tumour confined to one region in one anatomic site.
    - T_{1b} : Tumour extending to two or more regions, but in one anatomic site.
  - T_2 : Tumour extending to more than one anatomic site, but confined to the larynx and without fixation of the vocal cords, e.g. glottic Ca, supraglottic Ca.
  - T_3 : Tumour confined to the larynx, but with vocal cord fixation.
  - T_4 : Extralaryngeal spread of tumour.
- Regional lymph nodes (N)
  - N_0 : No evidence of regional lymph node involvement.
  - N_1 : Single ipsilateral mobile lymph node.
  - N_2 : Ipsilateral involvement of multiple lymph nodes, but all less than 6 cm in diameter and all mobile.
    - N_{2a} : Multiple ipsilateral mobile lymph nodes (< 6 cm).
    - N_{2b} : Bilateral mobile lymph nodes (< 6 cm).
    - N_{2c} : Contralateral mobile lymph nodes (< 6 cm)
  - N_3 : Fixed regional lymph nodes or a mobile lymph node, which is more than 6 cm in diameter.
- Distant metastases (M)
  - M_0 : No evidence of distant metastases.
  - M_1 : Distant metastases present.

Spread

- Direct spread to adjacent tissues, e.g. pyriform fossa, base tongue, etc.
- Haematogenous spread—Late to occur.
- Lymphatic spread to jugular group of lymph nodes. Vocal cord Ca has poor lymphatic drainage as compared to other portions of larynx, hence spread is late.

Pathology

- **Gross:** It is seen as an ulcerative or a proliferative growth in the larynx and extending to adjacent tissues, e.g. pyriform fossa, etc. There may be areas of slough and necrosis. The surrounding tissues may be indurated due to microscopic invasion.
- **Microscopic:** The commonest is squamous cell carcinoma (95%). Sometimes, the tumour may be an adenocarcinoma, sarcoma, or basal cell carcinoma.

Clinical features

- **Symptoms**
  - Inspiratory dyspnoea occurs early in subglottic carcinoma due to the fact that this is the narrowest portion of the lumen.
  - *Change of voice:* This symptom is seen to occur early in glottic carcinomas. In supraglottic malignancy, there is a characteristic 'hot potato speech'.
  - Stridor.
  - Dry cough.
  - Constant irritation in the throat.
  - Bloodstained sputum.
  - Dysphagia, if a posterior commisure growth has involved the cricopharyngeal sphincter.
  - Swelling in the neck due to lymphnode metastases.
  - Odynophagia may occur as an early symptom in Ca involving the epiglottis.
  - History of coughing and choking, when swallowing food or water (aspiration), is also seen in Ca involving epiglottis preventing proper closure of the laryngeal inlet or in Ca pyriform fossa involving the superior laryngeal nerve and resulting in loss of sensory supply to larynx.
  - Referred ipsilateral otalgia (via Xth cranial nerve).
- **Signs**
  - Halitosis is usually present.
  - Indirect laryngoscopy is used to visualise the larynx clinically: Stagnation of saliva (pooling) may be seen in the pyriform fossa. An ulcerative or proliferative growth will be seen with areas of slough and necrosis. Adjacent tissues appear oedematous due to infilteration by tumour. Leukoplakia or erythroplakia may be seen on larynx. Vocal cord movement may be restricted or the cord may be immobile (fixed vocal cord).
  - Presence of enlarged cervical lymph nodes due to regional metastases. These are hard and separate and may be fixed or mobile.
  - Laryngeal crackle is checked by moving the larynx on the cervical vertebrae in the transverse direction. Absence of this crackle indicates involvement of the prevertebral space. (extralaryngeal spread).

Clinical staging of the Ca according to the TNM classification

T				N				M		Stage	
1	2	3	4	0	1	2	3	0	1		
+				+				+		I	$T_1 N_0 M_0$
	+			+				+		II	$T_2 N_0 M_0$
+						+		+			$T_1 N_1 M_0$
	+					+		+		III	$T_2 N_1 M_0$
		+		+				+			$T_3 N_0 M_0$
		+				+		+			$T_3 N_1 M_0$
			+			+	+		+	IV	Any T_4 or N_2 or N_3 or M_1

Investigations

- **Routine investigations include**
  - Haemoglobin (Hb), complete blood count (CBC), blood sugar, serum electrolytes, and electrocardiogram for the overall fitness of the patient, as these patients are usually emanciated and malnourished.
- **Biopsy** of the growth with histopathology is diagnostic. Biopsy is performed by direct laryngoscopy or microlaryngoscopy, if growth involves only glottis.
- **Direct laryngoscopy** helps to detect the exact site of involvement, the extent of the growth and also in examination of other adjacent tissues.
- **Radiological investigations**
  - X-ray chest–PA view to rule out coexisting tuberculosis or presence of secondary metastases.
  - X-ray soft tissue neck (lateral view), will also help to detect extent of the growth.
- **Venereal disease research laboratory (VDRL) test** is performed as syphilis may predispose or coexist with Ca larynx.
- Computed tonography (CT) scan is not much in use for Ca larynx, as most of the information regarding extent and mode of treatment and prognosis is obtained from direct laryngoscopy.

Differential diagnosis

- Tuberculous laryngitis.
- Syphilitic laryngitis.
- Vocal nodules.
- Vocal cord polyps.
- Vocal cord palsy.
- Chronic laryngitis.
- Leukoplakia of larynx.
- Vocal cord granuloma.

Management

This includes:

- Surgery.
- Radiotherapy.
- Chemotherapy.
- Palliative treatment.
- Rehabilitation

Choice of treatment depends upon:

- Stage of tumour.
- General condition of the patient.
- Occupation of the patient should be kept in mind while deciding on the treatment but, cure is of utmost importance.

Surgery for Ca Larynx   Both, partial and total laryngectomy can be performed with or without a radial neck dissection.

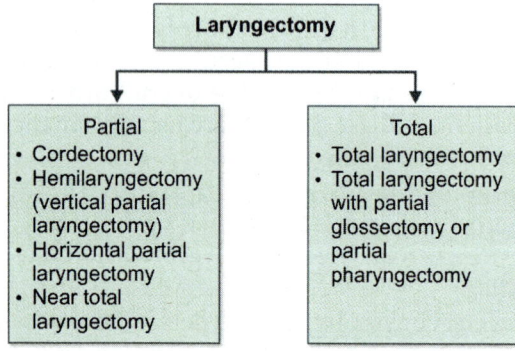

Surgery is recently performed using laser. This helps in haemostasis and wound healing.

Radiotherapy   External beam radiotherapy is given using cobalt 60 as the source. The dose is 6000–7000 rads, which is divided into small doses of 200 rads daily for 5 days a week over 6–7 weeks. The cervical spine is to be protected using shields.

Chemotherapy   It is given only as palliation to reduce the size of tumour and pain.

Palliative treatment   This includes:

- Ryle's tube feeding or a gastrostomy for dysphagia.
- Analgesics to relieve pain.
- Tracheostomy to relieve respiratory distress.
- Antibiotics to control infection.
- Chemotherapy.
- Palliative radiotherapy.

Rehabilitation after laryngectomy   See Chapter 43, rehabilitation after laryngectomy.

CHOICE OF TREATMENT

- *Stage I*   :   Radiotherapy is curative and preserves function of the larynx.
- *Stage II*   :   Surgery or radiotherapy, both give good results.
- *Stage III*   :   Surgery with or without radiotherapy, which is given either before or after surgery.
- *Stage IV or poor general condition of the patient*: Radiotherapy and/or chemotherapy for palliation.

Presence of cervical lymph node metastases are usually treated by a radical neck dissection or can be treated by radiotherapy.

CHAPTER 43

Rehabilitation after Laryngectomy

Rehabilitation after total laryngectomy includes the following:
- Voice rehabilitation.
- Management of permanent tracheostoma.
- Counselling.
- Job rehabilitation.

VOICE REHABILITATION

- Oesophageal speech.
- Surgical reconstruction.
- Prosthesis.
- Artificial speech.

After a total laryngectomy, the patient loses laryngeal speech. The methods of acquiring speech in these patients include the following:

Oesophageal speech   Simplest. No additional surgery is required. Easy to learn.

Surgical reconstruction
- Neoglottis.
- Asai technique.

Requires an additional surgery, which may not be possible in a cancer patient, who is already debilitated due to disease. However, results are better than oesophageal speech.

Voice prosthesis
- Blomsinger's voice prosthesis.
- Panje Button.

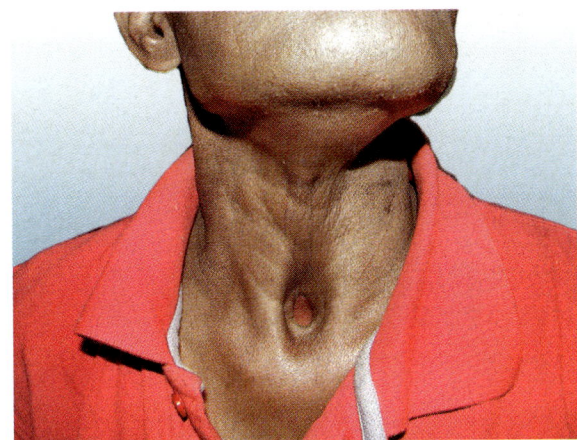

Fig. 43.1: Permanent tracheostoma

Results are good. No major surgery is required. However, these are expensive and need to be replaced at regular intervals due to wear and tear.

Artificial larynx
- Electrolarynx.
- Pneumatic larynx.

Bulky, expensive, not much in use nowadays.

MANAGEMENT OF PERMANENT TRACHEOSTOMA

Following a total laryngectomy, a permanent tracheostoma is created. It has to be maintained in the following manner:
- Tincture benzoin in steam inhalations 3–4 times daily for humidification of inhaled air.

- A thin cloth mask is tied around the neck, at all times to prevent entry of foreign bodies into the lower respiratory tract (as the larynx is no longer present, the protective cough reflex is lost in these patients and insects, etc., may enter through the tracheostoma).
- Regular cleaning of the tracheostoma with suction and instillation of 0.5 mL of sodium bicarbonate into the tracheostoma prior to each suction, so as to liquefy the crusts.

COUNSELLING

Counselling is to be given to the patient as well as to the relatives. A professional psychotherapist is preferred to deal with social problems and personal problems associated with the realisation of cancer and the problems associated with laryngectomy.

JOB REHABILITATION

This is a very important aspect of patient care, as the patient should not be made to feel useless. He should be given a change of job and should not be made to sit at home. Jobs suited for laryngectomy patients include manning a telephone booth or a newspaper stall or some such small industry, where the patient is independent.

Care of the Terminally Ill Patient

This is of utmost importance in improving the quality of life in patients who have disease, which has progressed beyond cure. It includes:

- Management of pain.
- Nutrition and airway.
- Chemotherapy.
- Care of the dying.
- Communication.
- Support of the family.
- Management of the final phase and bereavement.

Management of pain

- Head and neck malignancy is often associated with severe pain.
- Empirical treatment of pain is carried out in most hospitals by using anti-inflammatory analgesics in mild cases or even narcotics (morphine), can be used in such patients as the life expectancy is limited.
- Destructive procedures of the nervous system include:
  - Peripheral nerve destruction, i.e. destruction of the fibres of the trigeminal, glossopharyngeal, vagus or upper four cervical nerves, as the head and neck area is innervated by branches of these nerves. Depending on the area involved, the fibres supplying that area are destroyed by percutaneous phenol lysis or by nerve section.
  - *Thalamotomy*: Destruction of the medial thalamic sensory nuclei, relief lasts for 3–6 months.

- Destruction of the pituitary, relief of pain lasts for few months.
  - Destruction of the trigeminal sensory nucleus and tract.
- Electrical stimulation of the brain, i.e. electro-anaesthesia.

Nutrition and airway

- Nutrition is maintained by a Ryle's tube or even a feeding gastrostomy.
- Airway is maintained by a tracheostomy in the later stages.

Palliative chemotherapy

- It is given with an aim to suppress symptoms.
- Methotrexate and cisplatin are effective in head and neck cancers.

Care of the dying Symptoms such as pain, dysphagia, dyspnoea, fungation of the tumour, sinus formation, infection, constipation, mouth care, bed sores, etc., should be taken care of.

Communication There should be a good communication between the patient, his family, and the professional team. Psychological problems should be dealt effectively.

The management of the final phase Includes relief from pain, breathlessness, restlessness, and accumulation of secretions with the use of proper drugs.

CHAPTER 45

Miscellaneous Conditions of the Larynx

Miscellaneous conditions of the larynx are as follows:
- Laryngeal foreign bodies.
- Laryngomalacia.
- Laryngeal web.
- Vocal cord nodules.
- Laryngeal injuries.
- Contact ulcers.
- Laryngeal stenosis.
- Laryngeal oedema.
- Laryngocoele.
- Vocal cord cyst.
- Vocal cord polyp.
- Reinke's oedema.
- Stridor.
- Hoarseness of voice.
- Speech disorders

LARYNGEAL FOREIGN BODIES

Foreign bodies which are accidentally aspirated, rarely lodge in the larynx. If they do so, they may be fatal even before the patient reaches hospital for help. Aspirated foreign bodies usually lodge in the bronchus.

Types of foreign bodies which may lodge in the larynx:

Dentures   Due to their wires, these usually get lodged at the glottis. Also, in most cases, there is enough free lumen for respiration.

Large coins   In a child, a large coin may not be able to pass the glottis and gets lodged along the anterioposterior diameter of the larynx. This is very dangerous as movement may change the position of the coin causing sudden complete obstruction and death due to apnoea.

Fish bone   This is a rare but known foreign body in the larynx and may lodge anywhere in the supraglottis or glottis. It rarely causes death.

Other foreign bodies include, marbles, pins, peanuts, etc., which are at times fatal.

Clinical features
- History of aspiration of foreign body.
- A bout of severe cough and choking.
- Dyspnoea.
- Inspiratory stridor.
- Hoarseness of voice or aphonia.
- Pain in throat.

Treatment
- The immediate treatment is to hold the child by his legs upside down and to slap his back. This usually dislodges the foreign body.
- Urgent admission and emergency tracheostomy for the following reasons:
  - To prevent aspiration of the foreign body further into the lower respiratory tract.
  - To relieve the respiratory distress.

- To administer general anaesthesia during removal of the foreign body.

    If an urgent tracheostomy is not possible, a crico-thyrotomy may be performed to maintain the airway. This is done by inserting a no. 16 wide bore needle into the larynx through the cricothyroid membrane.

- Removal of the foreign body under general anaesthesia (to prevent injury to the vocal cords), using a direct laryngoscope or microlaryngoscope is performed.
- Antibiotics, anti-inflammatory analgesics and steroids are given till the pain and oedema subside. Tracheostomy tube can be removed after 7–10 days.

LARYNGOMALACIA

Synonyms   Congenital laryngeal stridor.

Definition   Laryngomalacia is a congenital condition seen in infants characterised by inspiratory stridor, which resolves spontaneously as the child grows.

Aetiology
- **Age:** It is common in infants.
- It occurs due to flabby tissues of the larynx, which get sucked-in during inspiration.
- The larynx is thought to be of an exaggerated infantile type.

Clinical features
- **Symptoms**
    - Inspiratory stridor present since birth, which increases on crying.
    - Rarely, there may be cyanosis.
    - Weak cry.
- **Signs**
    - Direct laryngoscopy reveals an infantile type of larynx.
    - The characteristic feature is that the condition is self-limiting and resolves spontaneously by the age of 2–5 years.

Treatment
- Reassurance to parents.
- No active treatment required.
- Very rarely, a tracheostomy may be required.

LARYNGEAL WEB

Definition   Laryngeal web is a failure of canalisation of the anterior commissure of the larynx resulting in obliteration of this commissure by a band of fibrous tissue.

Classification
- Congenital.
- Acquired.
    - Trauma.
    - After infection, e.g. syphilis, scleroma, and tuberculosis.

Clinical features
- A small web may be asymptomatic.
- Hoarseness of voice is a predominant symptom.
- Inspiratory stridor may be present.
- Direct laryngoscopy reveals a fibrous tissue band (web) between the anterior one-third of both vocal cords with a concave posterior border (Fig. 45.1).

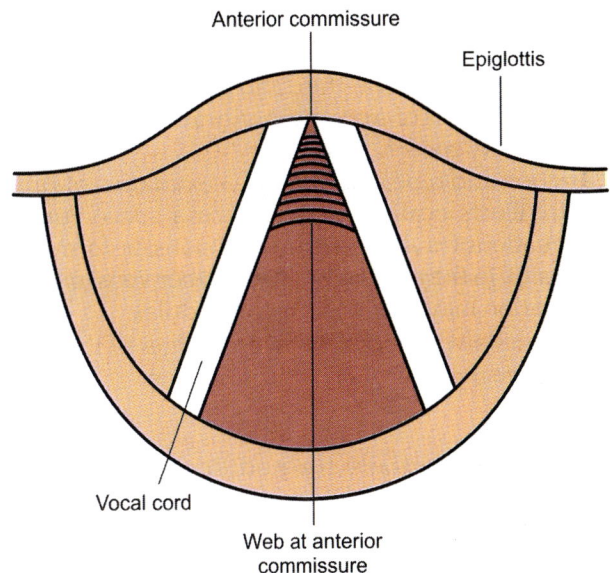

Fig. 45.1: Laryngeal web

Treatment
- If asymptomatic, no treatment is required.
- Microlaryngoscopy with surgical excision of web under general anaesthesia is done for symptomatic cases.
- **Recent advance:** The use of laser with microlaryngoscopy for excision.
- Rarely, tracheostomy is required.

VOCAL CORD NODULES

Synonym   Singer's nodes.

Definition   It is the localised hyperplasia of the epithelium of the free edge of both the vocal cords, at the junction of the anterior one-third and posterior two-thirds.

This condition is *always bilateral*.

Aetiology
- **Age:** It can occur at any age group, but is common in the second and third decades of life.
- **Sex:** Usually, more in females than males.
- Misuse or overuse of voice.
- **Occupation:** It is commonly seen in certain people, like teachers, hawkers, singers, who do not sing properly and housewives who shout at their children.

Pathology
The vocal cord can be divided into two main parts. Anterior two-thirds which is fibrous and posterior one-third which is cartilagenous. Vibrations are much more in the fibrous portion. When a person misuses his voice, there are excessive vibrations of the anterior two-thirds. The point of maximum vibration is the midpoint of the anterior two-third segment (i.e. the junction of anterior one-third and posterior two-third). This is the point of maximum vibration and friction during faulty speech.

Friction and repeated trauma → exudation of fluid, which collects locally in the submucosal space. Further continuation of faulty speech → fibrous tissue formation at this site. In the presence of still further vocal misuse, calcification may take place in the nodules.

Nodules always occur at the free edges of the cords as these are the sites of maximum friction.

Stages
- **Reversible:** Initially the nodules are reversible, with medical line of treatment and voice rest, when they appear clear and translucent containing only exudate.
- **Irreversible:** Later, there is fibrin deposit in the nodules making them opaque white in colour and irreversible. Further, there is a calcification in the nodules making them appear chalky white in colour.

Clinical features
- **Symptoms:**
  - Hoarseness of voice which worsens towards the end of the day due to vocal fatigue.
  - There is no pain or cough. History of vocal misuse is usually present.
- **Signs:** Indirect laryngoscopy shows presence of vocal cord nodules (Fig. 45.2) on both vocal cords at the junction of the anterior and middle one-third of the vocal cords. They may be translucent or whitish or chalky white in colour. Vocal cord movements are normal.

Differential diagnosis
All causes of chronic laryngitis.

Treatment
- Voice rest.

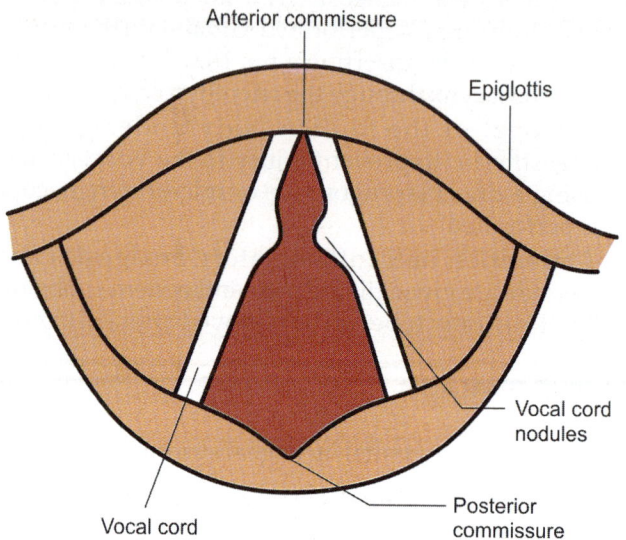

Fig. 45.2: Vocal cord nodules

- **Microlaryngoscopy (MLS)** under general anaesthesia to diagnose the stage.

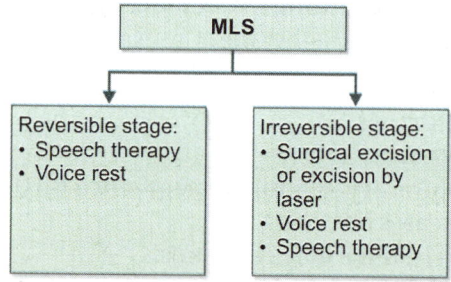

- **Prevention** is with speech therapy to correct the faulty use of voice.

LARYNGEAL INJURIES

Laryngeal injuries are classified as follows:

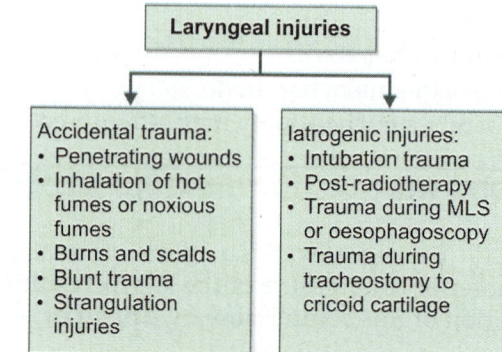

Intubation trauma   This occurs during endotracheal intubation.
- Aetiology
  - Improperly performed intubation can damage mucosa or even dislodge an arytenoid cartilage → vocal cord immobility.
  - Prolonged intubation beyond 48 hours can cause reactive granuloma formation on the vocal cords.
  - If the cuff of the endotracheal tube is in the glottis when inflated, it can result in damage to vocal cords.
  - Tubes made of red India rubber are more prone to cause trauma and irritation than those of portex or silicone.
- Clinical features
  - Hoarseness of voice on extubation.
  - Rarely dyspnoea or inspiratory stridor may occur due to oedema.
- Treatment
  - Voice rest.
  - Steroids to reduce oedema.
  - Excision of granulation tissue.
  - Rarely tracheostomy to relieve dyspnoea.
  - Dialatation of stenosis or plastic surgical correction of stenosis is performed.
- Reactions to radiotherapy of neck: This can cause oedema of mucosa, necrosis and slough formation of mucosa and in severe cases, it can result in cartilage necrosis with suppuration.
  - *Treatment*
    - Steroids.
    - Antibiotics.
    - Tracheostomy.
    - Rarely, in the case of unresolving cartilage necrosis, a laryngectomy is performed.
- Trauma during MLS or oesophagoscopy includes abrasion of mucosa leading to oedema or even dislocation of the arytenoid cartilage.
- During a high tracheostomy, the cricoid cartilage may be damaged resulting in subglottic stenosis at a later date.
- Penetrating wounds/open injuries occur due to stabs, cuts or gunshots and are characterised by:
  - Pain and haemorrhage.
  - Dyspnoea.
  - Hoarseness of voice.
  - Oedema of mucosa and submucosal haemorrhages with a swelling over the neck.
  - Subcutaneous emphysema with crepitations.

- Inhalation of steam or fumes result in a severe mucosal oedema with necrosis and fibrosis resulting in stenosis at a later date.
- Blunt trauma/closed injuries include blow to neck or strangulation. This causes injury to soft tissues of neck, laryngeal cartilages, and mucosa. Clinical features are similar to those of penetrating injury to larynx.
  - *Treatment includes*
    - Tracheostomy.
    - Antibiotics.
    - Steroids.
    - Anti-inflammatory analgesics.
    - Wound exploration and suturing.
    - Rarely, if there is irrepairable destruction, laryngectomy is required.

CONTACT ULCERS

Contact ulcers occur due to vocal abuse, but is very uncommon.

Also known as 'Cup and saucer' ulcer, characterised by ulceration (saucer) on the vocal process of one arytenoid and granulation (cup) on the vocal process of the other arytenoid. The granuloma of one side fits into the crater on the other side.

Patients present with hoarseness of voice and have a history of chronic voice abuse.

Treatment
- Voice rest.
- Excision of the lesion with MLS.
- Speech therapy after surgery to enable fast healing and prevent recurrence.

LARYNGEAL STENOSIS

Definition   It is a condition characterised by a narrowing of the lumen of the larynx.

Commonest in the subglottis, since it is the narrowest portion of the larynx, and any fibrosis at this site can cause symptomatic stenosis early.

Aetiology
- Stenosis
  - *Congenital*
    - Laryngeal atresia.
    - Laryngeal web.
  - *Acquired*
    - *Trauma:* Iatrogenic injuries.
      Accidental trauma.

- *Infection:* Laryngitis.
- *Tumours:* Ca larynx.
- *Miscellaneous:* Impacted foreign body.

Clinical features
- Hoarseness of voice.
- History of trauma/infection.
- Dyspnoea.
- Inspiratory stridor.

Treatment
- Treat the cause.
- Tracheostomy.
- Dialatation of stenosis.
- Laryngoplasty for reconstruction.

LARYNGEAL OEDEMA

Aetiology
- Laryngeal oedema
  - *Trauma*
    - Accidental.
    - Iatrogenic.
  - *Infection:* Laryngitis.
  - *Allergic:* Angioneurotic oedema due to allergy to dust, food, drugs, etc.
  - *Tumours:* Carcinoma can cause oedema due to infection or lymphatic obstruction.
  - *Miscellaneous:* Foreign body → may lead to oedema due to chemical irritation and physical trauma.

Clinical features
- History of causative factor may be present.
- Dyspnoea.
- Hoarseness of voice.
- Inspiratory stridor.
- Pain.

Treatment
- Treat the cause.
- Antibiotics.
- Steroids.
- Anti-inflammatory analgesics.
- Tracheostomy, if there is severe respiratory distress.

LARYNGOCOELE

Definition   Laryngocoele is defined as an aircontaining outpouching (sac) of the ventricle and saccule of the larynx.

Classification   Types of laryngocoele are shown in Fig. 45.3.

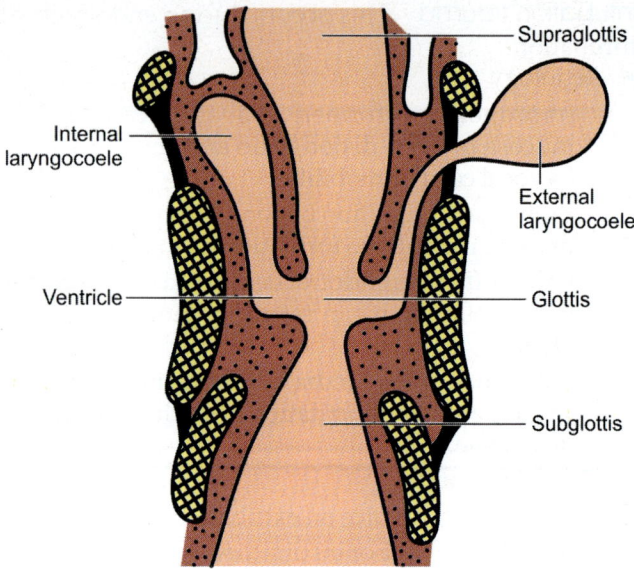

Fig. 45.3: Internal and external laryngocoele

- External laryngocoele: The sac lies outside the larynx.
- Internal laryngocoele: The sac lies outside the lumen but inside the cartilages of the larynx.
- Sometimes, it may be a combination of both internal and external.

Aetiology
- Congenital.
- Acquired.

Rise in intraglottic pressure may at times, cause this out-pouching, e.g. in asthamatics, or glass-blowers or musicians using wind instruments.

Clinical features
- Asymptomatic.
- Hoarseness of voice.
- Cystic swelling in the upper portion of the neck to one side of the midline which is reducible and reappears on coughing. This is characteristic of an external laryngocoele.

Investigations   A laryngogram is diagnostic (X-ray of larynx with use of contrast medium). The X-ray is repeated during cough/valsalva manoeuvre to see the sac.

Treatment
- If asymptomatic, no treatment is required.
- Excision via the neck, i.e. external approach, if symptomatic.

VOCAL CORD CYST

Definition   Vocal cord cyst is a formation of a cystic swelling on the vocal cord.

Sites

- It is commonly seen in anterior commissure or any one vocal cord or in the supraglottic larynx.
- They are usually unilateral and solitary and can be pedunculated or sessile.

Aetiology

- Mucous cysts.
- Congenital cysts.
- Cystic degeneration in a fibroma, vocal cord nodules or a polyp.

Clinical features

- Asymptomatic.
- Hoarseness of voice: This may be intermittent, if the cyst is pedunculated, i.e. it produces hoarseness only when it comes in between the phonating vocal cords.

Treatment

- Asymptomatic: No treatment.
- Symptomatic: Excision using microlaryngoscopy and surgical instruments (conventional) or laser (recent advance).

VOCAL CORD POLYP

Definition   It is a smooth, sessile, or pedunculated swelling arising from the vocal cord.

Types/Classification

- Unilateral—common
- Bilateral—very rare
- Pedunculated—common.
- Sessile—occasionally.

Treatment   Excision using microlaryngoscopy with surgical instruments (conventional) or laser (recent advance).

REINKE'S OEDEMA

Definition   Rinke's oedema is a condition characterised by the accumulation of oedema fluid in the submucosal space.

Aetiology   It occurs due to unresolved infection or trauma to vocal cords (Reinke's space of the vocal cords).

Clinical features   It is also known as polypoid degeneration of the vocal cords.

There is a bilateral smooth symmetrical swelling along the entire length of the vocal cords.

Treatment   Stripping of the vocal cords using microlaryngoscopy and surgical instruments or laser.

STRIDOR

Definition   Stridor is a noisy respiration due to obstruction to passage of air through the respiratory tract. It is a symptom and not a disease.

Classification/Types

- Inspiratory: It is seen in lesions of upper airway, i.e. nose, pharynx, and larynx.
- Expiratory: It is seen in lesions of lower airway, i.e. bronchi.
- Mixed: Both inspiratory and expiratory seen in tracheal lesions.

Aetiology   See Table 45.1.

Management plan

- History.
- Clinical examination.
- Investigations.
- Treatment.

TABLE 45.1: Aetiology of stridor					
	Congenital	Traumatic	Inflammatory	Neoplastic	Miscellaneous
Causes in the respiratory tract	• Web • Stenosis • Laryngomalacia • Cyst	• Accidental trauma • Iatrogenic trauma • Burns, fumes	• Laryngitis • Epiglottitis • Laryngeal diphtheria • Oedema	• Papilloma • Carcinoma	• Foreign body • Vocal cord palsy
Causes outside the respiratory tract	• Pierre-Robin syndrome • Vascular loops by aberrant vessels around the trachea or bronchi	• Trauma to neck or chest	• Ludwig's angina • Retropharyngeal abscess (acute or chronic)	• Enlarged thymus • Metastatic lymph nodes in mediastinum • Cystic hygroma	• Foreign body in cricopharynx especially in children

A patient who presents with stridor is treated as an emergency.

Even before taking a history, the patient is admitted to the hospital and an emergency tracheostomy or an endotracheal intubation (if possible) is performed to maintain an airway. The patient is administered humidified oxygen.

- **History:** A detailed history is taken to detect the cause:
  - Whether congenital or acquired,
  - History of fever and type of fever,
  - History of sore throat,
  - History of swelling in neck,
  - History of change of voice,
  - History of foreign body aspiration with coughing and choking.
- **Clinical examination:** This is performed with an aim to diagnose the cause:
  - Examination of the nose, nasopharynx, oral cavity, oropharynx, hypopharynx and larynx to rule out any cause in the upper airway,
  - Examination of the respiratory system,
  - Examination of the cardiovascular system for any anomalous vascular loops,
  - Examination of the neck.
- **Investigations:** These include:
  - Radiological examination of the neck (soft tissue) and chest,
  - CT scan of the involved site,
  - Direct laryngoscopy and bronchoscopy–using a fibroptic or rigid scope to confirm the diagnosis.
- **Treatment:**
  - Admission to hospital.
  - Emergency tracheostomy or, if possible, endotracheal intubation to relieve the respiratory distress.
  - Humidified oxygen.
  - Treatment of the cause with medical (antibiotics, steroids and anti-inflammatory analgesics) or surgical mode of treatment.

HOARSENESS OF VOICE

Definition   Hoarseness of voice is the change of voice from normal to one that is coarse and rough.

It occurs due to a pathology affecting the vocal cords or the glottis.

Pathogenesis   Any pathology affecting the movements of the vocal cords, approximation of the free edges of the vocal cords, tension of the vocal cords and the size of the vocal cords can cause a hoarseness of voice. Hoarse voice should be differentiated from a muffled and a breathy voice.

- A hoarse voice is rough and unpleasant.
- A muffled voice is due to a supraglottic or hypopharyngeal mass. It is also known as 'hot-potato speech'. The vocal cords are not involved and the pathology is above the level of the vocal cords.
- A breathy voice is more like a whiper and is due to lack of proper approximation of the vocal cords and escape of air during phonation. It is commonly seen in bilateral abductor vocal cord palsy.

Aetiology

- **Causes in the larynx and hypopharynx:**
  - *Congenital*
    - Laryngeal web.
    - Cysts.
  - *Infections*
    - Acute laryngitis.
    - Chronic laryngitis.
  - *Traumatic*
    - Vocal misuse.
    - Accidental injuries.
    - Iatrogenic injuries, e.g. intubation.
    - Radiation.
  - *Neoplastic*
    - Benign tumour.
      - Polyps.
      - Papilloma.
      - Cysts.
      - Fibroma.
      - Chondroma.
    - Ca larynx.
  - *Miscellaneous*
    - Vocal cord nodules.
    - Laryngeal oedema.
    - Stenosis of larynx.
    - Unilateral vocal cord palsy.
    - Functional hoarseness.
    - Laryngocoele.
- **Other causes**
  - Ca oesophagus → recurrent laryngeal nerve palsy.
  - Ca thyroid → recurrent laryngeal nerve palsy.
  - Pulmonary tuberculosis (TB) or Ca → recurrent laryngeal nerve palsy.
  - Diabetes.
  - Syphilis.
  - Cardiac, thyroid, or renal diseases.

Management plan
- History
- Investigations
- Clinical examination
- Treatment
- **History:** A detailed history is taken to detect the cause of hoarseness, e.g. age of patient, onset of hoarseness—sudden or gradual, since birth or not, history of trauma, other associated symptoms, etc.
- **Clinical examination:** Detailed clinical examination is required to arrive at a diagnosis for the cause of hoarseness.
  - With indirect laryngoscopy
    - Examination of the oropharynx
    - Examination of the larynx
  - Examination of the neck
  - Systemic examination–CNS, CVS, RS, etc.
- **Investigations**
  - Haematological–Hb, TC, DC, ESR, VDRL.
  - Radiological
    - X-ray chest to r/o tuberculosis and malignancy.
    - X-ray soft tissue neck to r/o malignancy.
    - X-ray of larynx with contrast laryngography.
    - Barium swallow to r/o Ca oesophagus.
  - CT scan of neck and chest.
  - Direct laryngoscopy under Ga for diagnosis, biopsy or swab examination.
  - Microlaryngoscopy under Ga for vocal cord pathology.
  - Panendoscopy which includes the following:
    - Nasopharyngoscopy.
    - Direct laryngoscopy.
    - Oesophagoscopy.
    - Bronchoscopy.
  - Mediastinoscopy which was performed previously is now not in use due to the advent of the CT scan.
- **Treatment**
  - Treatment of the cause.
  - Voice rest.
  - Antibiotics.
  - Anti-inflammatory analgesics.

- Steam inhalation using soothing agents like tincture benzoin, menthol or eucalyptus.
- Speech therapy.

SPEECH DISORDERS

Disorders of Voice

Disorders of intensity
- **Aphonia** due to hysteria, bilateral vocal cord paralysis or laryngectomy.
- **Dysphonia** due to phonation by venticular bands (dysphonia plica ventricularis), or puberty dysphonia (puberphonia).

Disorders of pitch
- High pitch.
- Low pitch.
- Breaks in pitch.

Disorders of resonance
- **Hypernasality** due to cleft palate, etc. (rhinolalia aperta).
- **Hyponasality** due to nasal obstruction, etc. (rhinolalia clausa).

Disorders of phonation
- **Harshness** of voice.
- **Hoarseness** of voice.

Disorders of Speech

Aphasia   Loss of speech due to lesion/pathology of the cortical speech centre.

Dysphasia   Disorder of speech due to lesion/pathology of the cortical speech centre.

Dysarthria   Speech disorder due to disorder of articulation.

Stammering   This is a functional speech disorder.

Treatment
- Treatment of the cause.
- Speech therapy.
- Psychotherapy (mental rehabilitation) of the child and parents to build confidence.

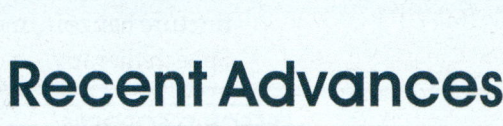

Recent Advances

CHAPTER 46

Hearing Aids

INTRODUCTION

A hearing aid can literally be any device, which can help a person to hear a sound better, though more technically, a hearing aid may be defined as:

'A device which helps to bring sound energy more effectively to the ear of a hearing impaired person'.

TYPES OF HEARING AIDS

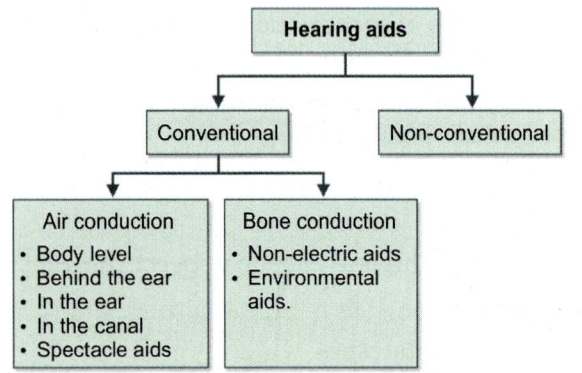

Conventional These are the most important ones. They are small electronic devices, which are worn by the patient, and help him/her in communication.

The following types, in ascending order of sophistication and development are available:

- Air conduction hearing aids
  - *Body level/worn:* The microphone, amplifier, and batteries are in a small body-worn box and a short

lead, called 'Y lead' connects it to earphones held in ear moulds (Fig. 46.1).

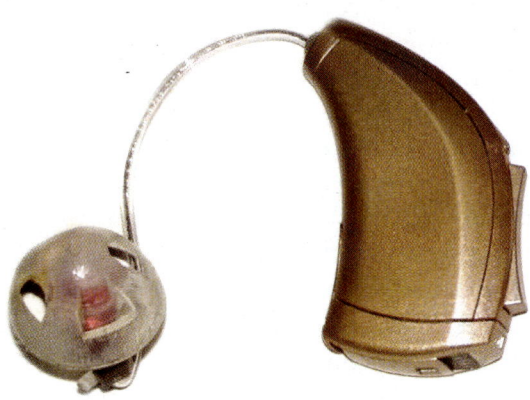

Fig. 46.1 : Body-worn/receiver in canal hearing aid

- *Behind the ear:* The hearing aid unit is worn behind the pinna and amplified sound is transmitted to the external auditory canal (EAC) via a plastic tube (Fig. 46.2).
- *In the ear:* The hearing unit is worn within the concha (Fig. 46.3).
- *In the canal:* The hearing unit is worn in the EAC invisible hearing aid / CIC (Fig 46.3).
- *Spectacle aids:* Behind the ear hearing aid is incorporated in the spectacle frame (Fig. 46.4).

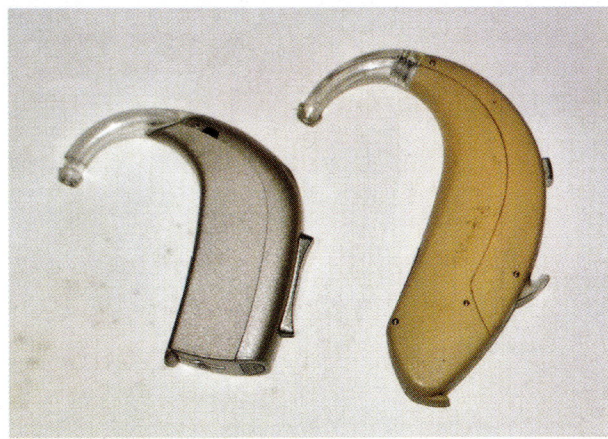

Fig. 46.2 : Behind the ear hearing aids

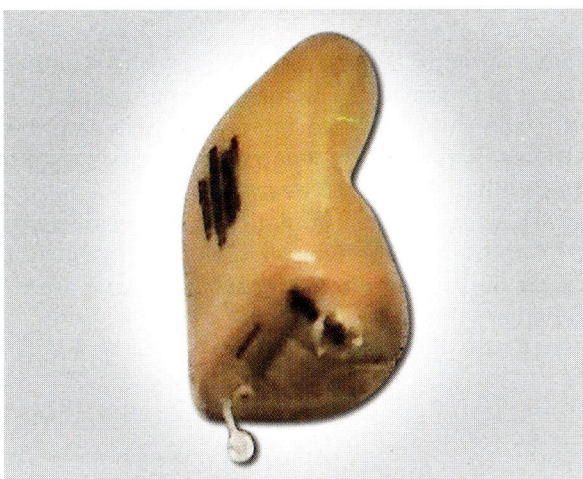

Fig. 46.3 : In the ear and in the canal

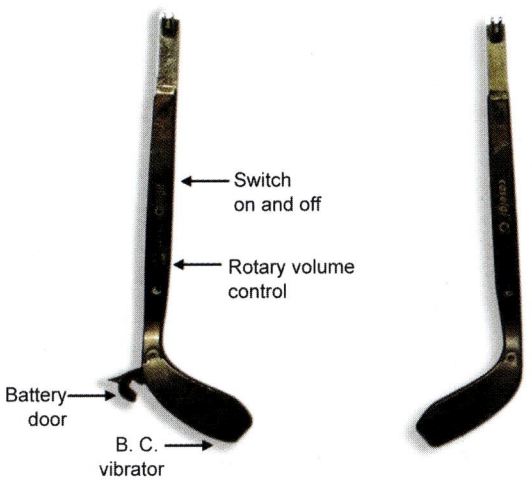

Switch on and off

Rotary volume control

Battery door

B. C. vibrator

Fig. 46.4 : Spectacle aids

- Bone conduction hearing aids:
  - Sound, instead of being transmitted via air to the tympanic membrane, is directly presented to the inner ear by means of a 'bone conduction vibrator', which is applied to the mastoid process.
  - They are useful in patients who have congenital malformations of external and middle ears and in continuously discharging ears.

Non-conventional aids

- Non-electric aids: Cupped hands, ear trumpet, conversation tubes.
- Environmental aids: Alerting devices help in recognising door bells, telephone ring, e.g. by the use of a flashlight system.

COMPONENTS

Components of a hearing aid are as follows (Fig. 46.5):
- Microphone: It converts sound to electrical impulses.
- Amplifier: It increases the amplitude of impulses generated by the microphone.
- Earphone: It converts amplified electrical energy back into sound.
- Earmoulds: These help to anchor the earphone to the concha.
- Battery: It supplies power to the amplifier.

INDICATIONS

- Sensorineural hearing loss due to:
  - Presbycusis.
  - Noise induced.
  - Ototoxic drug induced.
- Conductive hearing loss patients unfit or who refuse surgery due to:
  - Otosclerosis.
  - Chronic suppurative otitis media (CSOM).
  - Congenital malformation.

CONTRAINDICATIONS

- Profound sensorineural hearing loss.
- Discharging ear (airconduction aids are contraindicated).

Special use of hearing aids in schools for the deaf includes the group-teaching hearing aids, which are used for communication between one teacher and many students and the desk model hearing aid for speech training of individual students.

Points to be noted in the use of a hearing aid:
- It is only of palliative value. It cannot cure deafness.

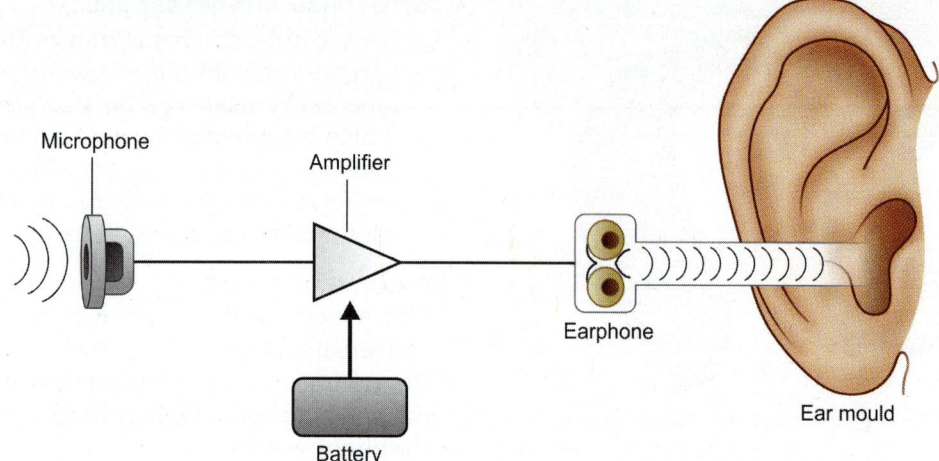

Fig. 46.5 : Diagrammatic representation of the components of a hearing aid

- It cannot restore hearing to 100% normal.
- It simply amplifies all frequencies within its range.

RECENT ADVANCE

Recently computerised hearing aids have flooded the market. These hearing aids are used with or without a remote switch. They are prefed information on particular sounds which they should amplify in a particular set environment, e.g. in the market, while seeing TV, or in a quiet room, etc. The most recent ones available are the computerised hearing aids, which can 'think for themselves', i.e. the wearer need not change the setting with a remote with every change of the environment. This hearing aid automatically changes its setting with a change in the wearer's environment. Both, these are only airconduction hearing aids and are very expensive.

Cochlear Implants

INTRODUCTION

Cochlear implant is the latest endeavour in man's pursuit of his battle against the handicap of deafness. It is an entirely new concept from conventional hearing aids, in that, it directly stimulates the cochlear nerve with electrical energy in a patient, who has lost his cochlear function, but still has an intact cochlear nerve.

FUNCTIONING

A cochlear implant (Fig. 47.1) consists of:
- Microphone to convert sound into electrical energy.
- Speech processor converts electrical impulses from the microphone into electrical signals, which stimulate the VIIIth cranial nerve endings in the cochlea in a pattern, which makes it easier for the patient to understand speech.

- Transmitter coil transmits these signals transcutaneously to the implanted receiver coil.
- Receiver coil is implanted into bone subcutaneously behind the ear to receive signals from transmitter coil.
- Electrodes are placed within cochlea, to stimulate the endings of the 8th cranial nerve.

TYPES

Number of channels
- Single channel: Only one electrode stimulates the nerve endings.
- Multichannel: Four to 22 electrodes may be used to stimulate the nerve endings.

Types of speech processer
- Analogue—older type.

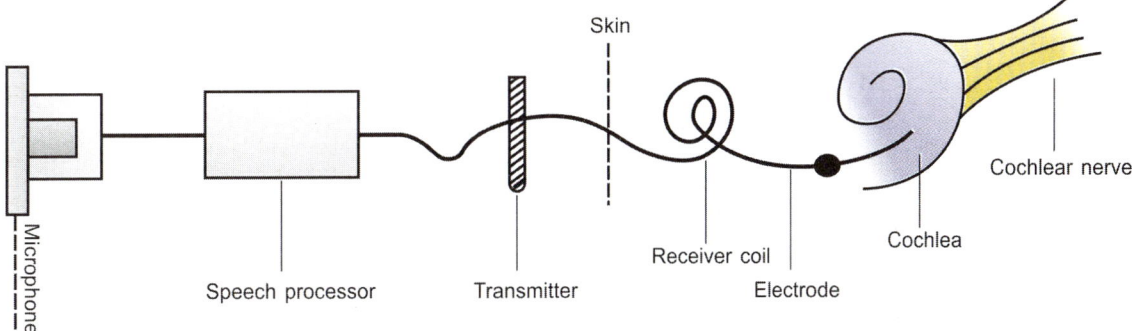

Fig. 47.1 : Diagrammatic representation of the cochlear implant

- Feature extraction: Selection of only those sounds, which are important for recognition of speech.

INDICATIONS

The following prerequisites must be satisfied:
- Congenital profound sensorineural (SN) hearing loss with no residual cochlear function (cochlear reserve).
- Intact VIIIth cranial nerve and central auditory function.
- Postlingual SN hearing loss.
- Parents/Patient should be prepared for an extensive, rehabilitation programme.

CONTRAINDICATIONS

- Useful cochlear function exists.
- Prelingual/Congenital deafness in children, who have already learnt other methods of communications (sign language, facial expressions)
- Malformations of cochlea.
- Central deafness.
- Unilateral hearing loss.
- Labrinthitis ossificans.

CONSEQUENCES

- Perception of sound by patient.
- Patient may not recognise the sound, i.e. normal sound perception is not attained 'Patient is told that sounds may not be the same again'.

- The patient and the parents are explained that post-surgery, extensive auditory verbal therapy (AVT) will be required. Sometimes this may take up to 2–3 years.

SURGERY

- Simple mastoidectomy is done with a posterior tympanotomy.
- Electrodes are inserted via round window membrane into the cochlea.
- Receiver is implanted in the bone behind the ear in a sort of a shallow cavity drilled into it.

COMPLICATIONS

- Damage to remaining neural elements.
- Stimulation of facial nerve may cause facial twitching.
- Labyrinthitis.
- Cerebrospinal fluid (CSF) leak.
- Meningitis.
- Abnormalities of taste due to stimulation of chorda tympani nerve.
- Device failure.
- Patient cannot undergo magnetic resonance imaging (MRI) investigation as the electric fields of the implant interfere with the magnetic fields of the imager.
- Nowadays with advances in technology, low-intensity MRI is possible using productive shields over the implant.

Recent Advances

CHAPTER 48

Nasal and Sinus Endoscopy

INTRODUCTION

Endoscopic procedures have revolutionised surgical care in virtually every field. Nowhere else has the impact of endoscopes been more, than in sinus surgery; owing to the intricate and inaccessable anatomy of the paranasal sinuses.

INDICATIONS

The indications can be broadly categorized into two categories. They are:
- Diagnostic.
- Therapeutic.

Diagnostic
- Office endoscopy for diagnosis of site of epistaxis.
- Biopsy of nasal mass or mass in the maxillary sinus.

Therapeutic
- Removal of foreign body from nose
- Functional endoscopic sinus surgery (FESS).
- Mucocoele of paranasal sinuses.
- Atticoantral and ethmoidal polyps.
- CSF rhinorrhoea.
- Endoscopic DCR (dacryocystorhinostomy).
- Vidian neurectomy.
- Optic nerve decompression.
- Orbital decompression.
- Transsphenoidal pituitary surgery.
- Choanal atresia or stenosis.

- Today endoscopes are being used to access regions within the cranial vault for surgical management of intracranial lesions. The ENT surgeons and the neurosurgeons work as a team using the expanded endonasal skull base approach to the cranial fossa.

CONTRAINDICATIONS

- Acute sinusitis.
- Sinusitis complicated by:
  - Intracranial extention.
  - Orbital complication.
- Invasive fungal infections (mucormycosis).
- Malignancy.

FUNCTIONAL ENDOSCOPIC SINUS SURGERY

Functional endoscopic sinus surgery is a new concept in the treatment of chronic sinusitis. It is based on the concept of minimal amount of intervention, sufficient to restore the functional capacity of the mucocilary transport system of the mucosa of the paranasal sinuses.

Pathophysiology   According to the new concept, the 'key area' in the pathogenesis of chronic sinusitis is an area called the 'osteomeatal complex (OMC)', which is situated within the middle meatus.

The OMC consists of the following structures:
- Uncinate process: A hook shaped projection in the lateral wall of the nose at the middle meatus.
- Bulla ethmoidalis: A bulge caused by the middle ethmoid cells.

- **Infundibulum:** A groove between the bulla and the uncinate process in which opens the:
  - Maxillary sinus ostium.
  - Ostia of the anterior ethmoid cells.
  - Frontonasal duct.

Chronic infection of the sinuses occurs whenever there is a breakdown of the mucociliary transport mechanism of the sinuses. The commonest site is the ethmoids, where stagnation of the secretions causes blockage of drainage of sinuses which drain via, OMC, i.e. the frontal, maxillary, and the ethmoid. Thus relief of obstruction at the OMC will cause resolution of maxillary and frontal sinus pathology, which are secondarily involved due to ethmoid pathology.

Procedure

- Preoperative CT scan of the paranasal sinus to know the anatomical boundaries, extent of pathology, and any anatomical anomaly (serves as a 'roadmap' during surgery).
- Local anaesthesia is preferable to general anaesthesia as there is less bleeding.
- However, today hypotensive general anaesthesia is preferred.
- If local anaesthesia is used, the patient's nose is sprayed with 10% lignocaine spray and packed with cotton neuropatties (pledgets) soaked in 4% lignocaine and 1:1,00,000 adrenaline solution. This is repeated once or twice after sedation to decongest and anaesthetise the nose. 2% lignocaine - adrenaline solution is used for infiltration and local anasthesia of the nasal mucosa.
- If general anaesthesia is used , cotton neuropatties soacked in solution of 1: 33,000 saline-adrenaline solution are used to decongect the nasal mucosa in the operation theater.
- If the septum is very deviated, causing obstruction, a septoplasty is performed endoscopically.
- Under endoscopic vision the uncinate process is removed, maxillary ostium widened and cleared of all disease. An anterior and posterior ethmoidectomy is performed. The frontal recess is cleared of all disease and the frontal sinus is cleared using saline washes. The spheroid ostium is identified, widened and the spheroid sinus is cleared of all disease.
- The nasal cavities are then packed with Merocel®/ Netcel® nasal packs and an anterior nasal dressing is given after achiving haemostasis.
- Then packs are removed after 48–72 hours.

Complications

- Adhesions in middle meatus area.
- Haemorrhage.
- Damage to:
  - Orbital structures.
  - Cribriform plate of the ethmoids.
  - Optic nerve.
- Epiphora due to damage to nasolacrimal duct.
- CSF rhinorrhoea.
- Dental neuralgia.

Recent Advances

CHAPTER 49

Laser

INTRODUCTION

Laser represents the 'State of the art' in otolaryngological surgery. It has opened up new frontiers of surgical technique and promises tantalizing possibilities, which uptil now were not possible with conventional surgery.

PHYSICS

Laser is an acronym for 'light amplification by stimulated emission of radiation'.

A laser beam is electromagnetic (EM) radiation which is produced by certain substances known as 'lasing mediums', when the electrons in them are excited to a higher energy level. When these electrons fall back to their normal state, they emit EM radiation known as 'Photons'. Millions of photons combine to produce the laser beam.

PROPERTIES OF LASER BEAM

The special characteristics, which make laser so useful are:

- ◆ *Monochromatic* : All rays are of one wavelength.
- ◆ *Collerant* : All waves are in same phase.
- ◆ *Collimated* : All the rays are parallel (therefore can be focused to a very small spot).

TYPES OF LASERS

Lasers are known by the type of lasing medium:

CO_2 Carbon dioxide gas is used as lasing medium.
- Properties: It is absorbed by the water contained in tissues and causes boiling and subsequent vapourisation of tissues. It is used to vapourise lesions or as a scalpel to cut through tissues.

Argon   Argon gas is used as lasing medium, which emits green light. Thus, it is selectively absorbed by blood, which is red in colour. It can pass through water and clear tissues, e.g. perilymph, cornea, etc., without damaging them. It has deeper penetration than CO_2.

Neodymium-doped yittrium aluminium garnet (Nd-YAG):
- Produces infrared light.
- It is the most powerful surgical laser.
- It has the greatest depth of tissue penetration.
- It can coagulate blood vessels up to 1.5 mm diameter.

Other less frequently used lasers are:
- Dye laser.
- Helium–Neon.
- Potassium titanyl phosphate (KTP).
- Metal vapour (gold, copper).

ADVANTAGES

- Precision because the laser beam can be focused to a very small point, it can offer amazing precision in surgery.
- Haemostasis: Laser seals blood vessels by coagulation thus offering an 'excellent operative field'.

- **Better visibility** due to clear operation field.
- **Minimal fibrosis:** Laser wounds heal with minimal tissue reaction and fibrosis, thus there is less post-operative scarring.
- **Healing:** Laser wounds heal faster due to minimal trauma to adjascent tissue.
- **Pain:** Laser wounds result in less post-operative pain.
- **Decreased morbidity** due to faster healing.
- **Immediate tissue destruction**—No seeding of cancer cells.
- **Minimal instrumentation** required.

DISADVANTAGES

- Expensive.
- Special training required.
- May injure operating surgeon/staff.
- Tissue is burnt or vapourised, so excised specimen is not available for histopathology, if the lesion is small.

USES

Otology

- Stapedectomy.
- Excision of tumours, like glomus or haemangioma.
- Acoustic neuroma.
- Welding of tympanic membrane graft in tympanoplasty.

Rhinology

- Coanal atresia.
- Haemorrhagic telengiectasis—Osler–Weber–Rendu disease.
- Excision of papilloma, rhinosporidiosis, and adhesions.
- Inferior turbinate resection.
- Vidian neurectomy.

Laryngology

- Juvenile laryngeal papillomatosis.
- Laryngeal webs.
- Laryngeal stenosis.
- Laser arytenoidectomy.
- Stage I and II malignancies of larynx.

Oral cavity

- Excision of
  - Leucoplakia.
  - Malignant growths.
  - Haemangiomas.
- Other surgeries like:
  - Pharyngeal pouch excision.
  - Surgery for tracheal stenosis.
  - Palliation of oesophageal and endobronchial malignancy.

PRECAUTIONS

- To prevent fire due to ignition of anaesthetic gases, the endotracheal tube should be:
  - Metallic or
  - Rubber or portex tube should be covered with aluminium foil.
- Instruments should have dull black finish (to prevent reflection of laser beam).
- Protection of eyes with goggels.
- Special laser room with doors, which lock automatically when laser is in use.

COMPLICATIONS

- Fire hazard due to:
  - Burning of endotracheal tube.
  - Explosion of anaesthetic gases.
- Damage to adjacent tissues by reflected beam.
- Injury to operating personnel.

EAR

Sodium bicarbonate eardrops
- Contents
  - Sodium bicarbonate : 6 g
  - Liquid phenol : 1 mL
  - Glycerine : 50 mL
  - Distilled water diluted to : 100 mL
- Actions: Softens the wax, which can be later removed by aural syringing.
- Uses
  - Impacted wax.
  - Crusts in the external auditory canal (EAC).
- Contraindication: It can never be used in presence of perforated tympanic membrane as it is ototoxic.
- Dose: 2–3 drops 4 times a day for 5–7 days.

Glycerine ichthammol eardrops
- Contents
  - Ichthammol : 12 g
  - Glycerine : 100 mL
- Actions
  - Glycerine, because of its hygroscopic action, reduces the oedema, and hence, pain in EAC.
  - Ichthammol acts as an antiseptic agent when placed in the EAC with a wick of ribbon gauze soaked in it. It helps to immobilise the cartilagenous portion of the EAC and reduce pain.

- Uses
  - Otitis externa.
  - Furunculosis.
  Can be used both as:
  - Eardrops or
  - Used with wick of ribbon gauze, soaked in it, to pack the EAC.
- Dose: Two drops 4 times a day. If wick is inserted in the EAC, it is changed on alternate days.

Gutta boric–spirit eardrops
- Contents
  - Boric acid : 2 g
  - Methylated spirit : 20 mL
  - Distilled water to make : 100 mL
- Actions
  - Antiseptic agent is boric acid.
  - Spirit has an astringent effect. It reduces the aural discharge.
- Uses: Chronic suppurative otitis media (CSOM).
- Dose: Two drops 4 times a day.

Glycerine-phenol eardrops
- Contents
  - Phenol : 2 g
  - Glycerine to make : 100 mL
- Actions
  - Glycerine reduces pain and oedema of inflammation due to its hygroscopic action.
  - Phenol is antiseptic.

- Uses
  - It is not commonly used.
  - It is instilled in acute otitis media prior to the stage of perforation.
  - Otitis externa.
  - Furunculosis.
- Dose: Two drops 4 times a day.

2% salicyclic acid eardrops
- Contents
  - Salicylic acid   : 2 g
  - Spirit   : 10 mL
  - Glycerine to make   : 100 mL
- Action
  - Salicyclic acid creates an acidic medium, which is unfavourable to fungal growth (antifungal action).
  - Spirit has astringent effect, thus, reducing local moisture.
- Uses: It is used in treatment of fungal infection of the ear (otomycosis).
- Dose: Two drops 4 times a day.

Trichloroacetic acid local application
- Contents: 40% trichloroacetic acid.
- Actions: It causes chemical cauterisation.
- Uses
  - Applied with a swab stick soaked in this solution over aural granulations, till blanching occurs for treatment of this condition.
  - Also the edges of a small tympanic membrane perforation, are cauterised with trichloroacetic acid to enable healing.

NOSE

Alkaline nasal douche
- Contents
  - Sodium bicarbonate   : 50 g
  - Sodium biborate   : 50 g
  - Sodium chloride   : 100 g
- Actions
  - Sodium bicarbonate—dissolves crusts.
  - Sodium biborate—antiseptic action.
  - Sodium chloride—makes the solution isotonic.
- Uses
  - It is used in atrophic rhinitis.
  - To clear the nasal cavity of crusts following surgery.
  - In case of nasal maggots (myiasis).
- Dose: Nasal washes 3 times a day with 1 teaspoon of this powder mixed in 1 pint of water. Nasal wash

is given with 20 cc syringe, attached to a red rubber catheter placed along the nasal floor.

Salicylic sulphur ointment
- Contents:
  - Salicylic acid   : 200 mg
  - Sulphur precipitate   : 200 mg
  - Paraffin   : 30 g
- Actions: Antiseptic and emollient.
- Uses: Ointment is applied in the nasal vestibule in the following conditions:
  - Dermatitis.
  - Nasal vestibulitis.

Bismuth–iodine and paraffin paste (BIPP)
- Contents and actions
  - *Bismuth* : Reduces oedema and inflammation by its hygroscopic action.
  - *Iodine*: Antiseptic action.
  - *Paraffin*: Emollient-lubricates the nasal cavity.
- Uses
  - Used for packing the nose with a gauze impregnated with this paste.
  - For packing the abscess cavity after inscision and drainage of mastoid abscess (BIPP pack).

PHARYNX/THROAT

Condy's gargles
- Content: Potassium permanganate crystals in distilled water in 1: 4000 ratio.
- Actions
  - Antiseptic.
  - For soothing local area of infection.
- Uses: For gargling in the following conditions:
  - Acute tonsillitis.
  - Chronic tonsillitis.
  - Post-tonsillectomy.
  - Pharyngitis.
  - Apthous ulcer.
  - After surgery in oral cavity, e.g. cleft palate.
  - After tooth removal.
  - After nasal surgery to prevent halitosis as patient breathes through the mouth.
- Dose: 1 tablespoon of the crystals in one pint of distilled water for mouth wash and gargles.

Mandl's throat paint
- Contents:
  - Iodine   : 1.25 g
  - Potassium Iodide   : 2.50 g
  - Distilled water   : 2.50 mL

- ◆ Oil of peppermint   :   0.60 mL
- ◆ Glycerine to make   :   100 mL
- Actions
  - ◆ Antiseptic.
  - ◆ Local soothing action.
- Uses
  - ◆ Granular pharyngitis.
  - ◆ Aphthous ulcers.
- Dose: Local application twice a day to the posterior pharyngeal wall with 2–3 swab sticks.

1% gentian violet
- Contents: 1% gentian violet.
- Actions: Antifungal.
- Uses: It is used as a local mucosal paint on a swab stick in case of fungal infections of the ear, nose, or oral cavity.

Tincture benzoin compound
- Contents: Compound of 1% tincture benzoin. 30 drops of compound of tincture benzoin is put in 1 litre of hot water and vapours are inhaled.
- Actions:
  - ◆ Humidifies the inhaled air.
  - ◆ Helps to liquify secretions and prevents crusting.
  - ◆ Local soothing effect.
- Uses: It is used as an inhaling agent in
  - ◆ Acute and chronic laryngitis.
  - ◆ Acute and chronic sinusitis.
  - ◆ After nasal surgery when nose is packed to humidify the inhaled air.
  - ◆ Patients on tracheostomy.
- Doses: Inhalation 3 times a day.

NOSE AND PARANASAL SINUSES

WATER'S VIEW (OCCIPITO-MENTAL)

The patient sits facing the X-ray plate with his nose and chin touching the plate. The head is extended till a position, where the orbito-meatal line makes an angle of 45 with the plate (horizontal plane) (Fig. 51.1).

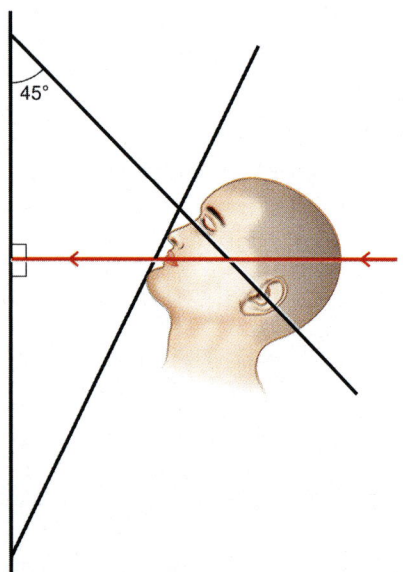

45°

Fig. 51.1: Position of the patient and X-ray beam for an X-ray PNS—Water's view

The various structures seen are:
- Maxillary sinuses on either side of the nasal cavities,
- Nasal septum,
- Frontal sinuses,
- Ethmoid cells,
- Sphenoid sinus through open mouth in water's view taken with mouth open,
- The odontoid process just below the mentum. This confirms adequate extension of the head.

Inference

- **Normal:** The odontoid process lies exactly below the mentum. The maxillary sinuses are seen as radiolucent cavities on either side of the nasal cavities. To label a maxillary sinus as pathological, it has to be more radio-opaque as compared to the orbit. Normal maxillary sinus is as radiolucent as the orbit.

- **Maxillary sinusitis:** A characteristic homogenous ground-glass haziness (radio-opacity) of the sinus is seen. The mucosa may show a soft tissue thickening in the antrum in chronic sinusitis. A fluid level is seen sometimes which has a concave superior margin. The final confirmation of the presence of fluid in antrum is done by repeating the X-ray in the lying down position which will result in obliteration of the fluid level (Fig. 51.2 A to I).

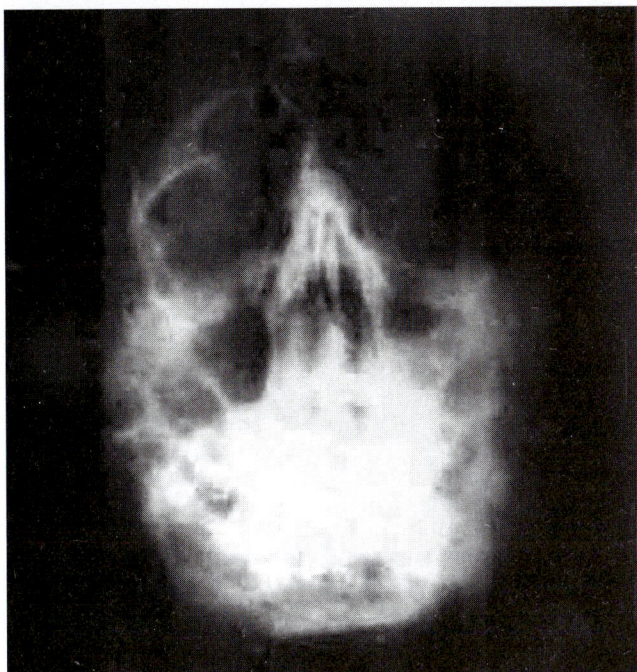

Fig. 51.2A: X-ray paranasal sinuses—Water's view: Both the maxillary sinuses show a characteristic 'ground-glass' haziness with a concave upper border indicating an air-fluid level which is characteristic of acute maxillary sinusitis or blood in the maxillary antrum following trauma. The frontal sinuses are normal

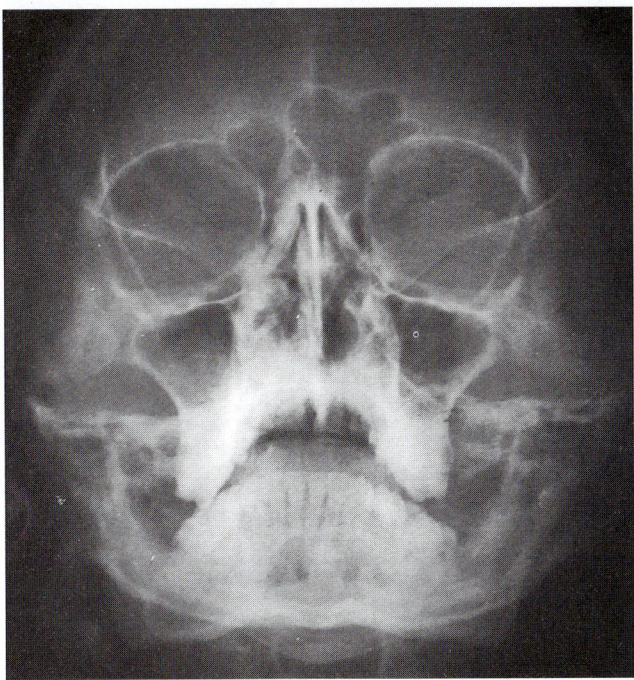

Fig. 51.2C: X-ray paranasal sinuses—Water's view showing evidence of soft tissue opacification in the right maxillary sinus with a convex upper margin, suggestive of a polyp/retention cyst in the right maxillary sinus

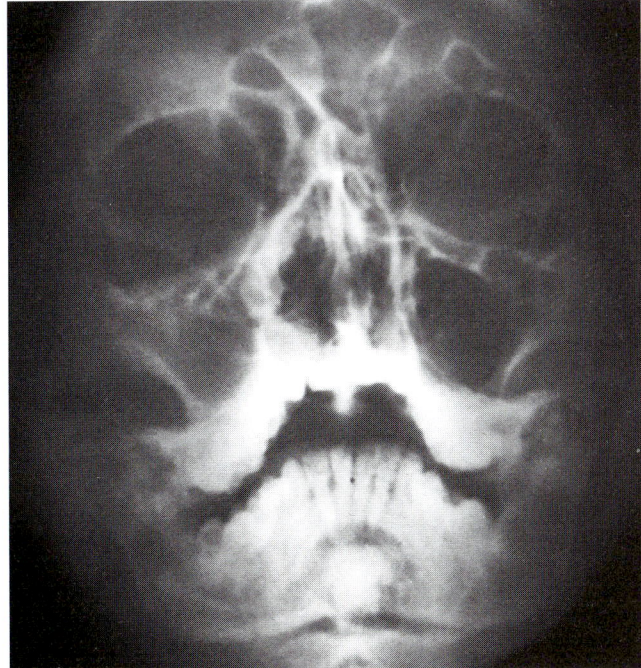

Fig. 51.2B: X-ray paranasal sinuses—Water's view showing complete opacification of the right maxillary sinus suggestive of right maxillary sinusitis

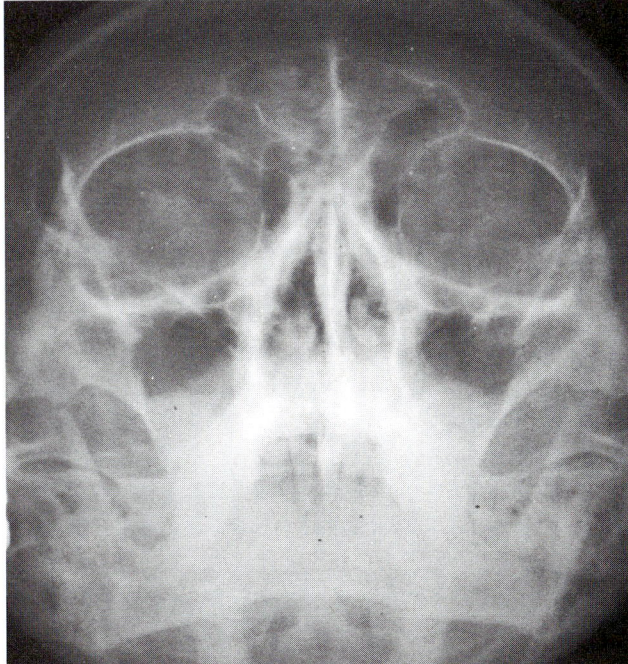

Fig. 51.2D: X-ray paranasal sinuses—Water's view showing bilateral maxillary polyps/retention cysts

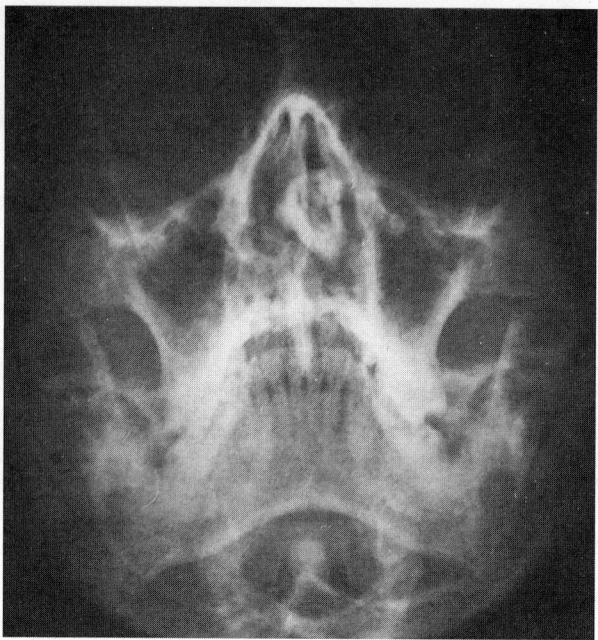

Fig. 51.2E: X-ray paranasal sinuses—Water's view showing a radio-opaque shadow in the nasal cavity suggestive of a rhinolith

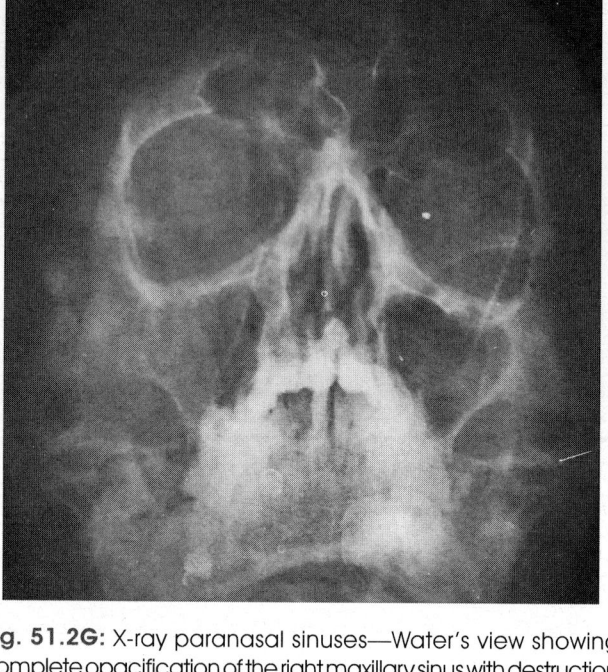

Fig. 51.2G: X-ray paranasal sinuses—Water's view showing complete opacification of the right maxillary sinus with destruction of its anterolateral wall suggestive of a malignancy involving the right maxillary sinus

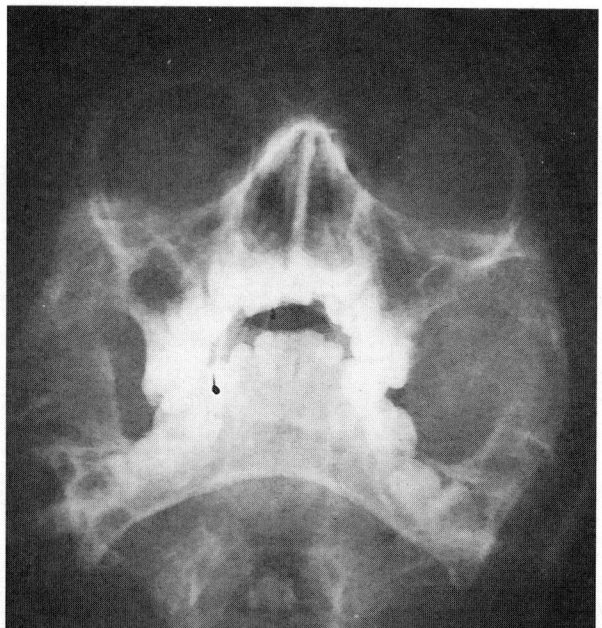

Fig. 51.2F: X-ray paranasal sinuses—Water's view showing opacification of the left maxillary sinus, with an increased distance between the anterolateral wall of the left maxilla and the coronoid process of the mandible on the left side (as compared to the right). This is a positive Handousa's sign suggestive of a mass in the infratemporal fossa (in this case probably arising from the maxillary sinus)

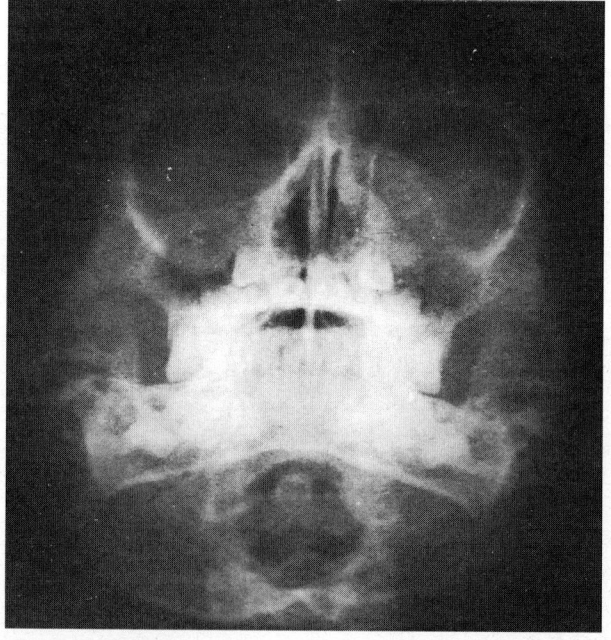

Fig. 51.2H: X-ray paranasal sinuses—Water's view showing ground glass haziness involving the left laxillary sinus and extending towards the left orbit and zygoma, suggestive of fibrous dysplasia

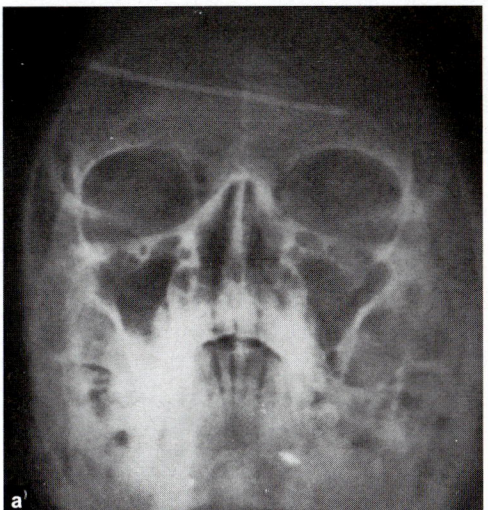
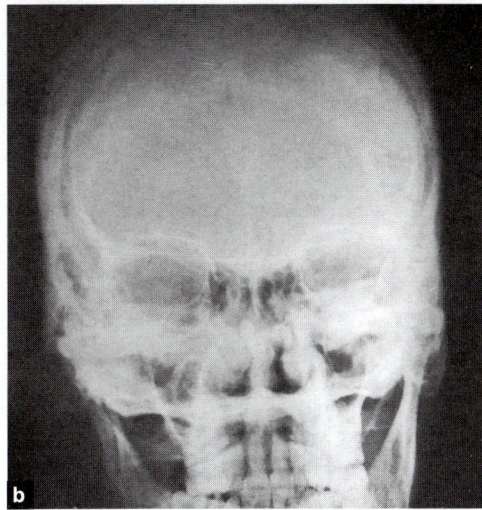

Fig. 51.2I: (a) X-ray paranasal sinuses—Water's view and (b) X-ray paranasal sinuses—Caldwell's view showing aplasia of the frontal sinuses

- Polyp: A soft tissue density shadow is seen in the maxillary sinus. The upper margin of this soft-tissue density shadow is convex. A repeat X-ray on lying down shows no shift in opacity.
- Malignancy: Heterogenous opacity of the entire sinus is seen. Destruction of the walls of the maxillary sinus is diagnostic of malignancy. The distance between the antero-lateral wall of the maxilla and the coronoid process of the mandible is measured. Increased distance on one side suggests widening of the infratemporal fossa due to involvement by the tumour (Handousa's sign positive).

CALDWELL'S VIEW (OCCIPITO-FRONTAL)

The patient is sitting up with his nose and forehead touching the X-ray plate and the X-ray beam makes an angle of 20° with the orbito-meatal line (Fig. 51.3A, B and C).

The various structures seen are:
- Frontal sinus,
- Ethmoid sinus,
- Orbits.

Nasal septum and the nasal cavities on either side.

Inference
- Normal: The normal frontal sinus is similar to the orbit in radiolucency. There is no constant pattern of pneumatisation. Therefore, there is an individual variation in size, shape and asymmetry of the paired sinuses, this should not be taken for a pathological state. Normally, the frontal sinus shows a radiolucent

shadow and individual cells are seen, giving it a scalloping (clove-like) appearance. Aplasia of the frontal sinuses is seen in kartagener's syndrome (with bronchiectasis and dextrocardia).

- Chronic frontal sinusitis: Characteristic 'Ground-glass' opacity of the frontal sinuses is seen with absence of normal scalloping. This is also seen with a mucocoele or pyocoele which is a complication of chronic frontal sinusitis.

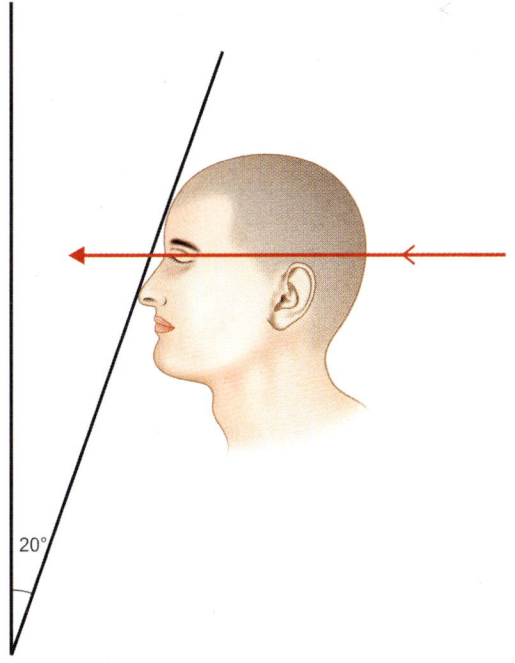

Fig. 51.3A: Position of the patient and X-ray beam for an X-ray PNS—Caldwell's view

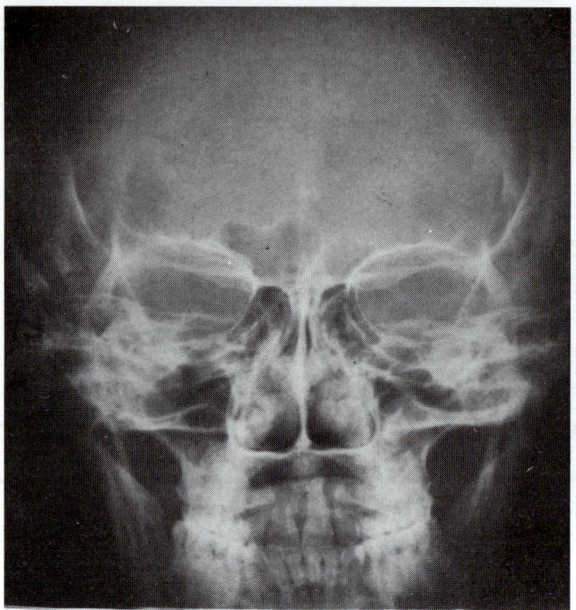

Fig. 51.3B: X-ray of the paranasal sinuses in the occipito-frontal view (Caldwell's view). Note that the frontal sinuses are usually asymmetrical

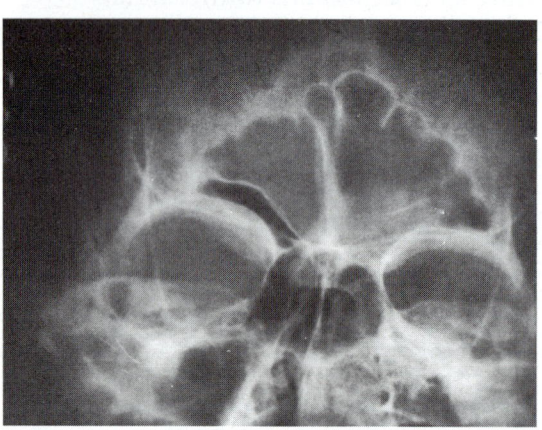

Fig. 51.3C: X-ray of the paranasal sinuses in the occipito-frontal view (Caldwell's view). Well pneumatised frontal sinuses usually show a scalloping appearance, which may be lost in mucoceles or tumours

- Osteoma: It appears as a well-defined opacity in the frontal sinus. The patient is usually asymptomatic and the finding is coincidental. An X-ray lateral view of the skull gives an idea of the exact extent of the osteoma. Gardener's syndrome (inherited as an autosomal dominant trait) comprises of osteomas, soft tissue masses and multiple colonic polypi.
- Pneumatization: Hypopneumatization of the frontal sinuses is seen in severe erythroblastic anaemia. Hyperpneumatization is seen in Sturge-Weber disease and acromegaly.

X-RAY MASTOID SCHULLER'S VIEW

The patient lies in the lateral position with the side to be radiographed in contact with the X-ray plate. The X-ray beam is directed at an angle of 30 to prevent overlap of the other mastoid bone. The internal auditory meatus overlaps with the external auditory meatus on the same side. In a lateral X-ray of the skull there is no angulation. This angulation of 30 enables us to visualise each mastoid process clearly. Left and right mastoids are taken separately (Fig. 51.4).

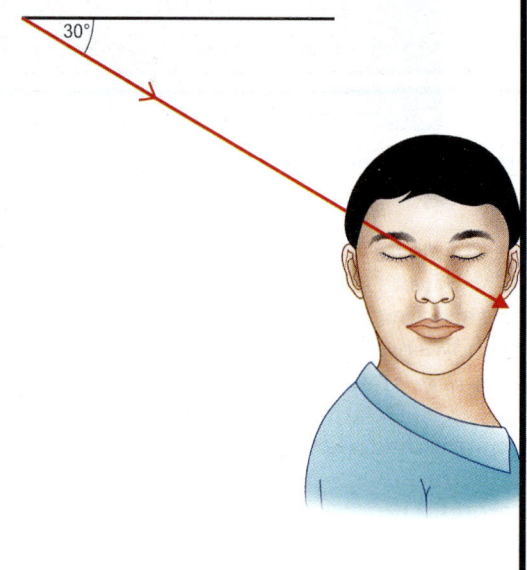

Fig. 51.4: Position of the patient and X-ray beam for an X-ray—mastoid-Schuller's view

Structures seen are:
- External auditory canal overlapping the internal auditory canal,
- Attico-antral region ('key-area' of the mastoid),
- Mastoid air cells,
- Dural plate,
- Sinus plate,
- Sino-dural angle,
- Dense bone of the labyrinth,
- Temporo-mandibular joint of the same side.

Types of mastoid
- Pneumatic mastoid: Air cells are seen filling the entire mastoid bone and also occassionally extending beyond the limits of the dural plate and sinus plate. Almost 80% of normal ears have a pneumatic mastoid (as seen in the X-ray).
- Sclerotic mastoid: There is an absence of air cells. The entire mastoid process is sclerotic (with marked

opacity) and small in size. This is a common feature in chronic otitis media. Sometimes, it is also seen in approx. 20% normal patients.

- Diploeic mastoid is characterised by presence of few air cells in the mastoid with areas of sclerosis.
- Mastoid with radiolucent cavity: Here a single radiolucent shadow is seen in an otherwise sclerotic

mastoid. To arrive at an accurate diagnosis, a clinical examination of the patient is required.

Differential diagnosis of radiolucent cavity in the mastoid
- Cholesteatoma (edges of the cavity are shaggy and irregular) (Figs 51.5–51.7)
- Operated mastoid cavity (edges of the cavity are usually smooth and regular),

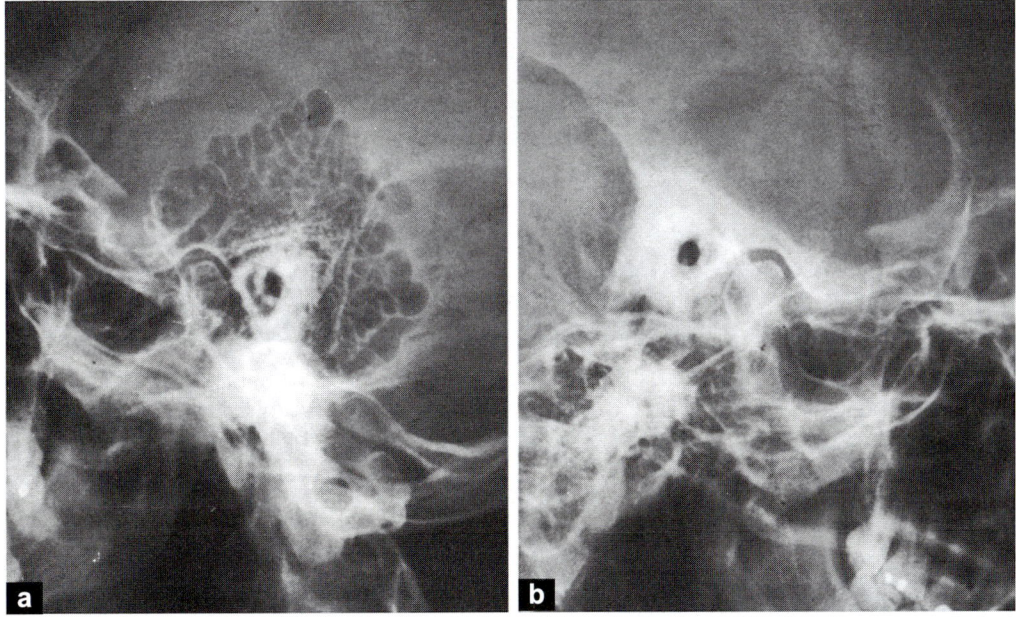

Fig. 51.5A: X-ray mastoid-Schuller's view showing (a) a pneumatised left mastoid and (b) sclerotic right mastoid

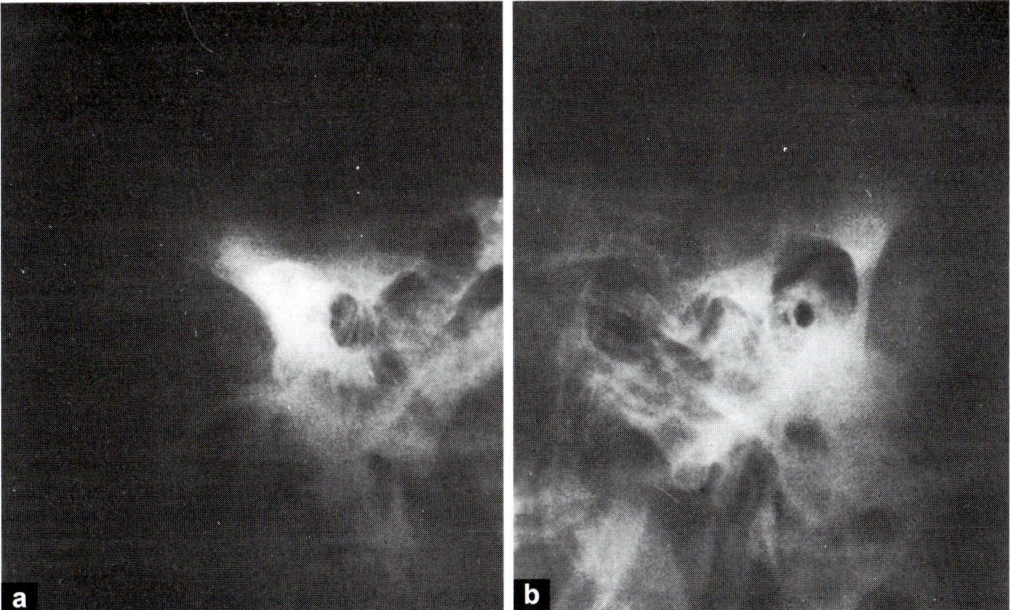

Fig. 51.5B: X-ray mastoid-Schuller's view showing (a) a radiolucent shadow in the left mastoid, with smooth walls and (b) no evidence of bony sclerosis, indicative of a postoperative cavity of a well performed mastoidectomy. Note the sclerosis of the right mastoid

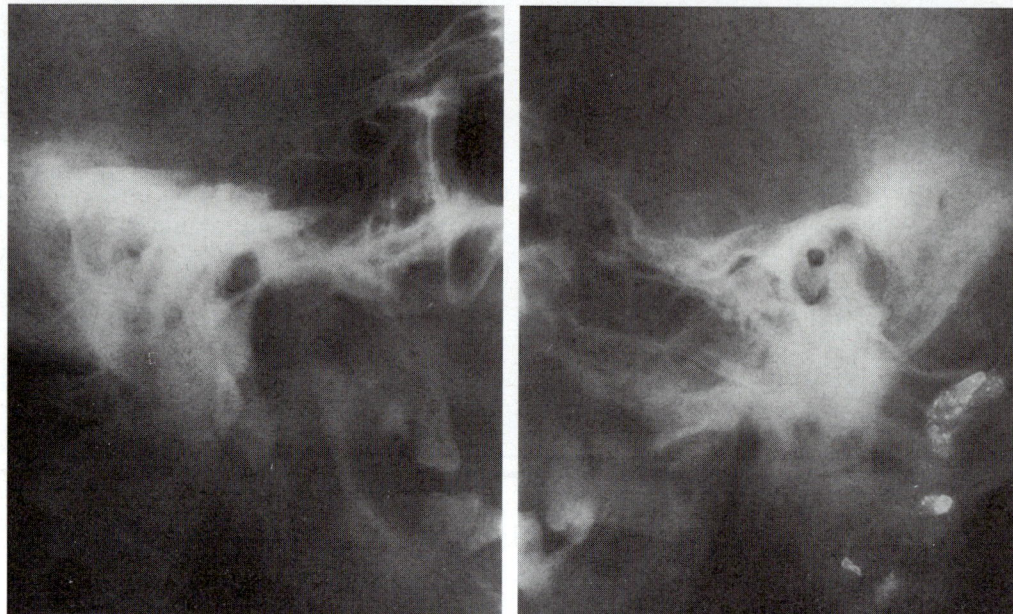

Fig. 51.6: X-ray mastoid-Schuller's view showing a radiolucent shadow in the left mastoid, with irregular walls showing bony sclerosis, with loss of integrity of the sinus plate suggestive of cholesteatoma/granulations/recurrent cholesteatoma after mastoidectomy/ poorly performed mastoidectomy cavity (D/D of an irregular/shaggy walled radiolucent shadow). Incidentally note the radiolucent shadow on the right side as well

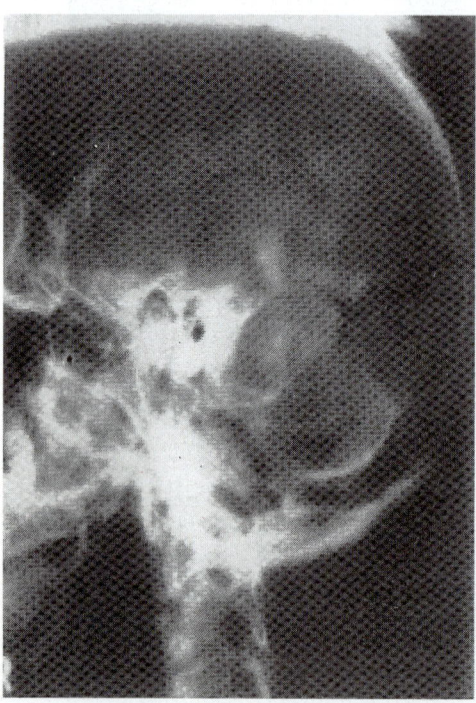

Fig. 51.7: X-ray mastoid-Schuller's view (right side) : The mastoid is sclerotic with a radiolucent shadow at the sinodural angle which is irregular and suggestive of cholesteatoma, granulations, etc. (D/D of radiolucent shadow in mastoid antrum)

- Large antral air cell,
- Large periantral air cell,
- Chronic mastoiditis with granulations,
- Eosinophilic granuloma,
- Tuberculoma or Tuberculous mastoiditis,
- Malignancy of the mastoid,
- Multiple myeloma,
- Secondary metastasis from malignancy of kidney, bronchus, breast, etc.

FRACTURE NASAL BONES

The patient sits erect and the X-ray beam is directed towards the root of the nose from the lateral aspect of the head. If the fragments are displaced, a reduction of the fracture is required. In the absence of dislocation, only a splint is required. (Figs 51.8 and 51.9) (Treatment of fracture nasal bones is described in Chapter 54)

X-RAY SOFT TISSUE NASOPHARYNX (LATERAL VIEW)

Normally the nasopharynx is occupied by air and hence seen as a radiolucent shadow postero-superior to the soft palate.

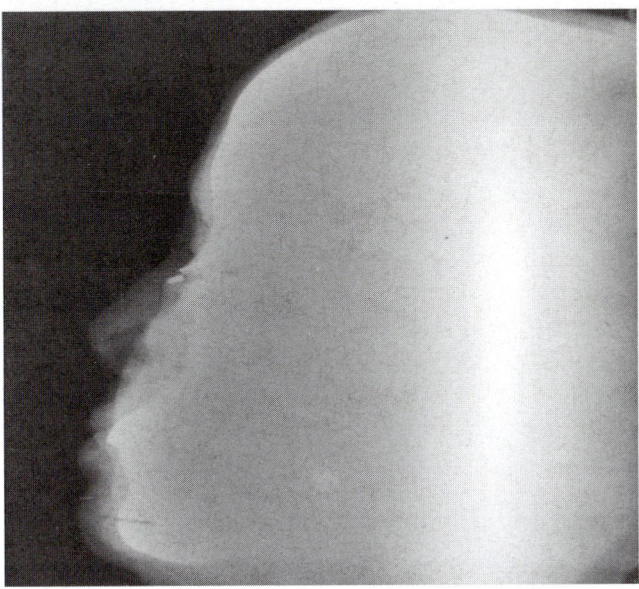

Fig. 51.8: X-ray nasal bone showing a depressed (dislocated) fracture of the nasal bones

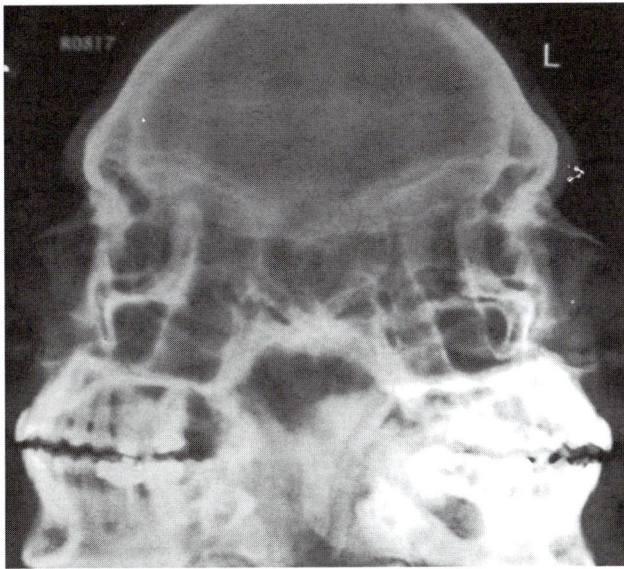

Fig. 51.9: X-ray of the nasal bones showing a fracture involving only the outer table of the nasal bone (akin to greenstick fractures)

- Obliteration of the air shadow anteriorly occurs with an antrochoanal polyp or a nasal mass as it extends into the nasopharynx from the choanae anteriorly. The air shadow is reduced to a small shadow around the free margin of the polyp (Crescent sign).
- Obliteration of the radiolucent shadow posteriorly is seen in the presence of adenoids (in children) or nasopharyngeal carcinoma (in adults) since both of them arise from the posterior wall and roof of nasopharynx.

X-RAY SOFT TISSUE NECK (LATERAL VIEW)

The diagnosis of a retropharyngeal abscess is made by (Figs 51.10–51.17):

- Marked increase in the area of the prevertebral space; i.e. it is more than three-fourths the size of the body of the vertebra.
- Air-fluid level—normally the retropharyngeal space is a collapsed structure not containing any air, hence presence of air indicates abscess.
- Loss of normal curvature of the cervical spine leading to straightening of the spine. This is due to reflex spasm of the prevertebral muscles occurring secondary to a retropharyngeal abscess.

Once the diagnosis is made, the vertebrae are seen for destruction of their bodies (tuberculous caries). Also the presence of any foreign body is to be ruled out. The commonest causes of retropharyngeal abscess are Koch's spine and foreign body in the pharynx (adults), or secondary to dental and tonsillar infection (children) (retropharyngeal abscess is described in detail in Chapter 34).

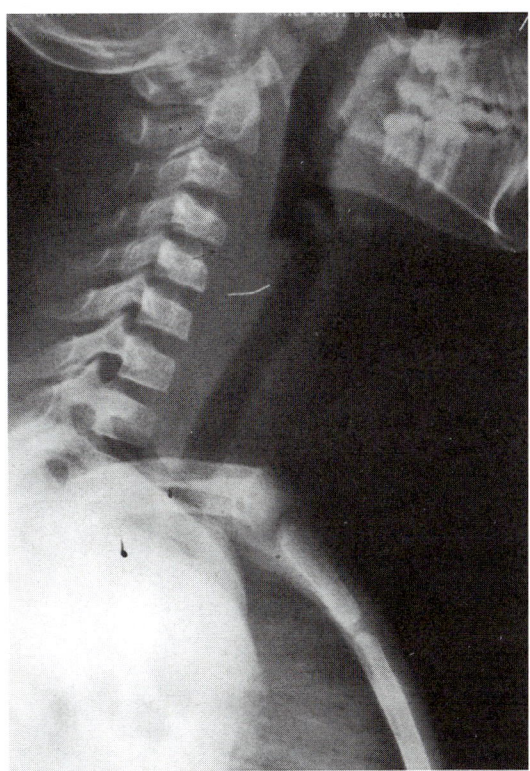

Fig. 51.10: Lateral X-ray of the cervical spine showing widening of the pre-vertebral soft tissue shadow, loss of cervical lordosis, and a sharp radio-opaque shadow indenting the prevertebral shadow, suggestive of a foreign body, which is the probable cause of the retropharyngeal abscess

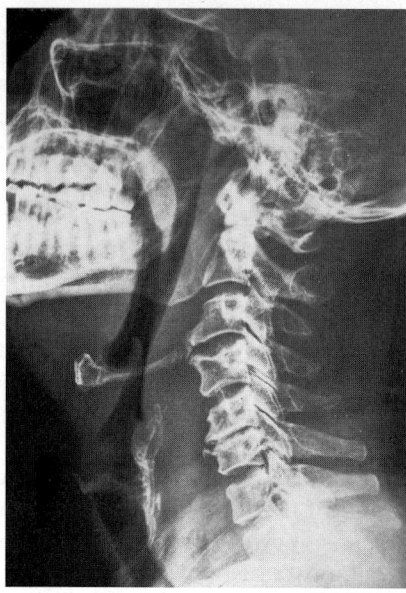

Fig. 51.11: Lateral X-ray of the cervical spine showing a retro-pharyngeal abscess caused due to tuberculosis of the spine. Note the advanced cervical spondylosis, osteophytes, erosion of the vertebral bodies, and collapse of the intervertebral disc space between C5 and C6

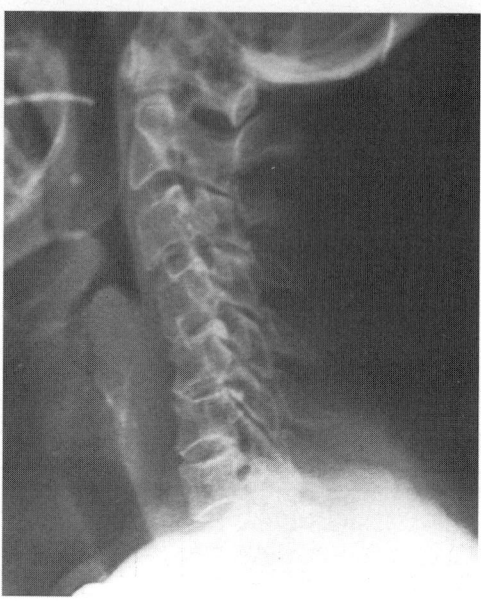

Fig. 51.13: Lateral X-ray of the cervical spine in a child showing thickening of the epiglottis (thumb sign) suggestive of acute epiglottitis. Note the straightening of the spine and forward protrusion of the head as the child displays air hunger

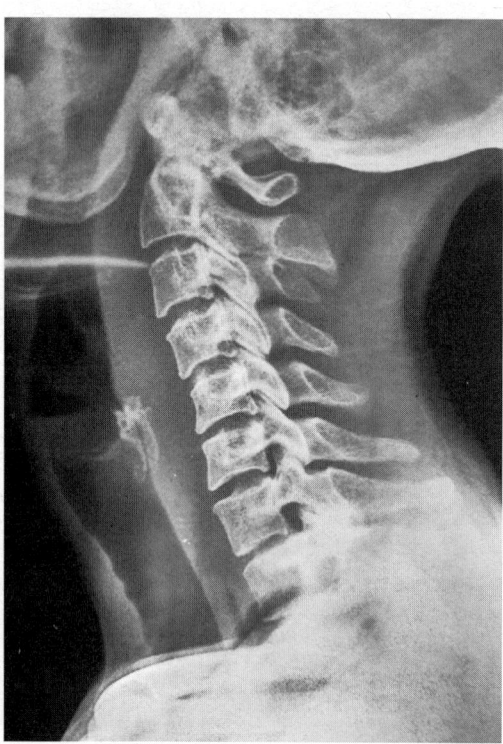

Fig. 51.12: Lateral X-ray of the cervical spine showing a minimal increase of the prevertebral soft tissue shadow, with marked loss of the normal cervical lordosis. This is a case of an early retropharyngeal abscess

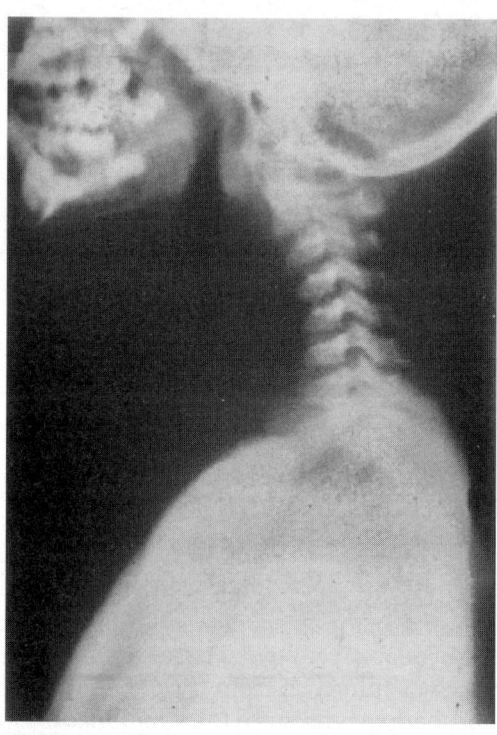

Fig. 51.14: X-ray of the soft tissues of the neck—lateral view: There is a widening of the soft tissues in front of the cervical spine with loss of normal curvature of the cervical spine (straightening). The vertebral bodies appear normal. This is diagnostic of a retropharyngeal abscess. The cervical spine is straightened due to spasm of the paravertebral muscles

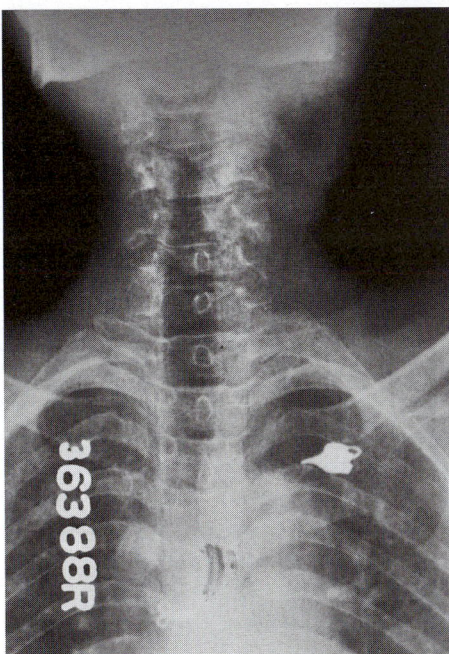

Fig. 51.15: Antero-posterior X-ray of the cervical spine showing a smooth narrowing of the airway shadow (steeple sign) in a case of acute laryngo-tracheobronchitis (croup). Note the air shadow below the mandible, suggestive of ballooning of the hypopharynx, which is commonly seen in these conditions due to excessive air intake by the child in an attempt to compensate for the narrowed airway

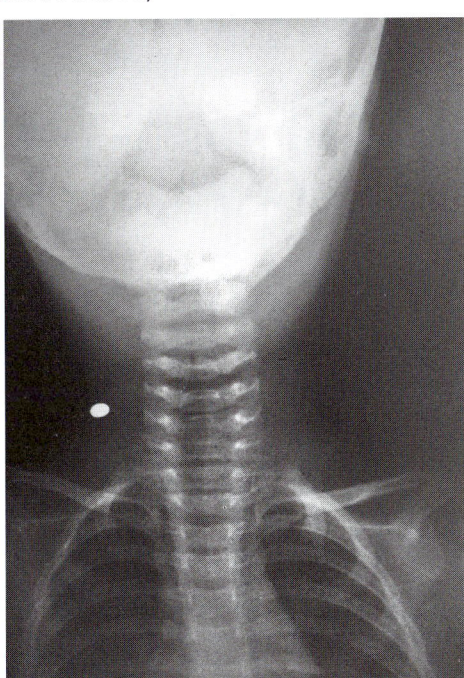

Fig. 51.16: Antero-posterior X-ray of the cervical spine in another case of croup, showing a more pronounced 'steeple sign' as compared to the previous X-ray

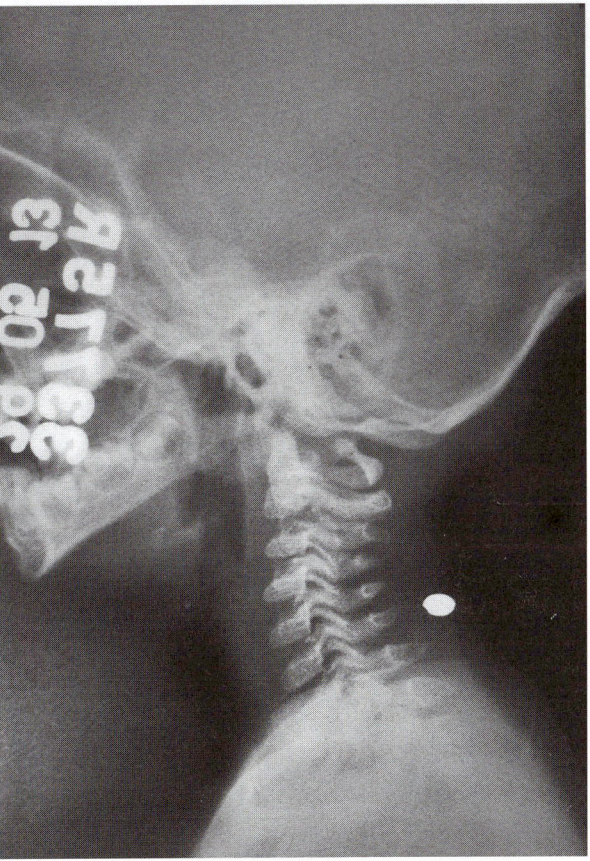

Fig. 51.17: Lateral X-ray of the same patient as in above, showing the ballooning of the hypopharynx

RADIOGRAPHS OF BARIUM SWALLOW

Radiographs of barium shallow are shown in **Figs 51.18–51.26).**

ACHALASIA CARDIA (CARDIOSPASM)

The following features are seen:
- Smooth and marked dilatation of the oesophagus,
- Fluid level in lumen,
- Abrupt stricture formation,
- No shouldering effect or rat-tail appearance,
- On administering methacholine, reverse peristalsis is seen.

One must also note that on plain X-ray of chest and abdomen the following features are seen:
- Presence of an air-fluid level in the oesophagus,
- Regular and marked dilatation of the oesophagus,
- Absence of air shadow in the fundus of the stomach,
- Lung abscess may be present due to aspiration,
- Mediastinal widening in late cases.

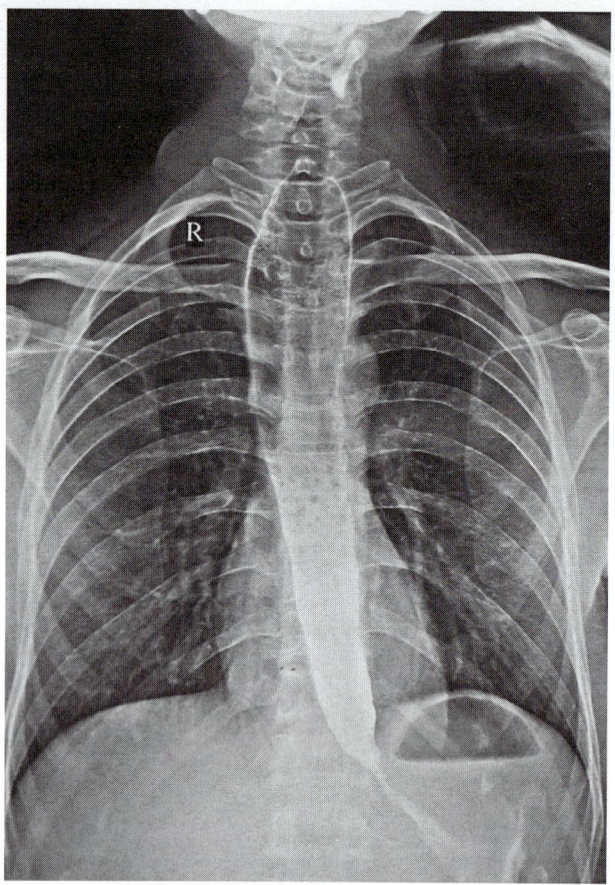

Fig. 51.18: Barium swallow showing another case of achalasia cardia with a narrowing of the distal oesophagus, with a smooth fusiform dilatation of the proximal part

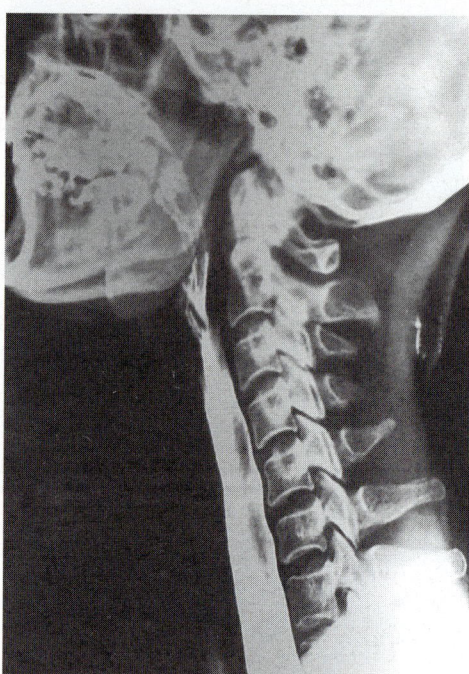

Fig. 51.19: Lateral view of a barium swallow showing a patient with loss of cervical lordosis and osteophytes, suggestive of cervical spondylosis, with multiple indentations of the oesophageal shadow. This is a case of 'cervical dysphagia'

OESOPHAGEAL VARICES

The following features are seen:
- Irregular filling defects, appearing like a 'string of pearls',
- Mainly seen in the lower one-third of the oesophagus,
- There is no evidence of any obstruction.

OESOPHAGEAL STRICTURES

The strictures of the oesophagus on a barium swallow can be classified as benign or malignant.

Benign strictures
- Multiple in number.
- Usually at the sites of the normal constrictions of the oesophagus.
- Mucosal regularity is maintained.
- Marked proximal dilatation of the oesophagus.

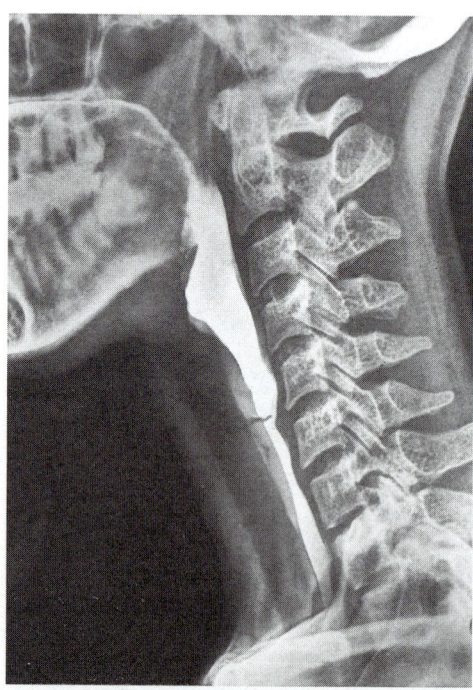

Fig. 51.20: Lateral view of a barium swallow in another case of cervical dysphagia, with an abrupt cut off of the barium shadow anteriorly at the level of C5 vertebra, with a normal barium shadow proximal and distal to it, suggestive of a cervical web

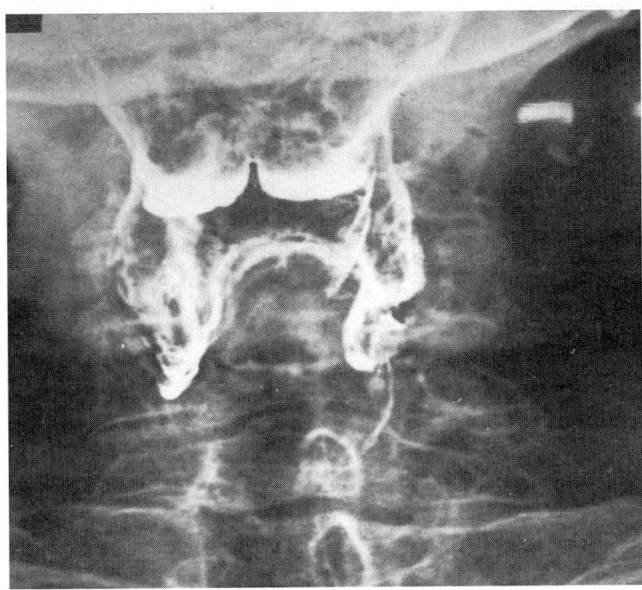

Fig. 51.21: Barium swallow of a patient, showing a filling defect in the lateral wall of the left pyriform fossa, as well as an apparent shortening (amputation) of the left pyriform fossa as compared to the right side, suggestive of a mass/growth in the left pyriform fossa

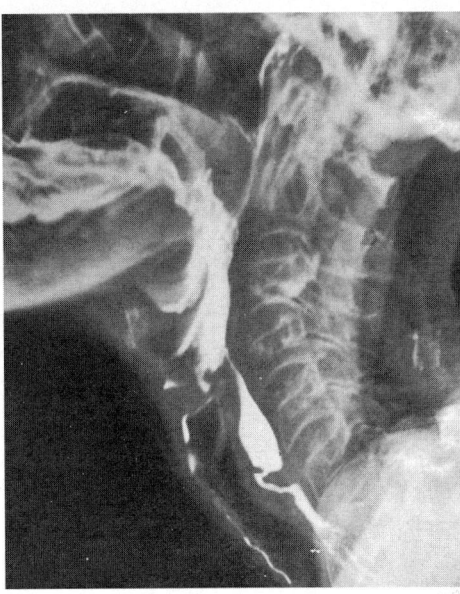

Fig. 51.22: Lateral view of a barium swallow of a patient showing a circumferential narrowing of the cricopharynx with an irregular outline at the level of C5 and C6, suggestive of a growth in the cricopharynx. Note the spillover of the barium into the airway, causing an outlining of the airway, suggestive of aspiration, which is probably due to the inability of the cricopharynx to allow food to pass through

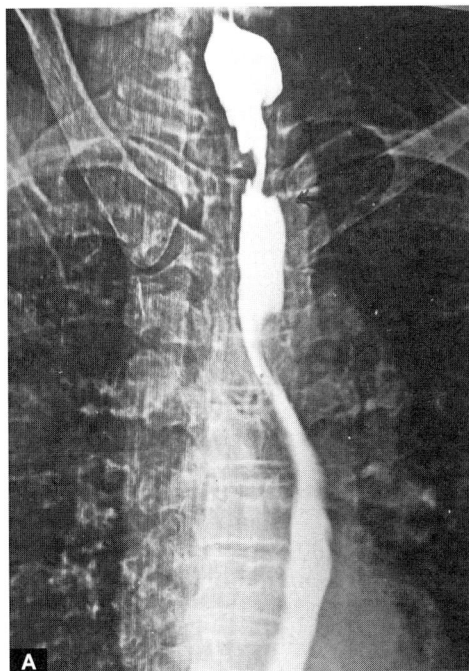

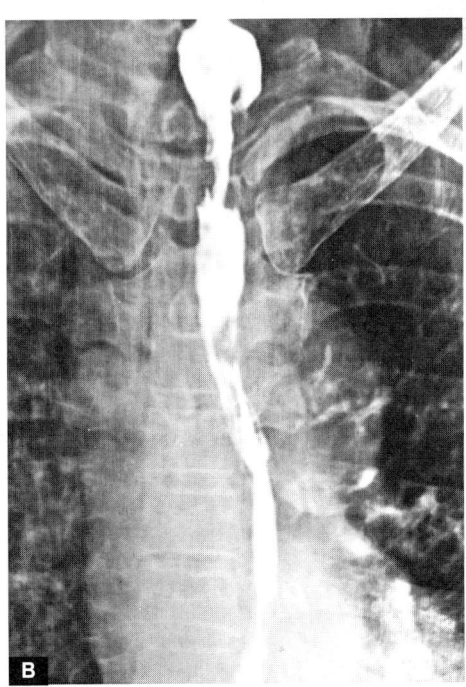

Fig. 51.23A and B: Barium swallow of a patient showing an 'apple core' appearance with a filling defect suggestive of a growth in the oesophagus

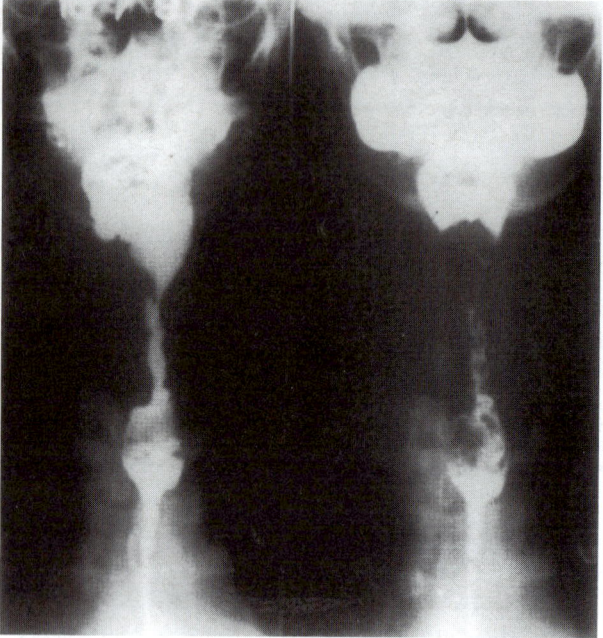

Fig. 51.24: Barium swallow showing the presence of a narrowing and irregularity ('apple-core appearance') in the smooth flow of barium in the upper one-third of the oesophagus with a 'shouldering defect' characteristic of a malignant stricture of the oesophagus

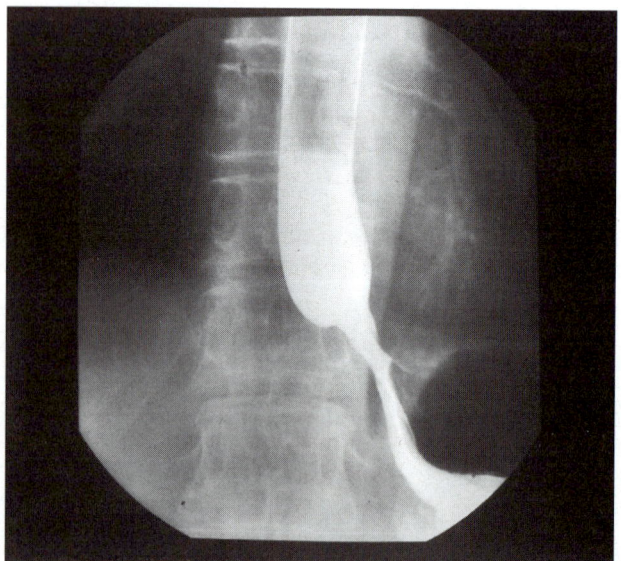

Fig. 51.25: Barium swallow of a patient showing an abrupt cut off of the barium shadow in the distal oesophagus, with a trickle of barium through the distal segment. This may represent either a normal peristaltic wave, or a growth in the distal oesophagus. Viewing serial/dynamic images will rule out the former, as the obstruction would not be fixed at one place, while a 'fixed' obstruction, with an irregular margin of the distal segment would suggest the latter (as is in this case) (Rat-tail appearance)

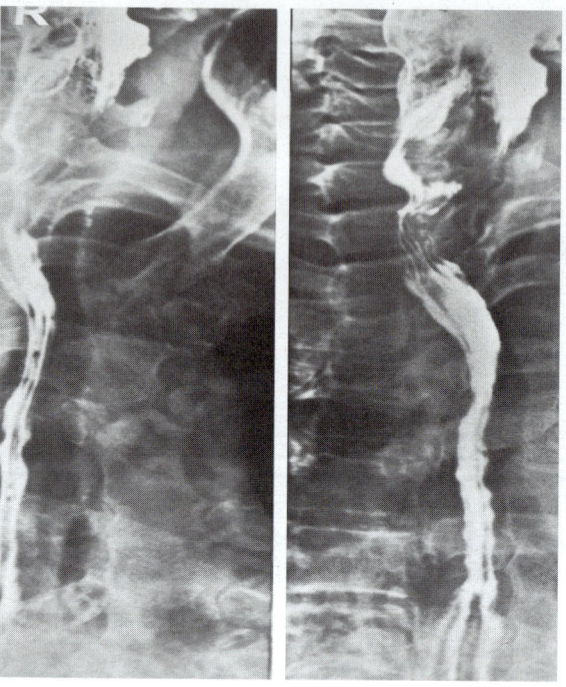

Fig. 51.26: Barium swallow of a patient showing multiple 'worm like' shadows/filling defects in the distal oesophagus, suggestive of oesophageal varices

Malignant stricture

- Usually single.
- Occurs at any site in the oesophagus.
- Mucosa appears irregular.
- No proximal dilatation is seen because of submucosal infiltration by the malignant tumour.
- 'Shouldering effect' is seen due to everted margins of a malignant ulcer causing an acute angle of the barium outline.
- 'Rat-tail' appearance is seen as the oesophangeal lumen becomes very narrow and only a thin streak of barium can pass through it.
- 'Apple-Core Appearance' is the term used to describe an extremely narrow and irregular stricture of the oesophagus with normal mucosa above and below.

OESOPHAGEAL FOREIGN BODIES

The commonest oesophageal foreign bodies (FB) are coins, marbles, or traumatic foreign bodies like a denture or pin (Figs 51.27–51.32).

The most common sites for lodgement are the normal constrictions of the oesophagus and radio-opaque foreign bodies can be seen easily in the plain antero-posterior (AP) and lateral views of neck and chest. An

AP and lateral view are both required in all cases as they help to confirm site of FB (trachea or oesophagus), shape of FB (coin or marble) and presence or absence of second FB.

Coin   They occupy a classical transverse position in the lumen of the oesophagus. This is due to the fact that the transverse diameter of the cricopharynx is much greater than the antero-posterior diameter. Therefore on an AP view of the neck-chest, the whole coin can be seen as a smooth round radio-opaque shadow.

A lateral X-ray is also taken to confirm the exact position of the foreign body and also to rule out a second foreign body if overlapping the first. On a lateral X-ray a vertical slit-like radio-opacity is seen. A foreign body which remains stationary for at least 6 hours is removed by oesophagoscopy which is performed under general anaesthesia.

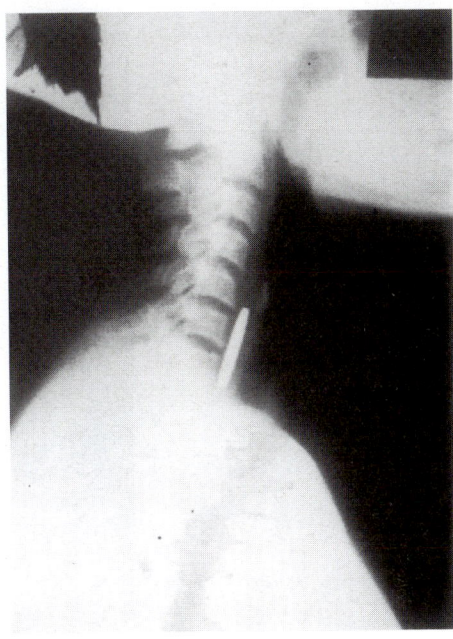

Fig. 51.28: X-ray neck and chest—lateral view showing a smooth flat radio-opaque shadow in the cervical oesophagus lying anterior to the C6 and C7 vertebral bodies and posterior to the tracheal air-shadow. This indicates the presence of this foreign body in the oesophagus at the level of the cricopharynx. When compared to the X-ray in Fig. 51.33. The FB seems to be a coin

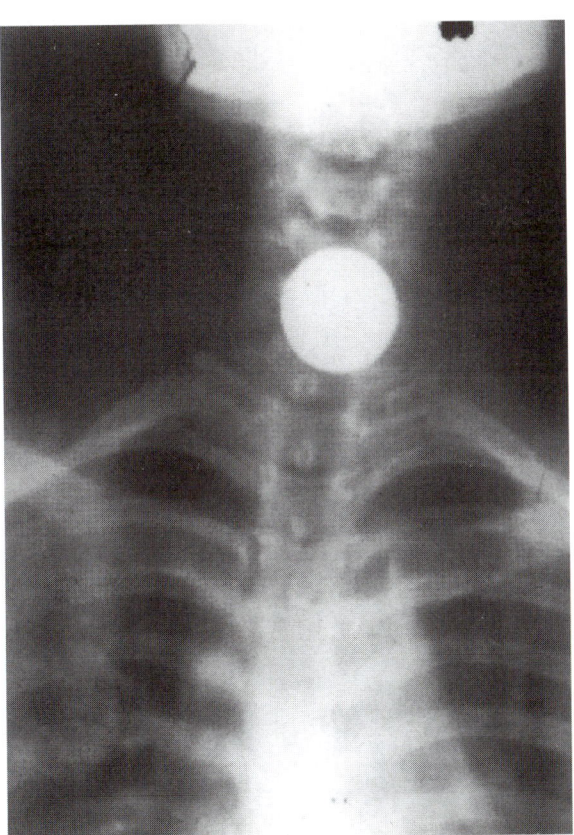

Fig. 51.27: X-ray neck and chest-AP view showing a smooth, circular, radio-opaque shadow in the neck indicative of a foreign body in the oesophagus or trachea. A lateral view is required for the following reasons: i) to know the site, ii) to know the shape of the FB (circular or spherical). iii) To know the number of foreign bodies since two FB of same shape may overlap each other in AP axis giving impression of only one FB. This is most important to decide the method of its removal

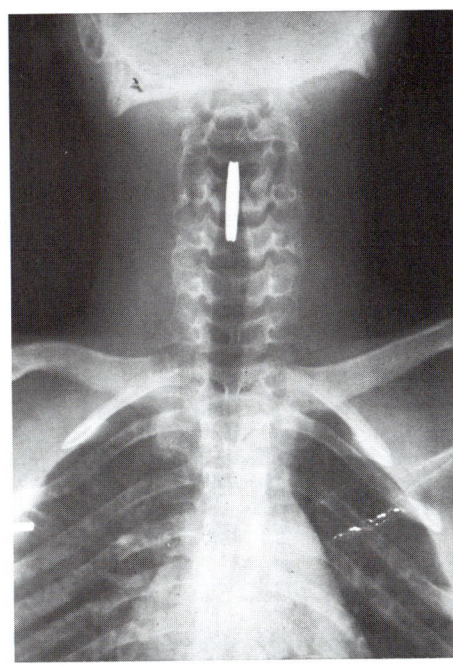

Fig. 51.29: Antero-posterior X-ray of the neck showing a smooth slit like radioopaque shadow suggestive of a foreign body in the oesophagus or trachea. The lateral view of the neck is mandatory to ascertain the site, shape, orientation and number of foreign bodies

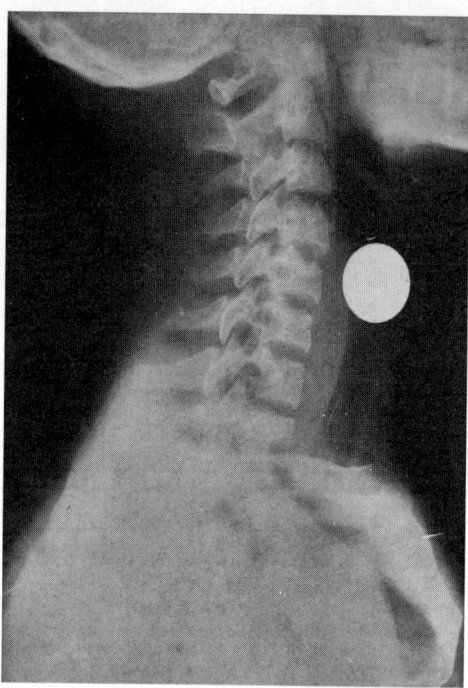

Fig. 51.30: The lateral view of the neck of the same patient reveals that the foreign body is circular and within the air shadow of the trachea. In addition, the orientation of the circular foreign body in the anteroposterior plane suggests that it is in the larynx/trachea and not in the oesophagus/pharynx

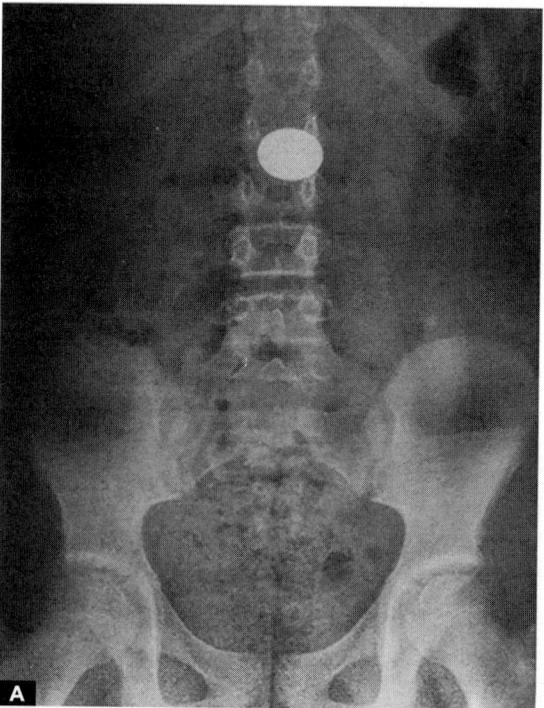

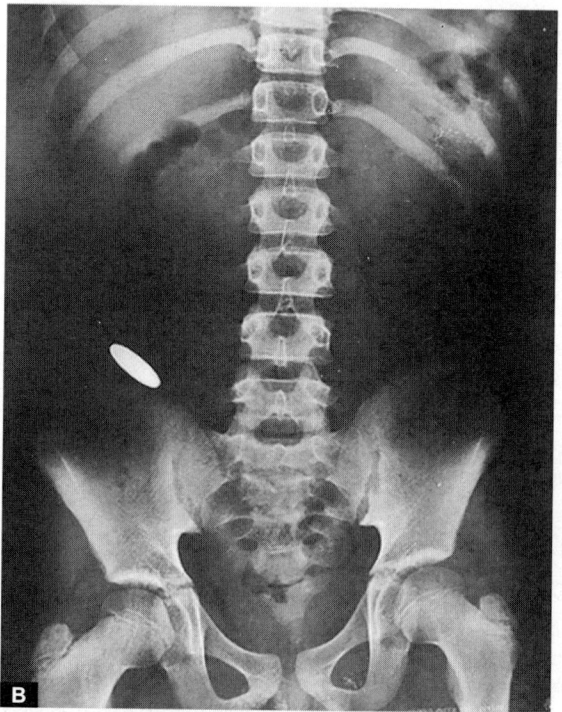

Fig. 51.31: It is always advisable to repeat the X-ray of a foreign body just prior to the planned removal. Often, it is seen that smooth foreign bodies such as coins migrate beyond the cricopharynx into the distal digestive tract. Usually once they have negotiated the cricopharyngeal sphincter (which is the narrowest part of the digestive tract) they tend to be passed out with the faeces. These two X-rays depict the presence of the foreign body in the (A) stomach and (B) colon.

Marble   It is seen as a radio-opaque shadow which is less dense as compared to a coin. On both AP and lateral X-ray film a smooth round foreign body is seen. This foreign body, requires to be removed only if it remains stationary (i.e. it stays at the same site on a repeat X-ray). A Foley's Catheter is passed distal to the foreign body then the balloon is inflated and the catheter is pulled out along with the marble. Also, a dormia basket may be used for its removal. A forceps is not used as it cannot grip the marble and may result in the marble slipping distally.

Traumatic foreign bodies   A sharp foreign body can cause a tear in the oesophageal wall during its removal. Commonly seen traumatic foreign bodies are either pins or dentures (with wires). Therefore certain precautions are taken to avoid damage to the oesophagus. For example, an open safety pin. An open safety pin can be in two positions:

- Favourable—the point of the open end is facing downwards.
- Unfavourable—the point of the open end is facing upwards.

An open safety pin can be removed by the following methods whichever applicable:

- If in favourable position, it is removed in the same position, by oesophagoscopy using a forceps.
- If in unfavourable position:
  - The pointed end is taken into the oesophagoscope and it is removed,
  - The pin in an unfavourable position can be pushed downwards into the stomach and rotated to a favourable position and then removed. (Gastro-version),
  - The pin can be cut with shears and each small piece removed,
  - The open pin can be closed with a Clerf-Arrowsmith safety-pin-closing forceps and then removed.

TRACHEO-BRONCHIAL FOREIGN BODIES

These foreign bodies may be life-threatening due to obstruction to respiration. Common tracheo-bronchial foreign-bodies are peanuts, marbles, seeds of fruits, pins, beads, etc.

Tracheal foreign-bodies are large in size because of which they cannot descend further. In case of a coin in the larynx (Fig. 51.33) unlike as seen in oesophageal foreign bodies, here the AP view shows a vertical opaque slit and lateral neck X-ray shows a

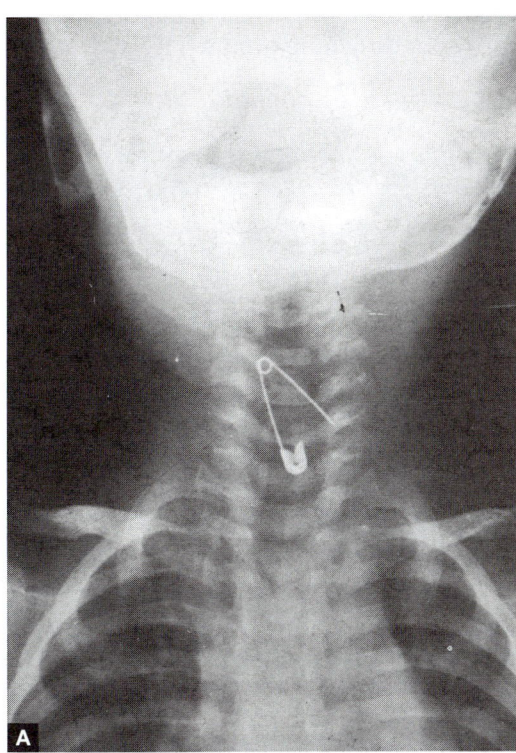
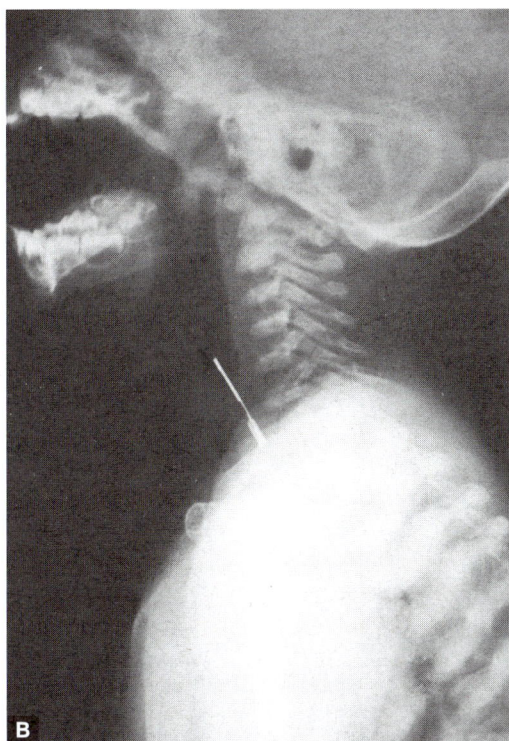

Fig. 51.32A and B: These two X-rays depict the presence of an open safety pin lodged in the neck. This is a favourable position of the safety pin, with its open end facing caudally

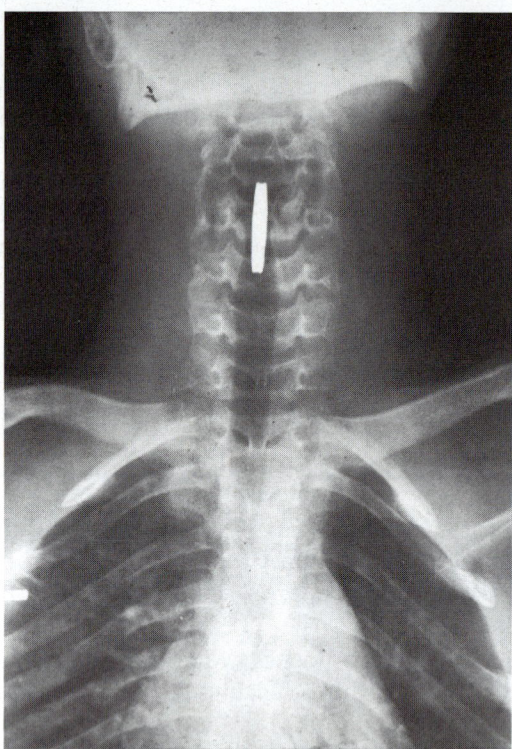

Fig. 51.33: Coin in larynx AP

complete coin (Fig. 51.34). This is because of the antero-posterior glottic inlet. Removal of the foreign body is done with a bronchoscope, keeping tracheostomy instruments ready if a tracheostomy is not already performed.

Three types of bronchial obstructions are seen clinically:

- Type I (Bypass-valve obstruction): The foreign body permits the passage of air in and out on inspiration and expiration so that no collapse or emphysema occurs distally. A wheeze is usually audible at the open mouth (the asthmatoid wheeze) (Fig. 51.35).

- Type II (Check-valve obstruction): The swollen mucosa retreats on inspiration owing to enlargement of the bronchial lumen. Promptly at the beginning of expiration the bronchial lumen diminishes sufficiently to bring the swollen mucosa into contact with the foreign body. This valve-like closure traps the air distally leading to a distal emphysema. This is termed as obstructive emphysema (Fig. 51.36A and B).

- Type III (Stop-valve obstruction): A foreign body embedded in swollen mucosa, completely obstructs the lumen in both phases of respiration. Absorption of the air distally soon results in a collapse. This is termed as obstructive atelectasis. If it is a main bronchus that is obstructed, massive collapse of the corresponding lung occurs (Fig. 51.37 A and B).

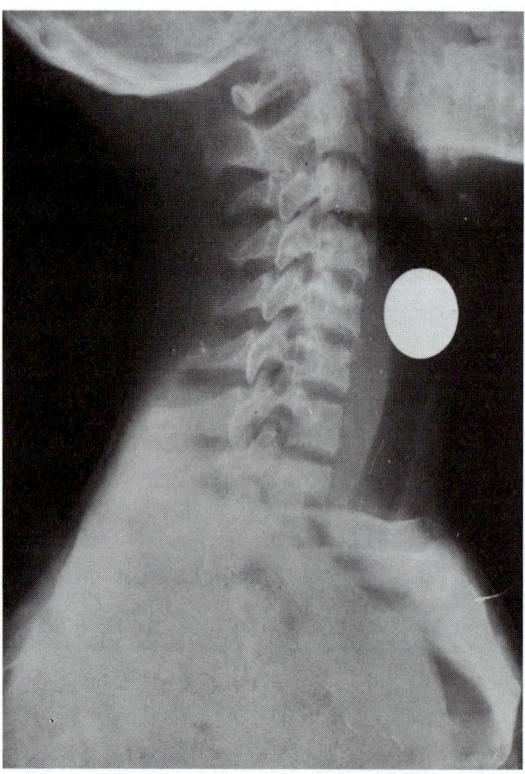

Fig. 51.34: Coin in larynx lateral

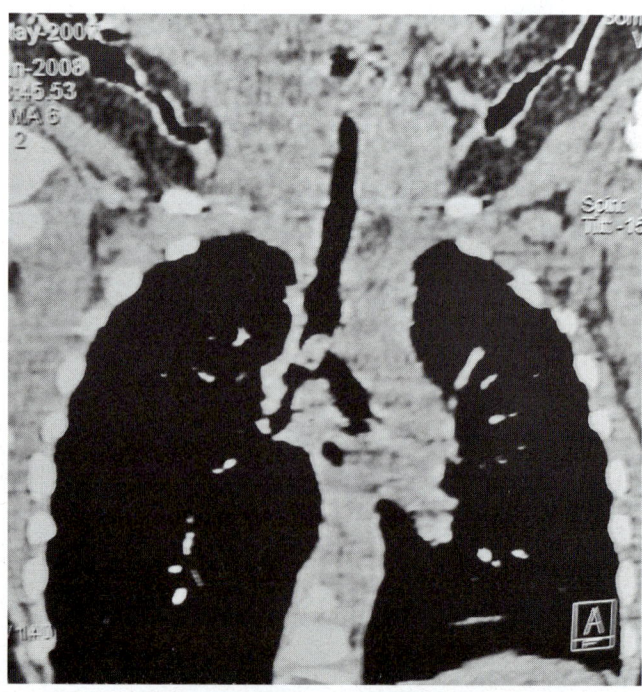

Fig. 51.35: Bypass-valve obstruction

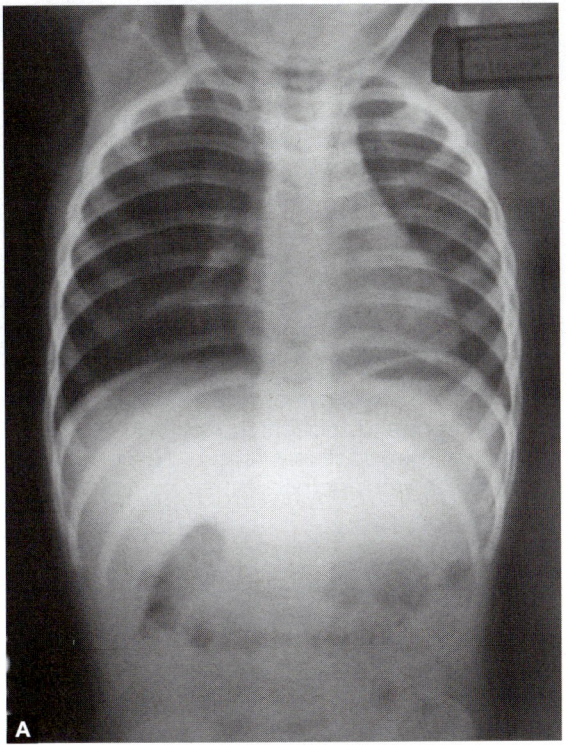
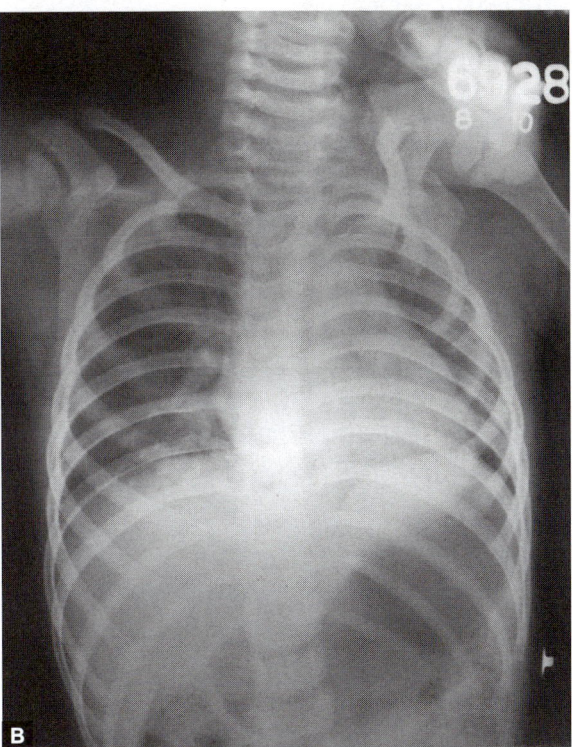

Fig. 51.36A and B: Check-valve obstruction

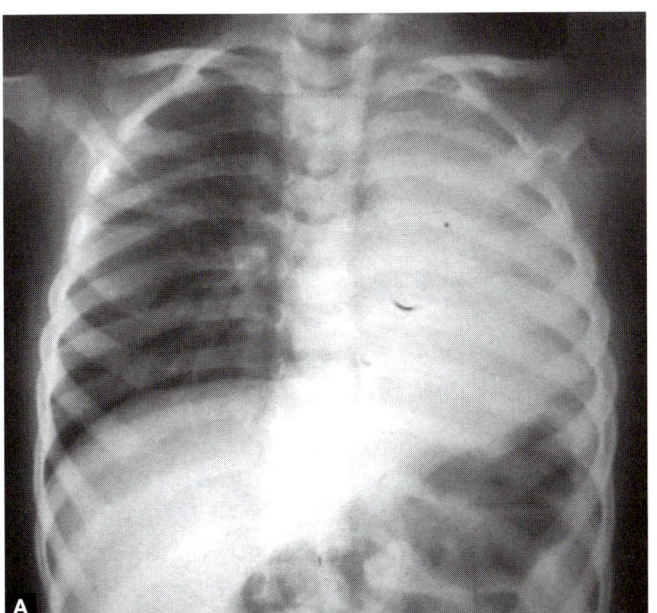
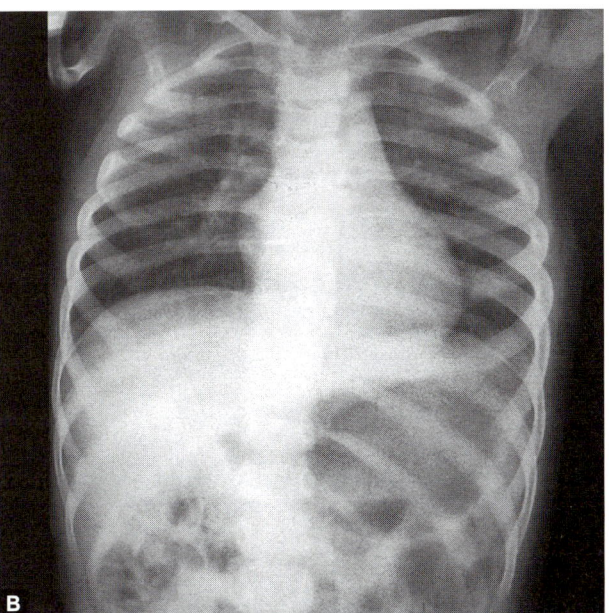

Fig. 51.37A and B: Stop-valve obstruction

ORTHOPANTOMOGRAM

Orthopantomogram (OPG) is also called as dental panoramic radiograph (DPR) is a panoramic scan, a type of dental X-ray to visualise the upper and lower jaws (Figs 51.38 and 51.39).

Images are taken in multiple planes, and a composite image is then made in a manner in which the jaws remain in focus, blurring out the surrounding structures.

The patient needs to remain still for a few seconds till the machine scans the entire dentition and jaws.

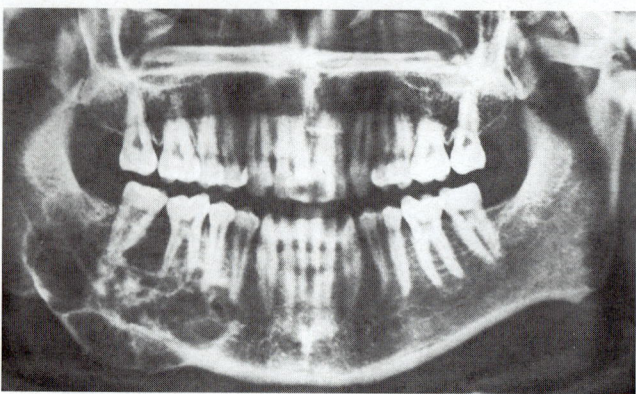

Fig. 51.39: Panoramic view (orthopantomogram) of a patient depicting an expansile radiolucent shadow in the right part of the lower jaw with a characteristic soap bubble appearance suggestive of an ameloblastoma

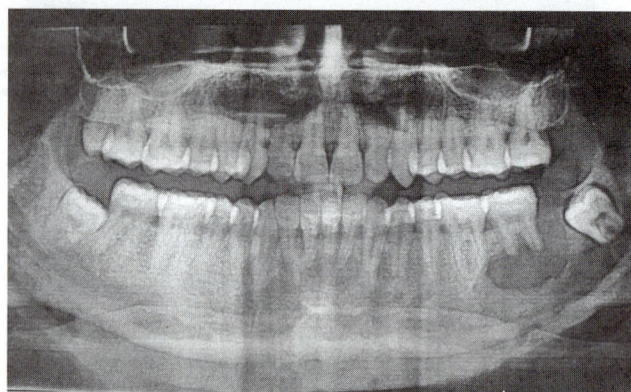

Fig. 51.38: Panoramic view (orthopantomogram) depicting a cystic radiolucent smooth shadow around the roots of the left lower second molar suggestive of a dental cyst

Indications

1. To look for impaced molar teeth
2. To look for inflammation around the teeth and their roots
3. Temporomandibular joint pathologies
4. Facial trauma
5. To see malignancies
6. To plan osteotomies
7. To plan for fitting of dental implants

GENERAL INSTRUMENTS

BULL'S EYE LAMP (Fig. 52.1)

- The light source which is used for ENT examination in the OPD
- Contains 100 watt white frosted bulb in the chamber which is black in color from inside. A convex lens is attached to the lamp which allows adequate dispersion of light. These rays of light fall on the head mirror used by the examiner.

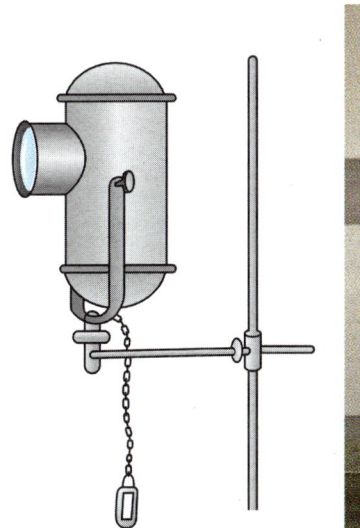
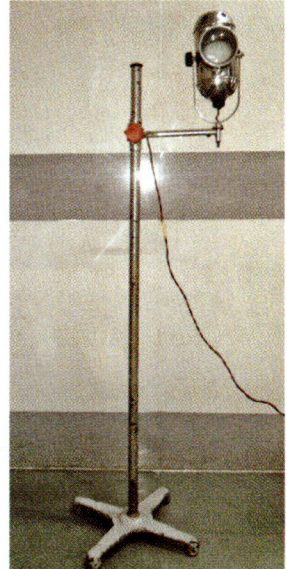

Fig. 52.1: Bull's eye lamp

HEAD MIRROR WITH ADJUSTABLE HEAD BAND (Fig. 52.2)

Consists of a concave mirror of:
- Focal length: 23.6 cm.
- Diameter: 9 cm.
- Central circular aperture: 2 cm.

Use For examination of ear, nose and throat by reflecting light from a light source (Bull's eye lamp). The head mirror is adjusted with the central aperture over the right eye.

Advantages
- Binocular vision is retained.
- The circular aperture coincides with the pupil of the right eye. The surgeon's gaze is parallel with the reflected beam of light, thus the part under examination is brilliantly illuminated and clearly visible.
- Both hands are free to carry out examination and procedures, e.g. aural syringing, antral puncture, indirect laryngoscopy, etc.

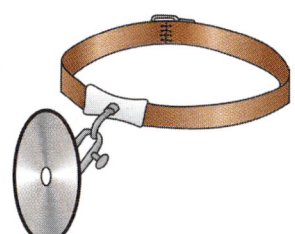
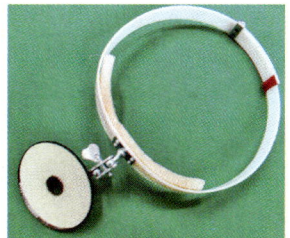

Fig. 52.2: Head mirror

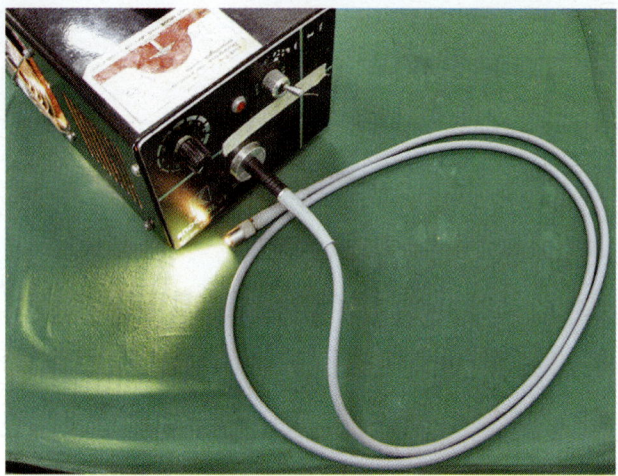

Fig. 52.3: Cold light fountain and fibre-optic cable

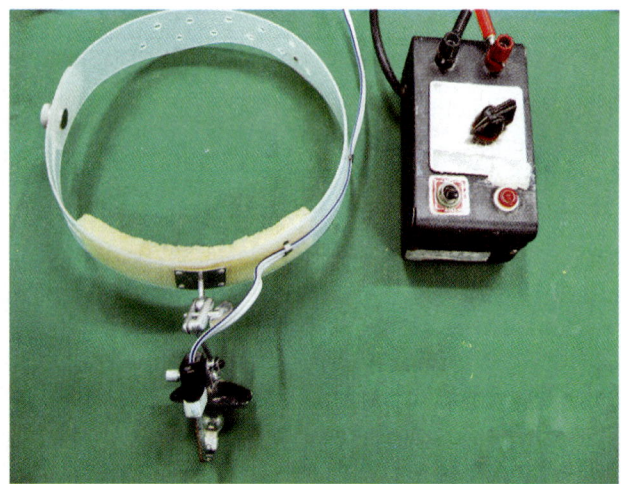

Fig. 52.4: Headlight

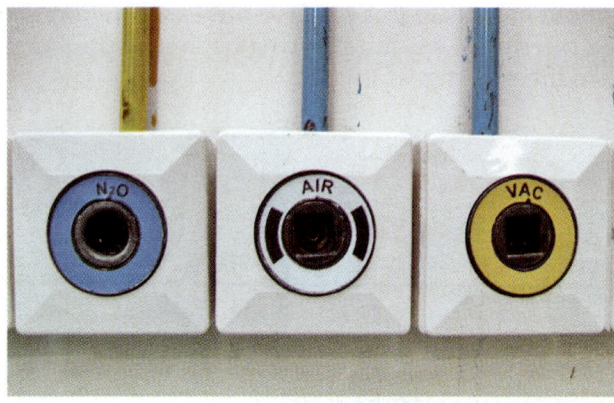

Fig. 52.5: Wall ports for nitrous oxide/ air vacuum suction

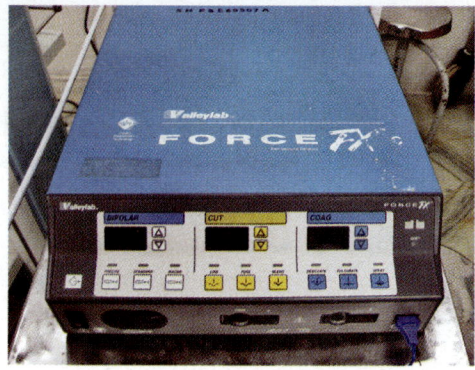

Fig. 52.6: Cautery machine

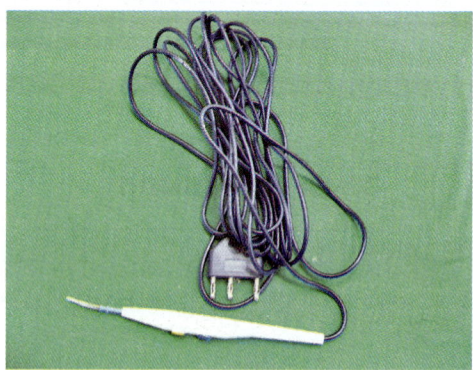

Fig. 52.7: Monopolar electrocautery

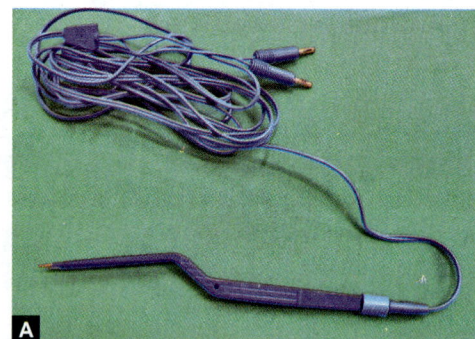

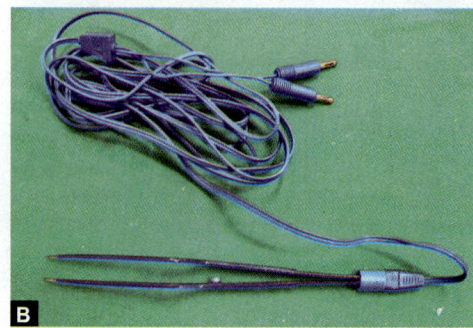

Fig. 52.8A and B: Bipolar electro-cautery (bayonet shaped)

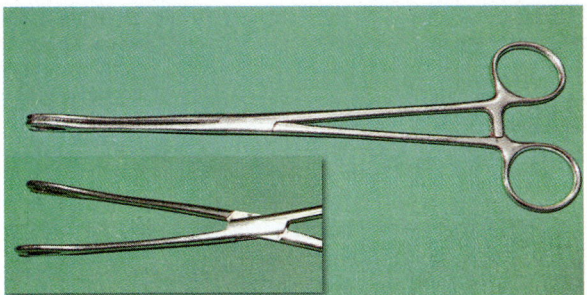

Fig. 52.9: Sponge holding forceps

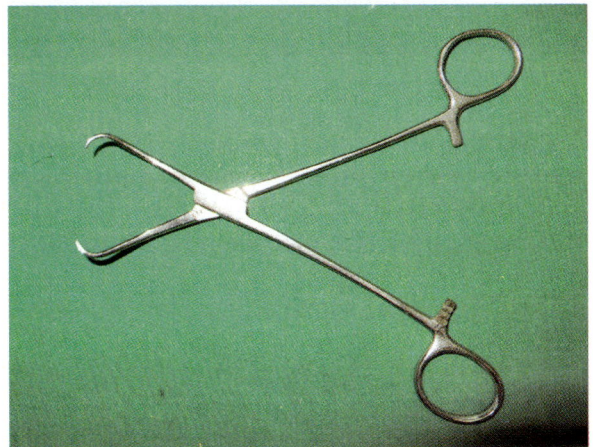

Fig. 52.10: Towel clip

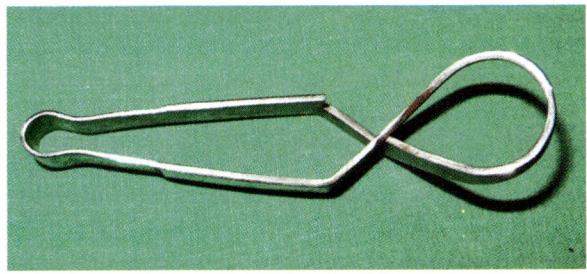

Fig. 52.11: 'Figure of 8' towel clip

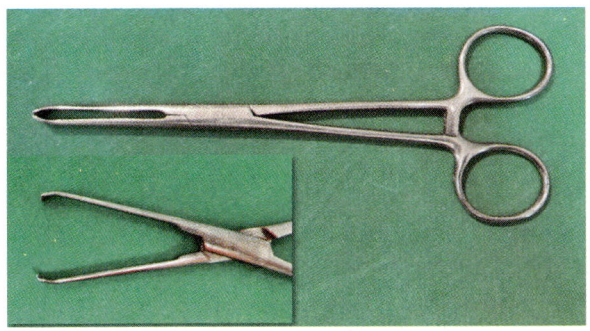

Fig. 52.12: Ellis forceps (tissue holding)

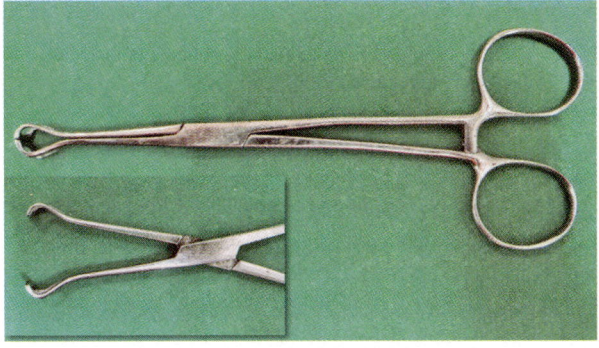

Fig. 52.13: Bab cock's forceps

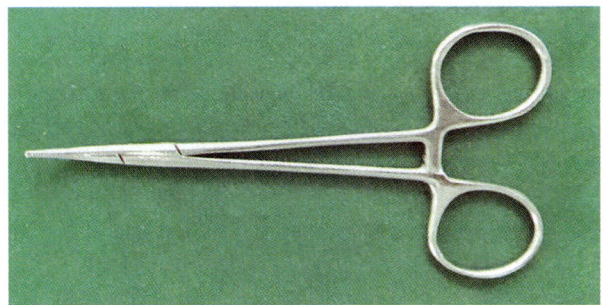

Fig. 52.14: Small curved haemostat

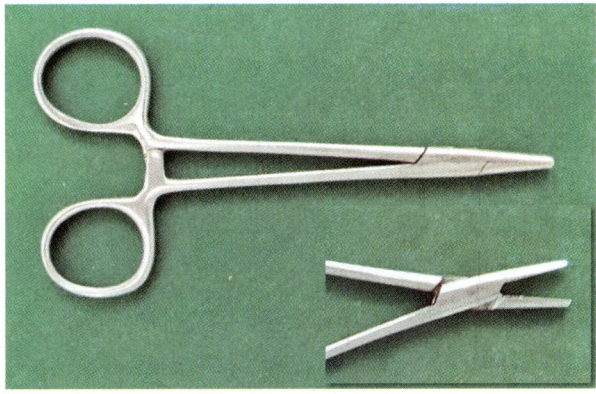

Fig. 52.15: Needle holding forceps

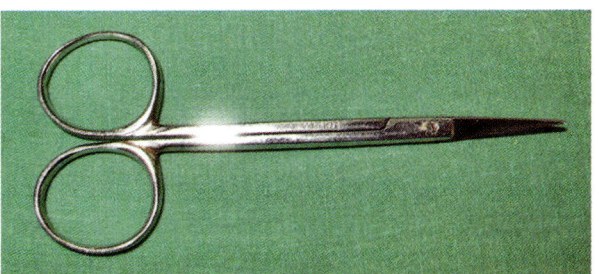

Fig. 52.16: Steele's fine scissors

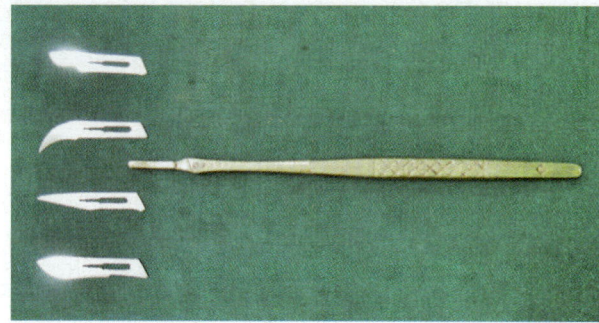

Fig. 52.17: Bard parker's handle with blades 10, 11, 12, 15

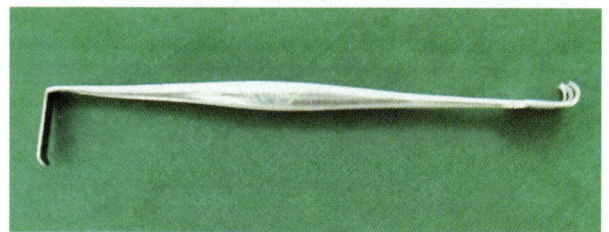

Fig. 52.18: Cat's paw with right angled retractor

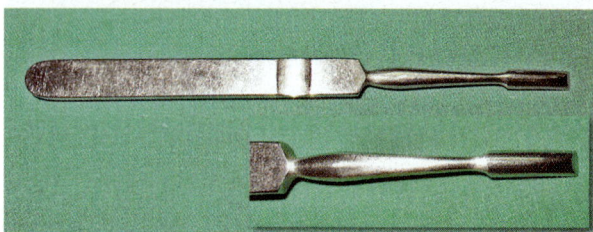

Fig. 52.19: Periosteal elevator

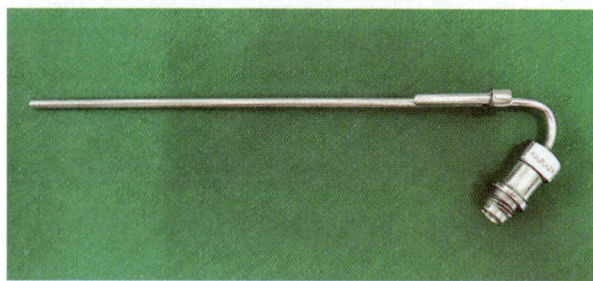

Fig. 52.20: Light carrier

EAR INSTRUMENTS

EUSTACHIAN TUBE CATHETER (Fig. 52.21)

Uses
- Diagnostic: To assess the patency of the Eustachian tube (ET) by catheterisation.

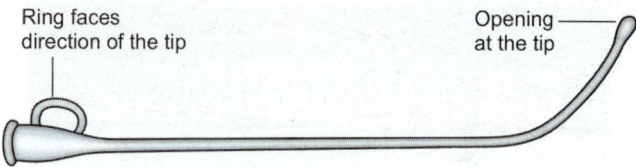

Ring faces direction of the tip

Opening at the tip

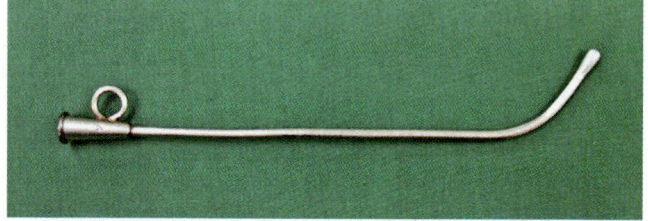

Fig. 52.21: Eustachian tube catheter

- Therapeutic
  - To inflate the middle ear and clear the Eustachian tube block.
  - Can be used in removal of foreign body from the nose.
  - Can be used as a suction canula for the nose.

Procedure   The catheter is introduced along the floor of the nasal cavity with the tip pointing downwards up to the posterior pharyngeal wall. It is then rotated through 90° medially and withdrawn anteriorly till it lies in contact with the posterior end of the nasal septum. Then, on rotating the catheter laterally by 180°, its tip fits into the Eustachian tube opening. Now, a politzer's bag is attached to the catheter and air is pushed in. Movement of the eardrum of the same side indicates no anatomical block in the ET.

Other methods for testing Eustachian tube patency:
- Valsalva's manoeuvre: Forced expiration on a closed glottis.
- Frenzel's manoeuvre: Voluntary contraction of floor of mouth (swallowing).
- Toynbee's manoeuvre: A swallow is made with the lips and nose closed.
- Tympanometry: Noting of middle ear (ME) pressure change on respiration.
- Instillation of sterile sugar solution in the ME if perforation is present and asking the patient to identify the sweet taste.
- Instillation of radio-opaque substance into the middle ear and visualising the Eustachian tube on a radiograph can be done only in presence of tympanic membrane perforation.
- Passage of a ligature material into the ET orifice during ear surgery and visualising it in the nasopharynx.

Eustachian tube blocks can be of two types:

- **Anatomical block:** A tumour or mass blocking the lumen of the Eustachian tube.
- **Physiological block:** Failure of aural secretion to drain into the nasopharynx via the Eustachian tube due to mucociliary defect in the mucosa lining the ET. There is no obvious mass obstructing the lumen.

TOYNBEE'S AURAL SPECULUM

The pinna has to be pulled upwards and outwards in adults and downwards and outwards in children before insertion of the speculum. This is to straighten the external auditory canal, i.e. align the cartilagenous EAC with the bony EAC. It is available in various sizes (Fig. 52.22).

Uses

- Examination of tympanic membrane and external auditory canal.
- Removal of wax, foreign body, fungus, etc.

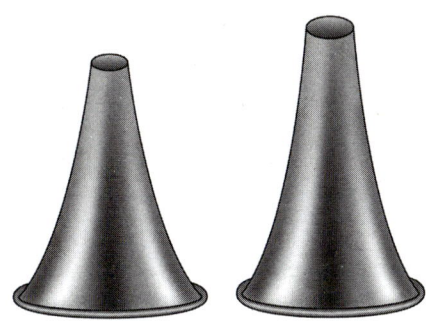

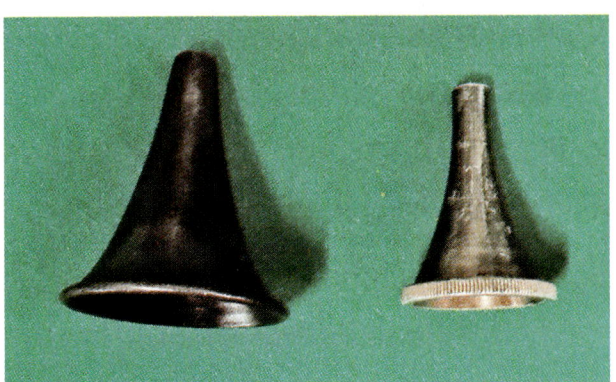

Fig. 52.22: Toynbee's aural speculum

- Procedures like myringotomy, polypectomy, granuloma removal, grommet insertion.
- For endomeatal incisions during surgery like stapedectomy, tympanic neurectomy, etc. A black aural speculum is used with the operating microscope during surgery to prevent reflection of the light in the surgeon's eye. The speculum is coated with a carbon alloy to make it black in colour.

- A metallic (non-carbonized) aural speculum is used in the OPD when using light reflected from a head mirror and falling eye lamp.

OTOSCOPE (Fig. 52.23)

Use   Examination of the external auditory canal and tympanic membrane.

Advantage over head mirror and Bull's eye lamp

- Magnified (2X) view of the eardrum and external auditory canal and better assessment of the aural pathology.
- Easy to handle.
- Direct vision.
- Battery operated (i.e. inbuilt light source), and hence easy to carry.
- Powerful illumination.

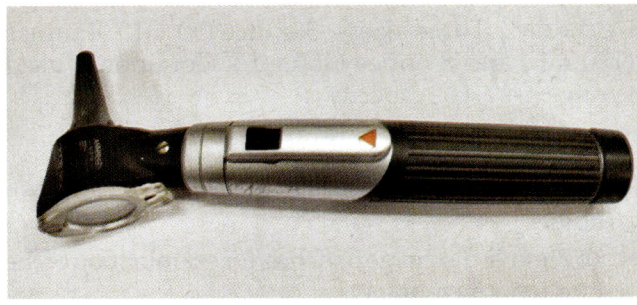

Fig. 52.23: Otoscope

JOBSON-HORNE'S COTTON-CARRIER WITH RING CURETTE (Fig. 52.24)

Cotton carrier   Ring curette

Fig. 52.24: Jobson-Horne's cotton carrier with curette

Uses

- Serrated probe end is used as cotton-wool carrier for aural toilet and to clean aural discharge.
- Probe can be used to trace a sinus tract or probe around an aural polyp.
- Used to apply antibiotic ointment into the external auditory canal.
- Curette is used to remove wax, foreign bodies and granulations from the external ear.

AURAL SYRINGE

This is a metal syringe. It has a cylinder with a piston that can push water with force through a nozzle (Fig. 52.25).

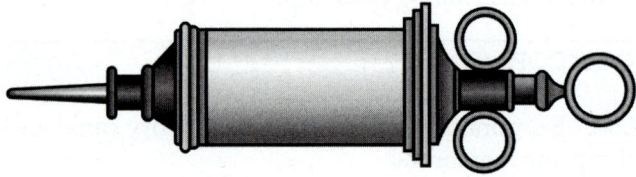

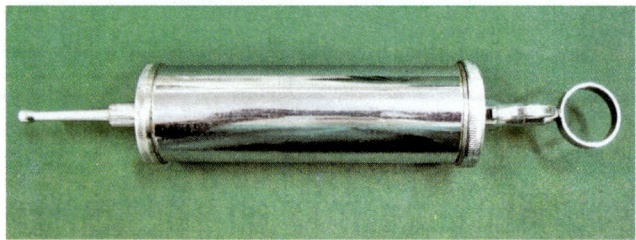

Fig. 52.25: Aural syringe

Capacity   Three sizes—3 ounce (90 mL), 4 ounce (120 mL) and 5 ounce (150 mL). Commonly used syringe has a 4 oz capacity.

Uses

- To remove wax and non-hygroscopic foreign bodies.
- To remove discharge or debris for examination of the tympanic membrane.
- It is preferably not used to clear fungus from the EAC since moisture will cause recurrence of this condition (otomycosis).

TUNING FORK

For testing hearing by Rinne, Weber and other tuning fork tests. Commonly used tuning forks are of 256, 512, 1024 Hz frequency (Fig. 52.26). The most useful is 512 Hz because:

- It falls in the mid-speech frequency,
- Tone decay is optimal (tone decay of 1024 Hz is faster),
- Stimulus given is auditory in nature rather than vibratory (256 Hz gives more of a vibratory stimulus),
- Overtones are minimal,
- Mild hearing loss is also detected.

It has a base, stem and 2 prongs which vibrate 'in phase', with each other to produce a 'pure tone', i.e. a single frequency tone.

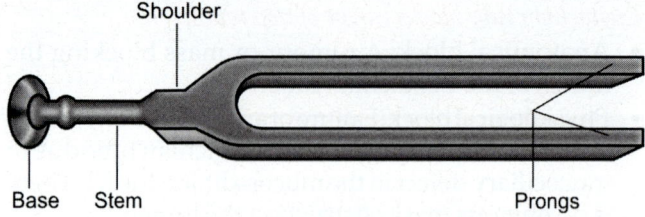

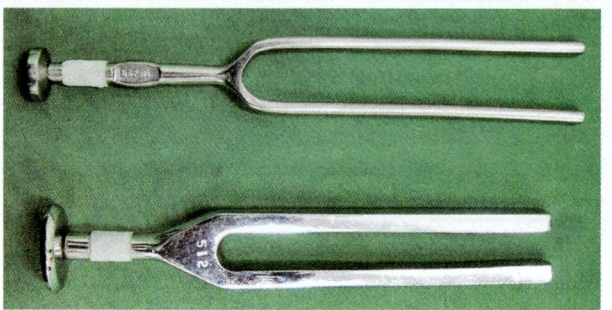

Fig. 52.26: Tuning fork

AURAL DRESSING FORCEPS (Fig. 52.27 A and B)

Types

- Hartman's forceps.
- Tilley's aural forceps.
- Hunter Tod's aural forceps.
- Fagge's aural forceps.

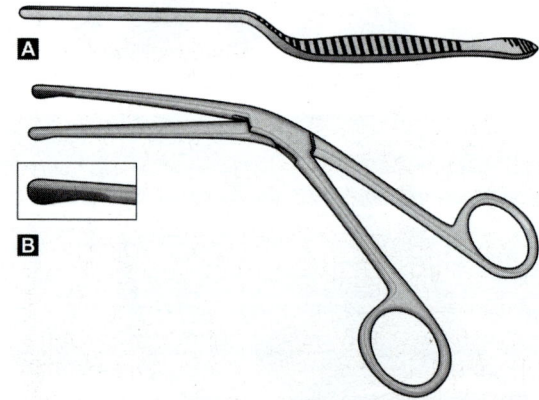

Fig. 52.27: Aural dressing forceps

Uses

- For inserting antibiotic soaked wick or a glycerine ichthyol pack in the external auditory canal in acute otitis externa.
- Removal of foreign bodies and crusts from the external auditory canal.
- In ear surgery for packing the EAC with gelfoam or gauze pack.

SIEGLE'S PNEUMATIC SPECULUM

Siegle's pneumatic speculum consists of aural speculum with magnification of 2X attached by a hollow rubber tube to a rubber bulb and is used to visualise the eardrum with a head-mirror and Bull's eye lamp (Fig. 52.28).

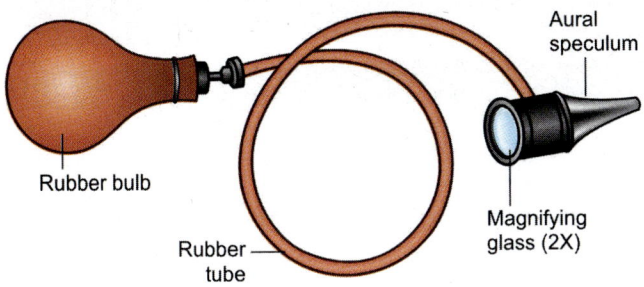

Aural speculum

Rubber bulb

Rubber tube

Magnifying glass (2X)

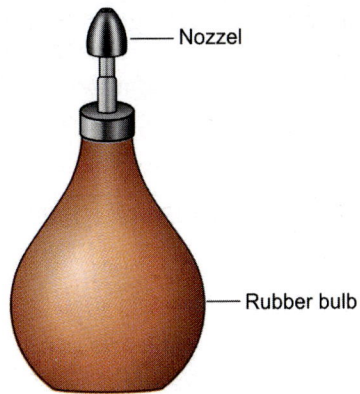

Nozzel

Rubber bulb

Fig. 52.29: Politzer bag

OPERATING MICROSCOPE

Operating microscope has great manoeuvrability and is a boon to the development of micro-surgery of the ear, nose and throat (Fig. 52.30).

It helps in improving surgery by magnification, illumination, identification and depth perception.

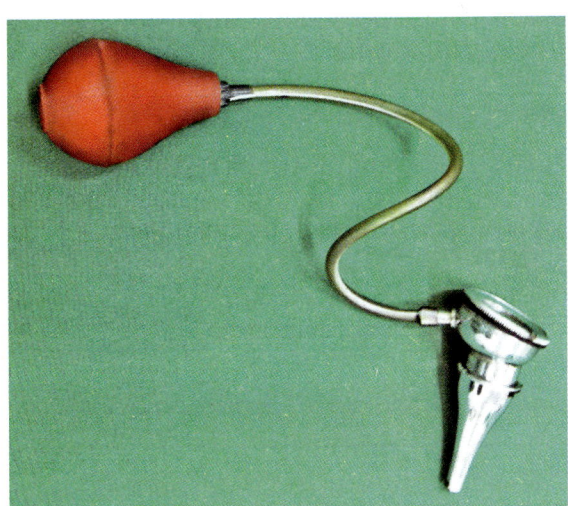

Fig. 52.28: Siegle's pneumatic speculum

Uses

- To obtain a magnified view (2X) of the tympanic membrane.
- To test for mobility of the tympanic membrane.
- To differentiate between a healed perforation and adhesive otitis media.
- For insufflation of medicaments in the ear.
- To clear secretions from the ear with a suction effect.
- To perform the fistula test which helps to detect a labyrinthine fistula.

POLITZER BAG

Politzer bag is used for testing the patency of the Eustachian tube by inserting its nozzel into one nasal cavity and also for inflating the middle ear after being connected to a Eustachian catheter (Fig. 52.29).

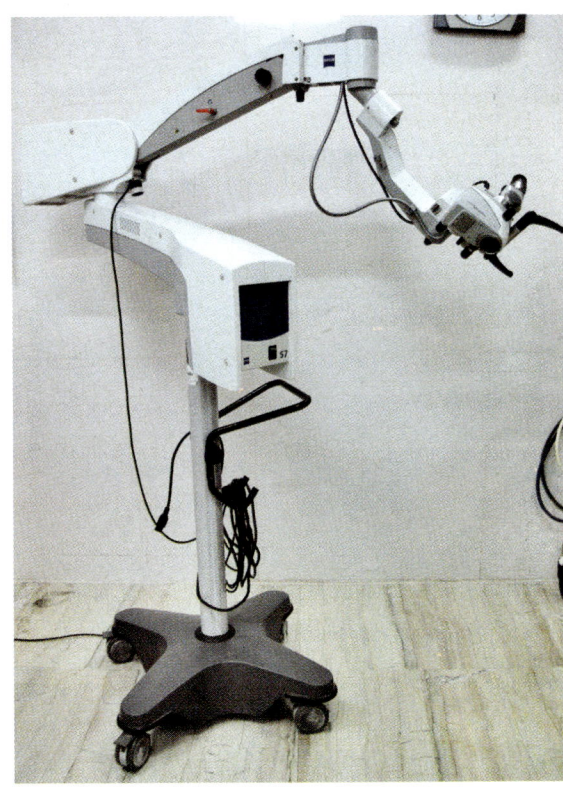

Fig. 52.30: Operating microscope

Uses

- For various micro-ear surgeries, i.e. myringoplasty, tympanoplasty, stapedectomy, etc.

- Used in micro-laryngeal surgery along with a micro-laryngoscope, e.g. excision of vocal cord nodules, etc.
- Used in operations of the nose and PNS where illumination and magnification are required, i.e. ethmoidectomy.

MOLLISON'S SELF-RETAINING HEMOSTATIC MASTOID RETRACTOR (Fig. 52.31)

Uses

- For removal of temporalis fascia as graft material.
- Two retractors are applied at right angles to each other during a myringoplasty, tympanoplasty or a mastoidectomy.
- Optic nerve decompression.
- Burr-hole operation or a craniotomy.
- Laryngofissure operation.
- External ethmoidectomy.

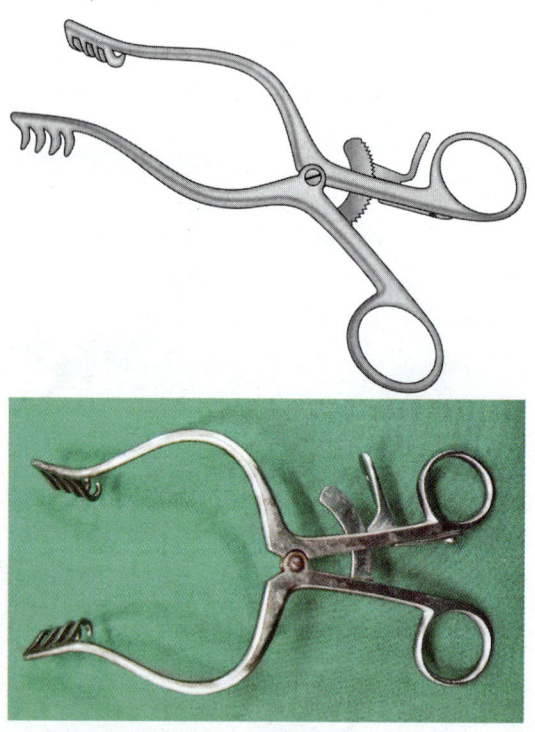

Fig. 52.31: Mollison's mastoid retractor

BONE GOUGE (JENKINS) (Fig. 52.32)

Used along with a hammer.

Uses

- Used previously to perform a mastoidectomy (Electric drill and burr is preferred nowadays).
- In Caldwell-Luc operation, to remove the anterior wall of the maxilla and gain access into the antrum.

- To remove osteoma or exostosis from the external auditory canal.

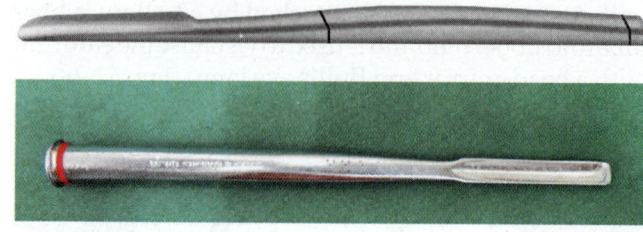

Fig. 52.32: Mastoid gouge

MYRINGOTOMY KNIFE (DAGGET'S MYRINGOTOME)

Used to make an incision in the tympanic membrane for treatment of secretory otitis media for insertion of a grommet or for performing only a myringotomy to treat acute otitis media.

STAECKE'S GUIDE AND PROTECTOR

Staecke's guide and protector is used to detect the aditus ad-antrum and protects the facial nerve, while removing the facial bridge in radical mastoid operation (Fig. 52.33).

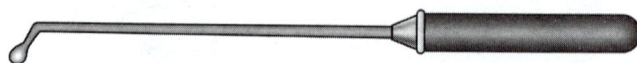

Fig. 52.33: Staecke's guide and protector

CHISEL

Used along with a hammer in lowering of the facial ridge in radical mastoid operation. Not used nowadays with the advent of the electric drill and burrs.

LEMPERT'S SCOOP

Used in different mastoid operations to curette diseased mastoid air cells and granulation tissue (Fig. 52.34).

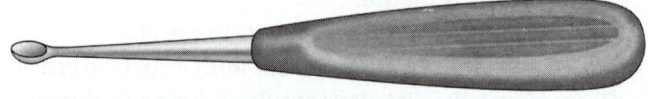

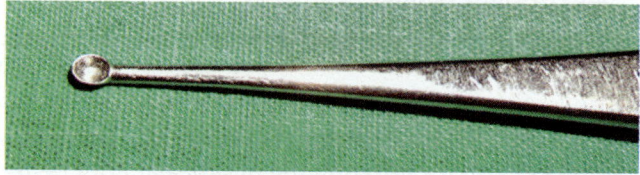

Fig. 52.34: Lempert's scoop

MAC-EWAN'S CELL SEEKER WITH CURETTE (Fig. 52.35)

Used for exploring the mastoid antrum and air cells. The other end is used as a mastoid curette to curette bone.

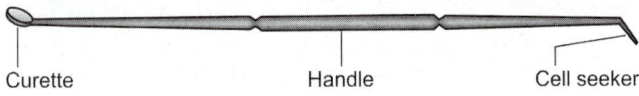

Curette   Handle   Cell seeker

Fig. 52.35: Mac-Ewan's cell seeker with curette

ELECTRIC DRILL AND BURR

These have largely replaced the traditional gouges and curettes in mastoidectomy. The burr cuts fast and neatly without leaving behind an irregular cavity. It prevents damage to the facial nerve. It is also used in middle ear surgery to operate on the ossicles (ossiculoplasty) (Fig. 52.36A to G).

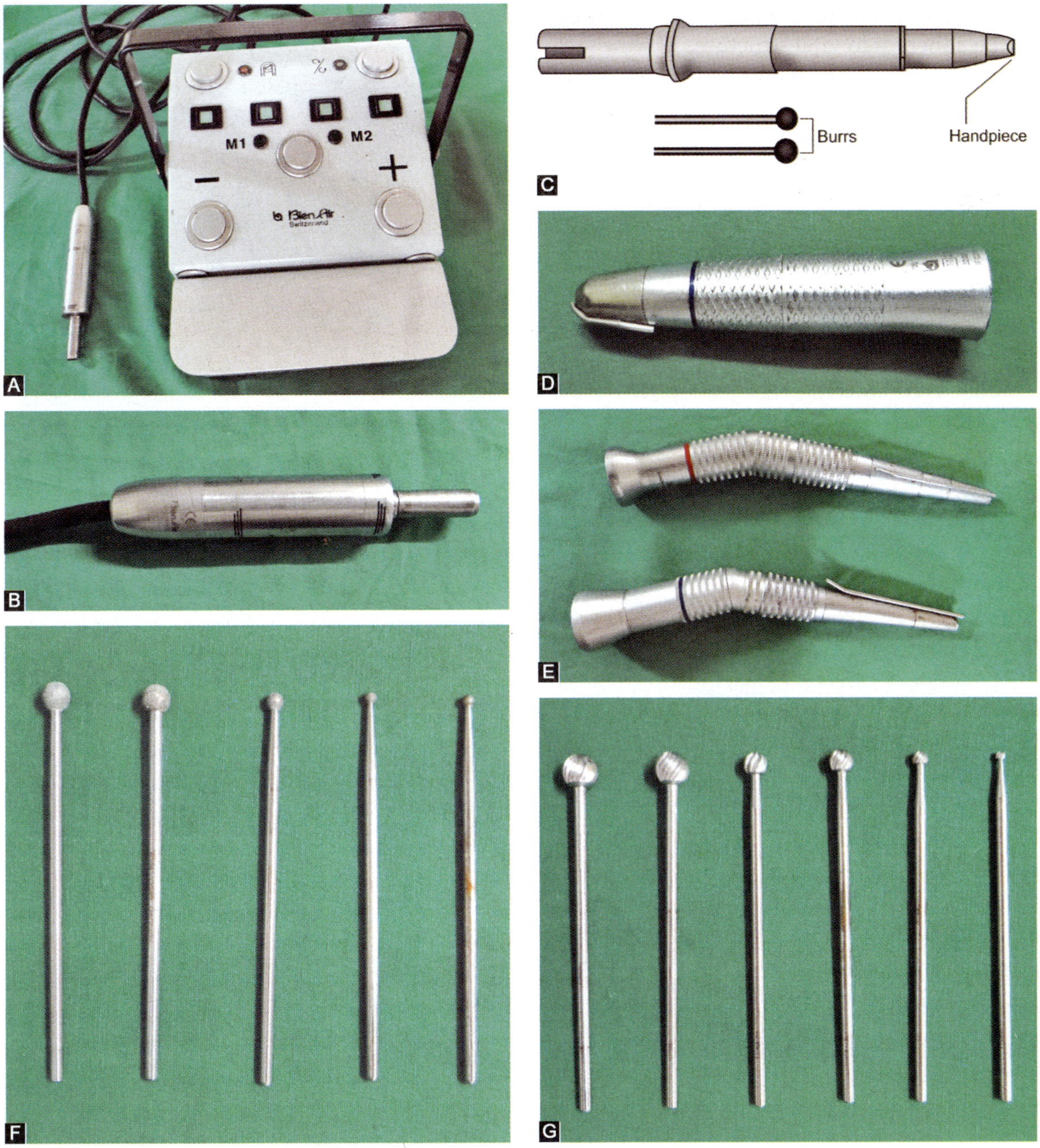

Fig. 52.36: Micro-motor drill with hand-piece and burrs

GROMMET

It is a ventilating tube used in secretory otitis media following myringotomy for drainage and aeration of the middle ear cleft.

AURAL SNARE (BALLANCE'S)

It is the smallest of all snares used in ENT. It crushes and cuts the pedicle of the aural polyp via the external auditory canal. An aural polyp should never be avulsed as it may be adherent to vital structures like the facial nerve, ossicles, or labyrinth and cause irreversible damage to them (Fig. 52.37).

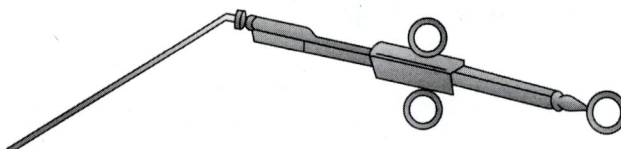

Fig. 52.37: Aural snare

OTHER INSTRUMENTS (Figs 52.38–52.55)

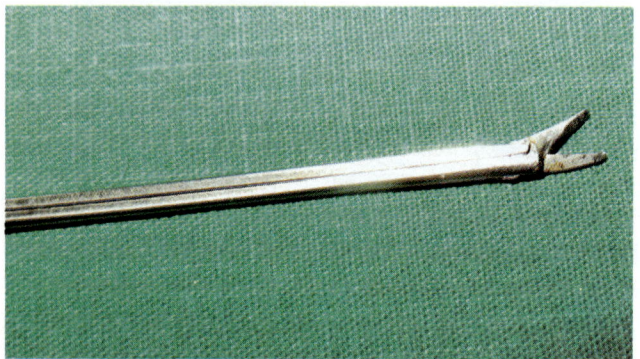

Fig. 52.38: Belluchi's scissors

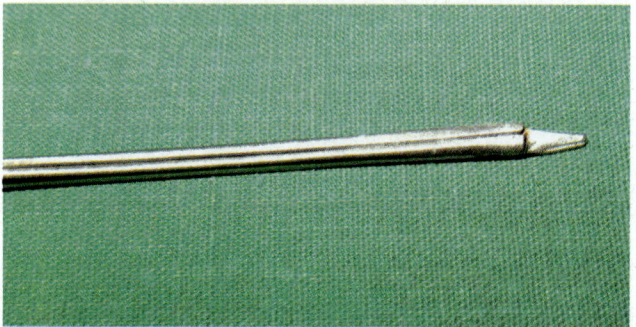

Fig. 52.39: Belluchi's scissors

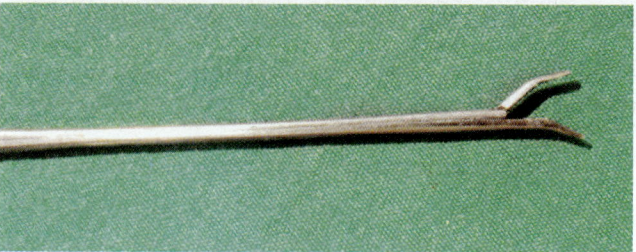

Fig. 52.40: Crimping forceps

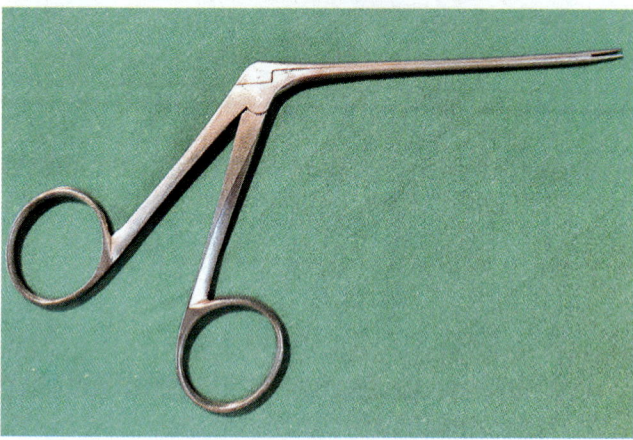

Fig. 52.41: Crocodile forceps

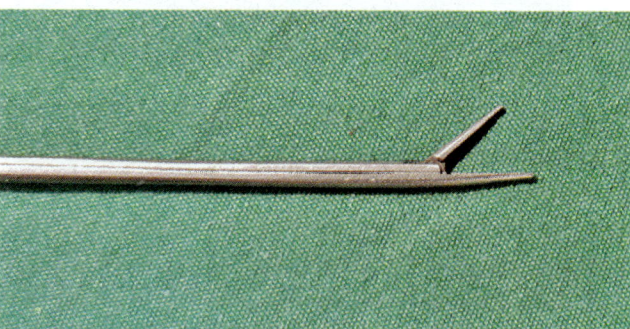

Fig. 52.42: Crocodile forceps

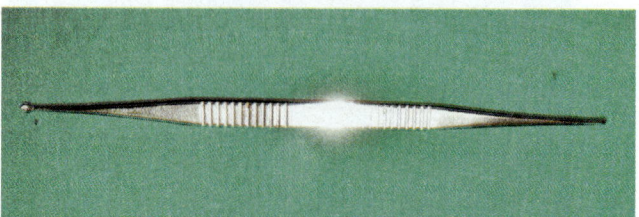

Fig. 52.43: Aural scoop

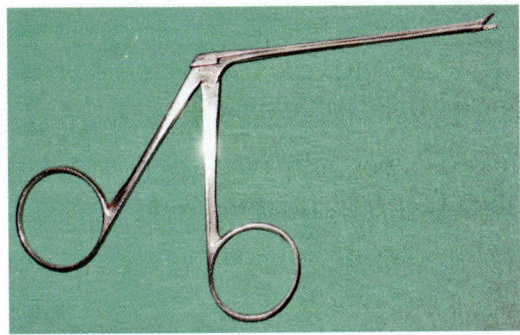

Fig. 52.44: Belluci's scissors used in micro-ear surgery

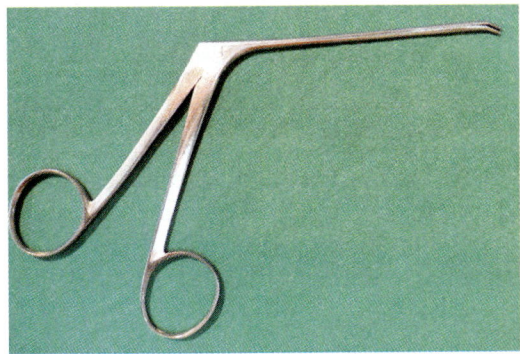

Fig. 52.45: Belluci's scissors used in micro-ear surgery

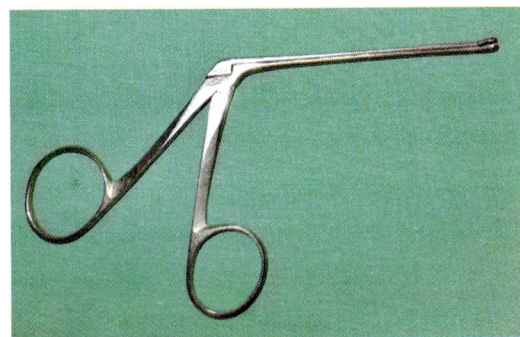

Fig. 52.46: Aural cup forceps

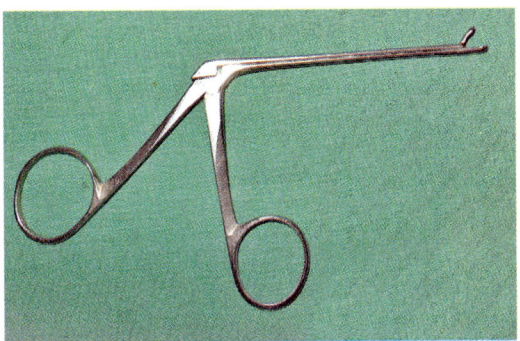

Fig. 52.47: Aural cup forceps

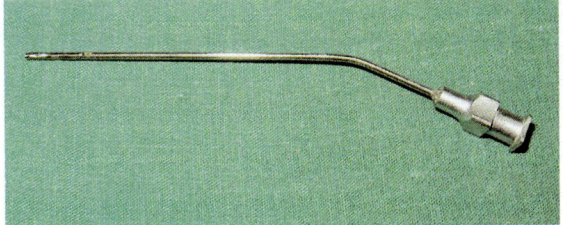

Fig. 52.48: Micro-suction cannula

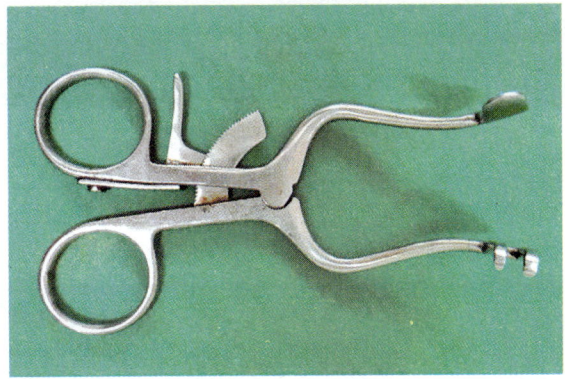

Fig. 52.49: Lempert's end-aural retractor

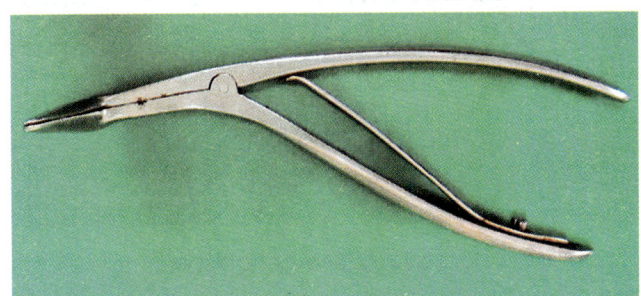

Fig. 52.50: End-aural speculam

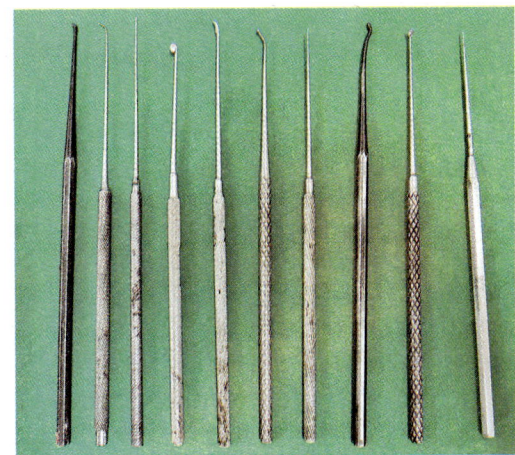

Fig. 52.51: Micro-ear surgery instruments

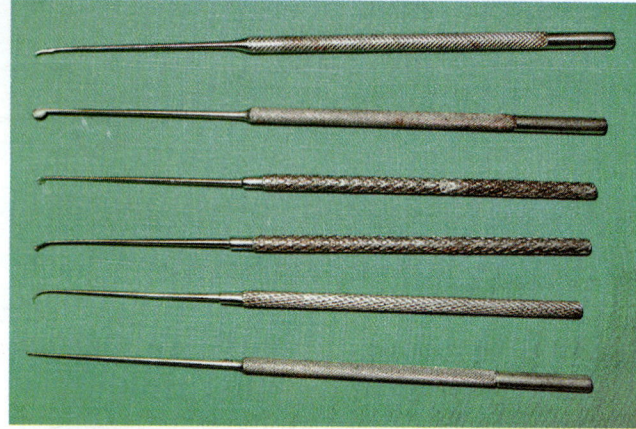

Fig. 52.52: Micro-ear surgery instruments

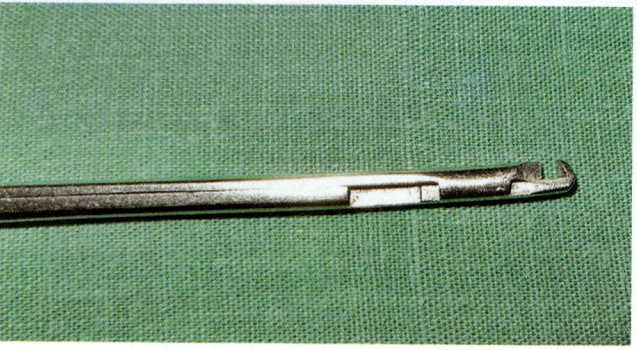

Fig. 52.55: Malleus head nipper

THROAT INSTRUMENTS

LAC'S TONGUE DEPRESSOR

The flat end is introduced into the oral cavity and the curved end is used by the examiner for holding the instrument (Fig. 52.56).

Uses
- In OPD
  - Examination of the oral cavity structures
  - For retraction of cheek and lip
  - To squeeze the tonsil for detecting pus from the tonsillar crypts
  - To test gag reflex
  - To check out loose teeth/hypersensitive teeth
  - In posterior rhinoscopy along with posterior rhinoscopy mirror

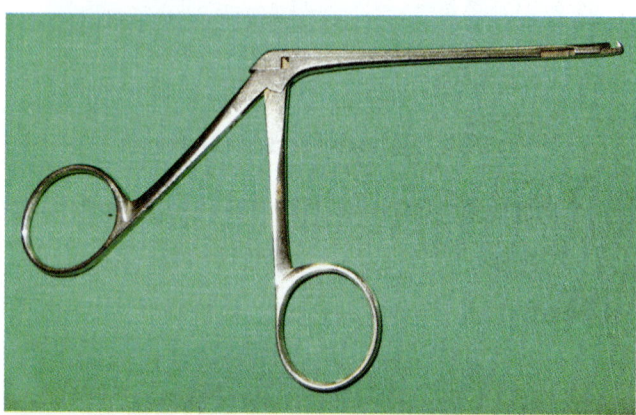

Fig. 52.53: Malleus head nipper

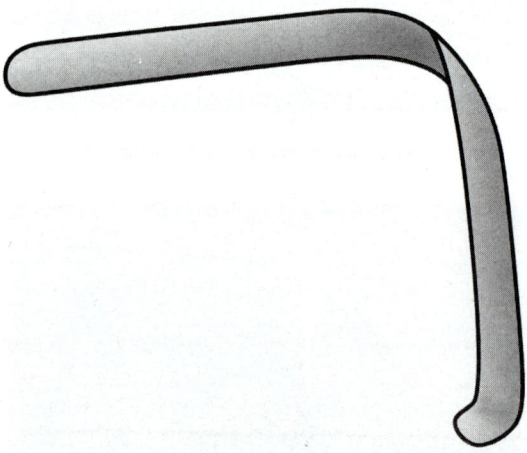

Fig. 52.56: Lac's tongue depressor

- To check air blast by seeing for misting on the tongue depressor to detect nasal obstruction or

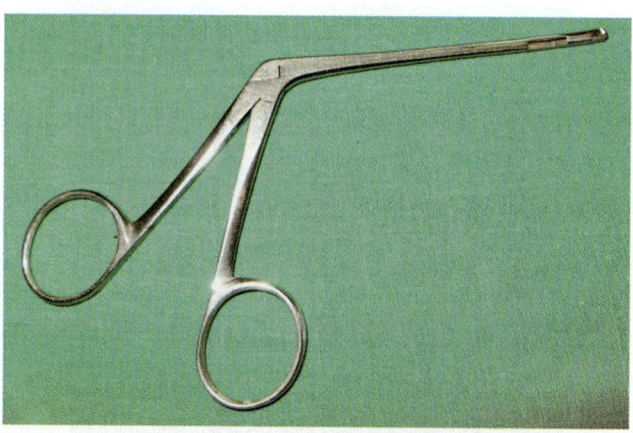

Fig. 52.54: Malleus head nipper

before and after septal or nasal surgery—'cold spatula test'.

- ◆ 'Spatula test'—to test for spasm of the masseter muscle in a suspected case of tetanus.
- In operation theatre
  - ◆ To check post-nasal bleeding in the throat after nasal surgery.
  - ◆ Operations of the throat like tonsillectomy, adenoidectomy, excision of buccal mucosal polyp/ papillomas, leukoplakic patch, etc. It is used with a Doyen's/Jening's mouth gag.
  - ◆ Quinsy drainage.
  - ◆ For taking biopsy from oral cavity lesions.
  - ◆ For removal of foreign body from the throat.
  - ◆ Simultaneous use of 2 tongue depressors with the curved end to lift the soft palate for visualising the nasopharynx.

GUILLOTINE (BALLENGER'S) (Fig. 52.57)

Use   Guillotine method of tonsillectomy operation. Not much used in recent years. It was used previously for tonsillectomy.

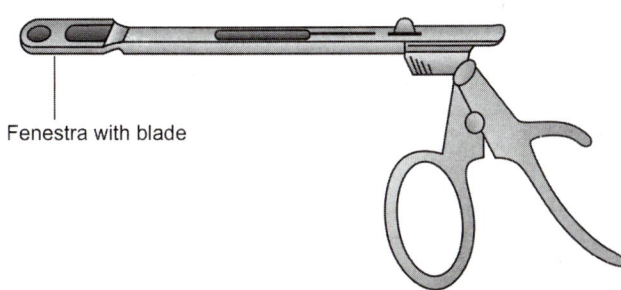

Fenestra with blade

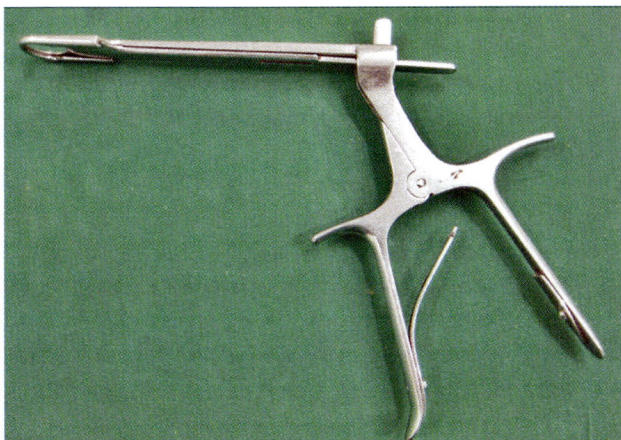

Fig. 52.57: Ballenger's gullotine

Disadvantages
- Only hypertrophied tonsils can be removed.
- Chances of tonsil tissue being left behind are high, i.e. incomplete removal.
- Difficult to achieve hemostasis.

MOUTH GAGS

Doyen's mouth gag   This type of mouth gag always has a piece of rubber tube covering the tips to prevent damage to the enamel of the teeth. It is placed over the second premolars or molars as they have two roots, thus being able to withstand pressure of the open mouth during surgery. It can be used only under general anaesthesia (Fig. 52.58).

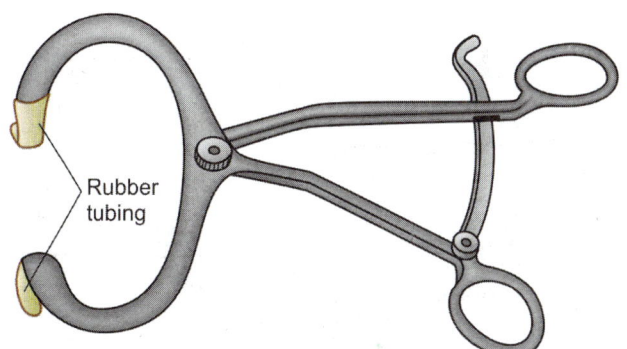

Rubber tubing

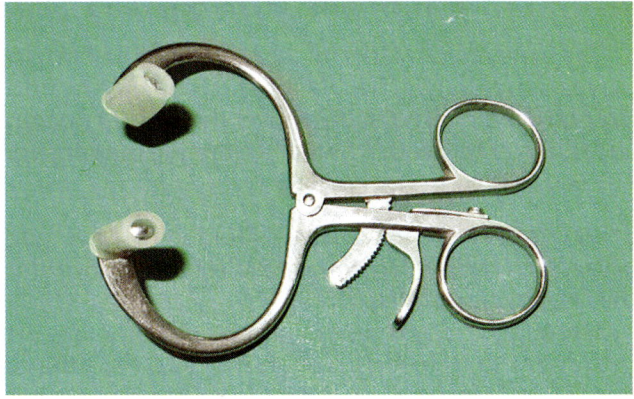

Fig. 52.58: Doyen's mouth gag

- Uses
  - ◆ During operations of tonsillectomy and adenoidectomy. (used with a Lac's tongue depressor).
  - ◆ Surgery of the floor of the mouth, e.g. excision of ranula, removal of Wharton's duct calculus, etc. (tongue–depressor is not used).
  - ◆ In an unconscious patient to prevent airway obstruction.

- ◆ Treatment of fibrous ankylosis of the temporo-mandibular joint.
  - ◆ Before a rigid nasopharyngoscope is introduced.
- Disadvantage: It cannot be used in edentulous patients since if rests on the teeth.

Jening's Mouth Gag   It can also be used in edentulous patients (unlike the Doyen's gag) as the blades rest on the gingiva and are atraumatic (Fig. 52.59).

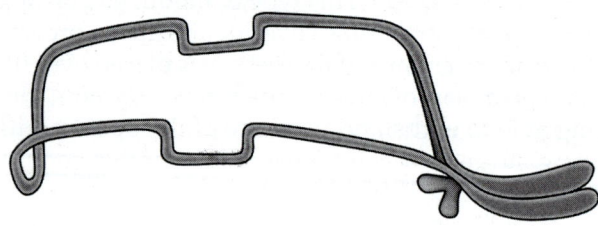

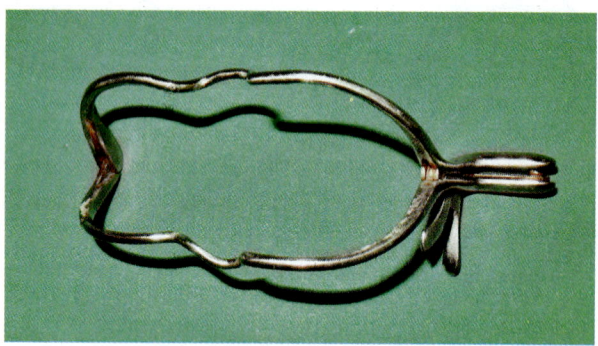

Fig. 52.59: Jening's mouth gag

The instrument works on the same mechanism as a Doyen's mouth gag, i.e. blades opens on closing and close on opening. The blades fit over the alveolar margin and not over the teeth. It is a self-retaining mouth gag.
- Uses: Similar to Doyen's gag.

Boyle Davis Mouth Gag   Boyle's blade and Davis' gag is used simultaneously for a tonsillectomy along with the Draffin bipods (Fig. 52.60).

The tongue depressor is inbuilt with the gag. It is brought to a closed position first and the tongue depressor is inserted in the mouth after depressing the lower jaw. The mouth gag is opened gradually and the mouth remains open because of the ratchet which makes the mouth gag self-retaining. This is attached to Draffin bipods which hold it in position. Always used under general anaesthesia.
- Advantages
  - ◆ The surgeon performs tonsillectomy from the head-end of the patient in a sitting position.
  - ◆ It does away with an assistant, as the tongue depressor is inbuilt with the gag.

- ◆ Other surgeries of the oral cavity, oropharynx and nasopharynx like repairing the cleft palate and transpalatal approach to the nasopharynx can also be performed using this mouth gag.

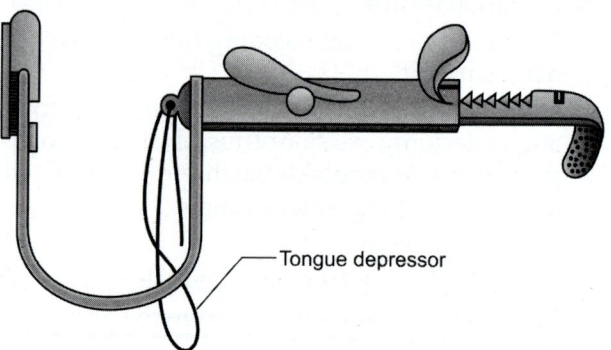

— Tongue depressor

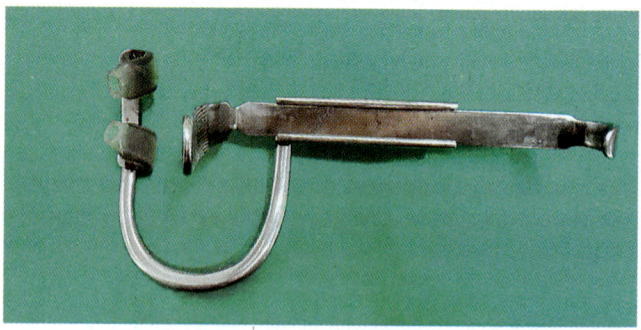

Fig. 52.60: Boyle davis mouth gag with tongue depressor

Dingman's Mouth Gag (Fig. 52.61)
- It is used specially for operations on the palate and the nasopharynx.
- It does not require an assistant as this instrument includes a tongue depressor, 2 cheek retractors and wire-spring on all 4 sides which help the palatal flaps to be held in position, with stay-sutures.
- Uses
  - ◆ Repair of cleft palate (palatoplasty operation).
  - ◆ Biopsy from nasopharynx and for nasopharyngeal surgery
  - ◆ For pharyngoplasty
  - ◆ Removal of angiofibroma
  - ◆ Surgery for choanal atresia
  - ◆ Transpalatal sphenoidectomy/hypophysectomy/vidian neurectomy
  - ◆ Can be used for oral surgeries like tonsillectomy
  - ◆ Any palatal surgery like fenestration operation, etc
  - ◆ For uvulo palatopharyngoplasty (UPPP) as a treatment for sleep apnoea.

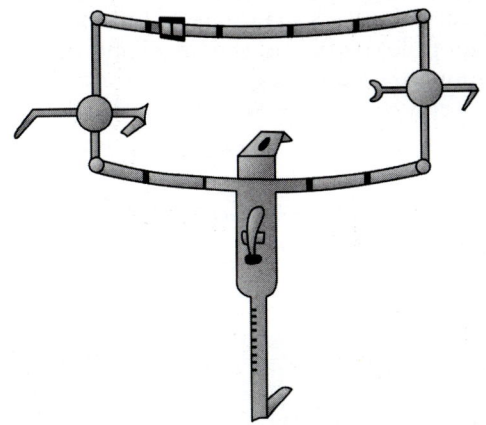

Draffin bipods are 2 rods with multiple rings in a row for fixing the Boyle Davis's mouth gag with neck of the patient in extended position. They rest on either side of the patient's head (Fig. 52.62).

Use   Used to fix Boyle-Davis mouth gag to perform oral surgery.

TONSIL HOLDING FORCEPS (DENIS BROWNE)

It has an alligator joint with fenestra on both the blades and teeth on the edge of the blades (Fig. 52.63).

Use   It is used to hold the tonsil firmly during tonsillectomy by the dissection method.

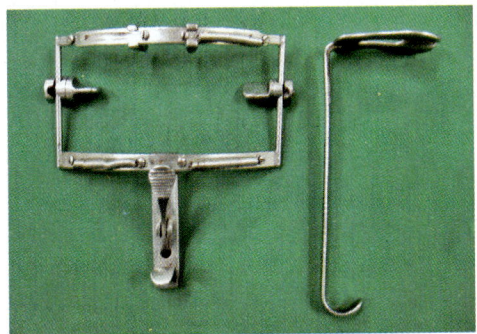

Fig. 52.61: Dingman's mouth gag

DRAFFIN BIPODS (BIPOD METALLIC STAND)

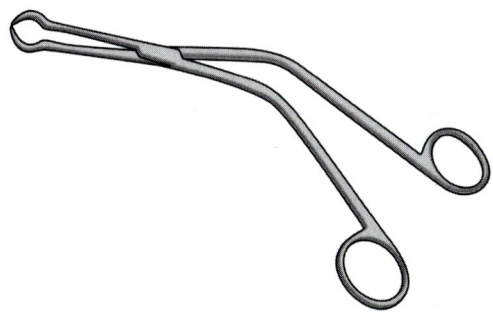

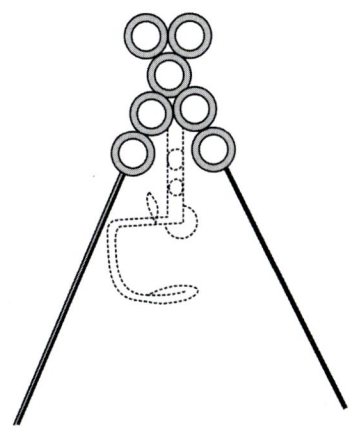

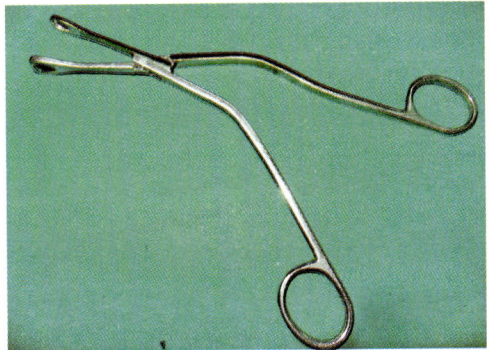

Fig. 52.63: Tonsil holding forceps

LONG DISSECTING FORCEPS (WAUGH'S)

Use
• It is used during dissection of the tonsil.
• Can also be used in catching bleeding vessels and packing the tonsillar fossa with gauze prior to ligating bleeding vessels.

TONSIL DISSECTOR WITH ANTERIOR PILLAR RETRACTOR (MOLLISON'S AND BEAVIS'S VARIETY) (Fig. 52.64)

Use   Used in tonsillectomy by the dissection method.

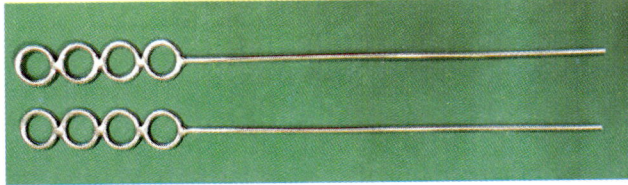

Fig. 52.62: Draffin bipod

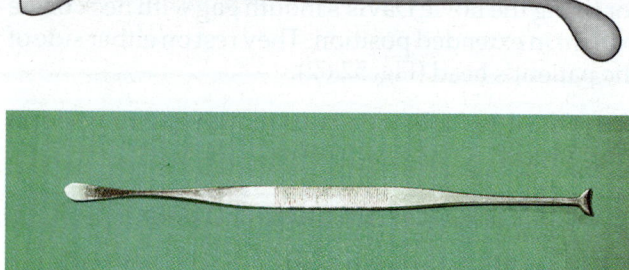

Fig. 52.64: Tonsil dissector with anterior pillar retractor

After making an incision the flat end (dissector) is used to separate the tonsillar capsule from its bed. The tonsillar fossa is the plane of cleavage.

The other curved end (anterior pillar retractor) retracts the anterior pillar after the tonsil is removed to inspect the tonsillar fossa for any bleeding vessel or remnant of tonsil tissue or any retained gauze pieces.

LONG SLENDER TONSIL ARTERY FORCEPS (TONSILLAR HAEMOSTAT: BIRKETT'S, NEGUS OR WILSON TYPES)

Use　Used to catch and ligate bleeding vessels after tonsillectomy by the method of cross-clamping.

This is a long (9 inch) and slender hemostat for better view while working at a depth and to avoid catching soft tissue with bleeding vessels (Fig. 52.65).

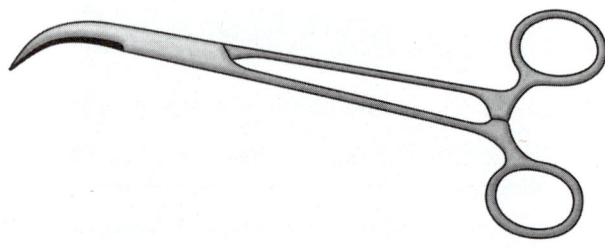

Fig. 52.65: Tonsillar haemostat

TONSIL SNARE (EVE'S) (Fig. 52.66)

Use　It is used to remove the tonsil by crushing and cutting the pedicle after dissection.

The blunt stainless steel wire of the snare 'crushes' the (lower pole) pedicle of the tonsil and then 'cuts', it thus achieving hemostasis.

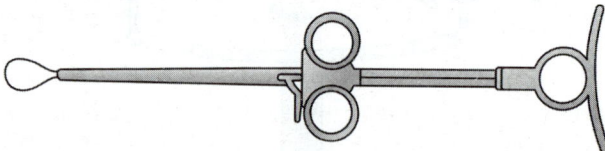

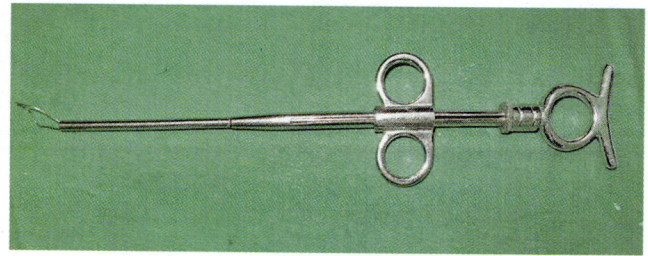

Fig. 52.66: Eve's tonsillar snare

The wire is 3 inches long and has a thickness of 28 gauge. It is made of stainless steel. The index and middle fingers are inserted into the 2 rings of the outer tube of the snare and the thumb is inserted in the ring of the central movable slide while engaging the tonsil pedicle into the loop. The loop of wire is withdrawn totally into the snare and this crushes and cuts the pedicle and provides hemostasis. During crushing and cutting movements the thumb is removed from its position in the ring and pressure is applied by placing the thenar eminence on the handle behind the ring.

Mechanism of action 'crush and cut'.

NEGUS LIGATURE CARRIER OR KNOT TIER

Use　It has a blunt forked end which helps to slip the ligature over the tip of the tonsillar hemostat during ligation of the vessels in the tonsillar bed following tonsillectomy (Fig. 52.67).

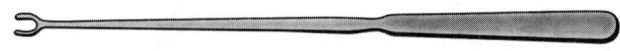

Fig. 52.67: Negus ligature carrier

TONSIL KNIFE (A NO. 12 'J' SHAPED BLADE WITH A BARD PARKER'S KNIFE HANDLE)

Use　Used for the submucosal incision on the anterior pillar (an inverted 'J') of the tonsil during the tonsillectomy operation.

TONSIL HAEMOSTATIC CLAMP (YORKE'S)

It has a circular platform on one blade which is covered with gauze and is inserted into the tonsillar fossa. The other blade has a concave rod which rests externally on the neck. It is used to compress the tonsillar fossa to achieve haemostasis (Fig. 52.68).

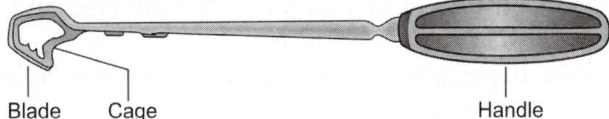

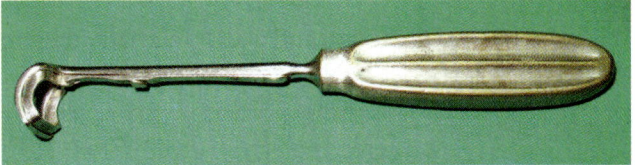

Blade   Cage   Handle

Fig. 52.70: Adenoid curette with cage

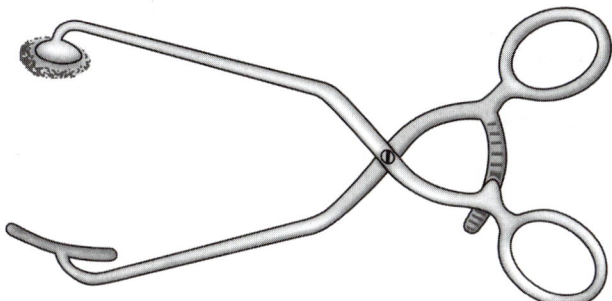

Fig. 52.68: Tonsil haemostatic clamp

Use This is not used anymore. In the early days this was used for haemostasis during reactionary and secondary haemorrhage. However, it should not be used for more than 15–20 minutes at a time.

QUINSY FORCEPS OR PERITONSILLAR ABSCESS FORCEPS (ST. CLAIR THOMPSON)

This is a bayonet shaped instrument and has a sharp trocar point with a shoulder for preventing deep entry (Fig. 52.69).

Use For draining a quinsy, the sharp trocar tip is introduced with the blades closed and the forceps is opened like a sinus forceps to drain the abscess, once it is inside.

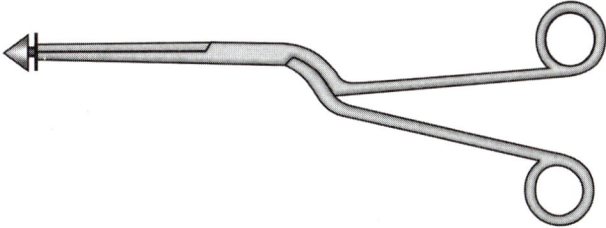

Fig. 52.69: Quinsy forceps

ADENOID CURETTE (ST. CLAIR THOMPSON)

They are of two types (Fig. 52.70):
- With cage (which has got fang like teeth to hold the adenoid tissues),
- Without cage.

The curette is held like a pen introduced into the oral cavity with the blades (cutting edge) facing down, till it reaches beyond the soft palate. It is then rotated by 180° and moved up till the blade touches the posterior end of the bony septum. The grip is then changed to that of a dagger and with a sweeping movement at the wrist joint the adenoids are shaved off the posterior nasopharyngeal wall. The cage prevents aspiration of adenoid tissue into the lower respiratory tract after its removal. The curette without a cage is relatively atraumatic and is used to gently remove tubal tonsils without damaging the openings of the Eustachian tubes.

YANKAUER'S NASOPHARYNGOSCOPE (Fig. 52.71)

Use For direct examination of the nasopharynx in tonsillectomy position under general anaesthesia and for taking biopsy.

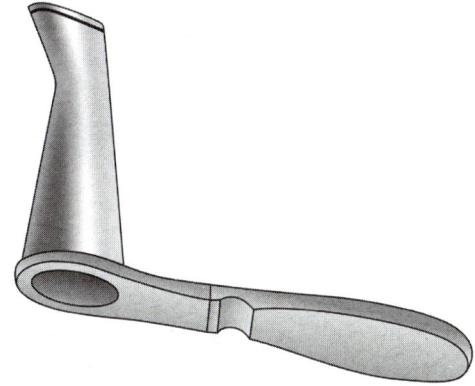

Fig. 52.71: Yankauer's nasopharyngoscope

It is not commonly used nowadays due to the advent of the flexible nasopharyngoscope. Other methods of visualising the nasopharynx:
- Flexible nasopharyngoscope.
- Sinus endoscope.

- With the help of two simple rubber catheters and a posterior rhinoscopy mirror.
- With the help of two Lac's tongue depressors to lift the soft palate.

VALSELLUM

It is used to hold the tonsil and pull it medially during dissection.

TONSIL NEEDLE

It is a sharp curved needle on a long handle. The needle is at a right angle to the handle (Fig. 52.72).

It is used for suturing the tonsillar pillars together for stopping reactionary haemorrhage which cannot be controlled by ligation with the tonsil artery forceps.

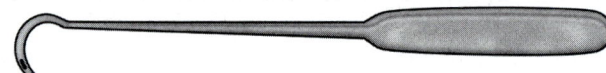

Fig. 52.72: Tonsil needle

YANKAUER'S TONSIL SUCTION (OROPHARYNGEAL SUCTION)

This instrument (Fig. 52.73) is different from other suctions by its:
- Long length,
- Tip is covered with a piece of rubber tube to prevent damage to oropharyngeal mucosa,
- The curve or bend is to prevent the instrument from obscuring the view,
- Large handle.

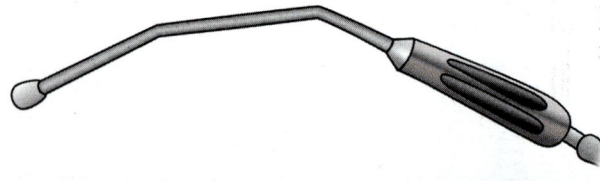

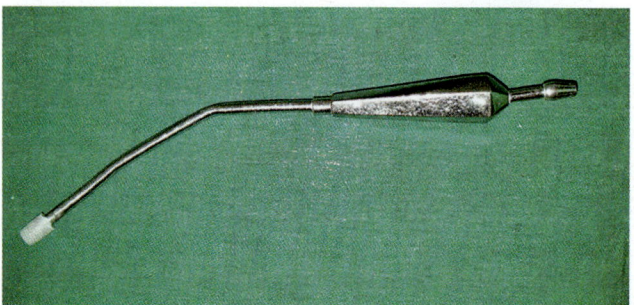

Fig. 52.73: Yankauer's tonsil/Oropharyngeal suction

Uses For removal of secretions and blood from the oropharynx by vacuum suction during surgery of the oral cavity, nose and pharynx.

LIP AND CHEEK RETRACTOR (Fig. 52.74)

Use Used in Caldwell-Luc operation to retract the mucoperiosteal flap—the shape of the instrument conforms to the architecture of the face thus preventing the assistant's hand from obscuring the site of operation.

The right angled curve is used for retraction of the lip and cheek.

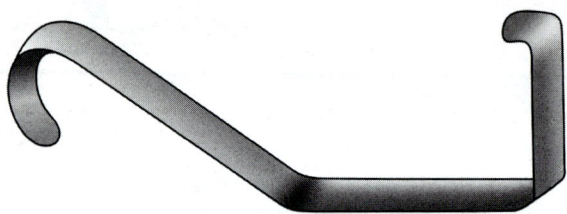

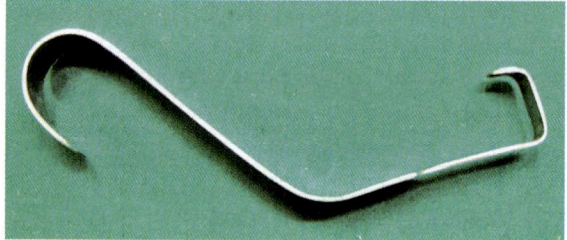

Fig. 52.74: Lip and cheek retractor

NASAL INSTRUMENTS

THUDICUM'S NASAL SPECULUM (Fig. 52.75)

Uses
- Diagnostic
  - For anterior rhinoscopy, i.e. examination of anterior part of nasal cavity. Structures seen are:
  - Nasal vestibule,
  - Little's area on the nasal septum,
  - Anterior part of septum,
  - Anterior part of inferior and middle turbinates.
  - Any pathological lesion can be observed in the above areas, e.g. polyps, atrophic rhinitis, foreign bodies, nasal mass like rhinosporidiosis, adhesions, etc.
- Therapeutic
  - Introduction of cotton pledgets for the purpose of local anaesthesia (4% xylocaine solution) before any nasal surgery.

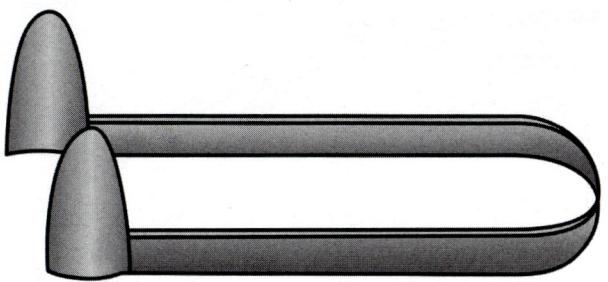

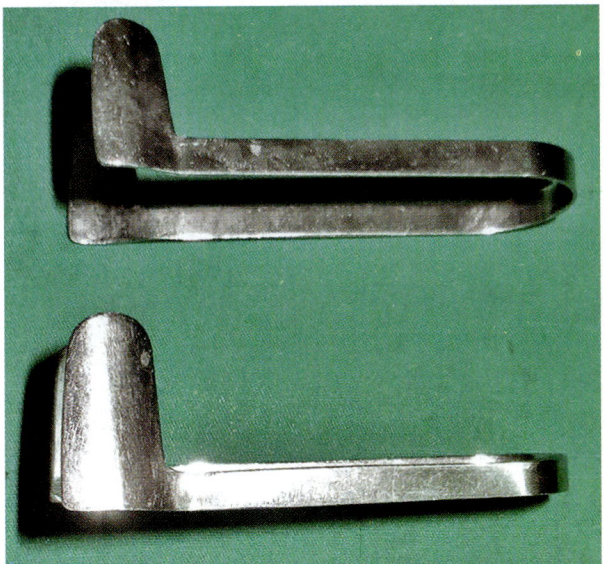

POSTERIOR NASAL OR RHINOSCOPY MIRROR (ST. CLAIR THOMPSON'S) (Fig. 52.76)

- This is used along with a tongue depressor to perform a posterior rhinoscopy.
- The step in the handle (bayonet shaped) allows a clear view of the area under examination as, the examiner's fingers do not obstruct vision.
- It is smaller in size than an indirect laryngoscope (IDL) mirror.
- The number on the metal surface indicates its size. (available in sizes 0–5).
- It has a plain mirror without any magnification.

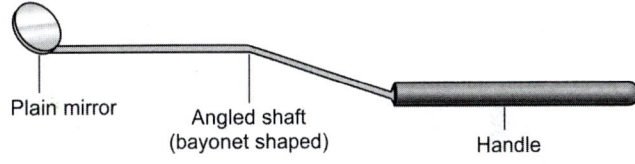

Plain mirror   Angled shaft (bayonet shaped)   Handle

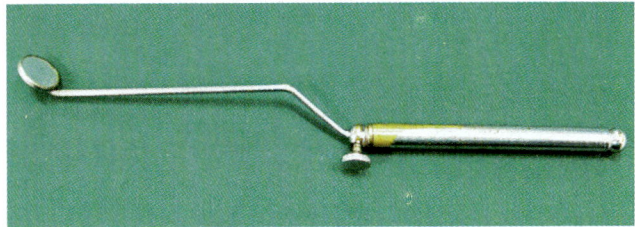

Fig. 52.76: Posterior rhinoscopy mirror

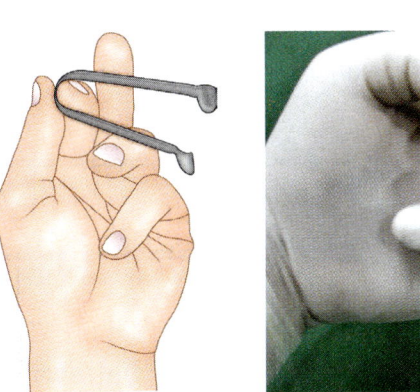

Fig. 52.75: Thudicum's nasal speculum

- Anterior nasal packing.
- Nasal foreign body removal.
- Three stick method of anaesthesia also known as 'Sludder's Method' prior to antral puncture.
- Various nasal operations—septoplasty, submucous resection (SMR), polypectomy, antral puncture, submucous cauterization, etc.

Uses   To perform a posterior rhinoscopy for examination or to detect or confirm presence of a pathology.

Structures seen on posterior rhinosopy:
- Choanal apertures,
- Posterior end of bony nasal septum,
- Posterior part of nasal cavities,
- Posterior end of inferior and middle turbinates,
- Eustachian tube opening,
- Fossa of Rosenmuller,
- Lateral nasopharyngeal wall,
- Superior surface of soft palate,
- Roof of the nasopharynx,
- Posterior nasopharyngeal wall,
- To visualise the nasopharynx for taking biopsy under local anaesthesia.

NASAL DRESSING FORCEPS (HARTMANN'S) (Fig. 52.77)

The instrument has a bend so that the surgeon's hand does not obstruct the view of the nasal cavity. The tip is diamond or olive shaped and has a groove in its centre.

Uses
- Removal of an anterior nasal pack.
- Removal of nasal foreign bodies.
- Introduction of cotton pledgets into the nose for the purpose of anaesthesia.

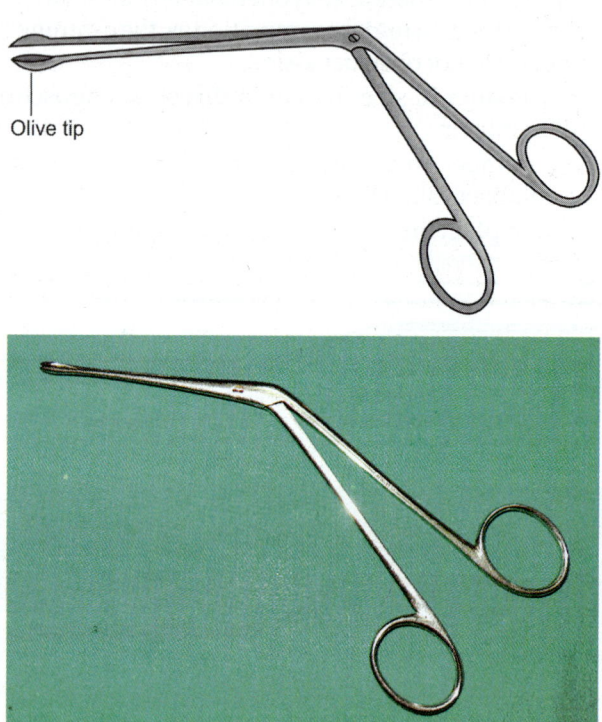

Fig. 52.77: Hartmann's nasal dressing forceps

- In all nasal surgeries for removal of bone chips, pieces of septal cartilage/bone, etc.
- Sometimes, for the removal of foreign bodies from the oral cavity and the oropharynx.

NASAL PACKING FORCEPS (TILLEY'S)

The tip of the instrument is straight with serrations thus having a poor grip. It is an angled instrument to prevent the surgeon's hand from obstructing the field of vision. It is not used for removal of foreign bodies (Fig. 52.78).

Use For anterior nasal packing, the indications being:
- After nasal operations for hemostasis, e.g. SMR, septoplasty, Caldwell-Luc etc.,
- Epistaxis,
- Along with posterior nasal packing.

Advantages During anterior nasal packing, the pack remains in place as it is arranged in layers when the instrument is removed out, since it has a smooth tip. A nasal dressing forceps may be entangled in the roller gauze due to its olive/diamond shaped tip.

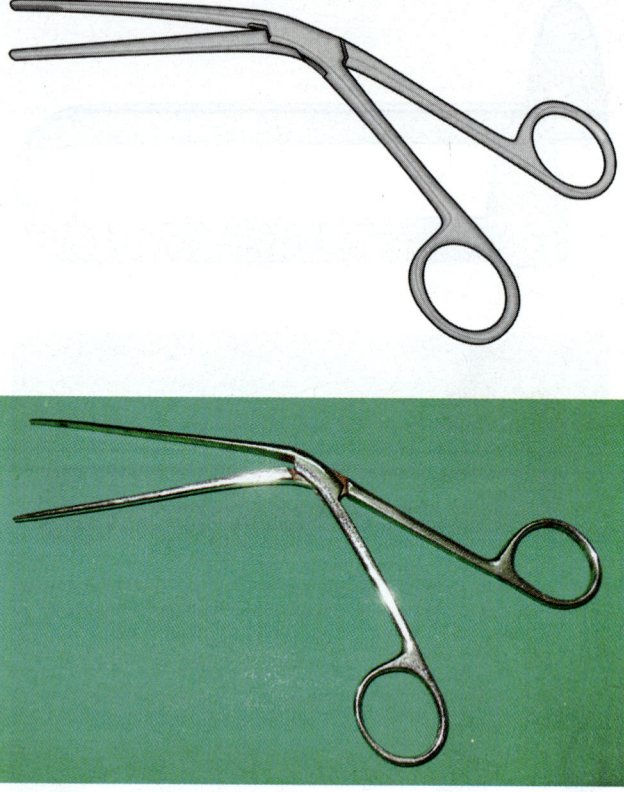

Fig. 52.78: Tilley's nasal packing forceps

TILLEY LICHWITZ ANTRAL PUNCTURE TROCAR AND CANNULA (Fig. 52.79)

Use Used for maxillary antral puncture along with a Higginson's syringe.

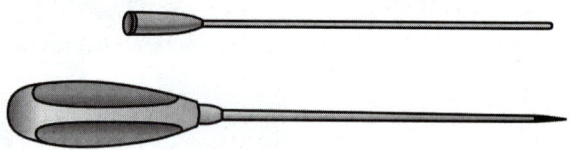

Fig. 52.79: Tilley lichwitz antral puncture trocar and cannula

The antrum is punctured through the inferior meatus, usually under local anaesthesia as this is the most accessible site for puncture. Returning fluid drains from the ostium of the maxillary sinus.

TILLEY'S ANTRAL HARPOON (Fig. 52.80)

Use It is used to puncture the medial wall of the maxillary antrum at the inferior meatus in the intranasal antrostomy operation for chronic sinusitis or along with the Caldwell-Luc operation.

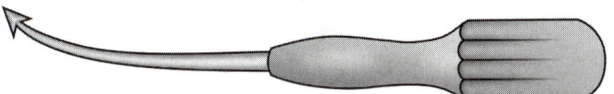

Fig. 52.80: Tilley's antral harpoon

It has a sharp tip which is introduced in the inferior meatus to create an opening in the medial wall of the antrum. After the opening has been made a Tilley's antral burr is introduced to smoothen out the antrostomy opening. The antrostomy is approximately 1.5 × 2 cm in dimension and situated in the inferior meatus as this is the most dependant site for enabling drainage of secretions by gravity.

ANTRAL BURRS (TILLEY'S)

Use   Used to dilate and smoothen the antrostomy opening following puncture by the Tilley's antral harpoon.

MUCOPERICHONDRIUM/MUCOPERIOSTEAL ELEVATOR
(Fig. 52.81A and B)

Uses
- For elevating the mucoperichondrial flaps in SMR and septoplasty operations of the nasal septum.
- For displacement of the inferior turbinate in antrostomy operation.
- For fracturing of turbinates.
- For removal of the maxillary crest in SMR.
- In mastoid operation for elevating the canal skin or soft tissues over the mastoid cortex—very rarely.

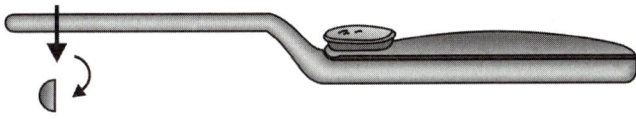

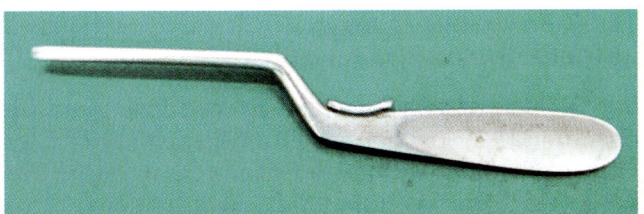

Fig. 52.81A: Killian's mucoperiosteal elevator

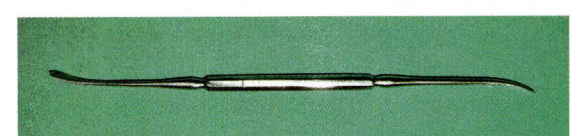

Fig. 52.81B: Freer's mucoperichondrial elevator

ST. CLAIR THOMPSON'S NASAL SPECULUM (LONG BLADED)

It is used in SMR and septoplasty operation to keep the mucoperichondrial flaps on either side of the nasal septum apart. The long blades protect the flaps from injury during trimming of the septum, otherwise there is a chance of septal perforation (Fig. 52.82).

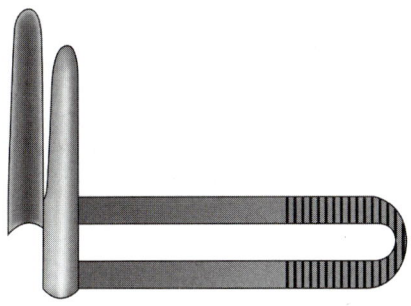

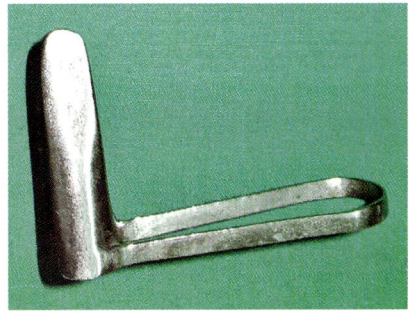

Fig. 52.82: St. Clair Thomson's long bladed nasal speculum

It cannot be used in the OPD as local anaesthesia is required before the long blades are introduced into the nasal cavity.

KILLIAN'S SELF-RETAINING NASAL SPECULUM (Fig. 52.83)

Uses
- Septoplasty
- SMR
- Nasal polypectomy

Advantages

- Long bladed, the distance between these blades can be adjusted and fixed with the screw during operation thus making it self-retaining and hence the surgeon has both his hands free to operate.
- Good visualization of structures deep in the nasal cavity minimises injury to mucosa.

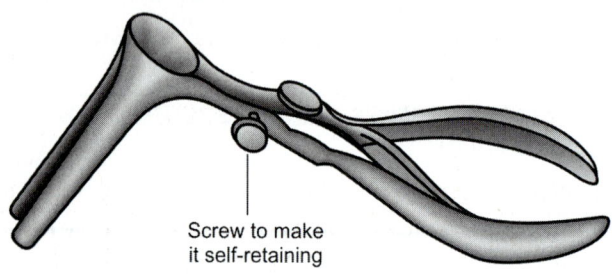

Screw to make
it self-retaining

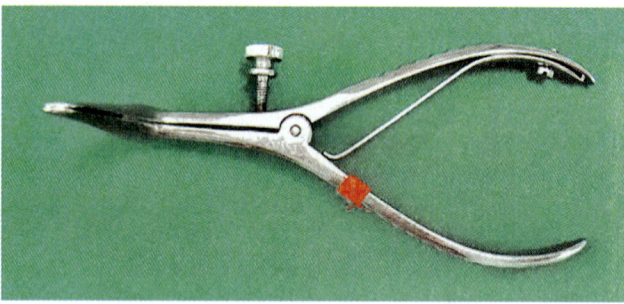

Fig. 52.83: Killian's nasal speculum

KILLIAN'S BAYONET SHAPED NASAL GOUGE

The tip is sharp and this instrument is used along with a hammer (Fig. 52.84).

Use   In SMR and septoplasty surgery to remove the maxillary crest and septal spur after elevation of the mucoperiosteal flaps.

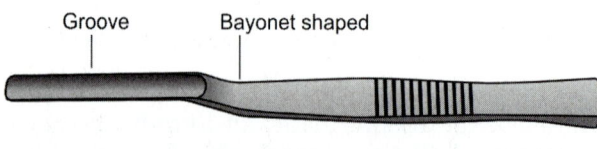

Groove   Bayonet shaped

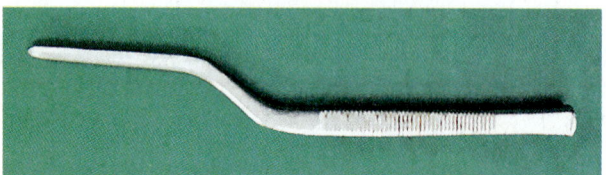

Fig. 52.84: Nasal gouge

LUC'S FORCEPS

It has a screw joint and 2 blades which have fenestrated and sharp ends which provides an excellent grip of the tissues during surgery. Also, the tissues bulge through the fenestra and are not crushed. This prevents alteration of tissues for histopathology (Fig. 52.85).

Uses

- In SMR and septoplasty for removal of cartilage or bone.
- In Caldwell-Luc operation to remove a polyp.
- To take punch biopsy from the oropharynx and nasopharynx.
- In tonsillectomy to hold the medial lip of the incision and tonsil tissue, only a blunt Luc's forceps may be used for this.

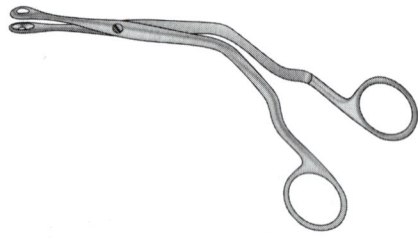

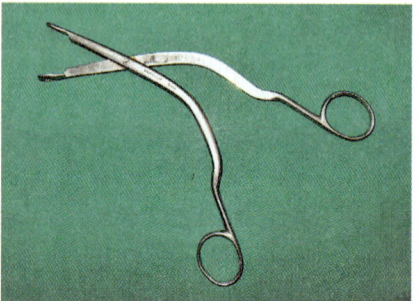

Fig. 52.85: Luc's forceps

- To remove the tags after adenoidectomy.
- Nasal polypectomy.
- For turbinectomy.

BALLENGER'S SWIVEL KNIFE

The blade can rotate through 360°. It is a bayonet shaped instrument with a blade at its tip (Fig. 52.86).

Use   It is used to cut the septal cartilage during an SMR operation after elevation of the mucoperichondrial flaps with leaving an adequate dorsal and caudal strut. The movement of the instrument is backwards, downwards and forwards. The cartilage is removed in a single piece and can be used later for rhinoplasty.

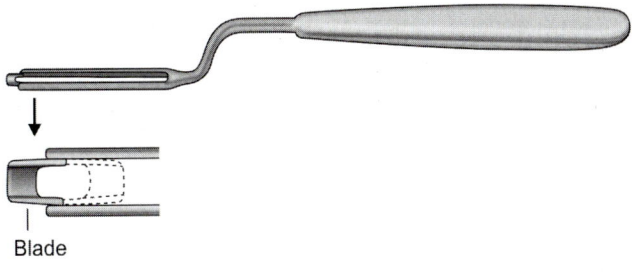

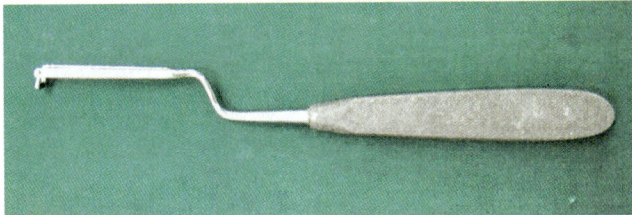

Fig. 52.86: Ballenger's swivel knife

NASAL FOREIGN BODY HOOK

It is used for removal of a foreign body from the nose especially in children.

MYLE'S RETROGRADE GOUGE

Used for making an opening in the inferior meatus during the intranasal antrostomy operation (like the antral harpoon).

WALSHAM'S FORCEPS

This is a straight forceps. A rubber tubing is used to cover one blade to protect the skin of the external nose (Fig. 52.87).

Use It is used for reducing the fracture of the nasal bones after dis-impacting them.

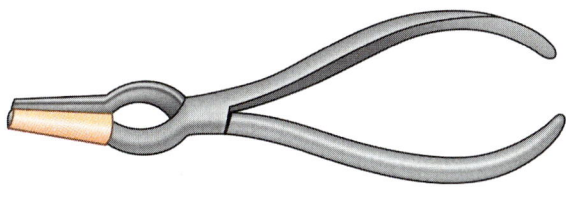

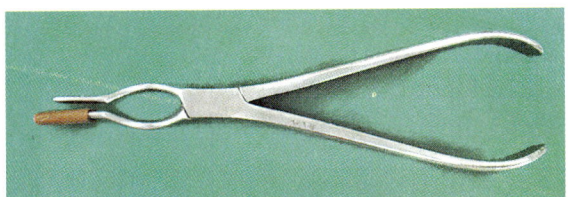

Fig. 52.87: Walsham's forceps

ASCH'S FORCEPS

This is used for reducing the fracture of the bony nasal septum by lifting the fragments of the nasal septum upwards and forwards (Fig. 52.88).

These forceps are bent at an obtuse angle. When the blades are closed, there is a gap between the blades to prevent the crushing of the nasal septum. It does not have rubber covering for the blades. There is a wider gap between the blades proximally to prevent damage to the columella.

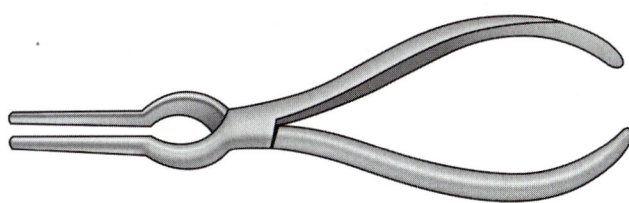

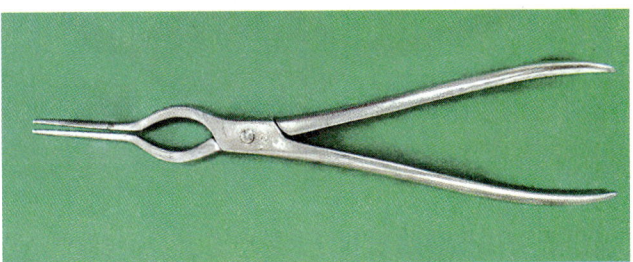

Fig. 52.88: Asch's forceps

GLEGG'S NASAL SNARE

Use In nasal polypectomy, it holds the pedicle of the nasal polyp and the polyp is removed by avulsion, i.e. the pedicle is held and the polyp is pulled out gently. The steel wires of this snare do not go completely into the shaft on closing. This is important to prevent cutting and help avulsion of the polyp. Mechanism of action— 'avulsion' (Fig. 52.89).

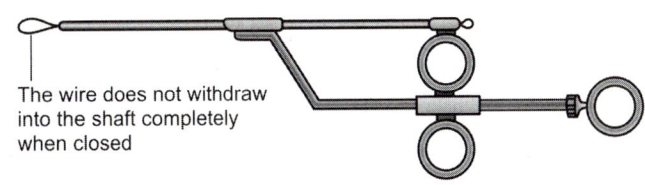

The wire does not withdraw into the shaft completely when closed

Fig. 52.89: Glegg's nasal snare

HIGGINSON'S SYRINGE

It is made of red India rubber. It has a central pouch (bulb) which is filled with saline or distilled water and a tube at either end. One end has a nozzel which fits into the Tilley Lichwitz antral puncture cannula and the other end has a one-way valve for allowing saline to enter into the bulb. There is a second one-way valve just 5–6 cm away from the nozzel, i.e. there are two one-way valves. It has a capacity of 3 oz (90 mL) (Fig. 52.90).

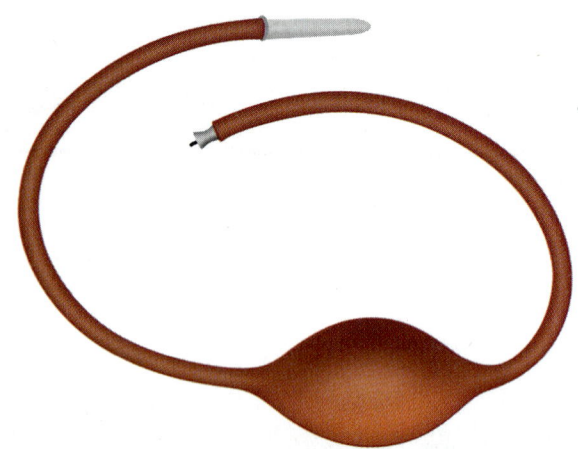

Fig. 52.90: Higginson's syringe

Use

• For giving maxillary antral washes following antral puncture and intranasal antrostomy either with saline or antibiotics as required.
• Can be used for nasal douching in atrophic rhinitis.

ROSE'S SINUS WASHING CANNULA

It is different from the Eustachian catheter in the following aspects (Fig. 52.91):
• Shorter in length,
• The opening of the cannula is situated at the side of the tip to prevent blocking by antral mucosa during its entry into the antrum.

Use   For washing the maxillary antrum through an antrostomy opening in a case chronic sinusitis. Used with a Higginson's syringe for this purpose.

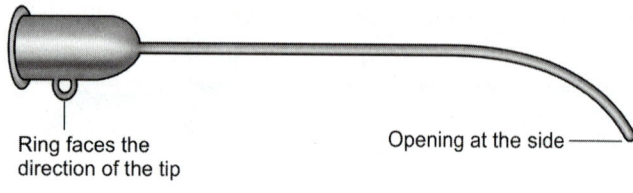

Ring faces the direction of the tip   Opening at the side

Fig. 52.91: Rose's sinus washing cannula

DOUBLE-ACTION BONE PUNCH (JENSON MIDDLETON'S)

It is called double-action because it has 4 joints with a double lever system to allow the blades to close and open to a limited extent in a narrow deep cavity. The double lever mechanism allows greater amount of force to be exerted at the tip of the instrument (Fig. 52.92).

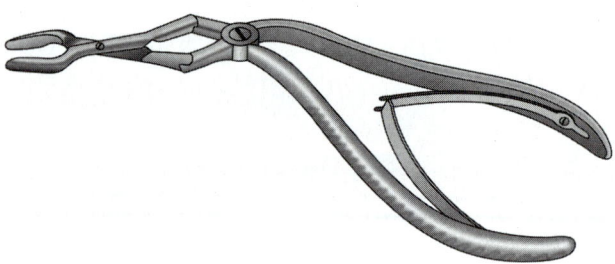

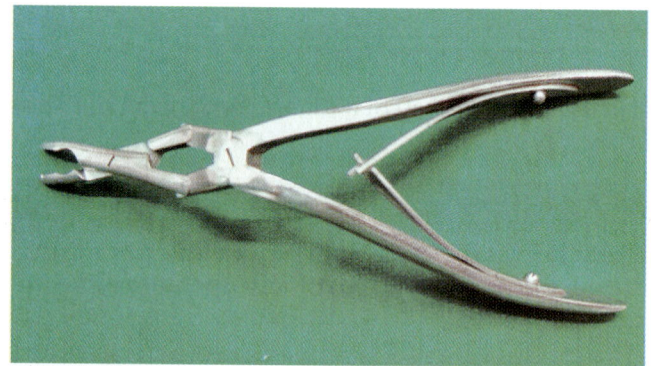

Fig. 52.92: Jenson-middleton's double action bone punch

Use   Used for removal of bony spurs during septal surgery.

Advantages   It simultaneously crushes the bone while removing it and thus achieves hemostasis.

HENCKLE'S ETHMOID PUNCH FORCEPS

It has crocodile jaws. It is used in nasal surgery. Its superior surface has markings to enable the surgeon to know the depth of the area reached during surgery thus preventing damage to important structures in relation to the ethmoid sinus, e.g. orbit, etc.

Uses

• Ethmoid polypectomy.
• Punch biopsy from the nasal cavity.
• Other surgeries of the posterior ethmoid sinus.

CITELLI'S PUNCH FORCEPS

It is a stouter instrument. It has no markings (Fig. 52.93).

Uses

- Sphenoidectomy.
- Intranasal antrostomy.
- Caldwell-Luc operation.
- External fronto-ethmoidectomy.

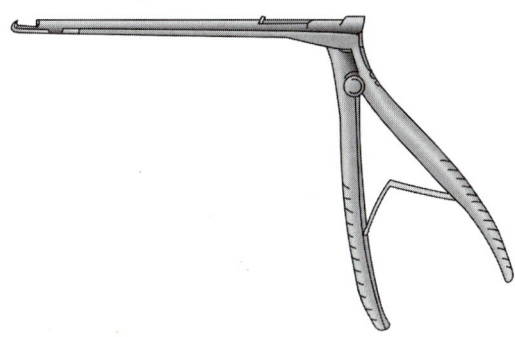

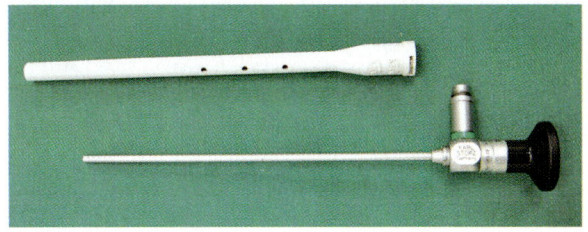

Fig. 52.94: Hopkins rigid 4 mm nasal endoscope (Green 0°)

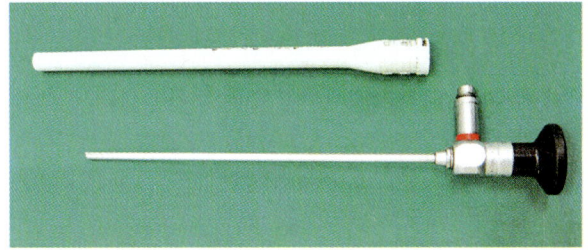

Fig. 52.95: Hopkins rigid 4 mm nasal endoscope (Red 30°)

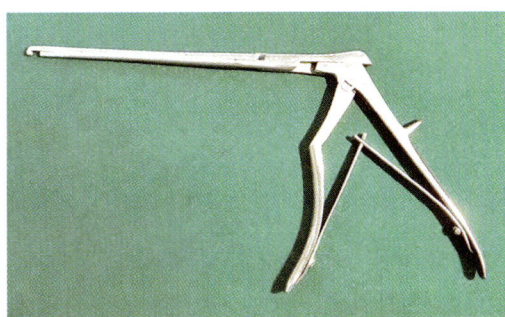

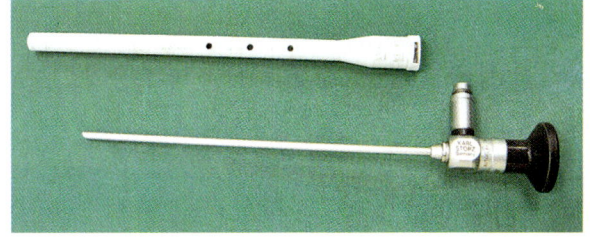

Fig. 52.96: Hopkins rigid 4 mm nasal endoscope (Black 45°)

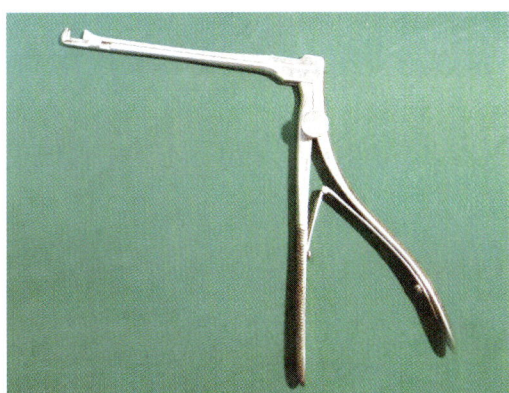

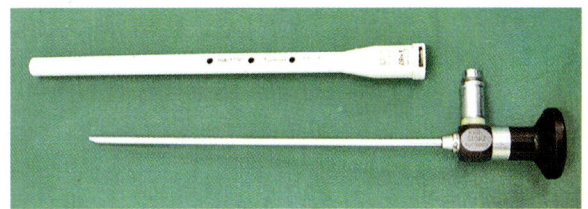

Fig. 52.97: Hopkins rigid 4 mm nasal endoscope (Yellow 70°)

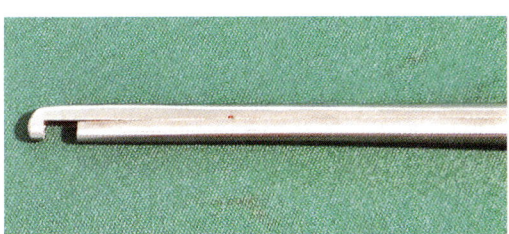

Fig. 52.93: Citelli's bone punch

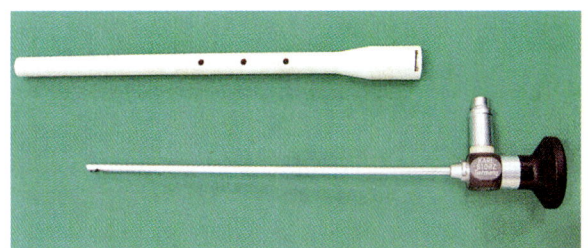

Fig. 52.98: Hopkins rigid 4 mm nasal endoscope (White 120°)

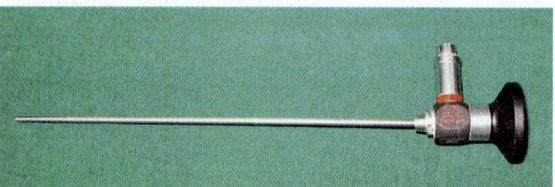

Fig. 52.99: Hopkins rigid 4 mm nasal endoscope (pediatric red 30°)

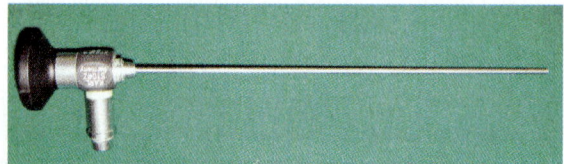

Fig. 52.100: Hopkins rigid 4 mm nasal endoscope (pediatric green 0°)

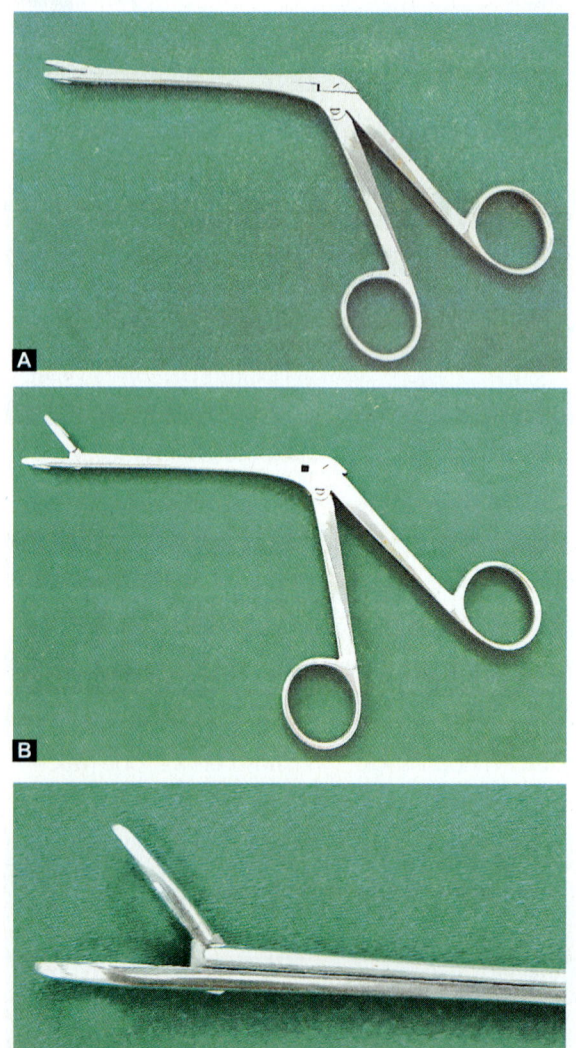

Fig. 52.101: A to C Blakesley weill grasping forceps

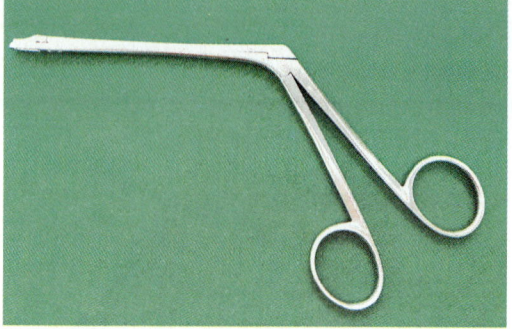

Fig. 52.102: Trucutting forceps

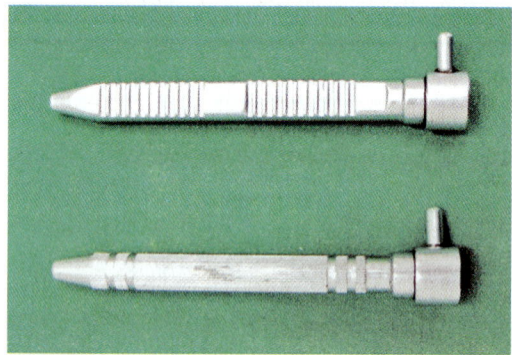

Fig. 52.103: Sheath for rigid nasal endoscope

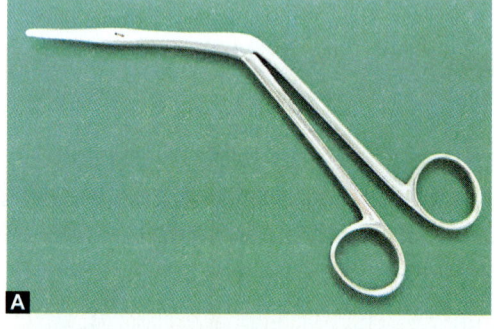

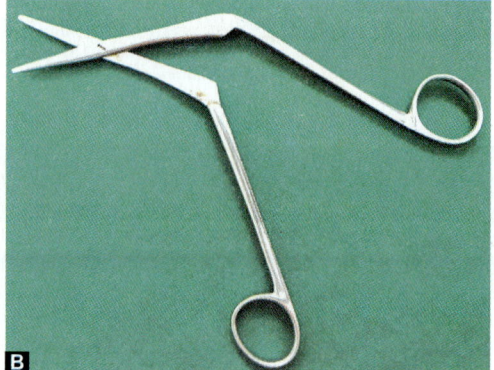

Fig. 52.104: Turbinectomy scissors

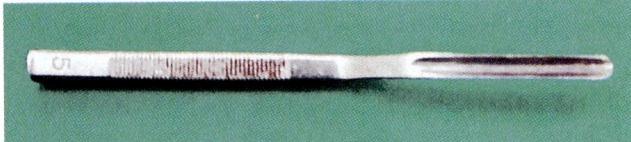

Fig. 52.105: Nasal gouge

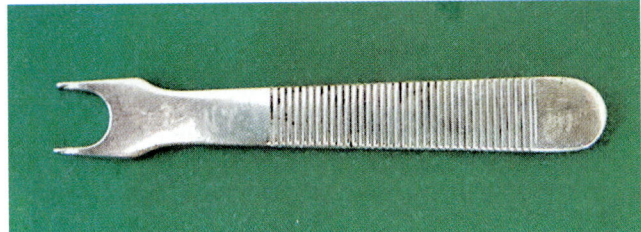

Fig. 52.106: Alar retractor

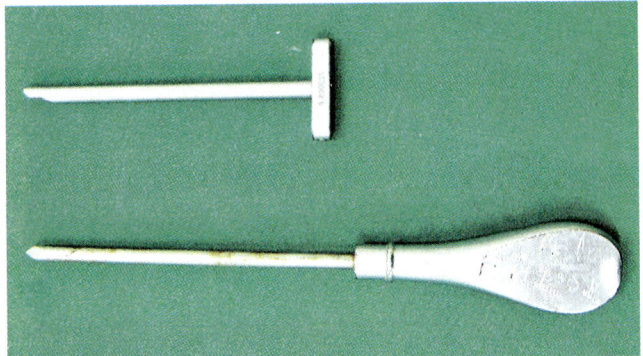

Fig. 52.107: Trocar and cannula for antrostomy

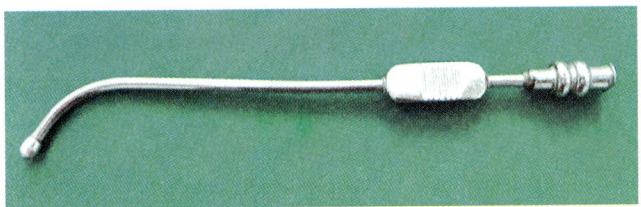

Fig. 52.108: Curved suction cannula

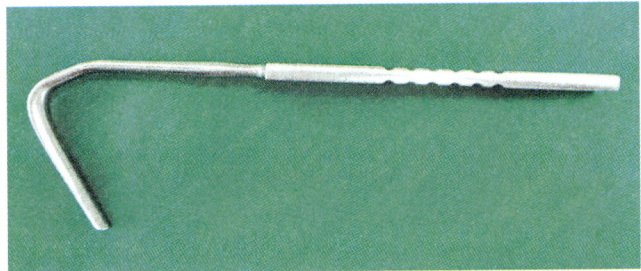

Fig. 52.109: Aufrich's specullum/retractor

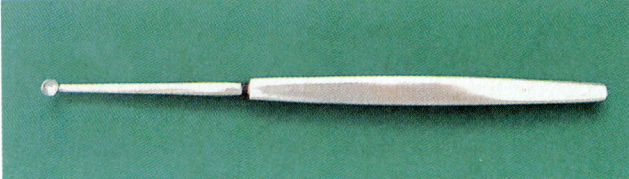

Fig. 52.110: Bone scoop

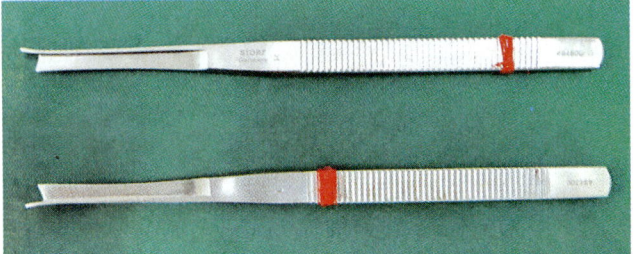

Fig. 52.111: Guarded osteotome

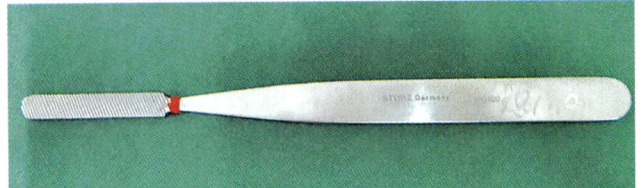

Fig. 52.112: Nasal rasp

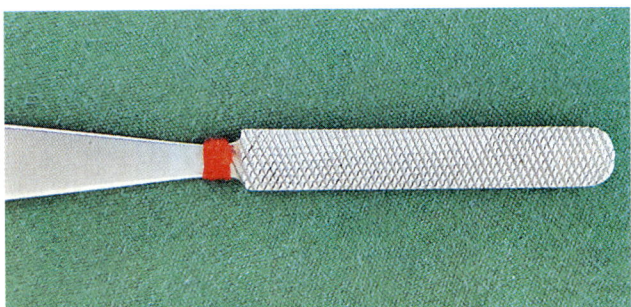

Fig. 52.113: Nasal rasp

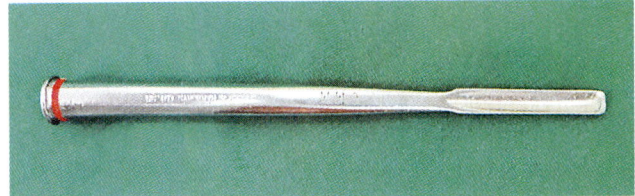

Fig. 52.114: Straight bone gauge

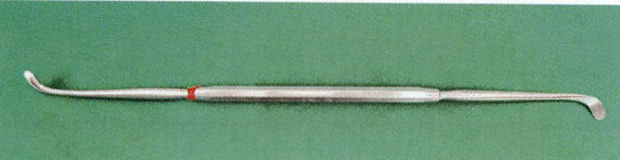

Fig. 52.115 : Cottle elevator

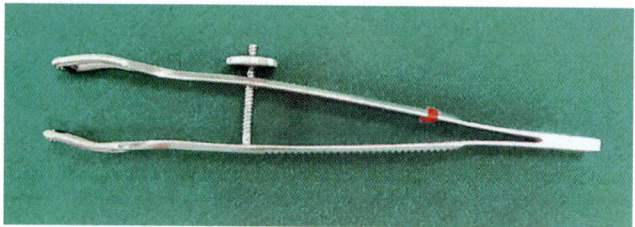

Fig. 52.116: Cottle columella clamp

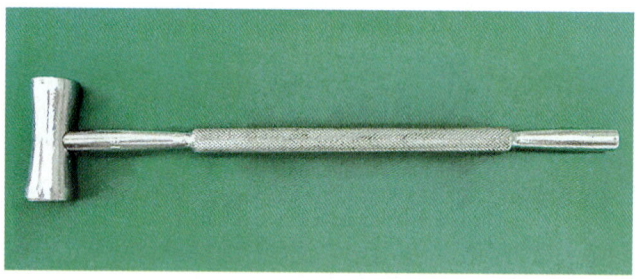

Fig. 52.117: Hammer/Mallet

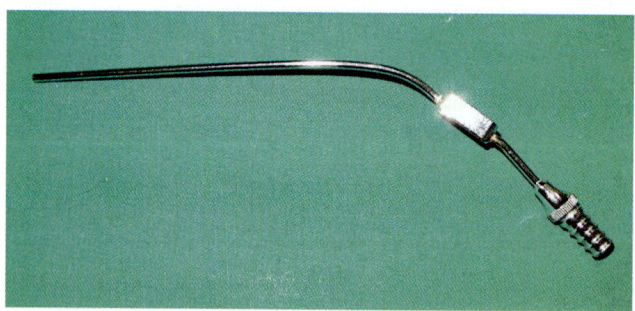

Fig. 52.118: Nasal suction cannula

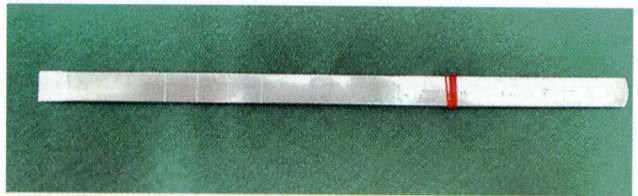

Fig. 52.119: Straight osteotome

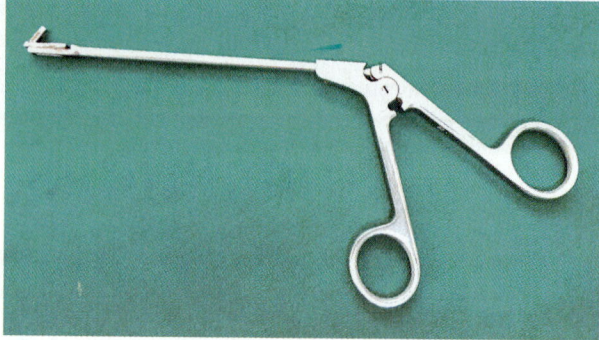

Fig. 52.120: Back-biting forceps (upward)

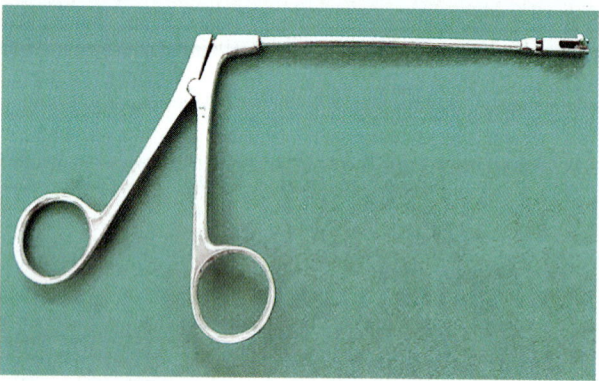

Fig. 52.121: Biting forceps (left)

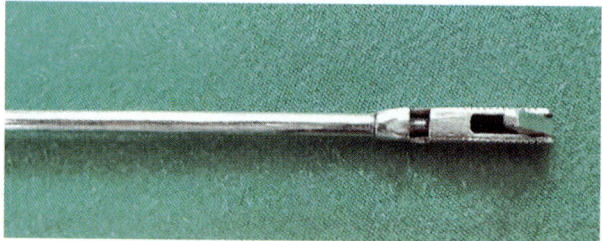

Fig. 52.122: Biting forceps (left)

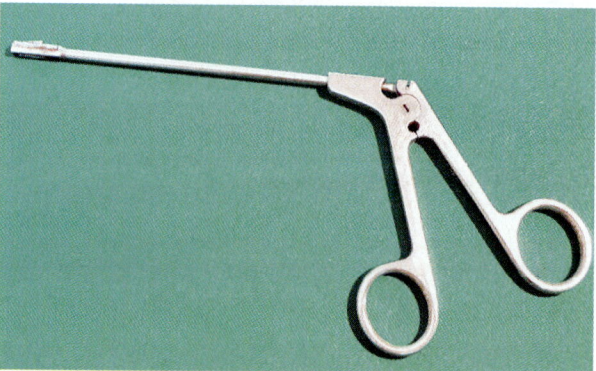

Fig. 52.123: Biting forceps (right)

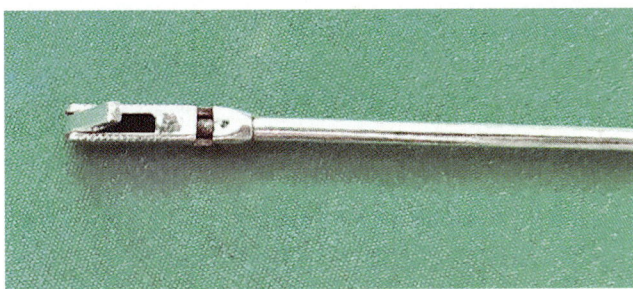

Fig. 52.124: Biting forceps (right)

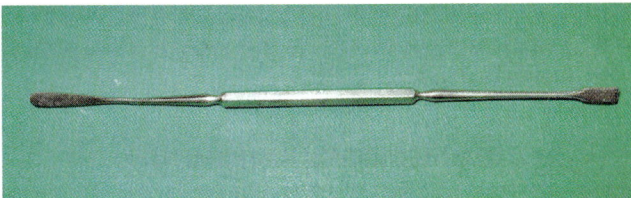

Fig. 52.125: Periosteal elevator

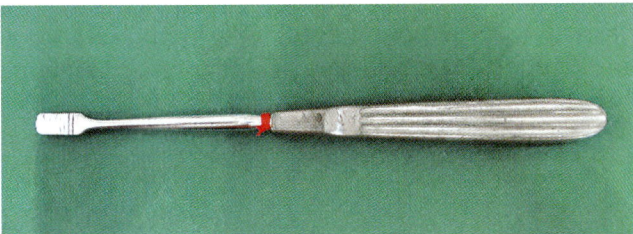

Fig. 52.126: Curved rasp

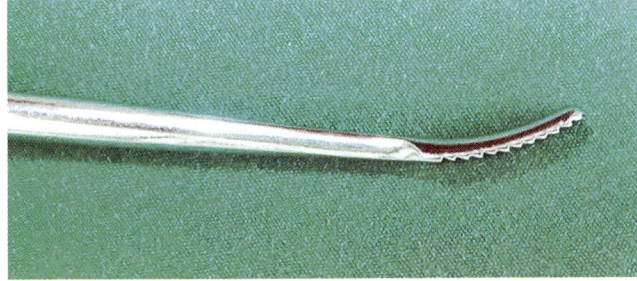

Fig. 52.127: Curved rasp

LARYNGEAL MIRROR

A long straight handle with the mirror placed at an angle. The mirror is a plane mirror without magnification (Fig. 52.128).

Uses
- In indirect laryngoscopy
  Structures seen are:
  - Base of tongue.

- Epiglottis (dorsal surface).
- Valecullae.
- Glosso-epiglottic folds.
- Aryepiglottic folds.
- Arytenoids.
- Interarytenoid region (posterior commissure).
- Pyriform fossa.
- Anterior commissure—sometimes.
- Vocal cords—true and false.
- Subglottis ⎤
- Few tracheal rings ⎦ Occasionally.
- To visualise oropharynx to remove foreign bodies like fishbone, etc., from oropharynx.

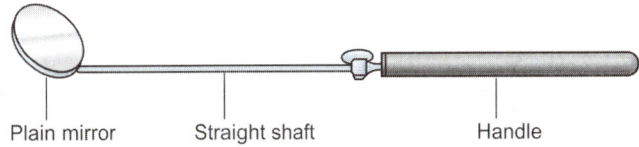

Plain mirror   Straight shaft   Handle

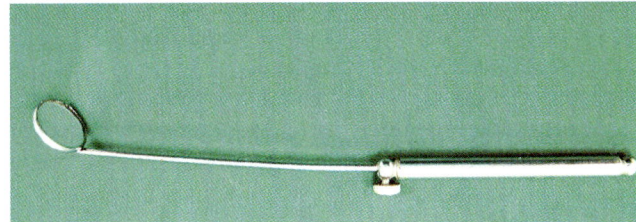

Fig. 52.128: Indirect laryngoscopy mirror (Laryngeal mirror)

- Application of cotton pledgets in the pyriform fossae which are dipped in 4% lignocaine for anaesthesia for direct laryngoscopy (i.e. blocking the superior laryngeal nerve) performed under local anaesthesia.

Structures not seen on IDL
- Post-cricoid region,
- Apex of pyriform fossa,
- Anterior commissure, (seen only in some patients on IDL),
- Ventricles,
- Laryngeal surface of epiglottis.

ENDOSCOPES

Chevalier Jackson's direct laryngoscope   It is used for direct laryngoscopy. The laryngoscope is 'U' shaped. It is made of German silver. The illumination is at the distal end and the handle is at a right angle. The illumination is by a fibre-optic light source. There is no magnification. It is used to visualize the hypopharynx and larynx.

- Uses
  - Direct laryngoscope is used.
  - It helps to visualise all areas of the hypopharynx and larynx not visible on IDL.
  - To assess the pathology and extent of the disease.
  - For taking biopsy from lesions of the hypopharynx or larynx.
  - For removal of foreign bodies.
  - The laryngoscope with a detachable blade is used to aid in a bronchoscopy.

Oesophagoscope   Used for visualisation of the oesophageal lumen. It is a rigid stainless steel instrument.

The following types of rigid oesophagoscopes are used:

- Jackson
- Negus

Jackson's oesophagoscope	Negus' oesophagoscope
• Distal illumination	• Proximal illumination
• Single bulb	• Double bulb
• Constant diameter	• Tapering distally
• No markings	• Marked

Illumination can be by a fibre-optic system or use of an electric bulb. The former is preferred as an electric bulb can fuse or explode due to getting over-heated.

- Use: Used for oesophagoscopy.

Microlaryngoscope (Kleinsasser's)   It is a stainless steel instrument and is made self-retaining, by fixing it on the anterior chest wall by means of a chest-piece to enable the surgeon to work with both hands. The procedure is performed under the magnification of an operating microscope. The micro-laryngoscope does not have any magnification by itself. The proximal aperture is wide for good visualisation and easy manipulation of instruments.

- Use: Used for micro-laryngoscopy.

Bronchoscope (Jackson)   It is a hollow metal tube with distal illumination similar to that of the laryngoscope. A fibre-optic light source is usually used. Nowadays a ventilating bronchoscope is used. At the distal end on its sides, the bronchoscope has holes called 'vents' (for ventilation) which permit ventilation of the lung through other bronchi in addition to the bronchus in which the bronchoscope has been inserted.

- Use: Used for bronchoscopy.

Fibre-optic flexible endoscopes   This includes naso-pharyngoscopes, laryngoscopes, bronchoscopes and oesophagoscopes. The illumination is by the fibre-optic system.

- Advantages
  - Gives minimum discomfort to the patient.
  - Performed only using surface anaesthesia.
  - May be performed as an OPD procedure.
  - Photography is easy.
  - Complications of anaesthesia are avoided.
  - Complications of rigid endoscopy like trauma, haemorrhage, etc., are avoided.
- Disadvantages
  - These are expensive.
  - Unsuitable for removing large foreign bodies.
  - Requires co-operation of the patient, as no anaesthesia is used.

TRACHEOSTOMY INSTRUMENTS

TRACHEAL DILATOR (TROUSSEAU'S)

It is used for dilating the incision made in the trachea prior to inserting the tracheostomy tube. Its tip is blunt and its blades spread out on approximating its handle (Fig. 52.129).

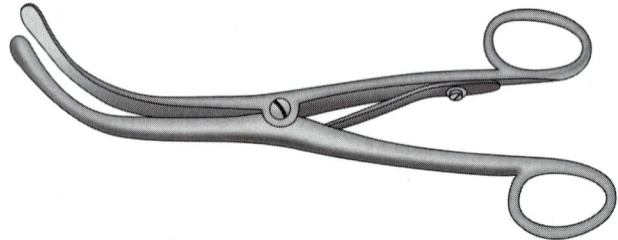

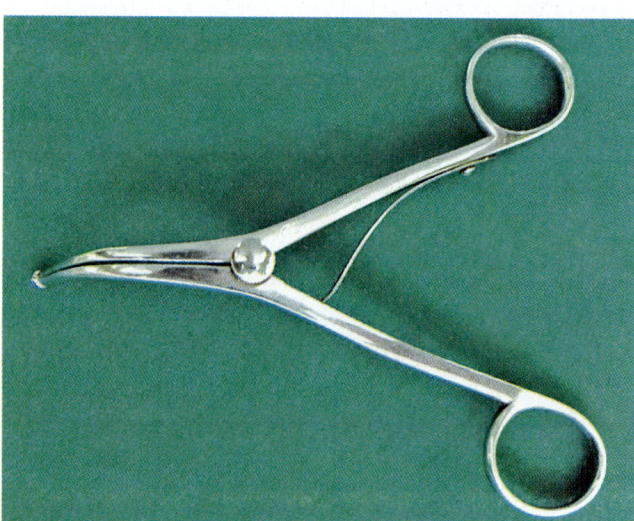

Fig. 52.129: Tracheal dilator

DOUBLE HOOK RETRACTOR

It is used to a retract skin, subcutaneous tissue and strap muscles of the neck on the two sides of the incision line during exposure of the tracheal rings. It is a blunt instrument (Fig. 52.130).

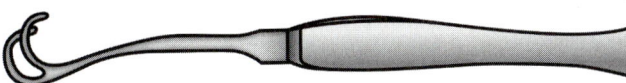

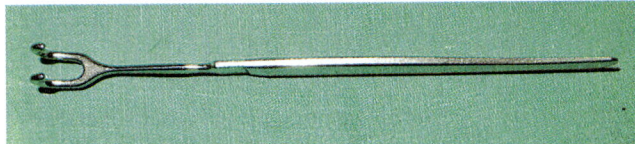

Fig. 52.130: Double hook retractor

SINGLE HOOK (SHARP) RETRACTOR

It is used to fix the larynx by retracting the cricoid cartilage superiorly prior to tracheal incision during the tracheostomy operation (Fig. 52.131).

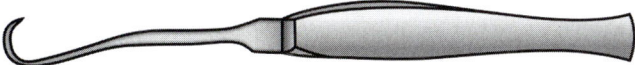

Fig. 52.131: Single hook retractor (sharp) (cricoid hook)

SINGLE HOOK (BLUNT) RETRACTOR

It is used for retraction of isthmus of the thyroid gland or midline soft tissue superiorly for exposure of the tracheal rings on the anterior wall in a mid or low tracheostomy operation (Fig. 52.132).

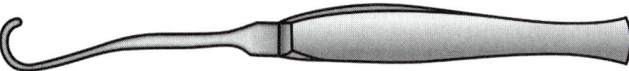

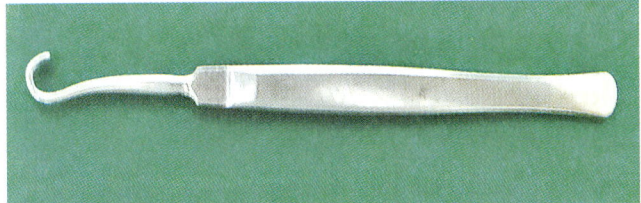

Fig. 52.132: Single hook retractor (blunt)

TRACHEOSTOMY TUBES (Fig. 52.133 A to C)

Chevaliar Jackson's tube It consists of an outer tube and an inner tube. Inner tube is longer than the outer so that when the tube gets blocked, the removal of the inner tube will restore patency and hence air-flow.

Traditionally, it is made of German silver which is non-irritant.

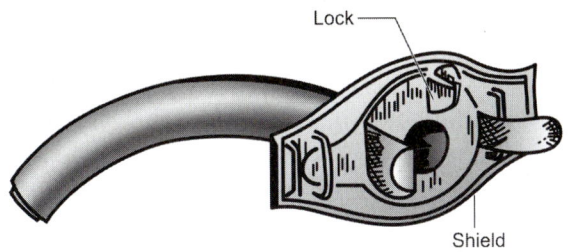

(A) Outer tube with inner tube in position

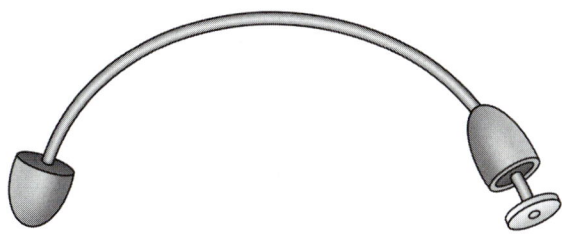

(B) Obturator

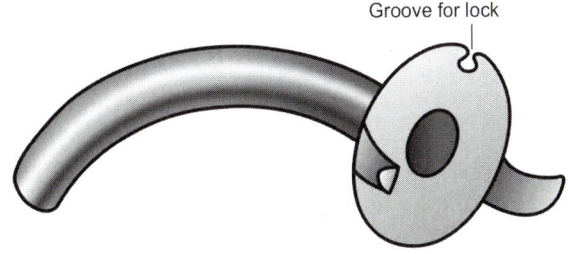

(C) Inner tube

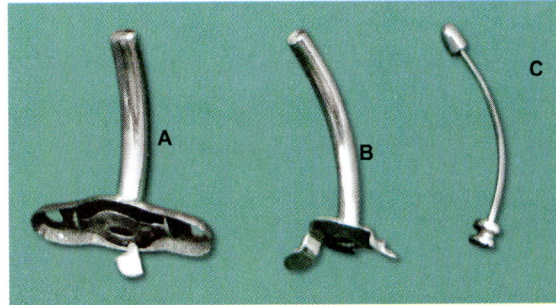

Fig. 52.133A to C: Chevalier Jackson's metallic tracheostomy tube

- Parts
  - *Outer tube*: Fits into the tracheostomy opening.
  - *Inner tube*: Fits snugly into the outer tube. But, protudes for approximately 2–3 mm beyond the outer tube.
  - *Shield*: It is attached to the proximal end of the outer tube and the tracheostomy tube is fixed to the neck by a linen tape threaded through the holes of the shield.
  - *Lock*: It is fitted on the shield and is meant to fix the inner tube inside the outer tube.
  - *Pilot*: It is a blunt ended curved obturator, which is inserted into the outer tube after removing the inner tube. It is used for inserting the tracheostomy tube in the tracheal opening as it makes the end atraumatic. As soon as the tube is inserted, the pilot is withdrawn and the patient starts breathing through the tracheostomy tube. Then, the inner tube is passed into the outer tube and fixed with the help of the lock.
- Other varieties
  - *Fuller's bi-valved tracheostomy tube*: Bivalve helps in introduction into tracheostome (acts as a dilator) without assistance of a tracheal dilator. The opening on the postero-superior wall of the inner tube helps in decannulation, i.e. determines whether normal air-passage is established on blocking the tracheostomy tube (Fig. 52.134).
  - *Edinburg type*: Movable shield with pilot.

Speaking valve   It is now possible for a tracheostomised patient to speak. (The speaking valve is attached to the inner tube.) This is one of the various procedures of speech rehabilitation in a laryngectomised patient.

Portex tracheostomy tube   Available with or without a cuff. It is a single tube (i.e. no inner tube) with a pilot and a blue line impregnated with a barium salt which makes the tube radio-opaque (Fig. 52.135).
- Advantages: (over the metal tube)
  - Less irritant.
  - Non-traumatic.
  - Can be used in patients who are on a respirator to give intermittant positive pressure ventilation (IPPV) due to presence of the cuff.
  - Does not come in way of radiotherapy.
  - Prevents aspiration, once cuff is inflated.
  - Can be used while giving general anaesthesia due to presence of the cuff which prevents leakage of anaesthesia gases.

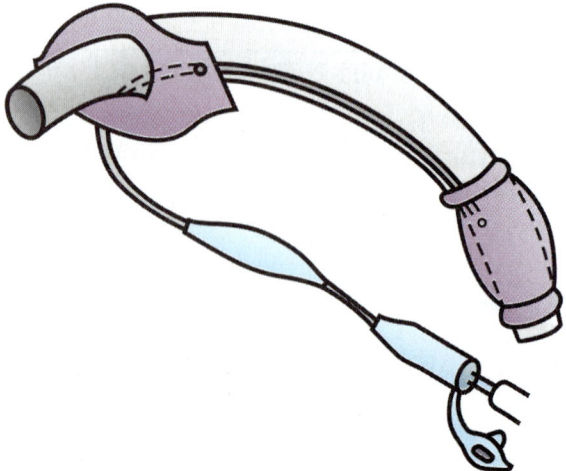

Fig. 52.135: Cuffed portex tracheostomy tube

LARYNX INSTRUMENT (Figs 52.136–52.143)

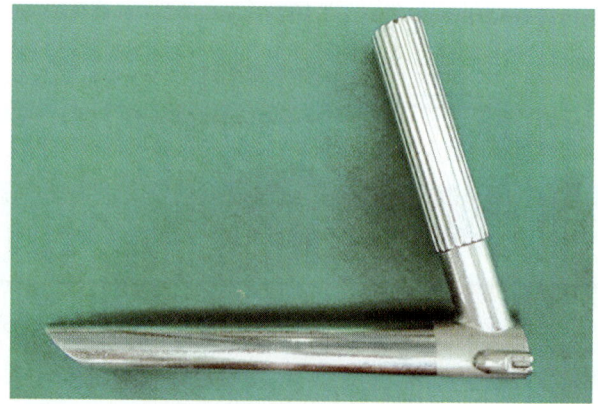

Fig. 52.136: Micro-laryngo scope

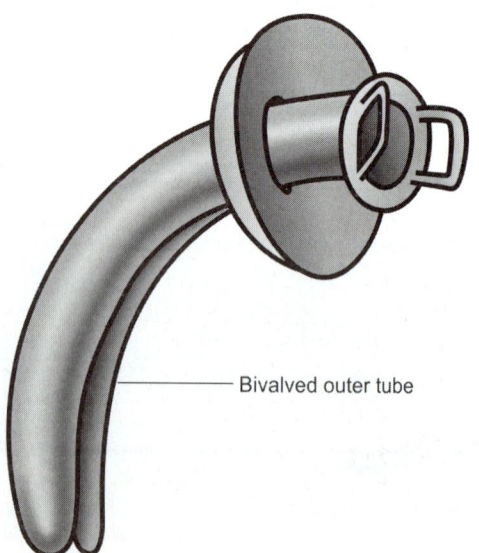

— Bivalved outer tube

Fig. 52.134: Fuller's bivalved tracheostomy tube

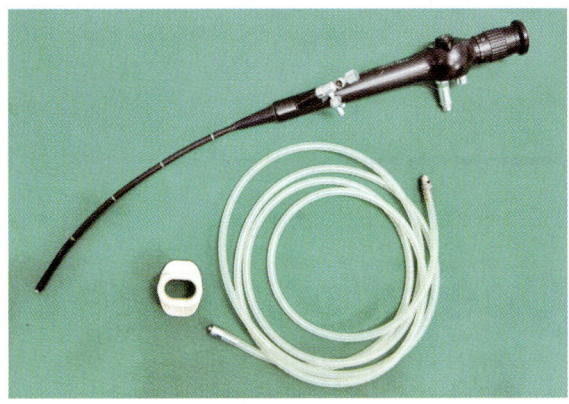

Fig. 52.137: Fiber-optic flexible laryngoscope

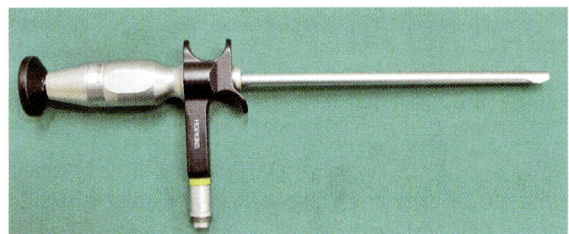

Fig. 52.138: 9 mm rigid Hopkin's telescope (laryngoscope)

Fig. 52.139: Micro-laryngeal cupped forceps

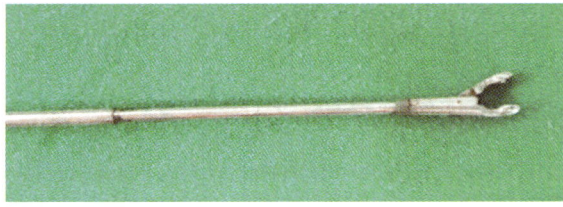

Fig. 52.140: Micro-laryngeal cupped forceps

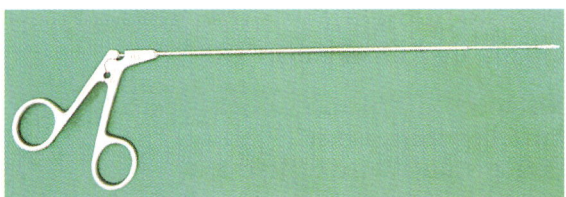

Fig. 52.141: Micro-laryngeal scissors

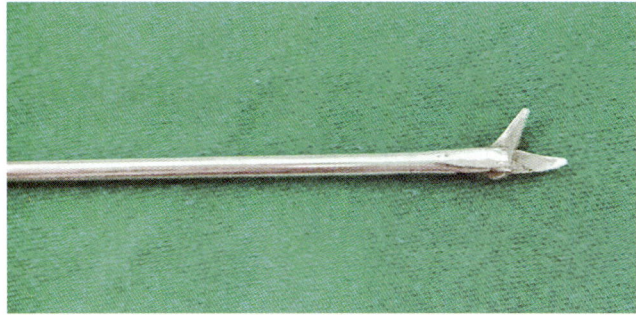

Fig. 52.142: Micro-laryngeal scissors

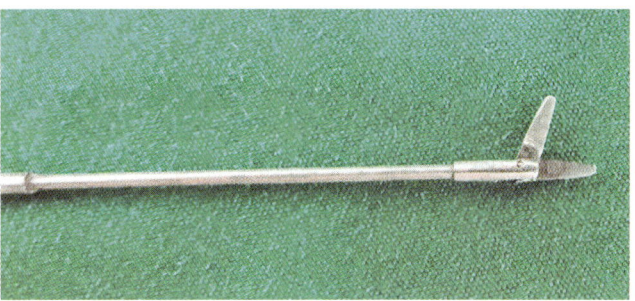

Fig. 52.143: Micro-laryngeal scissors

HEADLIGHTS IN ENT

CLAR'S HEADLIGHT

It has a 2-inch mirror which reflects light from a bulb attached to it and an adjustable head band.
It is usually electrically operated.

Uses   In all ENT operations. The mirror focuses the light to the site of the operation.

KASCHE'S HEADLIGHT

It has binocular vision and a magnification adjustable to 2X, 4X or 6X.

Use
- In minor ear surgeries like myringotomy, etc.
- In mastoid surgery.
- Facial nerve decompression.
- In OPD for diagnostic examination of ear diseases.
- It can be used for examination or operations on the nose and throat also.

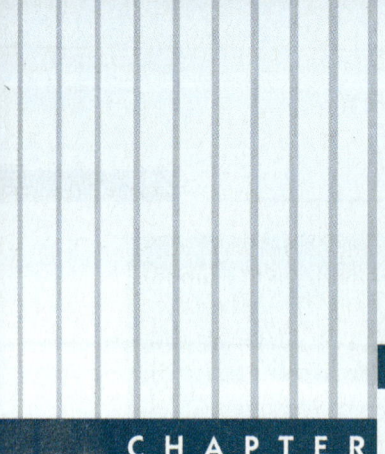

CHAPTER 53

Operations of the Ear

STAPEDOTOMY

Definition Stapedotomy is the surgery by which the fixed stapes footplate is by-passed using a prosthesis, so as to restore ossicular mobility. When the surgery was first described, the entire posterior half of the fixed stapes footplate was removed and the piston was placed on a connective tissue (fat/vein-graft/fascia), covering this opening and, hence was termed stapedectomy. Nowadays, only a fenestra of size 0.6–0.8 mm is made in the posterior half of the fixed stapes footplate. Hence, the term stapedectomy is more appropriately used.

Aim/Principle The immobile/fixed ossicular chain is made mobile, thus enabling sound waves to be transmitted into the inner ear.

Indications Stapes footplate fixation due to otosclerosis.

Contraindications
- Presence of infection, e.g. otomycosis: This surgery results in creating a fistula between the inner ear and middle ear. In the presence of any infection, transmission of infection into the inner ear can result in irreversible sensorineural hearing loss due to labyrinthitis.
- Medical contraindications like hypertension, diabetes, etc.
- Very young patients (age less than 16 years), since in these patients, there may be a congenital fixation of the stapes footplate and not otosclerosis. A congenital fixation is usually accompanied by other abnormalities, like a large cochlear aqueduct, etc., which have to be ruled out by a CT scan.
- Active otosclerosis (otospongiosis): Surgery in these cases is associated with bleeding and exacerbation of this condition.
- Pregnancy: The disease is usually in the active stage during pregnancy.
- Paget's disease.
- Cochlear otosclerosis: If the disease has involved the cochlea, improvement in hearing is not possible.
- Tympanosclerosis.
- Tinnitus and vertigo: This indicates involvement of the vestibular labyrinth and is usually associated with sensorineural loss, which cannot improve with surgery.
- Other ossicular pathologies, like congenital ossicular fixation, fixed malleus-incus syndrome, etc.
- Only hearing ear: Hearing aid is preferred over surgery.
- Unilateral otosclerosis.
- Tympanic membrane perforation: In such cases, a myringoplasty is performed first, followed by stapedotomy after 3–4 months.

Anaesthesia Local anaesthesia is usually preferred for the following reasons:
- Intraoperative bleeding is less.
- Hearing improvement is tested immediately on the operating table.
- Patient being adult is always cooperative.

Position Patient is supine with the ear to be operated up and head turned to opposite side.

Procedure

- The operating microscope is used for this surgery.
- Incisions: The various incisions used for stapedotomy are:
  - *Rosen's endomeatal incision:* On the posterior bony external auditory canal (EAC) from 6 O'clock to 12 O'clock position, 6 mm away from the annulus. Incision is bone deep (Fig. 53.1).
  - *Lempert's endaural incision:* The incision at the 12 O'clock position (roof) in the external auditory canal extends from the annulus to about 1–2 cm in front of the tragus. The 6 O'clock incision extends from the annulus to the junction of bony and cartilagenous EAC and a horizontal incision on the bony EAC joins the two.

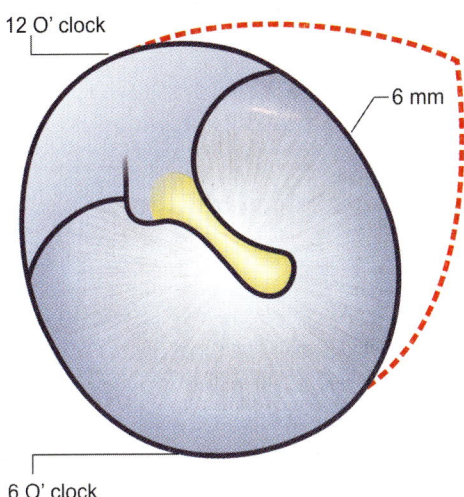

Fig. 53.1 : Rosen's endomeatal incision

- *Wilde's post-aural incision:* The incision extends from the superior end of the pinna to the mastoid tip about 0.5 mm behind the post-aural groove.
- The tympanomeatal flap (comprising the tympanic membrane and meatal skin), is elevated and reflected forward, so as to visualise the ossicular chain.
- The incudostapedial joint is visualised clearly including the stapes footplate. The posterosuperior bony overhang, needs to be either curated/drilled out until the base of the pyramidal process is seen.
- Presence of stapes footplate fixation is confirmed by testing ossicular mobility.
- The stapedius tendon is cut near its origin from the pyramidal process, to prevent adhesion forming which can impede mobility of the ossicular chain.

- The incudostapedial joint is dislocated and the stapes suprastructure (head, neck, and both crura) is removed.
- A small fenestra is made on the fixed footplate, using a stapes footplate perforator, a skeeter drill (attached to a microdebrider console) or even LASER. Sometimes the otosclerotic footplate may need to be thinned out using a diamond burr, in case of obliteration otosclerosis, prior to making a fenestra, thus exposing the inner ear, i.e. a window is created between the inner and middle ear.
- A teflon piston is placed between the long process of the incus and the fenestra on the stapes footplate.
- Now, when the ossicular chain moves, the mobility is transmitted into the inner ear via the piston (Figs 53.2 and 53.3).
- The tympanomeatal flap is now replaced.
- Hearing is tested on the operation table.
- The EAC is packed with gelfoam soaked in antibiotic drops.
- If the incision is endomeatal, no sutures are required; if the endaural incision is used, sutures are taken and a dressing is given.

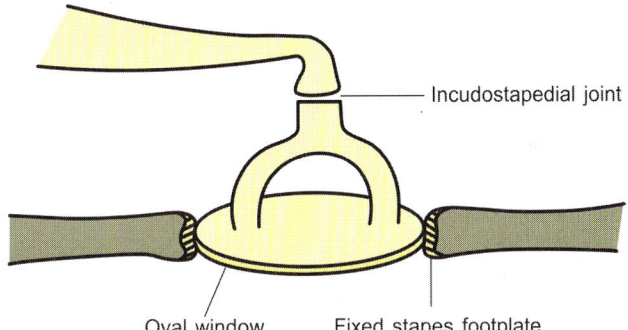

Fig. 53.2 : Otosclerotic stapes footplate

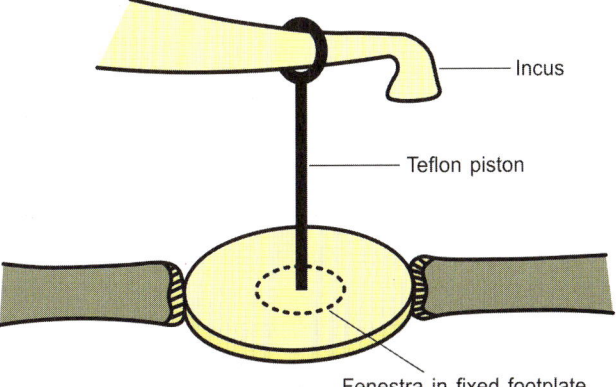

Fig. 53.3 : Teflon piston in position

Complications

- **Complications of anaesthesia:** Arrythmias, hypotension, or hypertension.
- **Perforation of the tympanic membrane,** if occurs, it is closed using a temporalis fascia graft.
- Dislocation of the incus from the malleus.
- **Sensorineural hearing loss** due to damage to inner ear while making the fenestra.
- **Labyrinthitis** due to infection resulting in sensorineural hearing loss.
- **Vertigo, nausea, and vomiting** due to stimulation of the labyrinth. Treated with labyrinthine sedatives.
- **Facial nerve palsy,** if the nerve is dehiscent and accidentally damaged.
- **Conductive hearing loss** due to dislocation of piston from incus or fenestra.
- **Perilymph fistula resulting in sensorineural loss** due to sudden straining, e.g. sneezing or vomiting, etc.

Postoperative care

- Antibiotics.
- Anti-inflammatory analgesics.
- Nasal decongestants.
- Avoid swimming or flying in unpressurised aircraft for 6 weeks.
- Avoid straining or lifting weights or sneezing.

FACIAL NERVE DECOMPRESSION

Definition   It is the surgery performed to relieve facial nerve of compression and, hence, treat facial paralysis due to this cause.

Relevant anatomy   Parts of the facial nerve along its course from the geniculate ganglion to the stylomastoid foramen include:

- Intracranial
- Extracranial
  - Intratemporal
  - Extratemporal

Temporal course includes the following parts:

- Petrous (in the internal auditory canal) part.
- Labyrinthine part.
- Tympanic or Horizontal part.
- Mastoid or Vertical part.

Extratemporal course includes the following parts:

- Preparotid.
- Course of the nerve in the parotid gland.
- Extra parotid course.

The facial nerve is more often prone to palsy than other cranial nerves, due to the following reasons:

- It has the longest course traversed by any nerve in a bony canal.
- Its course is altered radically at the first genu, second genu and on its exit from the stylomastoid foramen.
- It is closely related to several important structures like the cerebellopontine angle, VIIIth cranial nerve, middle ear, mastoid, and parotid gland. Pathology involving any of these, leads to involvement of the facial nerve.

Indications

- Bell's palsy, where conservative/medical line of management has failed even after a trial for 6–9 months or where the palsy progresses.
- Post-traumatic facial palsy.
- Iatrogenic facial palsy after ear surgery (tympanoplasty/mastoidectomy/stapedectomy) or parotid gland surgery.
- Facial palsy due to cholesteatoma.
- Facial palsy due to acute otitis media or secretory otitis media.

Anaesthesia   It can be done under general or local anaesthesia.

Position   Patient is supine with the ear to be operated facing up.

Procedure

- The operating microscope is used for this operation.
- A postaural (Wilde's) incision is taken.
- A simple/cortical mastoidectomy is performed.
- Landmarks to delineate the facial nerve:
  - Short process of incus.
  - Lateral semicircular canal.
  - Tympanic annulus.
  - Tympanomastoid suture line.
  - Digastric ridge.
  - Stapes footplate.
- The facial nerve is exposed by using a diamond burr over the fallopian canal.
- Once the facial nerve is exposed and pressure is relieved, any pathology, e.g. cholesteatoma or bone spicules are removed.

The sheath is not incised in case of infectious pathology, i.e. cholesteatoma and usually incised in case of Bell's palsy.

Complications

- Complications of anaesthesia.
- Ossicular dislocation resulting in conductive hearing loss.

- Infection resulting in perichondritis.
- Labyrinthine damage resulting in sensorineural hearing loss.
- Tympanic membrane perforation.

ENDOLYMPHATIC SAC DECOMPRESSION

Definition   It is the surgery performed for decompression of the endolymphatic sac in a case of Meniere's disease (endolymphatic hydrops).

Mechanism of action/Principle   In endolymphatic hydrops, there is an increase in the endolymphatic pressure within the endolymphatic sac, which results in symptoms, like nausea, vomiting, and vertigo. By decompressing the sac, this pressure is relieved and symptoms do not occur.

Anaesthesia   Local or general anaesthesia is used.

Position   Patient lies supine with ear to be operated uppermost.

Technique   A postauricular incision is taken and a simple mastoidectomy is performed using an operating microscope. All the three semicircular canals are delineated in their bony coverings,(Blue lining of semicircular canal). The endolymphatic sac lies in this region is now drilled using a diamond burr, so as to expose the endolymphatic sac, which gets decompressed as the bone over the sac is removed. This relieves the pressure in the sac and treats the cause of the symptoms.

Other surgeries useful in Meniere's disease:

- Cervical sympathectomy: It helps by reducing the production of endolymph.
- Vestibular neurectomy: The vestibular division of the VIIIth cranial nerve is sectioned and the labyrinth is denervated with relief of symptoms.
- Labyrinthectomy: The labyrinth is destroyed and symptoms are relieved. It is done by ultrasound or cryosurgery or by surgery.

Endolymphatic sac surgery is preferred as it reduces symptoms, is easy to perform and does not affect hearing.

AURAL POLYPECTOMY

Definition   It is the operation performed for the removal of an aural polyp.

Indications

- Aural polyp.
- Aural granulations.

Contraindications

- Infection in the EAC.
- Bleeding polyp (e.g. glomus tumour).
- It is important to get an audiological assesment of hearing post-polypectomy done by pure tone audiometry prior to surgery, to confirm the hearing loss and document for medicolegal purposes. Also to compare with postpolypectomy hearing.

Anaesthesia   It can be done under general or local anaesthesia.

Position   Patient is in the supine position with the ear to be operated uppermost.

Procedure   The operating microscope is used for this surgery with an aural speculum. The polyp is visualised under magnification and using a suction cannula, the site of origin of its pedicle is detected. A microear surgery scissors (Balluchi scissors) is used and the pedicle is gently cut holding the polyp taut with a suction cannula. A cup forceps is not preferred to hold the polyp, since the polyp may arise from or may be attached to an important structure in the middle ear (e.g. facial nerve, stapes footplate, etc.), which may be damaged, if the polyp is avulsed or pulled. Hence, since the pressure exerted by a suction cannula is moderate in degree, it does not avulse the polyp and damage to underlying tissues is prevented.

After the entire polyp is excised from its pedicle, the site of its origin is noted along with the pathology in the tympanic membrane (perforation or cholesteatoma).

The EAC is now packed with gelfoam dipped in antibiotic with steroid eardrops (Betnesol N or Neosporin H), which slowly dissolves over several weeks.

Complications

- Complications of anaesthesia.
- Pulling or avulsing the polyp will result in damage to important structures in the middle ear to which it may be adherent, e.g. facial nerve palsy, if it arises from the facial nerve, sensorineural hearing loss, if it arises from the stapes footplate, etc.
- Massive haemorrhage, if the history and examination is not done accurately, a glomus tumour can be mistakely excised resulting in torrential bleeding. Packing of the ear is required with a CT scan and proper excision at a later date.
- Damage to tympanic membrane, if polypectomy is done by an inexperienced surgeon.

AURAL SYRINGING

Definition   It is the procedure, whereby the external ear is cleared of debris, wax or foreign body using water or normal saline in a metallic aural syringe.

Indications   It is performed for removal of:
- Wax, after it is softened with sodium bicarbonate eardrops.
- Non-hygroscopic foreign body.
- Debris in the EAC.
- Clearing discharge from the EAC.

Contraindications
- Impacted wax removal is very painful and never complete.
- Hygroscopic foreign body, it will swell and get impacted.
- Perforation of the tympanic membrane.
- Cerebrospinal fluid (CSF) otorrhoea.
- Bleeding from ear.
- Otomycosis: Residual moisture will further aggravate this condition.

Other methods of foreign body/wax removal:
- Using a wax hook.
- Using a vectis.
- Using suction apparatus.
- Discharge and very soft wax can also be removed using a swab stick.
- Using a cup or crocodile forceps under the operating microscope.

Anaesthesia   Aural syringing is an OPD procedure, painless and does not require any anaesthesia. Small children are held by their parents/relatives or an assistant/nurse, for this procedure. Only, if the patient is very uncooperative, general anaesthesia is required for removal of wax or foreign body under an operating microscope. However, syringing is always an OPD procedure.

Position   Aural syringing is performed with the patient in the sitting position, facing the side opposite to the ear to be syringed, i.e. the ear to be syringed faces the surgeon who is seated in front of the patient. He visualises the EAC using a head-mirror and a Bull's eye lamp.

Procedure
- The aural syringe is a metallic syringe, which is held in the right hand of the examiner. The index and middle fingers are inserted into the two side rings

and the thumb is inserted into the central ring on the piston. The left hand of the examiner retracts the pinna, so as to straighten the EAC.
- Tap water boiled and then cooled to body temperature is used. Normal saline can also be used. If the fluid used is below or above body temperature, it can result in stimulation of the labyrinth and severe vertigo with nausea and vomiting.
- The nozzle of the syringe is directed towards the roof, anterior wall or posterior wall of the EAC i.e. away from the tympanic membrane, as it can get damaged.
- The piston is gently pushed, so that the water flows into the EAC at a moderate force and the wax flows out. Forceful syringing can result in damage to the eardrum or can result in abrasion of the EAC.
- If at times, the wax occludes the EAC completely, a small chink can be made using a vectis or wax hook, as it enables the water to enter the EAC behind the wax and force it out.
- After syringing is complete, the external ear and tympanic membrane are examined and the EAC is cleaned with a cotton swab dipped in spirit, so as to dry the ear and prevent otomycosis, which may develop due to the presence of moisture.
- Gutta Boric Spirit (GBS) eardrops are given in the dose of 2 drops twice daily for 3–5 days to keep the ear dry.

Complications
- Trauma to tympanic membrane or the EAC.
- Vertigo, if the water used is above or below the body temperature, as this results in stimulation of the labyrinth.
- Infection of the external ear; if the water used is unsterile or infection may occur in the middle ear, if there is a perforation of the eardrum and unsterile water enters the middle ear.
- Otomycosis may occur, if the ear is not cleaned dry with a swab stick after syringing, to remove the residual moisture.

Care after syringing
- Anti-inflammatory analgesics are given orally for 3 days to relieve pain and congestion.
- Gutta boric spirit drops are advised twice a day for 3–5 days keep the ear dry completely, and prevent infection or otomycosis.

MYRINGOTOMY

The details of myringotomy operation are described in the Chapter 9 'acute suppurative otitis media (ASOM)'.

However, myringotomy can be performed either with or without insertion of a grommet or ventilation tube.

Types of grommet
- Synonym: Ventilation tube.
- Classification
  - *Short-term ventilation tubes*
    - Shepard tube.
    - Donaldson tube.
  - *Mid-term ventilation tubes*
    - Shah grommet.
    - Reuter bobbin.
- Armstrong bevelled tube.
- Paparella type-I tube.
- Feuerstein split tube.
- JS Knight split tube.
- Linderman Silverstein arrow tube.
  - *Long-term ventilation tubes*
    - Per-Lee tube.
    - Goode T-tube.
    - Paparella type-2 and 3

Difference in myringotomy performed for ASOM and SOM   Differences between ASOM and SOM on the basis of myringtomy performed are given in Table 53.1.

TABLE 53.1: Differences in myringotomy performed for ASOM and SOM		
Myringotomy	*ASOM*	*SOM*
• Anaesthesia	• Always general anaesthesia, as local anaesthesia does not act effectively in the presence of acute infection.	• Local anaesthesia in adults. • General anaesthesia in children.
• Site of incision	• Posteroinferior quadrant.	• Anteroinferior.
• Type of incision	• 'J' shaped, as it cuts across the radial fibres and does not close soon.	• Radial, as grommet is to be inserted.
• Insertion of grommet	• Not done.	• Always done.

CHAPTER 54

Operations of the Nose and Paranasal Sinuses

FRACTURE NASAL BONE REDUCTION

Definition   Fracture nasal bone reduction is a reduction of the dislocated fragments of the fractured nasal bones.

Indications   Fracture of the nasal bones with dislocation of the fragments, *only if seen within 48 hours of injury* as later on, oedema sets in.

In case of fracture without any dislocation, no reduction is required.

Anaesthesia   Local or general anaesthesia is required. Local anaesthesia is usually preferred unless the patient is uncooperative or a child.

Position   The patient lies supine on the operation table.

Procedure
* The Asch forceps is used for reduction of the dislocated nasal septum and the Walsham forceps are used for reduction of the dislocated nasal bones.
* Initially, the Walsham forceps is used on either side to separate the dislocated fragments. Then, the Asche forceps is used to reduce the fractured nasal septum. Following this, now the Walsham forceps is used on either side to reset the displaced fragments of the nasal bones.
* If the patient comes after 48 hours but within 4 weeks of fracture, antibiotics and anti-inflammatory analgesics are used to reduce the oedema and then reduction of the fractured fragments is performed.
* If the patient comes after 4 weeks of injury, a rhinoplasty is required, as by this time, new bone formation occurs.

LATERAL RHINOTOMY

Definition   Lateral rhinotomy is not an operation but an approach, which gives access to the following regions:
* Nasal cavities.
* Ethmoids.
* Nasopharynx.
* Sphenoid.
* Pterygopalatine fosse.

Incision
* The incision passes along the lateral border of the nose. It starts just at the level of the medial canthus and ends just around the alar margin (Fig. 54.1).
* The incision is also cosmetically very acceptable.

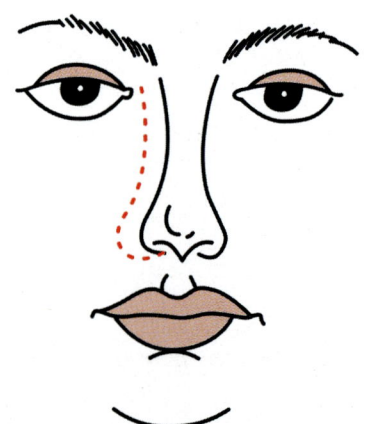

Fig. 54.1 : The lateral rhinotomy approach

Common indications

- Excision of rhinosporidiosis.
- Nasopharyngeal angiofibroma.
- Frontoethmoidal mucocoele or pyocoele.
- It can be combined with an anterior craniofacial approach.
- Malignant melanoma of the nose.
- Inverted papilloma of the nose.

MAXILLECTOMY

Definition Maxillectomy is an operation performed for removal of the maxillary bone.

Indications Malignant tumour of the maxilla confined to the maxilla without any metastasis.

Procedure

- Always under general anaesthesia.
- Weber Ferguson incision with a palatal incision. (Figs 54.2 and 54.3).
- After elevating the soft tissue flaps, the maxilla is exposed.
- The maxilla is freed with osteotomies through the following bones:
  - Zygoma.
  - Palate.
  - Frontal process of maxilla.
  - Pterygoid plates.
  - Ethmoid labyrinth.
  - Lateral orbital wall.

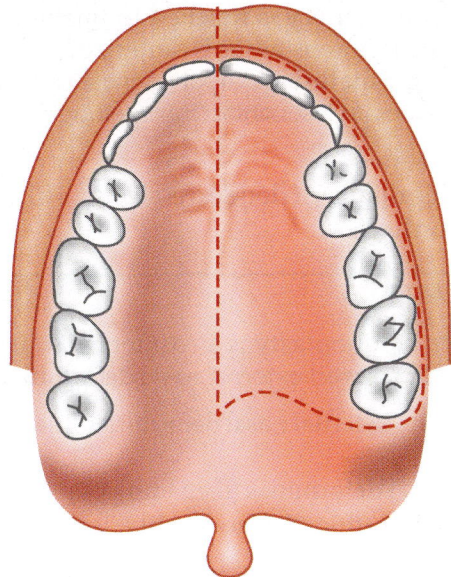

Fig. 54.3 : Weber Ferguson incision

Rehabilitation

- Principle: To give a minimal cosmetic and functional defect.
- The cavity is fitted with a temporary prosthesis soon after surgery and it is replaced by another prosthesis after 10 days. A permanent final prosthesis is given in the next 4–8 weeks.

SUBMUCOUS CAUTERIZATION OF TURBINATES

Indications Enlarged or hypertrophied inferior turbinates causing nasal obstruction.

Causes of turbinate hypertrophy

- Allergic rhinitis.
- Compensatory hypertrophy on the side of the concavity in severe deviated nasal septum (DNS).

Procedures for reducing the size of the inferior turbinate

- Submucous cauterization using electrocautery.
- Surface cauterization using chemical cautery like 25% silver nitrate.
- Turbinectomy.
- Laser.
- Cryocautery.

Procedure

- It is performed under local anaesthesia.
- Patient is supine.
- Thudicum's or Saint Claire's long bladed nasal speculum is used to visualise the turbinate.
- A long polythene sheathed needle is introduced into the submucosa of the inferior turbinate.

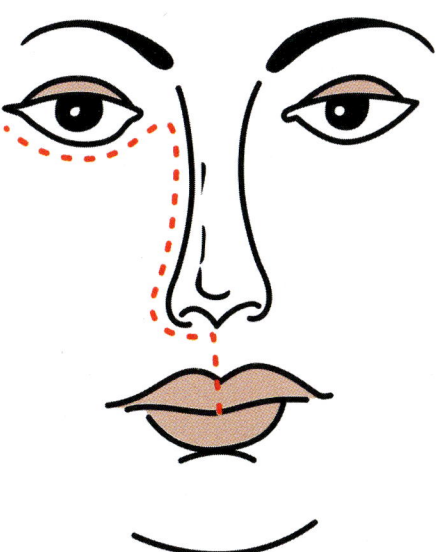

Fig. 54.2 : Weber Ferguson incision

- The electrocautery is touched to this needle and submucous fibrous tissue is cauterized, resulting in shrinking of the turbinate (polythene sheath insulates other tissues in close contact from getting cauterized).

Complications
- Atrophic rhinitis, if done excessively.
- Haemorrhage.

RHINOPLASTY

Definition   Rhinoplasty is a cosmetic nasal surgery performed to correct external nasal deformities.

Indications   External nasal deformities due to:
- Trauma.
- Congenital deformities like a hump.
- Deformities due to diseases like leprosy (saddle nose).
- Following previous nasal surgery, e.g. SMR.
- Can be combined with a septoplasty in case of a co-existing DNS; when it is known as septorhinoplasty.

Types
- External, where the incision is taken on the face.
- Internal, where the incision is taken inside the nasal cavity.
  Materials used for rhinoplasty are listed in Table 54.1.

TABLE 54.1: Materials used for rhinoplasty	
Homografts	*Prosthesis*
• Septal cartilage or bone	• Silicone
• Iliac crest bone	• Teflon
• Rib bone and cartilage	
• Calvarial bone	

Homografts are preferred, as they are easily available, inexpensive, and have a good success rate as seen on follow-up.

NASAL POLYPECTOMY

Definition   Nasal polypectomy is a surgery performed for the removal of nasal polyps.

Types of nasal polyps/Classification
- Antrochoanal polyp which originates from the maxillary antrum.
- Ethmoidal polypii which originate from the ethmoidal air cells.

Anaesthesia   Local or general anaesthesia.

Position   Patient lies in the supine position on the operation table.

Procedure
- If the patient is under general anaesthesia, the throat is packed around the endotracheal tube with a roller gauze pack to prevent aspiration of blood and secretions.
- The polyp is visualised using a Killian's self-retaining nasal speculum to widen the nasal cavity.
- The pedicle of the polyp, if possible, is visualised.
- The polyp is removed by avulsion using either a nasal snare or a Luc's forceps to grasp it, from the pedicle. If the pedicle is not visualised, as is common in case of large or multiple polypii, the polyp is grasped as near to the pedicle as possible and avulsed.
- Haemorrhage is controlled by packing the nasal cavity for 15–20 minutes with gauze dipped in saline-adrenaline solution (1: 200000 dilution).
- After haemostasis, both the nasal cavities are packed with roller gauze packs dipped in liquid paraffin.
- The packs are removed after 48 hours.

Postoperative care
- No oral feeds for 4–6 hours.
- Watch for bleeding through nose or postnasal bleeding.
- As patient has to now breathe through his mouth, Condy's gargles and tincture benzoin inhalations are given 4 times a day, for oral hygiene and humidification of air respectively.
- Antibiotics orally for 5–7 days.
- Anti-inflammatory analgesics orally for 5–7 days.
- Antihistaminics in case of ethmoidal polypii, where allergy is commonly an aetiological factor.

Complications
- Complications of anaesthesia.
- Haemorrhage (epistaxis).
- Incomplete removal and recurrence.
- Synechiae (adhesions) formation.
- Atrophic rhinitis, if the nasal cavity is too roomy after polypectomy.

SURGERY OF FRONTAL AND ETHMOIDAL SINUSES

Frontoethmoid surgery
- Conservative
  - Frontal sinus trephination
  - Intranasal ethmoidectomy
  - Transantral ethmoidectomy (Jansen-Horgan)
- Radical
  - *External frontoethmoidectomy*
    - Lynch Howarth's operation.
    - Patterson's operation.

- Killian's operation.
- *Osteoplastic flap*
- Macbeth's.
- *Osteoplastic flap with obliteration of frontal sinus*
- Montgomery's.
- *Sinusectomy*
- Riedl's

INTRANASAL ETHMOIDECTOMY

Definition   Intranasal ethmoidectomy is procedure used for removal of diseased mucosa from the ethmoidal sinuses via the nasal route.

Types
- Using an operating microscope.
- Using a sinus endoscope.

Anaesthesia   Preferably done under general anaesthesia where the nose is packed with cotton pledgets soaked in a solution of saline-adrenaline (1:100000 dilution).

If under local anaesthesia, the nose is packed with cotton pledgets soaked in 4% lignocaine-adrenaline (1:100000 dilution).

Aim   Removal of all diseased ethmoidal air cell mucosa through the middle meatus route.

Limitations of the procedure
- Aggar nasi cells (anteriormost ethmoidal air cells) cannot be reached.
- Only 80% of air cells are removed.
- Recurrence of polypii or disease may occur.
- It is a relatively blind procedure and hence complete removal is not possible. Also, complications are more likely to occur.

Complications
- Damage to orbit, proptosis and blindness.
- Damage to optic nerve.
- Damage to anterior cranial fossa dura and cerebrospinal fluid (CSF) rhinorrhoea.
- Haemorrhage.
- Infection and meningitis.

TRANSANTRAL ETHMOIDECTOMY

Synonym   Jansen-Horgan's Operation.

Definition   Transantral ethmoidectomy is a procedure used to clear the maxillary sinus and the adjacent ethmoidal labyrinth of all diseased tissue.

Indications
- When the maxillary sinus and the ethmoid air cells are to be cleared of disease through the same approach.
- Orbital decompression in 'malignant exophthalmos'.

Procedure   After a Caldwell-Luc operation is performed and the maxillary antrum is opened, the ethmoidal air cells are opened through the antrum by passing a forceps through the superomedial region of the antrum in the superior, medial, and posterior direction, i.e. towards the opposite parietal eminence.

Complications   Same as those for Caldwell-Luc and intranasal antrostomy.

EXTERNAL ETHMOIDECTOMY

Definition   External ethmoidectomy is clearance of disease from the ethmoidal sinuses via the external approach.

Synonym   Extranasal ethmoidectomy.

Indications
- Recurrence of disease (sinusitis or polyposis), after intranasal ethmoidectomy.
- Mucocoecle of ethmoid sinuses.
- Pyocoele of ethmoid sinuses.
- To detect and cauterise or ligate the ethmoidal artery in case of epistaxis.
- As an approach for:
  - Repair of CSF rhinorrhoea.
  - Optic nerve decompression.
  - Dacryocystorhinostomy.
  - Sphenoid sinus surgery.
  - Surgery of pituitary gland.

Incision   Howarth's incision.

Advantages over intranasal approach
- Complete removal of disease is possible.
- Less chance of complications, as it is performed under vision.

INTRANASAL ANTROSTOMY

Definition   Intranasal antrostomy is an opening made in the medial wall of the maxillary antrum for the purpose of antral washes and drainage.

Unlike the antral puncture, where the opening closes almost immediately after the removal of the cannula, this opening is larger and hence remains patent for a longer period of time. It facilitates long-time drainage of the maxillary antrum.

Indications

- Chronic maxillary sinusitis not responding to three repeated antral punctures.
- With a Caldwell-Luc operation.
- For a biopsy in case of Ca maxilla.
- To facilitate healing of an oroantral fistula.
- To facilitate drainage of an antral haematoma.
- For elevation of a depressed fracture of the maxilla.
- For elevation of a blow out fracture of the orbit.
- In patients, where repeated sinus endoscopic examination of the antrum is required.
- In cases of allergic rhinitis and sinusitis, it is performed with submucous cauterization of the inferior turbinates.

Procedure

- It is performed under local anaesthesia using 4% lignocaine soaked cotton pledgets placed in the inferior meatus for 10–15 minutes.
- The patient lies supine.
- Using the Tilley's antral harpoon, an opening is made in the inferior meatus, which is approximately 1 cm 2 cm in dimensions at the anterior end of the inferior meatus.
- The edges of the antrostomy are smoothened using the Tilley's antral burr.
- Antral washes can be given at regular intervals through the antrostomy using a Rose's antral wash cannula attached to the Higginson syringe with sterile water or saline.

However, this operation is preferably performed in association with a Caldwell-Luc operation in resistant cases of chronic maxillary sinusitis, which fail to respond to conservative treatment and if three consecutive antral punctures fail to resolve the condition.

NASAL FOREIGN BODY REMOVAL

Definition Nasal foreign body removal is the procedure by which a foreign body in the nose is removed. Common types of foreign bodies seen in the nasal cavities are:

- Non-living
  - *Organic*
    - Peas.
    - Seeds.
    - Pulses-like grams.
    - Groundnuts.
  - *Inorganic*
    - Beads.
    - Buttons.
    - Paper.
    - Chalk pieces.
    - Eraser.
- Living: Maggots.
- Iatrogenic
  - Cotton pledgets.
  - Small gauze piece or a small piece from a roller pack.

Complications

- The foreign body may give rise to infection or granuloma formation.
- It may slip backward into the tracheobronchial tree resulting in respiratory obstruction.
- Rhinolith formation may occur over an old foreign body.

Aetiology

- Age: It is commonly seen in children between 1–5 years of age as they tend to insert objects in the nose and forget.
- Seen in mentally retarded patients.
- Routes of entry
  - Anterior nares—commonest route.
  - Posterior nares: Food particles may get lodged into the nasal cavity during vomiting, rarely seen.
  - Direct entry through penetrating wounds, e.g. bullet, etc.
  - Sequestration of bone in situ may occur and act as a foreign body.

Clinical features

- Symptoms
  - History of insertion of foreign body into the nose may occasionally be present.
  - Nasal obstruction—unilateral.
  - Blood stained unilateral nasal discharge.
  - Unilateral purulent nasal discharge.
  - Foul smell from nasal cavity.
  - Sneezing.
- Signs
  - Foul odour emnating from patient's nose.
  - Anterior rhinoscopy shows any of the following findings:
    - The foreign body may be visualised.
    - Unilateral nasal discharge.
    - Granulation in the nasal cavity or surrounding the foreign body which is seen partly.

Investigations

- No investigations are usually required, as anterior rhinoscopy is diagnostic.

- X-ray of nose will reveal only a radio-opaque foreign body.

Differential diagnosis
- Nasal diphtheria: It is bilateral, accompanied by other manifestations and shows excoriation spreading beyond the nasal cavities.
- Sequestra of bone.
- Rhinolith.

Treatment   Removal of the foreign body is performed usually in OPD carefully, if it is easily visualised in the nasal cavity.

The child is held properly, so as to prevent movement of the head. A nasal dressing forceps, vectis, a wax hook or even an Eustachian tube catheter is used and inserted gently so as to pass beyond the foreign body. Then the vectis is brought into contact with the nasal floor and pulled out. The foreign body usually comes out with this manoeuvre.

- If:
  - The child is very uncooperative,
  - It is difficult to hold a mentally handicapped child steady.
  - The foreign body is impacted due to granulations.

  General anaesthesia is required for removal. A nasal dressing forceps can be used to grasp the foreign body and remove it.

ANTRAL PUNCTURE

Definition   Antral puncture is procedure performed for drainage of and giving washes to the maxillary antrum.

Indications   Indications are shown in Flowchart 54.1.

Flowchart 54.1: Indications of antral puncture

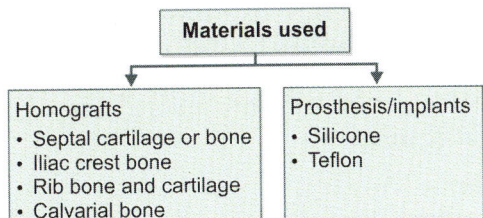

Contraindications
- Age: It is not performed under the age of 7–8 years as the patient is not cooperative and the maxillary antrum is not yet fully developed, hence, chances of false passage formation are more.
- Acute maxillary sinusitis: If antral puncture is performed, it will result in exacerbation of inflammation and osteomyelitis or excessive haemorrhage (epistaxis).

- Bleeding disorders: These can cause torrential haemorrhage (epistaxis).
- Diabetes mellitus.
- Hypertension.

Anaesthesia
- Local anaesthesia is preferred, using 4% lignocaine solution, as a surface anaesthetic agent at the site of puncture in the inferior meatus.
- General anaesthesia is used for small children, uncooperative patients, or mentally retarded patients. Usually, an intranasal antrostromy is preferred under general anaesthesia.

Premedication and preoperative preparation
- Patient is kept nil by mouth (no oral feeds) for 4 hours before the procedure.
- Injection atropine 0.6 mg IM ½ hour before the procedure is administered to prevent vasovagal attack.
- Injection tetanus toxoid 0.5 mL intramuscular is administered routinely before the procedure.
- Written informed consent of the patient is taken.

Position   The patient is in the sitting position, if under local anaesthesia and in the supine position, if under general anaesthesia.

Procedure
- Local anaesthesia is given using three swab sticks dipped in 4% lignocaine with adrenaline (1: 200000) placed at the following sites for 10 minutes:
  - *Inferior meatus*: For anaesthesia of the superior alveolar nerve.
  - *Middle meatus*: For anaesthesia of the spheno-palatine ganglion and its branches.
  - *Roof of the nose*: For anaesthesia of the anterior ethmoidal nerve.
- The Tilley-Lichtwitz trocar and cannula is introduced gently into the inferior meatus and passed backwards and upwards in the direction of the medial canthus of the eye, along the meatus.
- About 2 cm behind the anterior end of the inferior turbinate, there is a resistance to the passage of the cannula. This is the site of attachment of the inferior turbinate to the lateral nasal wall and is the weakest portion of the medial wall of the maxillary antrum.
- At this site, the trocar is pushed into the cannula so that the tip protrudes out and the direction of the trocar and cannula is changed, so as to be towards the lateral canthus of the eye.
- By a gentle rotating motion, the trocar and cannula are pushed, so as to enter the maxillary antrum

through its medial wall. There is a sudden feeling of give-way indicating that the trocar and cannula are in the maxillary antrum.

- To confirm that the trocar and cannula are in the antrum, the trocar should be withdrawn and the cannula is (rotated) moved in all directions. If the movement is free and without resistance, it indicates that the cannula is in the maxillary antrum and not in any soft tissue false passage.
- A Higginson rubber syringe is filled with sterile normal saline or lukewarm boiled water and one end of the syringe is fitted to the cannula.
- The patient is asked to bend forwards with his/her mouth open and explained to let the returning fluid run out through his nose and mouth.
- The antrum is now washed with the normal saline, which is introduced from the syringe into the antrum through the cannula. The fluid returns through the maxillary ostium and flows out through the nose and mouth of the patient and is collected in a kidney tray.
- The washing is continued till the returning fluid is clear. Then, the cannula is removed and the nose is packed with a cotton pledget or a roller gauze to prevent epistaxis. This is removed after 10–15 minutes.
- The same procedure is repeated on the other side, if required.

Postoperative care
- **Oral antibiotics for 7 days:** Capsule ampicillin (500 mg) QDS 7 days.
- **Nasal decongestants:** Ephidrine or Xylometazoline nose drops, 2 drops in both nostrils 4 times a day for 7 days.
- Anti-inflammatory analgesics for 3 days.

Complications
- **Complications of anaesthesia:** Vasovagal attack, hypotension, cardiac arrest.
- **Haemorrhage** (epistaxis) from local blood vessels or due to abrasion of mucosa, if procedure is performed by inexperienced person.
- **Formation of a false passage** due to wrongly inserted trocar and cannula into the soft tissues of the cheek or into the orbit.
- **Proptosis** due to pushing the water/saline into the orbit.
- **Air embolism** rarely occurs, if air is pushed into the maxillary sinus and if it enters a ruptured vein.
- **Infection.**

Difficulties encountered
- Inability to penetrate bone with the trocar and cannula: This occurs due to the bony wall being thickened and is seen commonly in atrophic rhinitis or long standing chronic sinusitis. Also, in atrophic rhinitis, it is difficult to find the site of puncture due to loss of anatomical landmarks.
- There is no returning fluid. This can be due to the following reasons:
  - Cannula is blocked.
  - Ostia of the maxillary sinus are blocked. A second cannula is introduced beside the first one to enable washes to be given.
  - Cannula may be abutting against the wall of the antrum preventing fluid from entering into the antrum. The cannula is withdrawn slightly and fluid flows in smoothly.
  - A false passage may have been created due to wrong introduction of the cannula. If water is pushed in forcefully, it will result in a swelling on the cheek or proptosis with severe orbital pain.
  - The tip of the cannula may be inside a polyp, thus preventing return of fluid.

CALDWELL-LUC

Definition   Caldwell-Luc is an operation in which an opening is made in the anterior wall of the maxilla via the canine fossa to visualise and remove disease from the maxillary sinus. This is followed by an intranasal antrostromy.

This operation was described simultaneously by Caldwell of Newyork and Luc of France.

Principles
- To remove the unhealthy irreversably damaged mucosa of the maxillary sinus.
- An inferior meatal antrostomy is performed to facilitate aeration and gravitational drainage of the maxillary sinus.

Indications
- **Chronic maxillary sinusitis:** Radical cure of chronic sinusitis is achieved by removal of part or whole of the diseased lining mucous membrane.
- Removal of foreign body, e.g. root of molar or pre-molar tooth and dental amalgam from the sinus cavity or removal of impacted bullet pellets.
- Inspection and biopsy of suspected maxillary antral malignancy.
- Closure of an oroantral fistula.
- Removal of dental cysts involving maxillary antrum.

- Removal of recurrent antrocoanal polyp.
- As an approach to:
  - The pterygopalatine fossa for:
    - Maxillary artery ligation.
    - Vidian neurectomy.
  - Sphenoid sinus.
  - Pituitary gland for hypophysectomy.
- Elevation and stabilisation of orbital floor fractures.
- For treatment of atrophic rhinitis:
  - *Raghav Sharan's operation:* Implantation of the maxillary sinus mucosa into the nasal cavity. This reduces the size of the roomy nasal cavity and also increases the secretory mucosal area, thus, treating atrophic rhinitis.
  - *Whitmack's operation:* Implantation of the Stenson's duct (parotid duct) into maxillary antrum in cases of atrophic rhinitis.
- Orbital decompression: Done only for malignant exophothalmus not responding to steroids.
- Jansen-Horgan's operation: Transantral ethmoid-ectomy with removal of disease from the ipsilateral maxillary sinus.
- Implantation of radioactive needles into the antrum in cases of malignancy of maxilla.
- Rarely to clear debris in osteoradionecrosis.

Contraindications

- Age below 12 years: As growth of the middle one-third of the face and dentition is not complete, any damage to growth centres will impede growth.
- Acute sinusitis: This procedure results in excessive bleeding and also dissemination of infection.
- Diabetes mellitus.
- Hypertension.
- Bleeding disorders.
- Recent trauma.

Anaesthesia and preoperative preparation

- Preoperative preparation is made by treatment of the nasal passage of the affected side with vasoconstrictors to help in haemostasis.
- Most surgeons prefer to carry out this operation under general anaesthesia with cuffed oral endotracheal intubation and pharyngeal pack to prevent aspiration of blood and secretions.
- However, Caldwell-Luc operation can be performed under local anaesthesia also.
  - *Local anaesthesia*
    - Surface anaesthesia is achieved by putting cotton strips impregnated in 4% xylocaine and adrenalene both above and below the inferior turbinate.
  - *Infiltration anaesthesia:* Two percent xylocaine with adrenaline is injected (1 in 2 lac) along the gingivobuccal sulcus in the region of the canine fossa. The infiltration is made from the first molar tooth to the central incisior tooth in the gingivobuccal and gingivolabial sulcii. Approximately, 6–8 mL is infiltrated.

Position of patient   Patient is in supine position with 15 head high. A semi-sitting position may be given in case local anaesthesia is used.

Procedure

- A bone deep incision is made 3 mm above and parallel to the gingivolabial fold in the canine fossa from the lateral border of the lateral incisor tooth to the lateral border of the molar tooth (3–4 cm in length).
- The mucoperiosteal flap is then gently dissected superiorly with a periosteum elevator to expose the anterior wall of the maxillary sinus up to the level of the infraorbital nerve. The periosteum is elevated by placing a piece of gauze in front of the periosteum elevator, so as to minimise risk of trauma to the infra-orbital nerve. The infraorbital nerve is identified and carefully preserved.
- The mucoperiosteal flap is retracted upwards exposing the anterior wall of the maxillary sinus. The direction of the pull should be away from the infraorbital nerve.
- Anterior wall of the maxillary sinus is opened in the region of the canine fossa. The opening into the maxillary sinus is made by using either a burr or a chisel and hammer. The opening is enlarged to a size of 1.5–2 cm in diameter by using either a rotating burr or a sphenoid punch forceps. Inferior extension of this opening may lead to damage to the teeth and their nerve supply. Lateral extension of the opening may result in hemorrhage from the terminal branches of the sphenopalatine artery. This should be avoided.
- Mucosa of the antrum is then incised, the sinus is examined and the diseased mucosa is removed. Removal of the mucous lining of the roof of the antrum must be done with care, since the infraorbital nerve may not have a bony covering in this region.
- Bleeding may be troublesome during the entire procedure. However, it stops when all the mucosa is removed. The success of this procedure depends on the complete removal of the diseased mucosa, so that an uninfected membrane lines the sinus post-operatively.

- A large antrostomy is made in the inferior meatus. Its size should be at least 1.5 2 cm. The antrostomy is made using Tilley's antral harpoon. Bony opening is enlarged with Hajek forceps in all the directions. The lower end of the opening should be upto the level of the floor of the antrum and the anterior end should be up to the anterior end of the inferior turbinate. (Fig. 54.4)

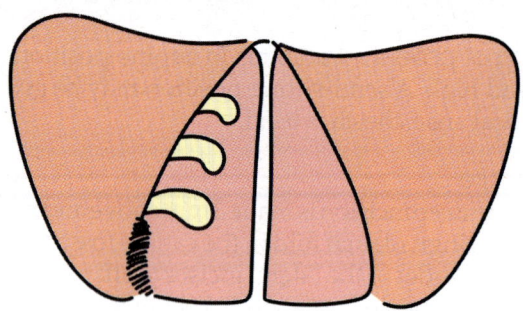

Fig. 54.4: Site for inferior meatal antrostomy

- Haemostasis is then achieved by packing the inferior meatus and the antrum with roller gauze soaked in bismuth iodoform paraffin paste (BIPP). The antrum must be packed in such a way that the roller gauze is easily removed through the nose.
- Closure of the buccal incision is done with 3–0 chromic catgut. Good approximation of the edges preserves gingivobuccal and gingivolabial sulcii. If this is obliterated, satisfactory fitting of artificial dentures may be difficult or impossible if required at a later date.
- Postoperatively, ice packs should be applied over the cheek for 24 hours to prevent oedema and hematoma formation. The nasal and antral packs are removed 48 hours after the surgery.

Complications Complications are shown in Flowchart 54.2.

Flowchart 54.2: Complications in Caldwell-Luc operation

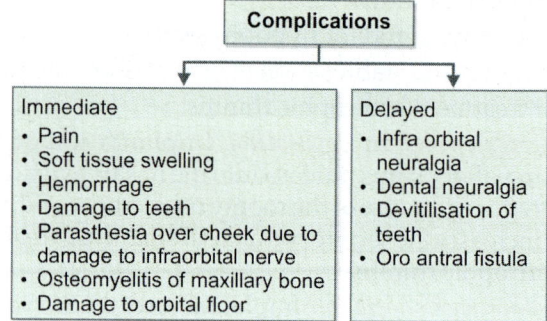

Modifications of Caldwell-Luc operation

- **Denker's procedure (1906):** The incision differs from Caldwell-Luc incision. It is extended medially up to the frenulum. This allows access into the nasal cavity and the maxillary antrum simultaneously. In all other ways, it is similar to the Caldwell-Luc operation.
- **Canfield's operation (1908):** Incision is made behind the nasal vestibule. Periostium is elevated laterally to expose the canine fossa. Anterior angle of maxillary sinus is chiselled off to expose the antral contents and the opening is continued posteriorly into an intranasal antrostomy.
- **Maxillary sinus obliteration (McNeill, 1966):** Mucous membrane of the sinus is removed completely. Antrum is then filled with abdominal fat.

CHAPTER 55

Tonsillectomy and Adenoidectomy

TONSILLECTOMY

Definition   It is an operation performed for removal of the palatine (faucial) tonsils.

Most commonly, it is done for chronic tonsillitis and hence done bilaterally except in some cases like embedded foreign body or excision biopsy for suspected neoplasm, when only one tonsil is removed.

Indications
- Local
  - Due to pathology in the tonsil
    - Chronic tonsillitis with recurrent acute attacks — More than 3–5 attacks a year. This is the commonest indication.
    - Following an attack of quinsy—Tonsillectomy is performed after 4–6 weeks.
    - Hypertrophic tonsils causing mechanical obstruction to swallowing and failure to grow in children.
    - Diphtheria especially, if the patient is a carrier,
    - Foreign body embedded in the substance of the tonsil.
    - Tonsillolith, which is symptomatic.
    - Huge tonsils causing respiratory obstruction.
    - Ulcer on the tonsil, which is suspicious of malignancy, the tonsil is removed for biopsy (excision biopsy).
    - Benign tumours or cysts of the tonsils.
  - As a treatment of sleep apnoea syndrome.
  - As an approach for:
    - Styloidectomy.
    - Glossopharyngeal neurectomy.
- Focal
  - When surrounding structures are infected by recurrent tonsillitis:
    - Persistent non-specific jugulodigastric lymphadenitis.
    - Tuberculous cervical lymphadenitis where the tonsil may be the portal of infection.
    - Eustachian tube catarrh due to recurrent tonsillitis resulting in secretory otitis media or even CSOM.
- General: When recurrent tonsillitis acts as a source of infection or sepsis for other tissues in the body:
  - *Respiratory system*: Exacerbation of asthma or chronic bronchitis.
  - *Cardiovascular system*: Focus of infection in subacute bacterial endocarditis or rheumatic heart disease.
  - *Kidneys*: Focus of infection in acute glomerulonephritis.
  - *Bones and joints*: Source of infection in rheumatic fever or rheumatic arthritis.
  - *Skin*: Exacerbation of urticaria, erythema multiforme, etc.
  - *Eyes*: Focus of infection in phylectenular conjuctivitis, choroiditis, etc.
  - *Failure to grow* adequately in children due to recurrent infection.

Indications for unilateral tonsillectomy

- Excision biopsy in suspected malignancy in case of ulcer on tonsil.
- Excision biopsy for lymphoma or tumour in case of unilateral enlarged tonsil.
- Foreign body embedded in the tonsil.
- Glossopharyngeal neurectomy in a case of glossopharyngeal neuralgia.
- Styloidectomy in a case of stylalgia (Eagle's syndrome)
- Tonsillar cyst.

Contraindications

- Acute tonsillitis: This increases the risk of primary and secondary haemorrhage.
- Upper respiratory tract infection, like rhinitis or pharyngitis.
- Below the age of 5 years, tonsillectomy is not performed for the following reasons:
  - Tonsils are important as immune defence mechanisms in very small children.
  - In very small children, anaesthesia is preferably avoided.
  - Surgery is difficult to perform as space for operation is smaller.
  - Blood loss is not tolerated well in very small children. Adenoidectomy is preferred in small children if required, followed by tonsillectomy at a later age.
- Granular pharyngitis: This should be treated prior to tonsillectomy, as the pharyngitis flares up after removal of the tonsils.
- Diabetes mellitus.
- Hypertension.
- Allergy and asthma.
- Blood dyscrasias and bleeding disorder.
- Pregnancy.
- Polio epidemic: Tonsillectomy is avoided during an epidemic of poliomyelitis, since they are important as immune defence mechanisms and their removal may result in bulbar poliomyelitis.

Preoperative investigations

- Routine haemogram with total count and differential count.
- Bleeding time and clotting time.
- X-ray chest PA view.
- Blood sugar and ECG, if required.

Methods of tonsillectomy

- Dissection.
- Guillotine.
- Electrocautery.
- Cryocautery.
- Laser.

Preoperative preparation (premedication)

- Written informed consent.
- Injection atropine 0.6 mg intramuscularly half an hour before the operation.
- Injection tetanus toxoid 0.5 cc intramuscularly on the day prior to surgery.
- Systemic antibiotics started a day or two prior to the surgery.
- Sometimes, calcium, vitamin C, and vitamin K may be given for 2–3 days prior to surgery, to aid in haemostasis.

Anaesthesia

- General anaesthesia with endotracheal intubation using a cuffed endotracheal tube with a tight throat pack of roller gauze is used. The cuff and throat pack prevent aspiration of blood.
- The endotracheal tube is passed transorally, if adenoidectomy is performed at the same time or transnasally, if adenoidectomy is not to be done, as this gives more operating space.
- Local anaesthesia is occasionally used only in adults with sedation using 1 cc fortwin and 1 cc phenergan given intravenously slowly. The peritonsillar tissues are infiltrated with 2%. Lignocaine solution with 1:100000 adrenaline for infiltration anaesthesia. It has the advantage of less haemorrhage and avoiding the complications associated with general anaesthesia.

Position

- Patient is in the supine position with neck extended by placing a sand-bag under the shoulders. Flexion of the cervical spine and extension of the atlantooccipital joint (Boyce's position). This position helps by giving a better view of the operating field and preventing aspiration.
- The surgeon stands on the right side of the patient or sits at the head end of the patient.

Procedure

- Dissection method: The mouth is kept open using a mouth gag (Doyen's, Boyle Davis' or Jenning's) and the tongue is depressed with a Lac's tongue depressor (Fig. 55.1). Under local anaesthesia, a mouth gag is not used, but the patient is asked to keep his/her mouth open and the tongue is depressed.
  - Incision: The anterior pillar is stretched by depressing the tongue and an inverted J-shaped

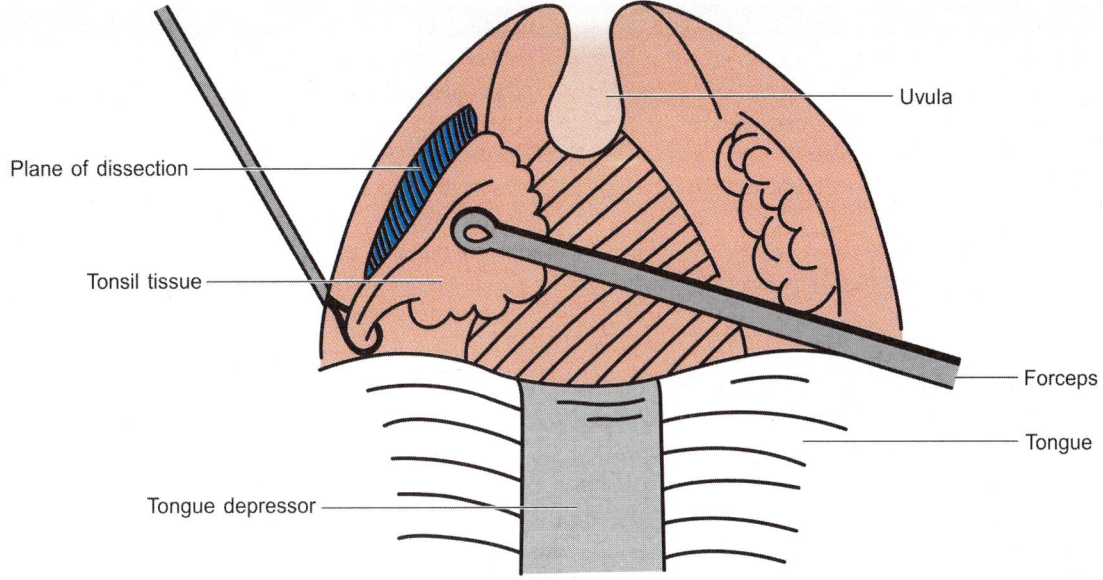

Fig. 55.1: Tonsillectomy

submucous incision is made using a knife with a no. 12 blade (tonsillar knife) along the edge of the anterior pillar from the base of the uvula to the lateral border of the tongue.

- The tonsil is dissected by blunt dissection along the plane of its capsule. The tonsil is held medially with a Denis-Brown tonsil holding forceps or a blunt Luc's forceps and the dissection is carried out in the plane between the tonsillar capsule and the tonsillar fossa using a Mollison's tonsil dissector and pieces of roller gauze. Blunt dissection prevents excessive haemorrhage during surgery.
- The tonsil is dissected free of its fossa except at its pedicle, which contains the insertion of the palatoglossus muscle in addition to its blood vessels and lymphatics. The Eve's tonsillar snare is used to crush and cut the tonsillar pedicle, while holding the tonsil with the forceps to prevent it from falling freely into the hypopharynx.
- The tonsillar fossa is packed with gauze under pressure for haemostasis.
- The same procedure is repeated on the other tonsil.
- The gauze in the fossa is removed and bleeding vessels are detected.
- Haemostasis in the tonsillar fossa is achieved by contraction and retraction of the blood vessels. However, a few bleeding vessels, which do not contract and retract after removal of the gauze are ligated using the method of 'cross-clamping' with the help of two tonsillar haemostats and linen or

silk (non-absorbable suture material). These are not to be removed, but slough off by the 7th or 10th day.

- **Guillotine method**
  - It is not performed nowadays. The instrument used is known as the 'Guillotine'. The name is derived from the French punishment of beheading a prisioner with the use of a Guillotine knife.
  - The technique includes the following steps:
    - *Insertion:* The guillotine is inserted along the Lac's tongue depresser into the oral cavity.
    - *Feeding:* The tonsil is 'fed' into the fenestra of the guillotine by applying pressure externally on the neck with one hand and feeding the now prominent tonsil into the fenestra by depressing the guillotine onto the tonsil. The handle of the guillotine faces the opposite cheek to enable adequate pressure to be applied.
    - *Excision:* When most of the tonsil is engaged into the fenestra, the blade is closed so as to cut the tonsil, taking care that the pillars and surrounding soft tissues are not caught in the fenestra.

Difference between dissection method and Guillotine method The differences between dissection method and Guilloine method are given in Table 55.1.

Postoperative care/Management

- **Position:** Patient is placed in the tonsillar position (Rose's), i.e. on one side with the knee and hip of the upper leg flexed and the lower arm flexed at the

TABLE 55.1: Differences between dissection method and Guillotine methods for tonsillectomy	
Dissection Method	*Guillotine Method*
• Can be done in all patients.	• Can only be done for patients with large tonsils.
• Time-consuming compared to Guillotine method	• Faster
• Excision of tonsillar tissue is complete	• Incomplete excision of tonsillar tissue is likely
• Damage to surrounding soft-tissues is uncommon	• Damage to the surrounding soft tissues is common
• Blood vessels are ligated.	• Haemostasis is achieved by pressure.
• Can be performed after quinsy.	• Contraindicated after quinsy.
• Can be done under local anaesthesia or general anaesthesia.	• Cannot be performed under local anaesthesia. Always to be done under general anaesthesia.

elbow and shoulder, and placed below the head of the patient. The upper hand is flexed at the elbow and placed in front of the patient and a pillow is placed behind him. This prevents the patient from rolling, under the effect of anaesthesia and also prevents aspiration in case of haemorrhage.

- Patient is kept nil by mouth for 6 hours following surgery.
- One hourly monitoring of pulse, temperature and respiration for 4 hours with maintenance of a temperature, pulse, respiration (TPR Chart).
- Dilute hydrogen peroxide gargles to clear the fossae on the first day after surgery.
- Injectable antibiotics.
- Injectable analgesics.
- Cold liquid feeds orally after 6 hours, e.g. ice cream or coconut water.
- Cold liquid feeds are given for 2–3 days followed by soft semisolid diet, e.g. soft bread dipped in milk, dal and rice, mashed potatoes, etc.
- Antibiotic syrup for 7 days, e.g. syrup ampicillin 1 tsp QDS for 7 days.
- Anti-inflammatory analgesic syrup for 7 days e.g. syrup combiflam 1 tsp TDS for 7 days.
- Condy's gargles (1 : 4,000 potassium permanganate) 3–4 times a day, as antiseptic for 7–10 days.
- The patient is asked to start semisolid feeds early, as this prevents stiffness of the pharyngeal muscles and helps in early recovery from pain. Some children may be asked to chew chewing-gum, as this helps to relieve pain by maintaining mobility of pharyngeal muscles.
- The patient is asked to follow up after 7 days.

Complications
- **Immediate:** During surgery or within 6 hours of surgery.
- **Delayed:** After 6 hours of surgery.
- **Immediate complications**

- *Complications due to anaesthesia*
  - Hypotension or hypertension.
  - Arrythmias.
- *Primary haemorrhage*: During surgery, it is controlled by pressure followed by ligation of the bleeding vessels.
- *Trauma* to surrounding structures like anterior or posterior pillars, tongue, teeth, lips, uvula or soft palate.
- Delayed complications
  - *Reactionary haemorrhage* occurs within 6–8 hours of surgery, but can occur up to 48 hours after surgery. It is due to:
    - Slipping of a loosely tied knot.
    - Dislodgement of a clot due to coughing/straining.
    - Failure to ligate all bleeding vessels.
    - Rise in blood pressure, as patient comes out of general anaesthesia can result in opening up of collapsed vessels in the postoperative period.
    - On removal of the mouth gag, the stretched faucial tissue relaxes and this results in bleeding from vessels.
    - Failure of a vessel to contract and retract after crushing the pedicle.
    - If surgery is under local anaesthesia, the vessels may dialate as the effect of adrenaline wears off.
    - *Clinical features*
      - Child is seen swallowing postoperatively even under the sedative effect after anaesthesia (children tend to swallow blood and hence, it is dangerous, if this is not kept in mind as the haemorrhage may not be detected and the child may collapse suddenly).
      - Sudden vomiting of a large amount of altered blood.
      - Child looks pale and in shock.
      - Tachycardia—fast, weak pulse.
      - Rise in respiratory rate.

- Raised temperature.
- Usually, adults or older children will spit out blood.
  - *Management*
    - Maintenance of airway by turning the child to one side and giving the tonsillar position.
    - The fossa is inspected.
    - If a clot is seen, it has to be removed with a forceps and a swab is held against the fossa for a few minutes. This usually helps to stop the haemorrhage.
    - If the bleeding is persistent, the child is taken back into the operation theatre and the bleeding is controlled by ligation of the vessel under general anaesthesia.
    - If the blood loss is severe, blood transfusion is to be given.
- *Secondary haemorrhage*: It usually occurs after 2–3 days following surgery. It is due to infection, which results in sloughing off of the walls of the ligated vessels. Commonly seen by the 6th or 8th postoperative days.
  - *Clinical features*
    - Rise in temperature.
    - Pain.
    - Patient spits out fresh blood or clots.
    - Tonsillar fossa shows slough and blood clots.
  - *Management*
    - Patient is admitted to hospital for observation.
    - Vital parameters are monitored.
    - The mainstay of treatment is to change the antibiotics to a higher generation. Intravenous administration of antibiotics is a must.
    - Intravenous fluids are administered.
    - Patient is kept on cold liquid diet.
    - Local pressure is given in the tonsillar fossa using swab on a tonsillar haemostat.
    - *Blood transfusion*: Fresh blood is preferred as it helps to replace factors of coagulation.
    - Local chemical cauterization of the fossa is performed using dilute trichloro-acetic acid, (TCA).
    - If the bleeding is yet not controlled, the anterior and posterior pillars are sutured together as a last resort, since the tissues are very friable and oedematous making ligation of bleeding vessels difficult.
- *Exacerbation of granular pharyngitis*: This occurs following tonsillectomy due to physiological rebound hypertrophy of pharyngeal lymphoid tissue.

- *Change of voice*: This occurs due to damage to the uvula or tonsillar pillars followed by fibrosis. The change of voice may range from nasal twang with nasal regurgitation to change in pitch. Speech therapy is required to treat this complication.
- *Recurrent or Residual tonsillitis*: It usually occurs due to a tag of tonsillar tissue left behind during surgery, which may get infected. Recurrence is impossible if the entire tonsil is excised.
- *Lingual quinsy*: The lingual tag left behind after tonsillectomy, may get infected resulting in ligual quinsy.
- *Aspiration* of a fragment of tonsillar tissue, may result in collapse of a segment of the lung or infection.

ADENOIDECTOMY

Definition   Adenoidectomy is operation performed for removal of the nasopharyngeal lymphoid tissue (adenoids).

Indications
- Enlarged adenoids with features of adenoid facies.
- Enlarged adenoids causing secretory otitis media by obstructing Eustachian tube openings.
- Enlarged adenoids causing recurrent upper respiratory tract infection.
- Recurrent adenoid and tonsillar infection causing failure to thrive in children.

It is usually performed along with a tonsillectomy operation. It can even be done in children below 5 years of age, where tonsillectomy is contraindicated.

Contraindications
- Acute upper respiratory tract infection.
- Cleft palate, especially in cases of submucous cleft palate, where enlarged adenoids help to close the incompetent nasopharyngeal sphincter.
- Bleeding disorders.

Adenoidectomy is performed *only* in children as adenoid tissue undergoes atrophy by the age of puberty.

Preoperative investigations
- Routine haemogram with total count and differential count.
- Bleeding time and clotting time.
- X-ray chest PA view.

Methods of adenoidectomy
- Using an adenoid curette.
- Using an adenotome.
- Finger dissection.

Preoperative preparation   Same as for tonsillectomy.

Anaesthesia   Always performed under general anaesthesia, as it is done in children.

Position   Supine position without extension of the neck. This prevents damage to the atlantooccipital joint, when the adenoids are curetted.

Procedure   The procedure for adenoidectomy is shown in Fig. 55.2.

- After application of a mouth gag, the adenoids are first palpated for the following reasons:
  - To detect the size,
  - To check for hypertrophy of tubal tonsils which are situated laterally,
  - To check for abnormal pulsations,
  - To push the tubal tonsils medially.
- Using a Lac's tongue depressor to depress the tongue, the adenoid curette is introduced into the oral cavity held like a pen with the blade towards the tongue.
- The blade of the adenoid curette is introduced in the oropharynx just beyond the soft palate but not touching the posterior pharyngeal wall.
- The curette is then rotated through 180 (the blade now faces superiorly) and introduced into the naso-pharynx. Now the curette is held like a dagger and

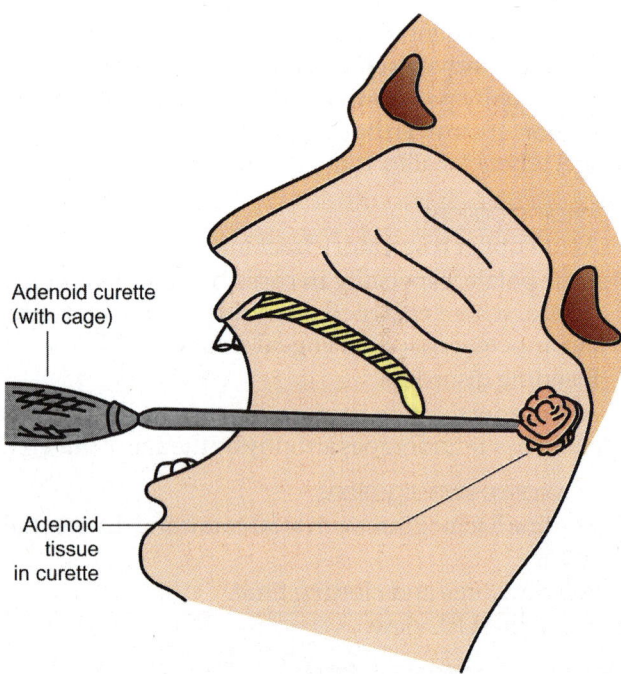

Adenoid curette (with cage)

Adenoid tissue in curette

Fig. 55.2 : Adenoidectomy

it is brought in contact with the posterior edge of the bony nasal septum to ensure that it is in the midline.
- With firm downward strokes, the blade of the curette shaves off the adenoid tissue from the roof and posterior wall of the nasopharynx.
- *The cage of the curette prevents fragments of the adenoid tissue from falling into the lower respiratory tract*, thus preventing aspiration.
- *Haemostasis* is achieved by application of pressure in the nasopharynx using a nasopharyngeal pack made of gauze for 4–5 minutes.
- The pack is removed and a digital palpation of the nasopharynx is performed for adenoid tags.
- Tags are removed using a small sized adenoid curette or a Luc's forceps or a conchotome. Following this, the pack is once again placed for a few minutes till complete haemostasis is achieved.

Complications
- Complications of general anaesthesia
  - Hypotension or hypertension.
  - Arrhythmias.
  - Vasovagal attack.
- Haemorrhage
  - *Primary*: Intraoperative bleeding is controlled by a pressure pack for 3–5 minutes. Failure of haemostasis after packing the nasopharynx for 3–5 minutes post-adenoidectomy can be due to:
    - Incomplete removal of adenoid tissue (tags).
      - Rx: Remove the tags.
    - Excessive curetting resulting in damage to the pharyngeal mucosa.
      - Rx: Repack for 10–12 minutes. Rarely, a postnasal packing, may be required for 48 hours.
  - *Reactionary haemorrhage*: Controlled by pressure packing for 3–5 minutes or even up to 10 minutes.
  - *Secondary haemorrhage*: Controlled by postnasal packing under general anaesthesia (as described for 'epistaxis') and high antibiotics.
- Trauma to soft palate, uvula, tongue, or Eustachian tube opening.
- Secretory otitis media due to stenosis of Eustachian tube orifice following trauma and fibrosis.
- Trauma to the altantoccipital joint, if neck is kept in extended position.
- Rhinolalia aperta: A nasal twang to voice develops, if this is performed in a patient having a submucous cleft palate.

CHAPTER 56

Tracheostomy

TRACHEOSTOMY

Definition   It is defined as a surgical opening made on the anterior wall of the trachea, so as to bypass the upper respiratory tract.

It is now frequently and correctly replaced by the term 'tracheotomy'.

Laryngotomy or cricothyrotomy is the emergency operation where the airway is opened through the cricothyroid membrane in case of acute respiratory obstruction, where there is no time for tracheostomy or inavailability of a competent surgeon to perform the tracheostomy. It is a relatively simple procedure and life-saving.

Relevant anatomy   The trachea is made up of approx. 16–20 'C' shaped rings of cartilage, of which 6–8 are in the neck. The upper part of the trachea is relatively superficial as compared to the lower part.

The thyroid isthmus lies at the level of the second and third tracheal rings. Tracheostomy is usually performed at the level of the third and fourth tracheal rings. The posterior wall of the trachea is closely related to the anterior wall of the oesophagus.

Classification

- (A)
  - ◆ Emergency.
  - ◆ Elective/Planned.
- (B)
  - ◆ Temporary.
  - ◆ Permanent.
- (C)
  - ◆ High.
  - ◆ Mid.
  - ◆ Low.
- Emergency tracheostomy is performed in a case of acute respiratory distress. Occasionally, an endotracheal tube can be passed in an emergency to tide over the crisis and if the tube is required for more than 48 hours, a tracheostomy is performed to prevent laryngeal damage (vocal cord granulomas, etc.) However, intubation may not be possible in every case of acute respiratory distress, e.g. in case of large malignancy of larynx, laryngeal papillomatosis, etc.
- Elective/Planned tracheostomy is performed whenever respiratory distress or upper respiratory obstruction is anticipated, e.g. prior to certain surgical procedures, such as hemimandibulectomy, hemiglossectomy, etc.
- Temporary tracheostomy is performed, if the causative factor can be removed or cured, e.g. laryngeal oedema, trauma, foreign-body larynx, etc.
- Permanent tracheostomy is performed, when the causative factor cannot be treated or removed, e.g. crush injuries of larynx, laryngectomy operation, etc.
- High tracheostomy is performed rarely, only in a dire emergency. It is performed at level of first or second

tracheal rings and has a very high risk of tracheal or subglottic (if cricoid cartilage is damaged), stenosis at a later date.

- Mid-tracheostomy is performed most commonly and it is at the level of third or fourth tracheal rings.
- Low tracheostomy is performed below level of fourth tracheal ring and is rarely done, e.g. in cases of tracheal stenosis, etc.

Principles /Functions of tracheostomy

- Bypasses the upper airway, thus, relieving obstruction.
- Reduces dead space by 30–50%.
- Reduces airflow resistance.
- Protects against aspiration.
- Assists in respiratory toilet or tracheobronchial suction.
- Assists in positive pressure ventilation.
- It physiologically separates upper airway from the tracheobronchial tree to avoid postoperative complications, such as aspiration or airway obstruction in planned surgery of the upper airway.
- Enables easy delivery of medication or humidification to lower respiratory tract.
- Relief of alveolar hypoventilation in pulmonary disease.
- Enables swallowing without reflex apnoea.

Indications

- Common indications of tracheostomy seen in practice
  - Foreign body in the larynx.
  - Malignancy of the larynx.
  - Tetanus.
- Head injury resulting in unconsciousness.
- Laryngeal diphtheria.
- Acute laryngotracheobronchitis.
- *Indications of tracheostomy*: These are shown in Flowchart 56.1.
- Indications due to pathology of the larynx (intrinsic)
  - *Congenital*
    - Laryngeal web.
    - Tracheo-oesophageal fistula.
    - Laryngeal stenosis.
  - *Traumatic*
    - Inhalation of fumes.
    - Swallowing of corrosives.
  - *Foreign body*
    - Impacted foreign body in the larynx or the trachea requires a tracheostomy to:
      - Bypass the airway obstruction.
      - Prevent further aspiration of the foreign body in the lower respiratory tract.
  - *Infective*
    - Laryngeal diphtheria.
    - Acute epiglottitis.
    - Acute laryngotracheobronchitis.
  - *Neurological*
    - Bilateral abductor cord palsy.
    - Tetanus.
    - Myasthenia gravis.
    - Bulbar poliomyelitis.
  - *Neoplastic*
    - Benign
      - Laryngeal papillomatosis.

Flowchart 56.1: Classification of endoscopies

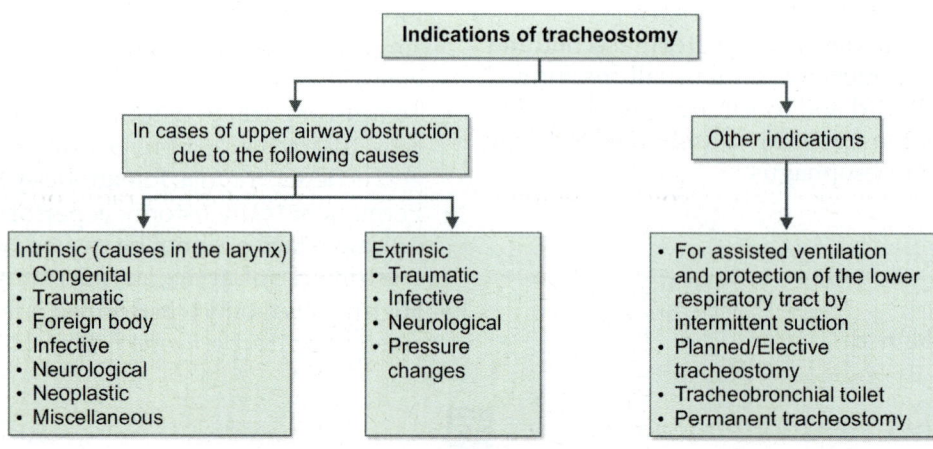

- Malignant
  - Carcinoma of oropharynx.
  - Carcinoma of larynx.
- Extrinsic indications
  - *Traumatic*
    - Cut-throat injury.
    - Crush injury to larynx.
    - Strangulation injury.
  - *Infective*
    - Ludwig's angina.
    - Retropharyngeal abscess.
    - Parapharyngeal abscess.
  - *Neurological*
    - Carcinoma of oesophagus involving the recurrent laryngeal nerve.
    - Carcinoma of thyroid involving the recurrent laryngeal nerve.
    - Metastatic mediastinal lymph nodes involving the recurrent laryngeal nerve.
    - Post-thyroidectomy trauma to both recurrent laryngeal nerves.
  - *Pressure changes*
    - Pressure compression of the trachea due to malignant thyroid tumour.
    - Tumour of the neck causing pressure on larynx or trachea.
- Other indications
  - *For assisted ventilation and protection of lower airway by intermittent suction:*
    - Unconscious or Comatose patient due to head injury, encephalitis, cerebrovascular accident etc.
    - Respiratory centre depression due to bulbar palsy, barbiturate poisoning, etc.
    - Lesions affecting the anterior horn cells and nerves controlling the muscles for respiration such as poliomyelitis, polyneuritis, myasthenia gravis, etc.
    - Lesions affecting the myoneural junction, such as tetanus.
    - Lesions affecting the chest wall such as multiple rib feactures, flail chest, etc.
    - Lung pathology, like fibrosis, collapse, emphysema, etc.
    - Grave injury to face, neck and chest, e.g. burns.
  - *Planned/Elective tracheostomy:* Usually done prior to major surgery of the head and neck to avoid aspiration after surgery and to maintain an airway e.g. prior to operations such as laryngofissure, hemiglossectomy, mandibulectomy, drainage of retropharyngeal abscess, operations for facio-maxillary injuries.
  - *Tracheobronchial toilet*, e.g. removal of secretions from the lower respiratory tract in diseases, such as chronic obstructive pulmonary disease (COPD) (emphysema, bronchiectasis).

Contraindications   There is no such contraindication to performing a tracheostomy, when required, as it is a life-saving procedure. However, only in cases of planned/ elective tracheostomy, relative contraindications, such as diabetes mellitus, hypertension, bleeding disorder, etc., may be controlled prior to performing the tracheostomy.

Types of tracheostomy tubes

- Metallic: Chevalier–Jackson tracheostomy tube:
  - Made of German silver. Has three parts:
    - Inner tube,
    - Outer tube, and
    - Obturator/Guide/Pilot.
  - The inner tube is longer than the outer tube by 2–3 mm, so that when the tube gets blocked, the blockage is cleared by removing the inner tube. It is fixed to the outertube by a locking mechanism and the outertube is fixed by a linen tape passed through the holes of the shield attached to the proximal end of the outer tube and tied around the neck. The obturator has a blunt olive tip and is passed through the outertube during insertion of the tracheostomy tube into the trachea, so as to make the distal end atraumatic. Once, the outer tube is in position, the obturator is removed and the inner tube is introduced and locked in position.
  - Available in sizes from no. 8 to 44 and only in even numbers, i.e. 8, 10, 12, etc.
  - Size used commonly for a:
    - Normal adult male—No. 34 or 36.
    - Normal adult female—No. 32 or 34.
- Portex tracheostomy tube
  - Made of portex.
  - It has a blue line running through the entire extent of the tube, which is impregnated with barium salt so as to make the tube radio-opaque.
  - Has 2 parts—The tube and the obturator.
  - No separate inner and outer tubes, since portex is not as rigid as metal, the walls of the tube are thick so as to maintain the patency and shape of the tube. The walls are 0.7–1.2 mm thick.
  - Available from sizes 3–10 inches increments of 0.5 i.e. 3, 3.5, 4, 4.5, etc.

- Size used commonly for a:
  - Normal adult male—No. 7.5 or 8.
  - Normal adult female—No. 6.5 or 7.
- All tubes of size no. 5 and below, are without a cuff and tubes no. 5.5 or above are available in two types: with or without cuff.
- The cuff is present at the distal portion of the tube and requires 2–3 cc of air for inflation. The pressure is indicated roughly by a small pilot bag attached to the flange/shield of the tube.
- *Advantages of cuff*: The cuff helps to make an airtight seal with the lower respiratory tract, i.e. air cannot escape between the tube and the lumen of the trachea due to the cuff, hence a cuffed tube can be used for:
  - Anaesthesia
  - Patients on Ventilator
  - Intermittent positive pressure respiration.
- The portex tracheostomy tube is kept in position by means of a linen tape passed through the shield/flange attached to its proximal end and tied around the neck. The cuff does not help to keep the tube in place.
- Silicone tracheostomy tube with or without a speaking valve
  - This tube is the most inert since silicone is least irritant. It is good for long-term use and has an inner as well as outer tube. The presence of a speaking valve is advantageous for patients who can use their larynx for speech (for example, in laryngotracheal stenosis).
- Salpekar's double-cuffed tracheostomy tube: It has two cuffs at the distal portion. This is useful in cases, where the cuff has to be kept inflated for a prolonged period continuously, e.g. comatose patient on ventilator. The advantage of two cuffs is that, one cuff is inflated for a while and the other is kept deflated alternately, so as to avoid pressure continuously, at one site on the trachea and, thus, avoid pressure necrosis.
- Fuller's bivalved tracheostomy tube: The tube consists of an inner tube and an outer tube. The outer tube is bivalved. The two cusps of the outer tube are compressed and the tube is easily inserted into the tracheal lumen without either a pilot or tracheal dialator. The inner tube is then inserted. The inner tube has an opening on the posterosuperior wall which helps in decannulation, i.e. patient can breathe through the upper respiratory tract on blocking the tracheostomy opening.

- Durham's tube: This has an adjustable shield/flange and, hence is very useful in patients with a short fat neck.
- Radcliff tube: This is a right angled tube and is used in patients with a short fat neck.

Also, tracheostomy tubes can be attached to a speaking valve, which is a one way Duck-Bill type of valve and helps the patient to speak. Valves available include Rusch valve, Disanti valve, and Tucker valve.

Procedure

- Preprocedure preparations
  - Written informed consent of patient and/or relative. In the event of an extreme emergency, this need not be done as tracheostomy is life-saving.
  - 0.5 cc injection tetanus toxoid intramuscularly.
  - 0.6 mg injection atropine sulfate intramuscularly ½ hour before the procedure.
  - Injection lignocaine test dose.
  - Tracheostomy tube, instruments, suction-machine, and good illumination should be checked, prior to the procedure.
  - Strict aseptic precautions are taken.
- Anaesthesia: It can be performed under general anaesthesia with endotracheal intubation or under local infiltration anaesthesia. The former is preferred in planned/elective tracheostomy and the latter is preferred in emergency tracheostomy.
- Position: Patient is in the supine position with full extension of the neck and head. This is obtained by placing a sand-bag or pillow under the patient's shoulders. Neck and head must be held in the midline. This position brings the cervical trachea forward in the neck and more tracheal rings are accessible in the neck.
- Steps
  - *Incision*: Midline vertical neck incision from lower border of cricoid cartilage to the suprasternal notch—commonly used.

    Horizontal neck incision midway between the lower border of cricoid cartilage and suprasternal notch—used rarely only in cases of elective tracheostomy.
  - A no. 11 surgical blade on a Bard–Parker handle is used.
  - The neck incision is deepened in the midline, cutting the superficial and deep cervical fascia and subcutaneous fat. The anterior jugular vein or transverse cervical veins may be encountered.
  - Dissection is carried out with a curved mosquito haemostat, strictly in the midline. The midline raphe between the two sets of strap muscles on

either side of the neck is encountered, dissected and strap muscles are retracted on either side by right-angled retractors or double-hook retractors.

- The thyroid isthmus is now exposed and it is retracted upwards with a single-hook retractor to expose the second and third tracheal rings. Some surgeons prefer to clamp and cut the thyroid isthmus, but this may cause bleeding and loss of precious time.
- The pretracheal fascia is incised with the surgical blade and dissected away from the tracheal rings with the curved mosquito haemostat.
- The tracheal rings are thus exposed and this is confirmed by palpation of the rings and aspiration of air from the trachea with a needle and syringe filled with 1 cc of 4% lignocaine solution. Once air bubbles are seen in the syringe, 0.5 mL of 4% lignocaine is instilled into the tracheal lumen to anaesthetise the mucosa and also prevent a vaso-vagal attack.
- With the surgical knife, an incision is made over the second and third tracheal rings on the anterior tracheal wall. There are various incisions, which can be used (Fig. 56.1).

The cruciate or circular incisions are commonly used. However, the horizontal incision does not pass through cartilage and, hence helps to minimize cartilage necrosis. This is preferred in children.

- The tracheal opening is dilated with a tracheal dialator and the tracheostomy tube is introduced with the obturator/guide in position.

- Following insertion, the obturator is removed and the presence of the tube in the tracheal lumen in confirmed by:
  - Airblast felt on the back of the hand.
  - Movement of a wisp of cotton placed near the opening of the tube.
  - Auscultation of chest for bilaterally equal air entry, and
  - If patient is on ventilator, then auscultation of chest after attachment of ventilator will confirm presence of tube in correct position.
- In case of metallic tube, the inner tube is placed into the outer tube and fixed in place with the locking mechanism.
- The tracheostomy tube is fixed in position by tying it to the neck with the help of linen tapes passed through the holes in the shield/flange.
- In case of cuffed portex tubes, the cuff is now inflated with 2–3 cc of air.
- A dressing is given in the form of a few sterile gauze pieces, cut and inserted between the shield of the tube and skin.
- Postoperative care
  - The following should be constantly by the patient's bed-side:
    - A set of tracheostomy instruments and a tracheostomy tube of the same size and type.
    - A bell to call the nurse and a piece of paper with pen for communication, if patient is literate.
    - Suction apparatus.
    - Oxygen.

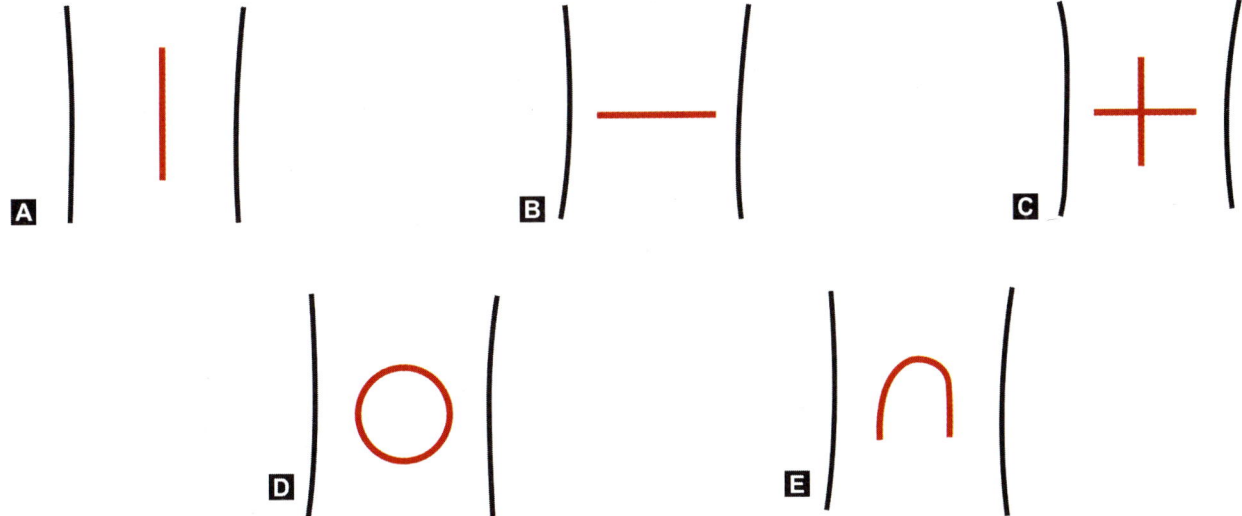

Fig. 56.1: Various incisions on the trachea

- Suction through the tube every half hourly and instillation of 0.5 mL of sodium bicarbonate into the tube prior to each suction. This helps to liquefy the crusts and aids in suction of secretions.
- In case of metallic tube, the inner tube should be removed, cleaned, boiled, and replaced every 4 hours or earlier if required.
- In case of a cuffed portex tube, the cuff needs to be deflated for 10 minutes, every 2 hours to prevent pressure necrosis of the tracheal rings.
- A single moist gauze piece is placed at all times, over the opening of the tracheostomy tube to help in humidification of air entering the lower respiratory tract and prevent entry of foreign bodies like insects, etc.
- The tracheostomy dressing is changed everyday using sterile gauze pieces.
- Steam inhalations twice or thrice a day to prevent excessive drying of secretions.
- Regular daily physiotherapy to avoid lower respiratory tract infection.

Sequelae

The problems faced by the patient following a tracheostomy are:

- **Inability to speak:** This is due to the larynx being bypassed.
- Difficulty in taking a shower or washing his head.
- Inability to swim.
- Inability to lift heavy weights.
- Difficulty in straining during micturition, constipation or childbirth. This is due to the fact that, there is a difficulty in increasing the intra-abdominal pressure required for these activities, as the thorax cannot be fixed.
- Anosmia, as the nose which contains the olfactory nerve endings is bypassed.
- Fifty percent of the dead space is eliminated by a tracheostomy, thus reducing airway resistance and making breathing easier.

Complications

- **Immediate:** During or immediately after the procedure.
- **Delayed:** Twenty-four hours after the procedure.
- **Late:** Occurring after a few weeks.
- **Immediate**
  - *Haemorrhage:* Primary haemorrhage may occur during the procedure, due to injury to the following:
    - Thyroid isthmus.
    - Transverse cervical vessels.
    - Strap muscles.

- High innominate artery especially in children.
- Carotid artery, if dissection is carried out more laterally, usually may occur in children.
- Jugular vein, may occur in children, if dissection is carried out more laterally.

  This can be avoided by meticulous dissection in the midline under good illumination.

- *Injury to the oesophagus* resulting in tracheo-oesophageal fistula.
- *Injury to the dome of pleura:* It is common in children.
- Injury to recurrent laryngeal nerve.
- *Injury to cricoid cartilage:* It is common in high tracheostomy.
- *Apnoea due to central respiratory failure:* Usually, may occur in a patient of prolonged dyspnoea. As soon as the trachea is incised, there is a carbondioxide washout. In such patients, hypoxia is the stimulus for the respiratory centre. This stimulus is lost suddenly, when CO_2 washout occurs and O_2 levels in the body rise, this results in apnoea.

  This can be treated by carbogen administration (95% oxygen and 5% carbondioxide).

- *Vasovagal attack, due to vagal stimulation:* This is prevented by instilling 0.5 cc of 4% lignocaine into the tracheal lumen before incising the trachea.
- Aspiration and lung collapse.
- Aerophagia, may occur in infants.

- Delayed complications
  - *Reactionary haemorrhage:* It occurs within 48 hours.
  - *Secondary haemorrhage:* It occurs on the 5th to 8th day usually, but can occur at anytime after 48 hours. Antibiotics should be administered and the wound should be explored to find the bleeding vessel which may have undergone necrosis.
  - *Surgical emphysema:* It occurs due to air, which leaks out from around the tracheostomy tube through the tracheal lumen, but cannot escape out due to tight suturing of the skin incision. Hence, this exhaled air is forced into the subcutaneous tissues of the neck and is characterised by crackling feel on palpation at the root of the neck followed by bloating up of the skin. It is prevented by taking care not to suture the skin wound too tightly around the tracheostomy tube. It can be treated by releasing the tight sutures. If untreated, it may involve the subcutaneous tissues of the entire body and require multiple punctures or small incisions over the skin. This can occur only in a non-cuffed portex or metal tube.
  - *Mediastinal emphysema:* It occurs due to escape of air from the tracheal lumen around the

tracheostomy tube under the pretracheal fascia into the pretracheal space, which communicates inferiorly with the superior mediastinum. This is prevented by incising the pretracheal fascia adequately and retracting it away from the site of the tracheal incision. This air leak can occur only in a metallic or non-cuffed portex tube.

- *Delayed tracheo-oesophageal fistula*: This occurs due to pressure necrosis of the tracheal wall, if the cuff is not deflated at regular intervals.
- *Tracheobronchitis*: It may occur as the lower respiratory track is exposed to the exterior or if septic precautions are not taken during change of dressing or suction of trachea.
- Pneumothorax and pyopneumotheorax.
- *Dysphagia*: This occurs due to the pressure of the cuff on the trachea in case of a cuffed portex tube, and due to a lack of positive subglottic pressure during deglutition.
- Blocking of the tube due to drying of secretions and crust formation.

- Late complications
  - *Tracheomalacia* occurs, if a large area of the tracheal wall has been removed during tracheostomy or if a cuffed tube has been used for prolonged period without deflation of cuff resulting in pressure necrosis of tracheal rings.
  - *Laryngeal stenosis*: In case of damage to cricoid cartilage in a high tracheostomy.
  - *Tracheal stenosis*: If the tracheostomy was badly performed, stenosis may occur at the site of the tracheostomy after decannulation or in case of prolonged use of cuffed tube, cartilage necrosis at the site of the cuff may result in stenosis after decannulation.
  - *Persistent tracheocutaneous fistula even after decannulation*: This may require surgical closure.
  - *Depressed scar*: It may occur at times following healing of the tracheostomy skin wound.

- *Difficulty in decannulation*: This may occur due to the following reasons:
  - Psychological dependence on the tracheostomy tube. This is common in children and occurs because of the patient gets accustomed to breathing without resistance as the upper respiratory tract (which gives a natural resistance to air flow), is bypassed. Hence, when decannulated, the patient gets breathless, even though the pathology which caused dyspnoea is cured.
  - Inadequate treatment of cause of dyspnoea which results in persistence of the obstruction and hence when decannulated, the patient may get breathless.
  - Presence of granulations in the tracheal lumen at site of tracheostomy.
  - Tracheomalacia.
  Hence, in such a case, one should first ascertain that the cause of dyspnoea is treated completely and absent. In case of psychological dependence the following is done.
  - Decannulate as soon as cure is achieved.
  - Partial blocking of the tube and gradual decannulation over a period of 2–3 days.

Tracheostomy in infants and children

- Should be avoided, if endotracheal intubation can be performed to maintain airway.
- Low tracheostomy should be avoided at all cost.
- Apical pleura, great vessels of the neck, and the innominate artery may be easily damaged in a child.
- Avoid excision of tracheal cartilage during opening the trachea. A vertical incision or a horizontal intercartilagenous incision is preferred.
- Avoid too deep an incision, as the tracheal lumen is narrow, and the incision may go through the oesophageal wall.
- Be prepared for decannulation problems, as psychological dependence is more common in children.

Endoscopies

The various types of endoscopics are as follows and their classification is shown in the Flowchart 57.1.

- Nasopharyngoscopy.
- Direct laryngoscopy.
- Microlaryngoscopy.
- Bronchoscopy.
- Oesophagoscopy.
- Fibreoptic endoscopy.

Flowchart 57.1: Classification of endoscopies

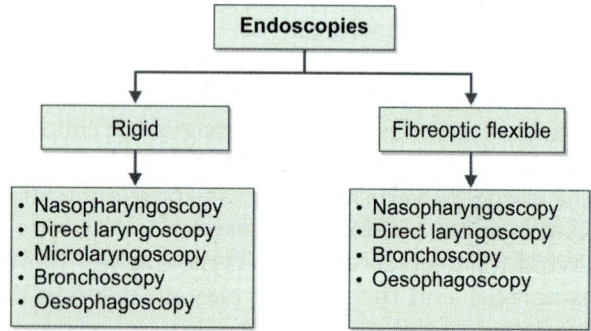

NASOPHARYNGOSCOPY

Definition   It is the procedure used for examination of the nasopharynx.

Types

- Rigid (using Yaunkauer's nasopharyngoscope).
- Flexible (using fibreoptic nasopharyngoscope).

Indications

- For early diagnosis of nasopharyngeal diseases, e.g. carcinoma, angiofibroma, etc.
- To detect site and cause of epistaxis.
- For biopsy of nasopharyngeal mass.
- To remove a foreign body from the nasopharynx.
- For supravital staining in early detection of malignant change.
- As a part of panendoscopy.

Methods of visualising the nasopharynx

- Retraction of soft palate using the curved end of the Lac's tongue depressor.
- Retraction of the soft palate using two soft red rubber catheters passed from the nose into the mouth.
- Using Yaunkauer's rigid nasopharyngoscope, which is inserted through the oral cavity.
- Using a flexible fibreoptic nasopharyngoscope, which is inserted through the nose.
- Using the rigid sinus endoscope (120), which is inserted through the nose to visualise the naso-pharynx.

In addition to visualising the nasopharynx, it is examined by finger-palpation.

Structures seen

- Choanae (posterior nares).
- Posterior edge of bony septum.
- Opening of the Eustachian tubes.
- Tubal tonsils.
- Adenoids.
- Roof of the nasopharynx.
- Posterior ends of inferior and middle turbinates.

Anaesthesia If the Yaunkauer's rigid nasopharyngoscope is used or if red rubber catheters are used, general anaesthesia is required.

If the flexible nasopharyngoscope or the sinus endoscope is used, local anaesthesia is required. Sedation using either injection calmpose or injection fortwin with phenargan is given in addition to a surface anaesthesia using either 4% lignocaine solution spray or 2% lignocaine gel for the oral cavity.

Position of patient Supine with minimal extension of neck or sitting comfortably in a chair.

Procedure If under local anaesthesia, using a flexible nasopharyngoscope, the patient is in the sitting position and the nose is sprayed with 4% lignocaine solution or may be packed with cotton pledgets dipped in 4% lignocaine solution for 10 minutes prior to the procedure. The procedure is explained to the patient and he/she is advised to breathe through the mouth to prevent fogging of the lens of the scope. The flexible scope is now passed along the floor of the nose and the nasopharynx is visualised. If required, a biopsy, supravital staining or a foreign body removal can be carried out.

If it is to be done under general anaesthesia, the patient is intubated with an endotracheal tube and the mouth is kept open using a mouth gag. The Yaunkauer's rigid nasopharyngoscope is introduced through the oral cavity and behind the soft palate to visualise the nasopharynx.

Complications
- Complications of anaesthesia
  - Hypotension or hypertension.
  - Arrythmias.
  - Vasovagal attack.
- Trauma to nasal mucosa.
- Trauma to oral mucosa, teeth, soft palate or tongue.
- Haemorrhage if biopsy is performed by an inexperienced surgeon.

DIRECT LARYNGOSCOPY

Definition It is the procedure by which the larynx and hypopharynx can be visualised using an endoscope.

Types
- Flexible direct laryngoscopy using a fibreoptic endoscope.
- Rigid direct laryngoscopy.

Direct laryngoscopy and microlaryngoscopy are described in detail in the Chapter 38 'examination of the larynx'.

BRONCHOSCOPY

Definition Bronchoscopy is a procedure used for direct endoscopic examination of the tracheobronchial tree.

Types
- Rigid bronchoscopy.
- Flexible fibreoptic bronchoscopy.

Indications Diagnostic and therapeutic indications of bronchoscopy are listed in Table 57.1.

TABLE 57.1: Diagnostic and therapeutic indications	
Diagnostic	*Therapeutic*
• Suspected foreign body.	• Foreign body removal.
• Malignancy for biopsy.	• Removal of broncholith.
• Vocal cord palsy.	• Aspiration of inspissated secretions.
• Sputum cytology for TB or malignancy.	• Removal of benign tumours, like papillomas or granulations.
• To detect spread of Ca from oesophagus or thyroid.	• Aspiration of lung abscess if it bursts into a bronchus.
• Biopsy of suspected mass in the tracheobronchial tree.	• Dialatation of bronchial stenosis.
• In cases of unexplained:	• In case of a difficult endo-tracheal intubation.
◆ Dyspnoea.	
◆ Haemoptysis.	
◆ Stridor.	
◆ Wheeze.	
◆ Chronic cough.	
• Rarely in dye studies for a case of tracheo-oesophageal fistula.	

Contraindications
- Any medical contraindications, such as active pulmonary kochs or diabetes or hypertension.
- Bleeding disorders.
- Trismus: However, a flexible bronchoscope can be used, as it is passed through the nose.
- Aortic aneurysm.
- Cervical spondylosis or fracture of cervical spine, Care is taken not to hyperextend the neck.
- Active haemoptysis or recent episode of massive haemoptysis.

Anaesthesia General anaesthesia using either a ventilating bronchoscope, where the Boyle's apparatus is connected to the bronchoscope or a jet ventilation by a Venturi, which supplies oxygen under high pressure in jets and intravenous anaesthetic agents are used.

Local anaesthesia of the nose and throat is required for a flexible fibreoptic bronchoscope.

Rigid bronchoscopy usually is done under general anaesthesia, but can be done under local anaesthesia also.

Position   Patient is in the supine position with extension of the head and flexion of the neck (Boyce's position).

Procedure

- The patient is hyperventilated using a mask for 3 minutes. The lips are retracted, mouth is opened, and upper teeth are protected by a piece of gauze placed on them.
- The scope is passed with the bevel facing down from the right corner of the mouth along the tongue gradually, till the epiglottis. The following structures are visualised: Base tongue, right vallecula, right tonsillar pillars, and right tonsil, and epiglottis.
- The scope is held in the right hand and guided by the left hand, which rests on the patient's mouth.
- The epiglottis is lifted up with the tip of the bronchoscope and the glottis is visualised as an anteroposterior chink between the two vocal cords.
- Now the scope is turned through 90 so that the bevel now faces the left vocal cord and lies in the axis of the glottic inlet. The scope is then passed under vision through the glottis into the trachea. Now, the scope is turned through 90 so that the bevel faces posteriorly or down.
- This step of entering the larynx and trachea is performed in a few seconds as until then, the patient is on intravenous anaesthesia but is not being ventilated.
- Once the scope is in the trachea, the anaesthesia apparatus (Boyle's machine) is attached to the ventilating bronchoscope or a Venturi needle is inserted into a non-ventilating bronchoscope. *Endotracheal intubation, as done for other endoscopies, cannot be used in a bronchoscopy as the scope passes through the same passage (trachea).* Hence, the scope is used for anaesthesia as well as by the surgeon.
- Now after the patient is well ventilated, the scope is introduced further into the trachea till the carina and the openings of the right and left primary bronchi are visualised.
- To enter the right primary bronchus, the patient's head is turned towards the left so as to align the trachea and the bronchus. Similarly, the patient's head is turned to the right to enter the left bronchus.
- The primary bronchi are inspected and the openings of the secondary bronchi are visualised.
- Unlike, the oesophagus, the tracheobronchial tree is not collapsible and the lumen can be visualised clearly for some distance distal to the scope. During removal of the scope, care is taken to turn the scope through 90 at the glottis so that the bevel faces the right vocal cord. Hence, both cords are also inspected.

- The scope is always removed under vision.
- In bronchoscopy, the surgeon and anaesthetist share the same passage and hence have to work in co-ordination.

Complications

- Complications of anaesthesia:
  - Cardiac arrhythmias,
  - Hypertension,
  - Hypotension,
  - Vasovagal arrest.
- Cardiac arrest or respiratory arrest due to the bronchoscope touching the carina resulting in vagal stimulation.
- Damage to lips, teeth, tongue or vocal cords.
- Dislocation of the arytenoid from the cricoarytenoid joint resulting in fixation of the vocal cord.
- Subglottic oedema and dyspnoea.
- Dislocation of cervical vertebra with resultant quadriplegia if done in a patient with diseased cervical spine.
- Tracheal or bronchial tear.
- Difficulty in removing a foreign body due to:
  - Difficulty in catching it e.g. small marble,
  - Foreign body slipping deeper into the tracheobronchial tree,
  - Disintegration of the foreign body on catching e.g. long-standing peanut,
  - Mucosal oedema and impaction of the foreign body,
  - Foreign body embedded in the wall of the tracheobronchial tree e.g. denture with wires.

OESOPHAGOSCOPY

Definition   It is a procedure used for direct endoscopic examination of the oesophagus.

Types

- Rigid oesophagoscopy.
- Flexible fibreoptic oesophagoscopy.

Indications   Indications are listed in Table 57.2.

TABLE 57.2: Diagnostic and therapeutic indications	
Diagnostic	*Therapeutic*
• Suspected foreign body.	• Foreign body removal.
• For detecting the cause of dysphagia.	• Dialatation of strictures.
• To detect the cause of haematemesis.	• Excision of benign tumours.
	Contd.

TABLE 57.2: Diagnostic and therapeutic indications (*Contd.*)

Diagnostic	Therapeutic
• As a part of panendoscopy done for detecting a primary malignancy in a patient, who has secondary metastasis in the neck nodes.	• Introduction of oesophageal feeding tube (Souttar tube) in patients with inoperable Ca oesophagus.
• To detect cause of vocal cord palsy.	• Injection of sclerosants into oesophageal varices.
• To take a biopsy to rule out malignancy.	• Repair of tracheo-oesophageal fistula.
	• Introduction of the Blomsinger's voice prosthesis after laryngectomy.
	• Endoscopic repair of a hypopharyngeal pouch (Dohlman's operation).

Contraindications

- Any medical contraindications, such as TB or diabetes or hypertension.
- Bleeding disorders.
- Trismus: A minimal mouth opening is required even for flexible oesophagoscopy, as the scope has to be passed through the oral cavity.
- Aortic aneurysm.
- Cervical spondylosis or fracture of cervical spine.
- Active haematemesis or a recent massive bout of haematemesis.
- Perforation of the oesophagus.

Anaesthesia   General anaesthesia with endotracheal intubation has to be used for rigid oesophagoscopy. It should never be attempted under local anaesthesia, as the oesophagus is a muscular structure with a collapsible lumen and can easily be damaged.

Position   Patient is in the supine position with extension of the head and flexion of the neck till the scope reaches the cricopharynx. After this, the head and neck are both extended till the scope reaches the aortic pulsations after which the patient's head projects beyond the table's edge and is supported by an assistant.

This change of position during the course of an oesophagoscopy is to align the oesophageal lumen with the axis of the rigid oesophagoscope.

Procedure   The oesophagoscope is held in the right hand and guided by the left hand and introduced from the right angle of the mouth. The scope is introduced with the bevel facing down along the tongue and the following structures are visualised   base tongue, anterior and posterior tonsillar pillars, tonsils, valleculae, oral surface of epiglottis, pyriform fosse, and

the posterior pharyngeal wall. Just inferomedial to the pyriform fossa, lies the cricopharyngeal opening, which when closed appears like a transverse slit in the mucosa. The scope is never pushed into the oesophagus but, gently glided into it, once the cricopharynx is relaxed. The cricopharyngeal sphincter is relaxed by either giving a muscle relaxant [Intravenous (IV)] succnyl choline given by the anaesthetist] or by gently touching the mucosa of the sphincter when, it reflexly opens (this is the mechanism of deglutition, i.e. the sphincter opens reflexly, when the food touches it). The bevel of the scope always faces down (posteriorly), in the oesophageal lumen and the scope is gently introduced, till the transmitted pulsations of the aorta are visualised on the oesophageal wall. Then, the patient's position is changed and the scope is further gently introduced till the cardiac end of the oesophagus.

The oesophagoscope is marked along its length to enable the surgeon to document accurately the site of the pathology in the oesophagus.

The scope is gently removed under vision.

Complications

- Complications of general anaesthesia:
  - Cardiac arrythmias.
  - Hypotension or Hypertension.
  - Vasovagal attack.
- Oesophageal perforation: The commonest site is the cricopharyngeal sphincter (it is hence, also known as the 'gate of tears') and occurs due to rough pushing of the scope against the closed contracted cricopharyngeal sphincter. However, perforations may occur due to not keeping the lumen in sight during scopy. The oesophagus, being muscular has mucosal folds and the lumen is not visibly patient like the air passages, thus, perforation is common, if the scope is pushed blindly forwards. Other causes of perforations are:
  - While removal of an impacted foreign body (as mucosa is inflamed and friable).
  - Biopsy of a growth, if a large chunk is forcefully pulled out.
  - Dialation of strictures very forcibly.
- Cardiac arrest due to vagal stimulation.
- Injury to lips, teeth, tongue and pyriform fossa mucosa.
- Dislocation of cervical vertebral column.
- Difficult oesophagoscopy due to trismus or stricture.

OESOPHAGEAL PERFORATION

Definition   It is defined as the perforation of the oesophagus and occurs as a dangerous and often life-threatening complication of rigid oesophagoscopy.

Site of perforation It commonly occurs at the crico-pharyngeal sphincter or it occurs in the thoracic oesophagus.

Aetiology

Site	Common cause
• Cervical oesophagus	• Inadequately relaxed cricopharyngeal sphincter and forceful pushing of the scope.
• Thoracic oesophagus	• During stricture dialatation or taking a punch biopsy.

Clinical features

Symptoms	Signs
• Severe shooting pain in the back between the scapulae	• Rise in temperature
• Fever	• Tachycardia
• Dyspnoea	• Respiratory distress
• Anxiety	• Surgical emphysema
	• Low blood pressure

Investigations

- X-ray chest PA view may show evidence of pneumo-mediastinum or pneumothorax.
- Dionosil dye studies for oesophageal swallow on radiology will reveal site of perforation. Barium is never used, as it can exacerbate the mediastinitis.

Treatment

- Strictly nil by mouth.
- Ryle's tube feeds or parenteral nutrition.
- Half hourly temperature, pulse, respiration (TPR) chart.
- Half hourly BP chart.
- IV antibiotics—ampicillin, gentamycin, and metronidazole.
- Intramuscular (IM) anti-inflammatory analgesics.
- Surgical repair of the perforation either through the neck or thorax, depending upon the site of the perforation.

CLEFT PALATE SURGERY

Definition   Cleft palate surgery is a surgery performed for the repair of a cleft palate deformity.

Types of operations
- Langenback's palatoplasty.
- VY pushback or Veau's palatoplasty.

If required, a pharyngoplasty is performed along with a palatoplasty to correct the defect in the nasopharyngeal sphincter.

Principles of surgery   These are shown in Figs 58.1 and 58.2. In both these operations, the mucosal flaps are based on the greater and lesser palatine blood vessels, which pass through the palatine foramina in the hard patate. Hence, while taking incisions or elevating mucosal flaps, care should be taken to prevent damage to the greater palatine artery on either side.

- Postoperatively: It is very important to give the patient, adequate and intensive speech therapy after 3 weeks of surgery for correct articulation.

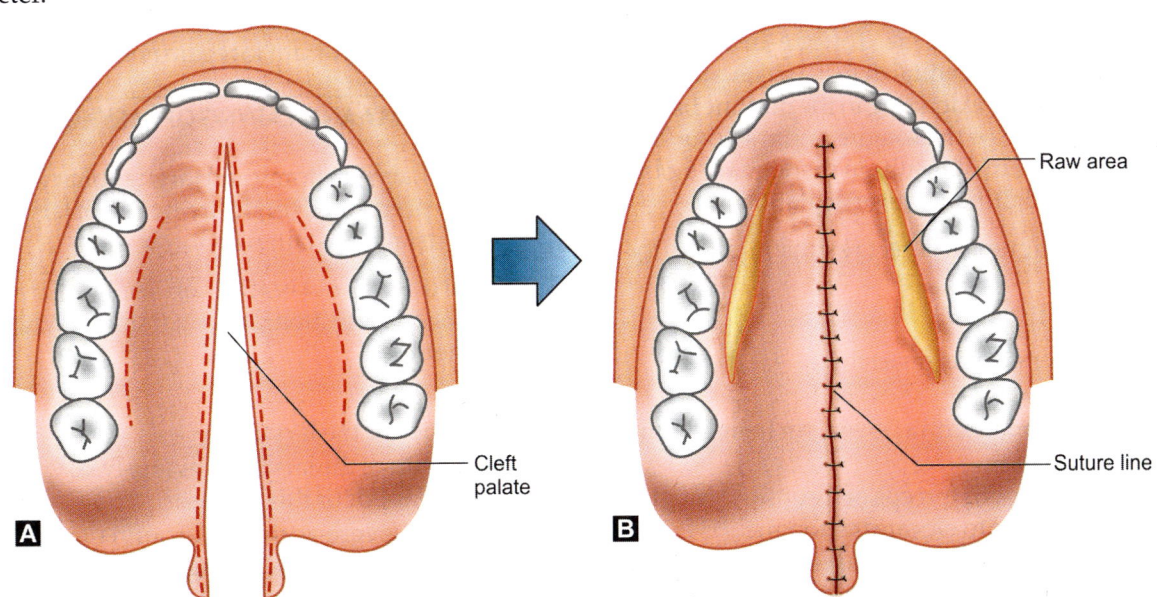

Cleft palate

Raw area

Suture line

A

B

Fig. 58.1 : Von Langenback's palatoplasty

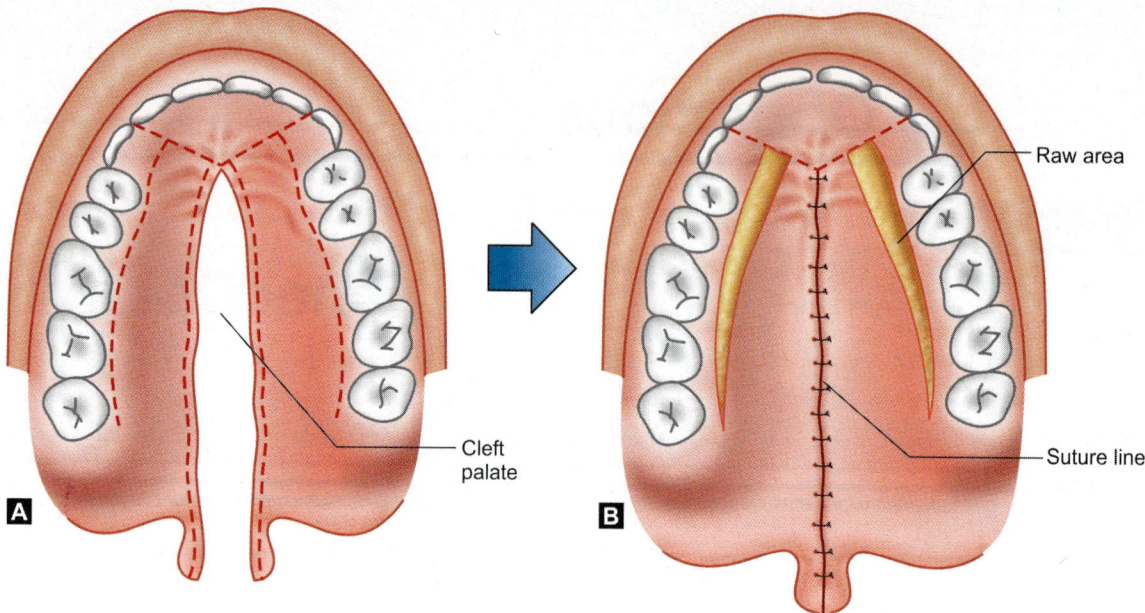

Fig. 58.2 : Veau's (V-Y pushback) palatoplasty

The raw areas on the hard palate are kept bare and heal by secondary intention (i.e. formation of granulations).

TONGUE-TIE RELEASE

Definition   Tongue-tie release is a surgery performed for the release of tongue-tie. Tongue-tie is the term used to describe a congenital defect, which presents as a fibrous tissue band extending in the midline between the ventral surface of the tongue and the floor of the mouth at the frenum. It results in inadequate mobility of the tongue and difficulty in articulation.

Indication   Tongue-tie defect results in difficulty in articulation.

Procedure
• Always under general anaesthesia.
• Patient lies supine.
• Mouth is kept open with a Doyen's or Jening's mouth gag.
• A towel clip, a tooth forceps or a suture through the tongue tip is used to elevate the tongue.
• The tongue-tie is visualised and released using a fine scissors taking care not to damage the lingual veins which run parallel to the frenum of the tongue, on either side.
• The cut edges are sutured in a vertical manner.

Complications
• Complications of anaesthesia.
• Haemorrhage, if lingual vein is accidentally damaged.
• Damage to the openings of the submandibular and sublingual salivary ducts on the floor of the mouth.
Postoperative speech therapy, after 2–3 weeks of surgery is most important to regain normal articulation.

LARYNGECTOMY AND LARYNGOPHARYNGECTOMY

Definition   Laryngectomy and laryngopharynectomy, is a surgery performed for the treatment of laryngeal or laryngopharyngeal malignancy.

Classification   For classification see Flowchart 58.1. A radical neck dissection can be combined with any of these surgeries.

Indications
• Malignancy of the larynx.
• Tuberculosis of the larynx, previously laryngectomy was performed for this disease.
• Following severe accidental trauma to the larynx with destruction of the laryngeal cartilages.
• Laryngeal cartilage necrosis due to infection or following radiotherapy.
• Rare tumours of the larynx, like chondrosarcoma, melanoma, and fibrosarcoma.

Flowchart 58.1: Classification of laryngectomy

```
                          ┌──────────────┐
                          │ Laryngectomy │
                          └──────┬───────┘
                 ┌───────────────┴───────────────┐
            ┌────┴────┐                      ┌────┴────┐
            │ Partial │                      │  Total  │
            └────┬────┘                      └────┬────┘
       ┌─────────┴─────────┐                      │
```

Vertical-partial	Horizontal-partial	• Total laryngectomy
• Cordectomy	• Epiglottectomy	• Total laryngectomy with partial pharyngectomy (laryngopharyngectomy)
• Hemilaryngectomy	• Supraglottic partial	• Total laryngectomy with partial glossectomy
• Frontal partial		

Anaesthesia Always performed under general anaesthesia.

Incision A transverse incision over the upper border of the cricoid cartilage extending from the anterior border of one sternocleidomastoid muscle to the other gives good exposure. A separate incision is taken for the tracheostomy.

Sequelae
- The patient has a permanent tracheostoma, after a total laryngectomy and, hence has to take care while bathing and in day-to-day life by adequately covering the stoma with a piece of clean cloth.
- Inability to speak.
- Inability to strain.
- Inability to lift heavy weights.
- Inability to swim.
  However, there is no dysphagia or aspiration, if healing is complete.

Postoperative care includes
- Care of tracheostoma.
- Voice rehabilitation.
- Counselling for job placement
- Regular follow up.

RADICAL NECK DISSECTION

Definition Radial neck dissection is a surgery performed to remove all lymph nodes, lymphatics, and fibroareolar tissue in the neck situated between the midline of the neck and the anterior border of the trapezius muscle and the lower border of the mandible and the upper border of the clavicle.

Indications
- Clinically, positive cervical lymph node metastases of head or neck malignancy.

- A fixed malignant neck mass that is resectable.
- Recurrent neck node metastases.
- Well-differentiated thyroid cancer.
- Malignant melanoma.
- Occult primary with neck node metastases.

Contraindications
- Presence of distant metastases.
- Inability to curatively treat the primary tumour.
- Involvement of the lumen of the carotid artery.
- Patient who is medically unfit for surgery.

Structures removed include
- All regional lymph nodes, lymphatics, and fibro-aerolar tissue.
- Two nerves—spinal accessory and greater auricular.
- Two muscles—posterior belly of the digastric and the sternocleidomastoid muscles.
- Two glands, submandibular salivary gland and parotid gland (partly).
- Internal jugular vein.

Complications
- **Intraoperative**
  - Injury to the brachial plexus or vagus nerve.
  - Haemorrhage from internal jugular vein.
  - Injury to thoracic duct.
  - Injury to subclavian vein causing air embolism.
  - Injury to pleura causing pneumothorax.
  - Pressure on carotid sinus can cause cardiac arrythmias.
- **Postoperative**
  - Haemorrhage due to slipping of ligature around internal jugular vein or posterior facial vein.
  - Necrosis of skin flaps.
  - Carotid artery blow out.
  - Wound infection.

- Shoulder droop.
- Shoulder pain.
- Chylous fistula more common if RND is performed on the left side.
- Intracranial complications occur with bilateral neck dissection.

PAROTIDECTOMY

Definition   Parotidectomy is the surgery performed for removal of the parotid salivary gland.

Types /Classification
- Partial or superficial.
- Total or complete.

Indications
- Chronic recurrent parotitis.
- Parotid sialolith (calculi).
- Parotid gland cyst.
- Parotid gland malignancy.
- Pleomorphic adenoma of the parotid gland.
- As a part of radical neck dissection (tail of parotid gland is removed).
- As a treatment for drooling—not very effective and not performed nowadays.

Incision   It is shown in Fig. 58.3.

Anaesthesia   Always under general anaesthesia.

Complications
- Complications of anaesthesia.
- Haemorrhage.
- Injury to facial nerve as it passes between the deep and superficial lobes of the gland.
- Recurrence of a benign neoplasm (pleomorphic adenoma).
- Gustatory sweating (Frey's syndrome).

SUBMANDIBULAR SALIVARY GLAND DISSECTION

Definition   It is an operation performed for the excision of the submandibular salivary gland.

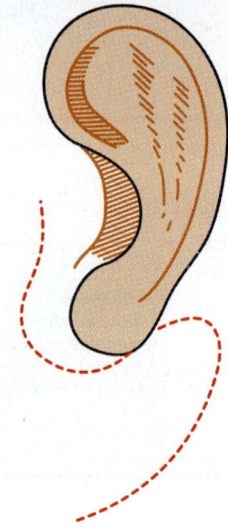

Fig. 58.3: Incision for parotidectomy

Indications
- Chronic recurrent submandibular sialadenitis.
- Submandibular sialolith (calculi).
- Tuberculosis of the submandibular salivary gland.
- Benign tumours of the submandibular salivary gland.
- As a part of radical neck dissection.
- Treatment for drooling or salivary fistula—not recommended nowadays.
- As an approach to the parapharyngeal space.

Anaesthesia   Always under general anaesthesia.

Incision   It is approximately 10 cm long and 2.5 cm below and parallel to the lower border of the mandible.

Complications
- Complications of anaesthesia.
- Injury to the mandibular division of the facial nerve resulting in deviation of the angle of the mouth.
- Injury to the lingual nerve.
- Injury to the hypoglossal nerve.
- Salivary fistula.
- Haemorrhage due to injury to the facial vessels, which lie in close relation to this gland.

Miscellaneous

CHAPTER **59**

CT Scan and MRI in ENT

COMPUTED AXIAL TOMOGRAPHY AND MAGNETIC RESONANCE IMAGING

COMPUTED AXIAL TOMOGRAPHY

Definition   Computed tomography is a radiographic technique that allows the measurement of small absorption differentials not recognizable by direct recording on X-ray films.

Principle   The computed tomographic scan is initiated at a chosen level, and the X-ray tube, collimated to a thin or pencil beam, rotates around the patient's immobilized head. The transmitted X-rays are picked up by detectors arrayed along the circumference of the tube trajectory, converted into electronic currents, amplified and transmitted to the computer for storage and processing. The computer analyzes the data and calculates the sum total of radiation absorbed per unit volume of tissue. Because different tissues absorb X-rays to different degrees it is possible to ascribe an absorption coefficient to them. The computer then develops an image on a dot matrix in which the brightness of each point is proportional to the absorption coefficient.

On the Hounfield scale water is zero, air is minus thousand units, dense bone is plus thousand units. Electrical and Musical Industry Ltd. (EMI) was the first to develop the CT scan. Water is zero and appears black on the screen. Because of their CSF content the ventricles, cisterns and sulci appear black. Fat has an absorption coefficient less than water whereas oedema, recent haemorrhage and tissue necrosis—brain tissue,

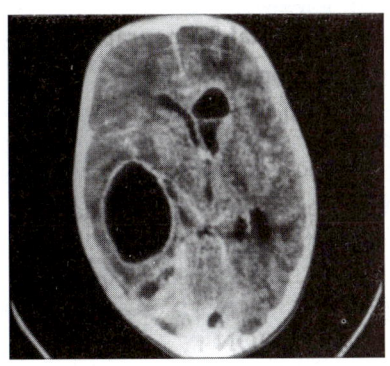

Fig. 59.1 : Contrast enhanced CT scan axial view showing ring enhancing lesion in the right temporal lobe suggesting of an intracranial (temporal) abscess. There is compression of the right lateral ventricle and air in the region of the left-lateral ventricle

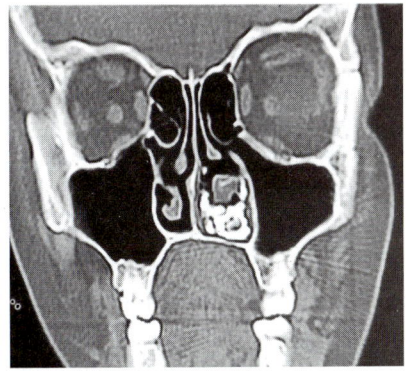

Fig. 59.2 : CT scan paranasal sinuses (plain) in the coronal plane depicting a radiodense opacity in the left nasal cavity and inferior meatus adherent to the left inferior turbinate, suggestive of a rhinolith or foreign body

concealed blood and calcification shade progressively through grey to white as the coefficient increases.

Advantages
- High contrast of the images is obtained
- Better recognition of bony structures and associated pathology
- Images easier to interpret because of lack of blurring
- It can be repeated after injection of contrast material

Disadvantages
- High cost
- Radiation exposure

Applications
- It is 95% effective in facial nerve tumours or meningiomas. CT scan is unlikely to demonstrate a tumour of less than 1 cm in diameter and even a tumour between 1–1.5 cm may occasionally be undetectable. False positive rate of 2–3% exists with the use of CT scan.
- CT scanning is of special value for the anatomy and pathologic conditions of:
  - Temporal bone including petrous apex and cerebello-pontine angle
  - Paranasal sinuses, naso pharynx and pterygo-palatine fossa
  - Nose and paranasal regions
  - Orbit and periorbital regions
  - Oropharynx, floor of mouth and parapharyngeal space
  - Larynx and hypopharynx
  - Facio-maxillary region
  - Intracranial region

High resolution CT (HRCT) scan is of particular value for the temporal bone. This is useful to visualise:
- Fractures
- Facial nerve anatomy
- Mastoid region

MAGNETIC RESONANCE IMAGING

Definition Magnetic resonance (MR) is an imaging modality, which is capable of producing cross section images of the human body in any plane without exposing the patient to ionizing radiation.

Principle The human body is a chemical composition made up of several elements such as hydrogen, carbon, nitrogen, sodium, etc. Atoms of some of these elements having protons in their nucleii possess magnetic resonance. The most abundant of these in the human body is the proton of hydrogen atom in the form of water and various other organic compounds.

The magnetic resonant signals have specific tissue characteristics. They are analyzed by a computer and reconstructed mathematically by a method called as 'Fourier transformation with sectional images of human body'.

Various types of images exhibit various tissue characteristics. Blood vessels usually appear in the MR images as areas of void or no signal because the stimulated protons of the circulating blood move out of the section before their emitted signals can be detected. Air, cortical bone and calcifications also appear as dark areas of no signal because they contain few free protons. MR demonstrates the pathologic processes whenever the hydrogen density and relaxation times of the pathologic tissues are different from those of the normal.

Advantages
- Non-invasive.
- 3–dimensional picture.
- No exposure to ionizing radiation.
- Greater potential for soft tissue density resolution.
- Can be repeated after injection of contrast material.

Disadvantages
- High cost
- Increased scanning time.

Applications
- Brain: cerebral infarcts, cerebello-pontine angle tumours.
- Spine: to differentiate between CSF, spinal cord, central canal and nerve roots.
- Infratemporal and parapharyngeal lesions.
- Musculo-skeletal system.
- Paediatric patients: Since no ionizing radiation is used.

Practical applications CT scan and MRI are mainly used for the following pathologies:
- HRCT: Temporal bone fractures, fallopian canal pathology.
- CT scan
  - Complications of chronic suppurative otitis media.
  - Tumours of nose, paranasal sinuses (PNS), naso-pharynx, larynx and internal auditory meatus.
- MRI
  - Cerebello-pontine angle tumours.
  - Para-pharyngeal space pathology.

NEWER RADIOLOGICAL MODALITIES

- Spiral CT scan.
- Fast spin echo.
- Fat suppression MRI.

Miscellaneous

CHAPTER 60

AIDS in Ear, Nose and Throat

INTRODUCTION

The human immunodeficiency virus (HIV) is the causative agent of acquired immunodeficiency syndrome (AIDS).

HIV

- A retrovirus.
- Ninety to 120 nm in diameter.
- Contains a single stranded RNA genome with a reverse transcriptase enzyme.
- Infects all cells bearing CD4 antigen and so infects principally the T4-lymphocytes (helper cells), thus affecting cell-mediated immunity.
- It is susceptible to all the common disinfectants and so standard washing procedures with detergents and hot water are adequate.
- For treatment of contaminated medical instruments, a 2% solution of glutaraldehyde is useful.

MODES OF TRANSMISSION

- Sexual intercourse: Anal, vaginal and oral.
- Blood and blood products: Blood transfusion, factor VIII tr.
- Tissue and organ donation: Semen, cornea, bone marrow and kidney.
- Infections and injuries
  - Shared needles by drug addicts.
  - Injection with unsterile needles and syringes.
  - Needle stick and other injuries to health staff.

- Mother to baby
  - Transplacental.
  - At birth.
  - After birth: Breastfeeding.

CLINICAL FEATURES OF HIV INFECTION

Acute infection with HIV

- Clinical features develop within a few weeks of infection with HIV—seen in 10–15% of patients.
- Low grade fever, malaise, headache, lymphadenopathy, rash, and arthropathy.

Asymptomatic infection

- Patients are symptomless from several months to years.
- Patient show positive HIV antibody tests.
- Patient are infectious.

Persistent generalised lymphadenopathy

- It is characterized by the presence of enlarged lymph nodes in two or more non-contiguous sites.
- Lymphoid tissue hyperplasia and hypertrophy is common in the head and neck region. It may involve both nodal and extranodal lymph tissue resulting in cervical lymphadenopathy, adenoid hypertrophy, lingual and palatine tonsillar hypertrophy.

This is due to polyclonal B-cell activation by infection with HIV or Ebstein-Barr virus or cytomegalovirus.

AIDS-Related complex

- Patient experiences all the constitutional symptoms, such as fatigue, unexplained fever, persistent diarrhoea, oral candidiasis, and marked weight loss.

AIDS

- It is the term used to describe the full blown end-stage disease.
- Patient is prey to progressive opportunistic infections and malignancies.
- Death ensues in months or years.

OPPORTUNISTIC INFECTIONS AND MALIGNANCIES COMMONLY ASSOCIATED WITH HIV INFECTION

Parasitic

- *Pneumocystis carinii.*
- Toxoplasmosis.
- Cryptosporidiosis.
- Isosporiasis.
- Generalized strongyloidiasis.

Mycotic

- Candidiasis.
- Cryptococcosis.
- Aspergillosis.
- Histoplasmosis.

Bacterial

- Mycobacterial infections—tuberculosis and non-tuberculous.
- Salmonellosis.
- Campylobacter.
- Nocardia and actinomycetes.
- Legionellosis.

Viral

- Herpes simplex.
- Cytomegalovirus.
- Ebstein-Barr virus (EBV).

Malignancies

- Kaposi's sarcoma.
- Lymphomas
  - Hodgkin's lymphoma (HL)
  - Non-Hodgkin's lymphoma (NHL)

AIDS IN EAR, NOSE AND THROAT

Ear, nose and throat (ENT) are as susceptible to AIDS, as any other organ. AIDS affects ENT in the following way:

Ear

- Acute otitis media mainly due to pneumocystis carinii infection.
- Otitis media with effusion: Effusion is due to increased incidence of upper respiratory tract infection (URTI), occasionally due to lymphoid tissue hypertrophy and rarely nasopharyngeal tumours.
  - *Treatment:* Myringotomy and ventilation tube insertion.
- Malignant otitis externa commonly seen in diabetic patients.
- Eustachian tube obstruction.
- External ear polyp due to pneumocystic carinii infection.
- Kaposis sarcoma of external auditory canal (EAC) and auricle and deposits in the VIII nerve.
- Otomycosis—Infection is invasive, causes severe pain and demands aggressive treatment.
  - *Treatment*
    - Surgical debridement.
    - Parenteral amphotericin-B.
- Ramsay hunt syndrome: Reactivation of herpes zoster due to suppressed CMI.
- Sensorineural hearing loss
  - Due to infection with viruses like cytomegalo; hepatitis B, *Herpes simplex*, and *Treponema pallidum.*
  - Due to ototoxicity of the drugs used for the treatment of oppurtunistic infections.
- Labyrinthine cryptococcosis
  - *Treatment:* Amphotericin B + Flucytosine followed by fluconazole.
- Herpes zoster oticus.
- Otosyphilis—tertiary syphilis in AIDS patients.
- Facial paralysis due to:
  - Herpes zoster oticus.
  - Progressive multifocal leucoencephalopathy.
  - Neoplasms.

Nose

- Seborrhoeic dermatitis: It commonly affects the face and especially the nasolabial folds. In AIDS, there is an abrupt onset, particularly severe and extensive which is seen as a red eruption with greasy scales.
- Rhinitis: It is often severe and signs like granular nasal mucosa and purulent discharge are seen.
- Acute and chronic sinusitis:
  - Generally diffuse and bilateral; mainly affect maxillary and the ethmoid sinuses.
  - They may cause pansinusitis and may develop a 'posterior sinus' disease.

- These are caused by opportunistic infections, like:
  - *Streptococcus pneumoniae, haemophilus influenzae*
  - Non-bacterial pathogens, like:
    - Cryptococcus neoformans.
    - Alternaria.
    - *Acanthamoeba castellani.*
- Epistaxis: It is a high infective risk for spread of HIV infection. Precautions to be taken while treating.
- Kaposi's sarcoma.

Oral and throat lesions

- Oral candidiasis: This is a common infection seen in HIV infection and is often a presenting sign, occurs as plaques of thrush.
- Clinical patients
  - Pseudomembranous.
  - Erythematous.
  - Hyperplasia.
  - Angular cheilitis.
- Treatment
  - Oral ketoconazale / fluconazole.
  - Clotrimazole troches.
  - Nystatin for local application.

Oesophagitis
It occurs due to candidiasis, crypto-megalo virus (CMV)/herpes.

- It is characterized by retrosternal pain, dysphagia, odynophagia
- Diagnostic investigation: Upper gastrointestinal (GI) endoscopy and barium swallow.
- Treatment
  - Candidiasis—fluconazole and amphotericin-B
  - CMV—gancyclovir and foscarnet
  - Herpes—acyclovir

Kaposi's sarcoma
It is characterized by lesions on the hard palate, oral mucosa and gingiva.

Recurrent aphthous ulcers present as:

- Minor aphthae.
- Major aphthae.
- Herpetiform aphthae.

Treatment

- Tablet acyclovir 200–400 mg 5 times a day.
- Tablet foscarnet.

Herpes simplex
It presents as oesophagitis and oro-labial lesions.

Stomatitis

Gingivitis

Acute necrotizing ulcerative gingivitis

Periodontitis

Necrotising stomatitis of periodontal origin

Oral hairy cell leukoplakia

- It presents as a whitish, verrucous and corrugated plaque commonly seen on the lateral surface of tongue.
- Caused by EBV.
- Treatment: High doses of acyclovir.

Salivary glands
Manifests as bilateral parotitis.

Sjogren's syndrome
Xerostomia sicca.

Osteomyelitis
It commonly affects the mandible.

Benign tumours
These occur due to human papilloma virus and are associated with papillomas, verruca vulgaris, and condyloma acuminata commonly found in oral cavity, and oropharynx.

Lymphomas
Non-Hodykin's lymphoma and high grade B-cell lymphoma are seen frequently affecting nasopharynx and palatine tonsil.

- Treatment: Systemic chemotherapy
- Risk of squamous cell carcinoma of the oral cavity, is increased in AIDS patients.

LABORATORY DIAGNOSIS

- Total leucocyte and lymphocyte count to demonstrate leucopenia. Lymphocyte count is usually below $2000/mm^3$.
- T cell subset assay: Absolute T4 cell count is usually less than $200/mm^3$ T4: T8 cell ratio is reversed.
- Platelet count will show thrombocytopenia.
- Raised immunoglobulin G and immunoglobulin A levels.
- Diminished CMI (cell-mediated immunity) as indicated by skin tests.
- p24 antigen detected in blood after about 2 weeks. Afterwards, the p24 antigen disappears from the circulation and reappears only, when clinical disease sets in.
- Enzyme-liked immunosorbent assay (ELISA) tests:
  - Standard screening test
  - Solid phase assay
  - Sensitivity 95%
  - Specificity: Not optimal
  - False positive results common

- Western blot test
  - Confirmatory tests
- Specific tests
  - Fujirebio agglutination tests
  - Karpas' test
  - Indirect immunofluorescence test

TREATMENT

- It is directed towards treating the opportunistic infections and used of antiretroviral drugs, which are reverse transcriptase inhibitors.
- Zidovudine
  - *Indications*
    - Patients with CD4 counts < 500/mL

- Treating patients with injury due to injection needles—treatment started within 2 hours of exposure, continued for 4–6 weeks.
- In pregnant females to reduce the incidence of maternofetal transmission of HIV infection.
  - *Standard dose*: 100 mg 5 times daily.
    Other regimens
    - 200 mg 3 times daily
    - 300 mg twice a day
- Didanosine
  - Dose: 200 mg BD for > 60 kg
    100 mg BD for < 60 kg
- Zalcitabine
  - *Dose*: 0.75 mg TDS.

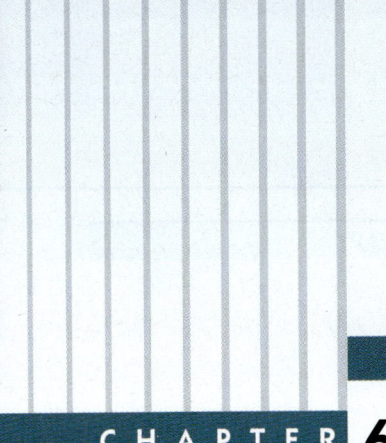

Miscellaneous

CHAPTER 61

Radiotherapy in Ear, Nose and Throat

INTRODUCTION

Modern cancer management in ear, nose, and throat (ENT) demands a multidisciplinary approach for improving the quality of life and survival of the patient. The three main modalities of cancer management, viz. radiotherapy, chemotherapy and surgery either alone or in combination achieve the best results.

DEFINITION

Radiotherapy is defined as the treatment modality which uses ionising radiation to achieve cure or palliation. The discovery of X-rays by Roentgen in 1895, laid the foundation for the development of radiotherapy. Radium discovered by Marie and Pierre Curie in 1898, was used within few years for the treatment of cancer.

PRINCIPLES OF RADIOTHERAPY

The principles of radiotherapy are based on the fact that radiotherapy has more chances of killing a malignant cell than a normal cell. Also cancer cells divide more frequently, as they have a shorter half life. Cancer cell repair less effectively.

FACTORS DETERMINING EFFICACY OF RADIOTHERAPY

- Cell type: The order of sensitivity to radiotherapy is:
  - Lymphoma → Carcinoma → Sarcomas
    (most sensitive)   (least sensitive)
  - Melanomas are least sensitive to radiotherapy.

- Extent of differentiation: Undifferentiated tumours are more susceptible to radiotherapy than differentiated tumours.
- Rate of division: Actively dividing cells are more susceptible to radiotherapy than differentiated tumours.
- Level of tissue oxygenation: Oxygenated cells are more radiosensitive, hence the use of hyperbaric O_2 and blood transfusion during radiotherapy.
- Hyperthermia: The cells are more radiosensitive, if ambient temperature is raised.

METHODS OF RADIOTHERAPY

Teletherapy   The source of radiation is away from the patient. Based on the energy level of radiation used, radiotherapy is classified as:
  - *Superficial*   :   100 kV
  - *Orthovoltage*   :   300 kV
  - *Megavoltage*   :   4–20 MV

Brachy therapy   Source of radiation is placed in and around the tumour.

Internal nuclear medicine using unsealed radio-isotopes.

Teletherapy or External beam radiotherapy is given by directing a beam of radiation by a machine to a tumour bearing part of a patient who is some distance away. The types of external beams used are:
- Photons (X-rays, γ-rays)

- Particles (photon, neutron and electron)
  - *Superficial radiations* have poor penetration and are now obsolete. They were used formerly for small skin tumours.
  - *Orthovoltage radiations* were used in treatment of advanced head and neck cancers. They have a disadvantage, that they cause laryngeal cartilage necrosis and osteoradionecrosis.
  - *Megavoltage radiations* are the main story of modern day radiotherapy. The advantages are:
    - Increased penetration.
    - Skin sparing.
    - Lesser damage to bone and cartilage.
    - Homogenous distribution.
    - Better precision.

Cobalt-60 and linear accelerator are the machines used to deliver megavoltage radiations.

Brachy therapy In brachytherapy, sealed sources of radioactive isotopes are either implanted in the tissue or placed in a natural cavity. Radionucleotides used in brachytherapy include radium, radon, caesium 137, iridium 192, iodine 125 and gold 198. The energy of photons emitted from radium and radon is very high and not used for brachytherapy. The main advantage of interstitial radiotherapy is that it enables very high radiation dose to be given to a very limited volume.

Internal nuclear medicine Unsealed radioisotopes can be used as drugs given orally or intravenously, e.g. treatment of differentiated follicular carcinoma thyroid with radiactive iodine.

Pretherapy assessment is a prerequisite to avoid unwanted complications. It include:
- Dental check-up
- Hemoglobin level and anemia management.
- Treatment of pre-existing infections.

SIDE EFFECTS OF RADIOTHERAPY

- Erythema of skin.
- Alopecia.
- Excoriation of skin.
- Stomatitis/glossitis.
- Bone marrow depression.
- Perichondritis.
- Osteoradionecrosis of tooth.
- Radionecrosis of mandible.
- Susceptibility to infection.
- Transverse myelitis of spinal cord.

RADIOTHERAPY SCHEDULE

- The SI unit of radiation absorbed is gray (Gy).
- Centigray = cGy = 0.01 Gy
- rad = cGy
- Conventional: 60 Gy (6000 rads) in 30 doses at 2 Gy (200 rads) per dose in 42 days.
- Hypofractionation: Smaller number of fractions each larger than 2 Gy.
- Hyperfractionation: Larger number of fractions each smaller than 2 Gy.

The dose of 200 rads/2 Gy is delivered to the tumour daily for 5 days a week with 2 days of rest, so as to enable normal cells to regenerate and acute mucosal reaction to settle.

Combination with other modalities Radiotherapy is combined with chemotherapy and surgery to achieve better treatment results. Surgery is easier and safer before radiotherapy, while radiotherapy works better with a good blood supply. Radiotherapy may be given preoperatively or postoperatively. The results of various series studied in literature marginally favour postoperative radiotherapy. Debulking surgery before radiotherapy, reduces the tumour load and increases efficacy of radiotherapy. Postsurgical radiotherapy can reduce the chances of recurrence in patients.

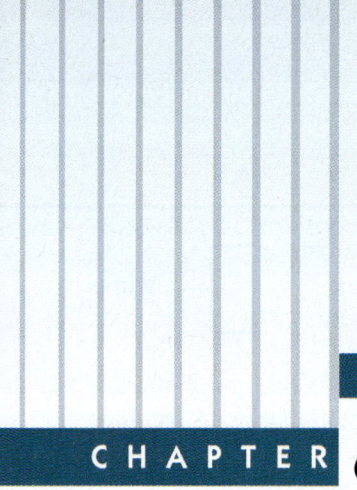

Miscellaneous

CHAPTER 62

Cryosurgery

INTRODUCTION

Cryosurgery is a technique, in which the tissues are exposed to extreme cold to produce intracellular irreversible cell damage. It is based on the idea of 'freezing surgery'.

CONCEPT

Alternate rapid freezing to a temperature of at least –20°C and thawing, causes multiple 'ice crystals' to form which are lethal to the cell. Thus, its main use is:
- Destruction of benign vascular lesions in the head and neck, e.g. hemangioma, angiofibroma and reduction of inferior turbinate hypertrophy.
- Palliation and relief of pain in uncontrolled or recurrent inaccessible cancers, e.g. Ca nasopharynx.

TECHNIQUE

A hollow probe is refrigerated by liquid nitrogen or pressurised nitrous oxide. Incorporated in the probe, is a rewarming device. Thus, tissues can be rapidly frozen and thawed as required.

The probe is applied to the tissue and freezing started, and when a 'tissue-ice-ball' has formed in the area to be treated, it is then immediately allowed to thaw. The process is repeated for 2–3 cycles to achieve maximum destruction.

PROBES

Probes could be open or closed.

- Open probe: Liquid nitrogen delivered, penetrates much deeper and more rapidly, but is not a precise instrument.
- Closed probe: It is a precise instrument. However, the accessibility is limited.

Probes are designed and modified as per the procedure and the accessibility of the tissue. Thus, there are various types:
- Cryoprobe
- Cryophake
- Cryopencil
- Cryoapplicator
- Cryostylet
- Cryopexie
- Cryocadet
- Cryoextractor

APPLICATIONS OF CRYOSURGERY IN ENT

Ear
- Meniere's disease: By cryosurgery, the vestibular end organ is selectively injured, while hearing is preserved. Transmastoid application of a cryoprobe cooled to –160 C to the lateral semicircular canals for three cycles of 2 minutes each, can control vertigo. The hearing is unaffected. However, there could be a delayed facial paralysis.
- Glomus jugularis tumours: Catheter embolization of the vessels feeding the tumour followed by cryosurgery within a few days helps in cure.

- Carcinomas of the auricle: Very satisfactory results are obtained.

Nose

- Inferior turbinate hypertrophy can be reduced by a cryoprobe and thus, treat hypertrophic rhinitis.
- Bleeding polypus of the septum/capillary angioma.
- Cavernous haemangioma—however, it tends to leave a depigmented noticeable scar.
- Vasomotor rhinitis and allergic rhinitis: Cryosurgery decreases the obstruction. However, allergic symptoms persist.
- Juvenile nasopharyngeal angioma.
- Epistaxis can be controlled.
- Nasal polyps can be removed. The polyp freezes and can be removed by fracturing the stalk.

Throat and oral cavity

- Tonsillectomy: Crytonsillectomy is indicated in patients with blood dyscrasias and chronic debilitating diseases. There is no bleeding, no pain, little discomfort and no damage to the pillars and peritonsillar tissue.
- Cryoadenoidectomy in patients of blood dyscrasias with recurrent middle ear infections.
- Cryoreduction of enlarged lingual tonsils, which occur as a delayed result of tonsillectomy mostly in adults.
- Granular pharyngitis.
- Leukoplakia of the tongue.
- Aphthous and herpetic ulcers.

- Juvenile laryngeal papillomatosis ⎤
- Multiple papillomas of larynx ⎬ V.imp.
- Adult bilateral papillomatosis. ⎦
- Lymphangioma.
- Cavernous hemangiomas.
- Multiple telengectasias (Osler–Rendu–Weber–Syndrome) for telengectasias of the face, lips, buccal mucosa and tongue—Cryo can be used.
- Basal cell carcinoma of face.
- Squamous cell carcinoma of the tongue.
- Epulis
- Ameloblastoma.

ADVANTAGES

- Bleeding is minimum and so can be used in patients and with blood dyscrasias.
- Pain is negligible.
- It can be used to reduce the bulk of the tumours, for relief of pain and bleeding.

DISADVANTAGES

- A need for special equipment.
- Efficacy is limited.
- Histopathology of the excised tissue is not possible due to destruction of the tissue by freezing.
- It leaves a depigmented scar.
- Unable to destroy all the tissue in one sitting.
- In larynx, may lead to postoperative edema and airway compromise.

1. Focal length of the head mirror is:
   (a) 20 inches
   (b) 20 cm
   (c) 20 feet
   (d) 20 meters

2. The otoscope has a magnification of:
   (a) 4X
   (b) 6X
   (c) 2X
   (d) 3X

3. The cone of light on the normal tympanic membrane is seen in the:
   (a) Anterosuperior quadrant
   (b) Posterosuperior quadrant
   (c) Posteroinferior quadrant
   (d) Anteroinferior quadrant

4. Eustachian tube is also known as:
   (a) Nasopharyngeal tube
   (b) Oronasal tube
   (c) Pharyngotympanic tube
   (d) Oropharyngeal tube

5. Promontory is formed by:
   (a) Basal turn of the cochlea
   (b) Apical turn of the cochlea
   (c) Bulge of the vestibule
   (d) Bulge of the semicircular canal

6. Stapes footplate covers the:
   (a) Round window
   (b) Oval window
   (c) Promontory
   (d) Facial nerve

7. The largest ossicle is:
   (a) Incus
   (b) Malleus
   (c) Stapes
   (d) Sulcus tympanicus

8. Chorda tympani nerve is a branch of:
   (a) Tympanic nerve
   (b) Facial nerve
   (c) Nerve to stapedius
   (d) Mandibular nerve

9. Suprameatal (MacEwen's) triangle is the surgical landmark for:
   (a) Facial nerve
   (b) Mastoid antrum
   (c) Hypotympanum
   (d) Stapes footplate

10. Valsalva's manoevure is used to test:
    (a) Patency of Eustachian tube
    (b) Cholesteatoma
    (c) Rhinitis
    (d) Hearing loss

11. A positive fistula test indicates presence of:
    (a) Tympanic membrane fistula
    (b) Labyrinthine fistula
    (c) Oroantral fistula
    (d) Pharyngotympanic fistula

12. Absolute bone conduction (ABC) test helps to detect the presence of:
    (a) Conductive hearing loss
    (b) Mixed hearing loss
    (c) Sensorineural hearing loss
    (d) Normal hearing

13. Dental abscess causing otalgia is due to referred pain through the:
    (a) VIth cranial nerve
    (b) Vth cranial nerve
    (c) Facial nerve
    (d) Glossopharyngeal nerve

14. Malignant otitis externa is due to:
    (a) Diabetes mellitus
    (b) Carcinoma
    (c) ASOM
    (d) Acute mastoiditis

15. Coalescent mastoiditis is a complication of:
    (a) CSOM
    (b) Cholesteatoma
    (c) ASOM
    (d) Furunculosis

16. Otomycosis is caused by:
    (a) Streptococcus and pneumoccus
    (b) Staphylococcus and pneumoccus
    (c) *Candida albicans* and *Aspergillus niger*
    (d) *Proteus mirabilis*

17. Eczematous otitis externa is a form of:
    (a) Allergic dermatitis
    (b) Viral infection
    (c) Fungal infection
    (d) Bacterial infection

18. Wax in the ear can be softened by:
    (a) 5% sodium bicarbonate eardrops
    (b) Condy's gargles
    (c) 2% salicylic acid eardrops
    (d) Gutta Boric Spirit drops

19. Vegetable foreign body in the ear, such as pea/seed is removed by:
    (a) Syringing
    (b) Saline
    (c) Wax hook or rectis
    (d) Putting eardrops

20. Uncomplicated acute suppurative otitis media (ASOM) which fails to resolve with medical treatment is treated by:
    (a) Mastoidectomy
    (b) Tympanoplasty
    (c) Grommet
    (d) Myringotomy

21. Safe variety of chronic suppurative otitis media (CSOM), is represented by:
    (a) Attic perforation
    (b) Central perforation
    (c) Marginal perforation
    (d) Granulations and cholesteatoma

22. Secretory otitis media is treated surgically by:
    (a) Myringoplasty
    (b) Myringotomy with grommet
    (c) Ossiculoplasty
    (d) Mastoidectomy

23. Complications are most commonly seen in a case of:
    (a) Safe CSOM
    (b) SOM
    (c) Unsafe CSOM
    (d) ASOM

24. Fixation of stapes is seen in:
    (a) Meniere's disease
    (b) Cholesteatoma
    (c) Otosclerosis
    (d) ASOM

25. Endolymphatic sac decompression is the treatment for:
    (a) Otosclerosis
    (b) CSOM
    (c) ASOM
    (d) Meniere's disease

26. Stapedectomy is the treatment for:
    (a) Meniere's disease
    (b) CSOM
    (c) ASOM
    (d) Otosclerosis

27. The osteomeatal complex lies in:
    (a) Inferior meatus
    (b) Superior meatus
    (c) Nasal septum
    (d) Middle meatus

28. Vestibule of the nose is lined by:
    (a) Skin
    (b) Mucosa
    (c) Olfactory epithelium
    (d) Respiratory mucosa

29. Little's area lies in the:
    (a) Vestibule
    (b) Columella
    (c) Septum
    (d) Middle turbinate

30. Infection from the dangerous area of the face may spread to:
    (a) Neck
    (b) Mediastinum
    (c) Scalp
    (d) Cavernous sinus

31. Capacity of the adult maxillary sinus is approximately:
    (a) 150 cc
    (b) 15 cc
    (c) 30 cc
    (d) 100 cc

32. While performing posterior rhinoscopy, after dipping the mirror in hot water, what is tested on the back of the examiner's hand ?
    (a) Mirror surface
    (b) Metal surface
    (c) Handle
    (d) Temperature of hot water

33. In addition to a posterior rhinoscopy mirror for performing a PRS examination, which one of the following is required ?
    (a) Lac's tongue depressor
    (b) Gauze piece to hold the tongue
    (c) Mouth gag
    (d) Mastoid retractor

34. When performing a PRS examination, patient is asked to:
    (a) Breathe through his/her nose
    (b) Not to breathe and hold the breath
    (c) Breathe through his/her mouth
    (d) Breathe normally

35. Which one of the following mentioned structures, is not visualised on PRS?
    (a) Choanae
    (b) Eustachian tube opening
    (c) Columella
    (d) Fossa of Rosenmuller

36. Rhinophyma is also known as:
    (a) Tomatonose
    (b) Potatonose
    (c) Cauliflowernose
    (d) Rhinoscleroma

37. The commonest cause of epistaxis in children is due to:
    (a) Nose-picking
    (b) Malignancy
    (c) Hypertension
    (d) Diabetes mellitus

38. The commonest site of epistaxis in children is:
    (a) Woodruff's plexus
    (b) Little's area
    (c) Anterior ethmoid artery
    (d) Root of nose

39. Turbinate hypertrophy secondary to a DNS towards the opposite side, is also known as:
    (a) Compensatory hypertrophy
    (b) Relative hypertrophy
    (c) Nasal polyp
    (d) Rhinoscleroma

40. The term 'impacted nasal septum' refers to:
    (a) DNS with spur
    (b) Mild DNS
    (c) Septal thickening
    (d) DNS touching the lateral nasal wall

41. Septoplasty is preferred over SMR as a treatment for DNS, because:
    (a) It is a conservative surgery
    (b) It is time consuming

(c) It causes more complications
(d) It is commonly done nowadays

42. In patients below 17 years of age, we prefer which one of these, as a Rx of DNS?
    (a) SMR
    (b) Septoplasty
    (c) Septal perforation
    (d) I and D

43. In a patient with right ear moderate conductive hearing loss and left ear normal hearing, Weber's test is lateralised to:
    (a) Left ear
    (b) Right ear
    (c) Centralised (no lateralization)
    (d) Both ears

44. In left ear sensorineural hearing loss and right ear, normal hearing Weber's test is lateralised to:
    (a) Left ear
    (b) Right ear
    (c) Both the ears
    (d) No lateralization

45. In a ear with moderate conductive hearing loss, Rinne test will be:
    (a) Positive
    (b) Negative
    (c) Either positive/negative
    (d) None of these

46. Nasal septal cartilage is preserved in:
    (a) SMR
    (b) Septoplasty
    (c) Both (a) and (b)
    (d) None of the above

47. Aetiology of antrochoanal polyps is:
    (a) Infective
    (b) Allergic
    (c) Viral
    (d) Fungal

48. Aetiology of ethmoidal polyps is:
    (a) Allergy
    (b) Infective
    (c) Viral
    (d) Fungal

49. Which nasal polyp is 'trifoliate' in appearance?
    (a) Ethmoidal
    (b) Antrochoanal
    (c) Both (a) and (b)
    (d) None of the above

50. FESS stands for:
    (a) Functional endoscopic sinus surgery
    (b) Flexible endoscopic sinus surgery
    (c) Fundamental endoscopic sinus surgery
    (d) Full removal of ethmoid sinuses

51. 'Ozaena' is another term for:
    (a) Allergic rhinitis
    (b) Atrophic rhinitis
    (c) DNS
    (d) Rhinitis medicamentosa

52. In 25% glucose in glycerine, nasal drops used for atrophic rhinitis, glucose acts by:
    (a) Hygroscopic action
    (b) Inhibiting the growth of proteolytic organisms
    (c) Empirical action
    (d) Placebo effect

53. 'Reservoir sign' is seen in:
    (a) Wax
    (b) Secretory otitis media
    (c) Otitis externa
    (d) Coalescent mastoiditis

54. Schwartz sign is seen in:
    (a) Otosclerosis
    (b) Meniere's disease
    (c) CSOM
    (d) Secretory otitis media

55. Young's operation is the surgical treatment for:
    (a) Allergic rhinitis
    (b) Atrophic rhinitis
    (c) Vasomotor rhinitis
    (d) Rhinosporidiosis

56. Cholesteatoma of the nose is a term used to denote:
    (a) Rhinitis sicca
    (b) Rhinitis caseosa
    (c) Hypertrophic rhinitis
    (d) Granulomatous rhinitis

57. Prolonged use of nasal decongestants results in:
    (a) Rhinitis sicca
    (b) Rhinitis caseosa
    (c) Rhinitis medicamentosa
    (d) Rhinoscleroma

58. Rhinosporidiosis is the infection of the nose by:
    (a) spore-bearing fungus
    (b) bacteria
    (c) virus
    (d) Lepra bacillus

59. Frisch bacillus is the causative organism for:
    (a) Rhinosporidiosis
    (b) Rhinoscleroma
    (c) Atrophic rhinitis
    (d) Tertiary syphilis

60. Syphilis of the nose results in septal perforation on:
    (a) Nasal bones
    (b) Cartilagenous septum
    (c) Bony septum
    (d) Membranous septum

61. A 'mulberry-like' or 'strawberry-like' nasal mass is seen in:
    (a) Rhinoscleroma
    (b) Rhinosporidiosis
    (c) Atrophic rhinitis
    (d) Tertiary syphilis

62. Leprosy or tuberculosis of the nose results in septal perforation in:
    (a) Cartilagenous septum
    (b) Bony septum
    (c) Membraneous septum
    (d) Nasal bonus

63. Autohaem therapy is used as a treatment for:
    (a) Allergic rhinitis
    (b) Atrophic rhinitis
    (c) Rhinosporidiosis
    (d) Rhinoscleroma

64. X-ray paranasal sinuses—Water's view is specific for:
    (a) Maxillary sinus
    (b) Frontal sinus
    (c) Sphenoid sinus
    (d) Mastoid antrum

65. X-ray paranasal sinus—Caldwell's view is specific for:
    (a) Maxillary sinus
    (b) Frontal sinus
    (c) Sphenoid sinus
    (d) Mastoid antrum

66. The characteristic term, given to the haziness of the maxillary sinus on X-ray, in a case of sinusitis is:
    (a) 'Ground glass' haziness
    (b) 'Ground-nut' haziness
    (c) 'Grounded' haziness
    (d) 'Grey-ground' haziness

67. 'Proof-puncture' is the treatment for:
    (a) Acute maxillary sinusitis
    (b) Acute frontal sinusitis

(c) Chronic maxillary sinusitis
(d) Pansinusitis

68. Mucocoele and pyocoele are commonest in:
(a) Maxillary sinus
(b) Ethmoid sinus
(c) Sphenoid sinus
(d) Frontal sinus

69. Lateral rhinotomy approach is for excision of:
(a) Antrochoanal polyp
(b) Ethmoidal polyp
(c) Turbinate
(d) Inverted papilloma

70. Painless loosening and falling-off of teeth is seen in:
(a) Maxillary sinusitis
(b) Ca maxilla
(c) Ca thyroid
(d) Glossitis

71. Maggots or myiasis of the nose is infestation of the nose by:
(a) Mosquitoes
(b) Larvae of a fly
(c) Bacteria
(d) Fungus

72. Lac's tongue depressor is used to depress:
(a) Posterior one-third of tongue
(b) Anterior two-thirds of tongue
(c) Soft palate
(d) Entire tongue

73. The palatine tonsils are also known as:
(a) Adenoids
(b) Faucial tonsils
(c) Tubal tonsils
(d) Lingual tonsils

74. The largest crypt running into the palatine tonsil is the:
(a) Big crypt
(b) Crypta magna
(c) Large crypt
(d) Big cleft

75. The faucial tonsil has:
(a) One pole
(b) Two poles
(c) Three poles
(d) Four poles

76. Anterior tonsillar pillar is formed by:
(a) Palatoglossus muscle
(b) Palatopharyngeus muscle
(c) Salpingopharyngeus muscle
(d) Pharyngeal muscles

77. Posterior tonsillar pillar is formed by:
(a) Palatoglossus muscle
(b) Palatopharyngeus muscle
(c) Salpingopharyngeus muscle
(d) Pharyngeal muscles

78. The main blood supply to the tonsil is:
(a) Tonsillar artery
(b) Lingual artery
(c) Palatine artery
(d) Ascending pharyngeal artery

79. The tonsillar pedicle contains the insertion of which one of the following muscles?
(a) Palatoglossus
(b) Palatopharyngeus
(c) Pharyngeal
(d) Musculus uvulae

80. Referred otalgia after tonsillectomy is via the:
(a) Hypoglossal nerve
(b) Vagus nerve
(c) Glossopharyngeal nerve
(d) Facial nerve

81. Quinsy is the synonym for:
(a) Peritonsillar abscess
(b) Tonsillolith
(c) Tonsillar cyst
(d) Parapharyngeal abscess

82. Haemostasis after tonsillectomy occurs by:
(a) Clot formation
(b) Blocking of blood vessels
(c) Contraction and retraction of blood vessels
(d) None of the above

83. The adenoid is also known as the:
(a) Palatine tonsil
(b) Nasopharyngeal tonsil
(c) Faucial tonsil
(d) Lingual tonsil

84. The main blood supply of the adenoids is via:
(a) Ascending pharyngeal artery
(b) Tonsillar artery
(c) Palatine artery
(d) Lingual artery

85. Killian's dehiscence is a potential gap between the two parts of the:
(a) Superior constrictor muscle
(b) Middle constrictor muscle
(c) Inferior constrictor muscle
(d) None of the above

86. Thornwaldt's bursitis is seen in the:
(a) Nasopharynx
(b) Oropharynx

(c) Hypopharynx
(d) Larynx

87. Passavant's ridge is formed by the fibres of:
(a) Palatopharyngeus muscle
(b) Palatoglossus muscle
(c) Musculus uvulae
(d) Cricopharyngeus muscle

88. Rathke's pouch is seen as a dimple in the:
(a) Hypopharynx
(b) Roof of nasopharynx
(c) Oropharynx
(d) Larynx

89. The fossa of Rosenmuller contains:
(a) Air
(b) Muscle
(c) Lymph node
(d) Venous sinusoids

90. Which one of these, is referred to as the surgeon's graveyard ?
(a) Gingivobuccal sulcus
(b) Tonsillolingual sulcus
(c) Gingivolabial sulcus
(d) Roof of month

91. The stylohyoid syndrome is also known as:
(a) Eagle's syndrome
(b) Brown's syndrome
(c) Neuralgia syndrome
(d) Pain syndrome

92. Vincent's angina or Trench mouth is caused by:
(a) Viral infection
(b) Fungal infection
(c) Gram negative fusiform bacilli and spiro-chaete
(d) Virus and fungal infection

93. Infectious mononucleosis is caused by:
(a) *Candida albicans*
(b) *Aspergillus niger*
(c) Spirochaete
(d) Epstein-Barr virus

94. Which one of these, is not a feature of 'Trotter's Triad'
(a) Pain on ipsilateral side of face
(b) Ipsilateral palatal palsy
(c) Ipsilateral conductive hearing loss
(d) Chronic cough

95. Plummer-Vinson syndrome is commonly seen in:
(a) Males
(b) Infants
(c) Females
(d) Children

96. Dysphagia Lusoria is the dysphagia occuring due to:
(a) An aberrant bronchus
(b) An aberrant blood vessel in the mediastinum
(c) Enlarged heart
(d) Achalasia cardia

97. In indirect laryngoscopy, the patient is asked to breathe through:
(a) His nose
(b) His mouth
(c) To hold his breath
(d) Both (a) and (b)

98. 'Thumb sign' is seen on X-ray lateral view of neck, in a case of:
(a) Acute epiglottitis
(b) Acute pharyngitis
(c) Chronic laryngitis
(d) Vocal cord nodules

99. Tuberculosis of the larynx usually tends to involve:
(a) Supraglottis
(b) Interarytenoid region
(c) Anterior commissure
(d) Subglottis

100. Scleroma of the larynx usually affects the:
(a) Subglottis
(b) Supraglottis
(c) Ventricle
(d) Glottis

101. Leucoplakia of the larynx is also known as:
(a) Laryngeal hyperkeratosis
(b) Singers nodules
(c) Laryngeal carcinoma
(d) Laryngitis

102. Functional aphonia is also known as:
(a) Bilateral adductor vocal cord (VC) palsy
(b) Bilateral abductor VC palsy
(c) Unilateral VC palsy
(d) VC nodules

103. Laryngomalacia is also called:
(a) Congenital laryngeal stridor
(b) Laryngeal web
(c) VC palsy
(d) Laryngitis

104. Laryngeal stenosis commonly involves the:
(a) Glottis
(b) Subglottis
(c) Supraglottis
(d) Trachea

105. Laryngocoele is an outpouching (sac) of this part of the larynx.
(a) Supraglottis
(b) Epiglottis
(c) Ventricle and saccule
(d) Subglottis

106. Reinke's oedema is characterised by:
(a) Submucosal oedema of vocal cords
(b) Epiglottitis
(c) Oedema of uvula
(d) Subglottic oedema

107. Noisy respiration due to obstruction to passage of air through the respiratory tract is known as:
(a) Dyspnoea
(b) Dysphagia
(c) Stridor
(d) Laryngeal web

108. The characteristic speech heard in a patient with a mass in the hypopharynx or supraglottis is termed as:
(a) Hot potato speech
(b) Hot tomato speech
(c) Blocked speech
(d) Rhinolalia

109. The term 'Laser' stands for:
(a) Light amplification by stimulated emition of radiation
(b) Low amplified and stimulated emitted radiation
(c) Lightly amplified smoothly emitted radiotherapy
(d) Low application of smoothly executed radiation

110. Glycerine ichthymmol eardrops is the treatment for:
(a) ASOM
(b) CSOM
(c) SOM
(d) Otitis externa

111. The X-ray used to visualise the mastoid air cell system is:
(a) Water's view
(b) Caldwell's view
(c) Anterioposterior (AP) view
(d) Schuller's view

112. The X-ray view to visualise the sphenoid sinus is:
(a) Water's view
(b) Caldwell's view
(c) Schuller's view
(d) Water's view with mouth open

113. 'Shouldering effect' and 'Rat-tail and Apple core appearance' of oesophagus on barium swallow is diagnostic of:
(a) Benign stricture
(b) Malignant stricture
(c) Oesophageal varices
(d) Achalasia cardia

114. The central aperture of the head mirror helps in:
(a) Better illumination
(b) Magnification
(c) Binocular vision
(d) Uniocular vision

115. The aural syringe has a capacity of:
(a) 4 Oz
(b) 7 Oz
(c) 2 Oz
(d) 6 Oz

116. The tuning fork of frequency 512 Hz is most useful because:
(a) It falls in mid-speech frequency.
(b) It is cheapest.
(c) It is easily available.
(d) It has two prongs.

117. Siegle's pneumatic speculum has a magnification of:
(a) 2X
(b) 3X
(c) 4X
(d) 5X

118. The advantage of Jening's mouth gag over Doyen's mouth gag is:
(a) It is smaller
(b) It is bigger
(c) It can also be used in edentulous patients
(d) It is made of stainless steel

119. The cage of the adenoid curette helps to:
(a) Add bulk to the instrument
(b) Prevent adenoid tissue from slipping into the respiratory tract
(c) Make the curette sharp
(d) Give a better grip to the surgeon

120. The mechanism of action of the Eve's tonsillar snare is:
(a) Cut
(b) Avulse
(c) Crush and avulse
(d) Crush and cut

121. The Glegg's nasal snare removes a nasal polyp by:
(a) Cutting
(b) Crushing

(c) Avulsion

(d) Cauterizing

122. The capacity of the Higginson's syringe is:
(a) 3 Oz
(b) 2 Oz
(c) 4 Oz
(d) 5 Oz

123. Aural syringing is done using:
(a) Normal saline
(b) Spirit
(c) Warm oil
(d) Antibiotic eardrops

124. Intranasal antrostomy is commonly done at which site:
(a) Superior meatus
(b) Inferior meatus
(c) Middle meatus
(d) Nasal septum

125. Denker's procedure is a:
(a) Modification of the Caldwell-Luc's operation
(b) Synonym for antral puncture
(c) Operation on the frontal sinus
(d) Type of tracheostomy

126. Tonsillectomy is performed as an approach for:
(a) Facial nerve
(b) Vagus nerve
(c) Glossopharyngeal nerve
(d) Trigeminal nerve

127. Unilateral tonsillectomy is an indication for:
(a) Ulcer on tonsil
(b) Hypertrophied tonsils
(c) Acute tonsillitis
(d) Granular pharyngitis

128. Cryotonsillectomy is recommended for:
(a) Acute tonsillitis
(b) Peritonsillar abscess
(c) Chronic tonsillitis in haemophilic patient
(d) Granular pharyngitis

129. The cuff of the tracheostomy tube helps:
(a) To keep it in position
(b) In radiotherapy
(c) To prevent aspiration
(d) To regain speech

130. Otosclerosis is associated with all of the following except one. Tick the one which does not apply to otosclerosis.
(a) Paracusis Willisi
(b) Bilateral conductive hearing loss
(c) Commoner in females
(d) Otorrhoea

131. Tick the one which does not apply to Meniere's disease.
(a) Vertigo
(b) Tinnitus
(c) Endolymphatic sac decompression
(d) Otorrhoea

132. A patient with cholesteatoma and otalgia with hectic fever (fever with rigors), is suggestive of:
(a) Facial palsy
(b) Sigmoid sinus thrombophlebitis
(c) Labyrinthitis
(d) Cerebral abscess

133. Simple mastoidectomy is also known as:
(a) Schwartz mastoidectomy
(b) Tympanoplasty
(c) Myringoplasty
(d) Schuller's mastoidectomy

134. Gradenigo's syndrome occurs due to:
(a) Mastoiditis
(b) Tumour
(c) Trauma
(d) Petrositis

135. The treatment for coalescent mastoiditis without any other complications is:
(a) Modified radial mastoidectomy
(b) Radial mastoidectomy
(c) Simple/Schwartz mastoidectomy
(d) Tympanoplasty

136. Haematoma of the pinna causing cartilage necrosis and deformity results in:
(a) Potato ear
(b) Tomato ear
(c) Bat ear
(d) Cauliflower ear

137. Which one of the following paranasal sinuses is absent at birth ?
(a) Frontal sinus
(b) Ethmoid sinus
(c) Sphenoid sinus
(d) Maxillary sinus

138. Bulla ethmoidalis occurs at which site?
(a) Superior meatus
(b) Middle meatus
(c) Inferior meatus
(d) Nasal septum

139. Kisselbach's plexus does not include, which one of the following blood vessels?
(a) Septal branch of the sphenopalatine artery
(b) Septal branch of the superior labial artery

(c) Greater palatine artery

(d) Posterior ethmoidal artery

140. Which one of the following is not an aetiological factor for oroantral fistula ?
    (a) Tooth extraction
    (b) Trauma
    (c) Ca maxilla
    (d) FESS

141. Which paranasal sinus is the commonest to develop malignant tumours?
    (a) Maxillary
    (b) Frontal
    (c) Ethmoidal
    (d) Sphenoid

142. Rhinosporidiosis is treated by:
    (a) Polypectomy
    (b) Topical nose drops
    (c) Systemic and topical antifungals
    (d) Excision with cautery of its base

143. Vacuum headache commonly occurs due to:
    (a) Meningitis
    (b) Head injury
    (c) Obstruction to frontonasal duct
    (d) Otitic hydrocephalous

144. Rhinosporidiosis is known to occur in:
    (a) Tropical climate areas
    (b) Dry and hot areas
    (c) Mountaineous terrain
    (d) Anywhere, irrespective of climate

145. Nasopharyngeal angiofibroma is commonly seen in:
    (a) Adolescent males
    (b) Middle-aged females
    (c) Newborn
    (d) Elderly males

146. Which artery is known as the 'artery of epistaxis'?
    (a) Anterior ethmoidal artery
    (b) Sphenopalatine artery
    (c) Posterior ethmoidal artery
    (d) Superior labial artery

147. The commonest aetiology of a cyst in the maxillary sinus is:
    (a) Nasal cyst
    (b) Orbital cyst
    (c) Ethmoidal cyst
    (d) Dental cyst

148. Osteoma is commonly seen in which paranasal sinus?
    (a) Frontal sinus
    (b) Ethmoidal sinus

(c) Sphenoid

(d) Maxillary sinus

149. The palatine/faucial tonsil has which one of the the following lymphatic drainage?
    (a) Preauricular lymph nodes
    (b) Paratracheal lymph nodes
    (c) Jugulodigastric lymph nodes
    (d) Retropharyngeal lymph nodes

150. The adenoids drain into
    (a) Preauricular lymph nodes
    (b) Retropharyngeal lymph nodes
    (c) Jugulodigastric lymph nodes
    (d) Paratracheal lymph nodes

151. Nasopharyngeal carcinoma is best treated by:
    (a) Surgery
    (b) Radiotherapy
    (c) Laser
    (d) Chemotherapy

152. The abductor muscle of the larynx is:
    (a) Transverse arytenoid
    (b) Lateral cricoarytenoid
    (c) Posterior cricoarytenoid
    (d) Vocalis

153. The cartilage which is 'signet ring' shaped in the larynx is:
    (a) Cricoid
    (b) Thyroid
    (c) Epiglottis
    (d) Arytenoid

154. The commonest cause of unilateral vocal cord palsy is:
    (a) Trauma
    (b) Tumour
    (c) Iatrogenic
    (d) Idiopathic

155. Which of these cancers has the best prognosis ?
    (a) Supraglottic
    (b) Glottic
    (c) Subglottic
    (d) Pyriform fossa

156. The presenting feature of glottic cancer is:
    (a) Dysphagia
    (b) Dypnoea
    (c) Hoarseness of voice
    (d) Neck swelling

157. The presenting feature of subglottic cancer is:
    (a) Dysphagia
    (b) Dyspnoea
    (c) Neck swelling
    (d) Hoarseness of voice

ANSWERS

1. b	26. d	51. b	76. a	101. a	126. c
2. c	27. d	52. b	77. b	102. a	127. a
3. d	28. a	53. d	78. a	103. a	128. c
4. c	29. c	54. a	79. a	104. b	129. c
5. a	30. d	55. b	80. c	105. c	130. d
6. b	31. b	56. b	81. a	106. a	131. d
7. b	32. b	57. c	82. c	107. c	132. b
8. b	33. a	58. a	83. b	108. a	133. a
9. b	34. a	59. b	84. a	109. a	134. d
10. a	35. c	60. c	85. c	110. d	135. c
11. b	36. b	61. b	86. a	111. d	136. d
12. c	37. a	62. a	87. a	112. d	137. a
13. b	38. b	63. a	88. b	113. b	138. b
14. a	39. a	64. a	89. c	114. c	139. d
15. c	40. d	65. b	90. b	115. a	140. d
16. c	41. a	66. a	91. a	116. a	141. a
17. a	42. b	67. a	92. c	117. a	142. d
18. a	43. b	68. d	93. d	118. c	143. c
19. c	44. b	69. d	94. d	119. b	144. a
20. d	45. b	70. b	95. c	120. d	145. a
21. b	46. b	71. b	96. b	121. c	146. b
22. b	47. a	72. b	97. b	122. a	147. d
23. c	48. a	73. b	98. a	123. a	148. a
24. c	49. b	74. b	99. b	124. b	149. c
25. d	50. a	75. b	100. a	125. a	150. b

151. b
152. c
153. a
154. d
155. b
156. c
157. b

Index